AN INTRODUCTION TO

Cardiovascular Physiology

FIFTH EDITION

J Rodney Levick DSc DPhil MA MRCP BM BCh(Oxon)
Emeritus Professor of Physiology
St George's Hospital Medical School
University of London, UK

HODDER
ARNOLD
AN HACHETTE UK COMPANY

First edition 1991, published in Great Britain by Butterworth Heinemann; reprinted 1992

Second edition 1995; reprinted 1996, 1998, also by Butterworth Heinemann

German translation *Physiologie des Herz–Kreislauf-Systems* by Fischer-Barnicol & Seller, published 1998 by Bath Verlag, Heidelberg

Third edition 2000 by Arnold, reprinted 2001

Fourth edition 2003 by Arnold, reprinted 2005, 2007

Fifth edition 2010 published in Great Britain by Hodder Arnold, a member of the Hodder Education, an Hachette UK company, 338 Euston Road, London NW1 3BH

British Library Cataloguing in Publication Data
A catalogue record for this book is available from the British Library

Library of Congress Cataloging-in-Publication Data
A catalog record for this book is available from the Library of Congress

ISBN 978 0340 942 048

3 4 5 6 7 8 9 10

Commissioning Editor: Joanna Koster
Project Editor: Francesca Naish
Editorial Assistant: Stephen Clausard
Production Controller: Karen Dyer
Cover Design: Amina Dudhia

Cover image © Science Photo Library
Typeset in 10.5/12 pt Bembo by MPS Limited, a Macmillan Company, Chennai, India
Printed and bound in Europe for Hodder Arnold, an Hachette UK company

What do you think about this book? Or any other Hodder Arnold title?
Please visit our website: www.hodderarnold.com

AN INTRODUCTION TO
Cardiovascular Physiology

To Charles Michel, following his retirement; in gratitude to my college tutor of many years ago, and an inspirational colleague and friend ever since

Contents

Website: www.hodderplus.com/cardiovascularphysiology

Additional references, chapter-by-chapter

Figures in electronic format

Sample questions and answers from companion self-assessment volume.

Please register on the website using the following access details:

Serial number: adkf47zsm3c9

Once you have registered, you will not need the serial number but can log in using the username and password you will create during registration.

Preface to fifth edition

An innovation for the 5th edition is the new website, which offers electronic versions of all the figures, references to original research papers organized by chapter (review articles are still listed under Further Reading in the main text) and a short selection of self-assessment questions and answers taken from a new companion volume, *Cardiovascular Physiology: Questions for Self Assessment*. The latter contains over 230 questions/problems in a variety of formats (multiple-choice predominating), organized under the same headings as the chapter of this textbook, with explanatory answers and figures.

Please visit the website at www.hodderplus.com/
    cardiovascularphysiology

The text of the 5th edition has been pruned wherever possible, to make way for new material from the *very* active field of cardiovascular research. New material includes accounts of cardiovascular embryogenesis, ion channel topography, vascular/endothelial TRP channels, Ca^{2+} sparks and waves, new drugs such as the cardiac 'funny' current blocker ivabradine, the glycocalyx-cleft model of endothelium, and insights from genetic knock-out mice. There are expanded accounts of exercise, angina, myocardial infarction, the ECG, hypertension and cardiac failure. This has, of course, required some new figures – 14 in all, plus substantial revisions to >30 figures. An error in the mean blood pressure figure, that had apparently escaped detection by all but one vigilant reader throughout four editions, has finally been corrected. This was a humbling reminder that textbooks are rarely, if ever, 100% correct! Along the same theme, I hope that most of the perennial 'factoids' of physiology have been weeded out – for example, the Starling principle of fluid exchange has been shown conclusively to operate in a rather different fashion from that taught to generations of students. After careful pruning, and the transfer of some peripheral material to the website, the 5th edition text is about the same length as the 4th edition – my aim being to restrict the book to a readable size.

Experts whom I would like to thank for valuable comments on the 5th edition include Dr Phil Aaronson (long-term BP regulation), Dr Kim Dora (EDHF), Professor Bren Gannon (endothelium), Professor William Large (vascular smooth muscle), Professor Graham MacGregor (clinical hypertension) and Professor Jeremy Ward (hypoxic pulmonary vasoconstriction). Hopefully, despite our ever-increasing knowledge of the complexities of cardiovascular function, the book may still fulfill its primary task – to provide an enjoyable, reasonably complete but not over-detailed account of the heart and circulation.

Rodney Levick
Physiology
St George's Hospital Medical School
January 2009

A note on active and problem-based learning

One may read a textbook and gain a primary level of understanding of its subject; but to master the subject thoroughly *active, 'hands-on' engagement with the subject matter is essential*. In other words *self-expression* is vital. One may think one knows the subject, but there is nothing like verbalising and answering questions to promote learning. To this end, learning objectives are given at the start of each chapter, and five clinical cases, with questions and answers, are included at the end of the book. The new website also provides a short selection of self-assessment questions with illustrated answers, taken from a new companion volume, *Cardiovascular Physiology: Questions for Self-Assessment*.

Using the learning objectives

Active learning is traditionally promoted by essay writing and question-and-answer tutorials. The *Learning Objectives* at the start of each chapter can be used as short-notes questions (e.g. 'Draw and explain a delayed after-depolarization', Chapter 3).

The sections containing the answers are cited after each learning objective. Another excellent way to learn actively is to write brief notes on each learning objective. The notes will prove invaluable when revising for examinations.

Problem-based learning

To encourage active learning and clinical relevance, medical schools increasingly base teaching on clinical cases – although this has serious drawbacks, as well as advantages, in the early years. Clinical cases are challenging, because they bring together many different topics and cut across many different chapters of the book. For example, heart failure (Case 1) involves altered cardiac excitation–contraction coupling (Chapters 3 and 18), Starling's law of the heart (Chapter 6), haemodynamics (Chapter 8), microvascular fluid exchange (Chapter 11) and extrinsic control of the circulation (Chapter 14). Clinical cases are therefore presented at the end of the book, with questions and answers linked to the main text.

CHAPTER 1

Overview of the cardiovascular system

Learning objectives

After reading this chapter you should be able to:

- Outline the distance limitation of diffusive transport and the roles of diffusion versus convection in oxygen transport (1.1).
- List the differences between the pulmonary and systemic circulations (1.3).
- Sketch out how blood pressure, velocity and total cross-sectional area change from the aorta to microcirculation to vena cava (Figure 1.9).
- Write down the basic law of flow (1.5) and apply it to work out the main source of vascular resistance.
- Sketch the structure of the blood vessel wall (Figure 1.10) and state the roles of endothelium, elastin, collagen and vascular smooth muscle.
- Name five main functional categories of blood vessel and state their roles (1.7).
- Define a 'portal circulation' and explain its functional value (1.8).

The heart and blood vessels evolved to transport oxygen, nutrients, waste products and heat around the body rapidly. This is crucial for tissue viability, so the cardiovascular system develops at an early stage in the embryo. Very tiny organisms, however, lack a circulatory system – their oxygen needs are satisfied by diffusion from the environment. Even large animals, such as humans, rely on diffusion for the transport of materials between the bloodstream and cells. Why, then, do we also need a cardiovascular system? The answer lies in the distance-limitation of diffusive transport.

1.1 Diffusion: its virtues and limitations

Diffusion is brought about by molecular 'drunkard's walk'

Diffusion is a 'passive' transport process, in the sense that it is driven by the rapid, random thermal motion of molecules, not by metabolic pumps. When a concentration gradient is present, the randomly directed step-movements of individual solute molecules result in a net movement down the concentration gradient, i.e. a net diffusive transport (Figure 1.1).

Distance dramatically slows diffusion

The rate of diffusive transport is important, because nutrient delivery must keep up with cellular demand. Fortunately, diffusive transport is very fast over short distances; for example, diffusion from a capillary to tissue cell, a distance of $\sim 10\,\mu m$, takes only ~ 50 milliseconds. Unfortunately, as Einstein showed, the time t that it takes randomly jumping particles to move a distance x, in one specific direction, increases as the square of the distance:

$$t \propto x^2 \tag{1.1}$$

As a result, diffusion is horribly slow over long distances (Table 1.1). Over 1 cm, which is the thickness of the human left ventricle wall, diffusion would take more than half a day. Sadly, nature often reminds us that Einstein's equation is correct. Figure 1.2 shows a section through a human heart after a coronary artery thrombus (clot) had blocked off the blood supply to the left ventricle wall. The pale area is cardiac muscle that died from lack of oxygen, despite the fact that the adjacent chamber is full of oxygenated blood. The patient died because a distance of just a few millimetres reduces the rate of diffusive oxygen transport to a level that is too low to support life.

Convection provides fast transport over long distances

For distances of >0.1 mm, a faster transport system is clearly needed. The cardiovascular system provides this (Figure 1.3). The cardiovascular system still

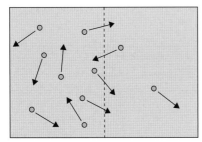

Time 1 (before random jumps):
concentration A = 8, concentration B = 2,
concentration difference $\Delta C = 6$

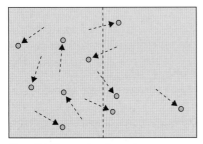

Time 2 (after random jumps):
concentration A = 6, concentration B = 4,
concentration difference $\Delta C = 2$

Figure 1.1 Spontaneous molecular steps in a random direction lead to a net movement of solute molecules (dots) down a concentration gradient. The probability of a randomly directed step from compartment A to B is greater than from B to A, because there are more solute molecules in A than B, per unit volume. Note that an individual molecule, such as the top one in B, may move 'uphill', i.e. into the more concentrated solution. Net diffusion is thus the result of unequal 'uphill' and 'downhill' fluxes.

Figure 1.2 Section of human left ventricle after a coronary thrombosis; myocardium stained for a muscle enzyme. Pale area is an 'infarct' – an area of muscle damaged or killed by lack of O_2. The pallor is due to the escape of enzymes from the dying muscle. The infarct was caused by a coronary artery obstruction, which halted the convective delivery of O_2. O_2 diffusion from blood in the main chamber (LV) is unaffected, yet only a thin rim of adjacent tissue (~1 mm) survived. (Courtesy of the late Professor M Davies, St George's Hospital Medical School, London.)

Table 1.1 Time taken for a glucose molecule to diffuse specified distance in one direction

Distance (x)	Time (t)[a]	Example *in vivo*
0.1 μm	0.000005 s	Neuromuscular gap
1.0 μm	0.0005 s	Capillary wall
10.0 μm	0.05 s	Capillary to cell
1 mm	9.26 min	Skin, artery wall
1 cm	15.4 h	Left ventricle wall

[a]Einstein's equation states $t = x^2/2D$, where D is solute diffusion coefficient (glucose, 0.9×10^{-5} cm^2 s^{-1} at 37°C; oxygen in water, 3×10^{-5} cm^2 s^{-1}, 37°C).
(Einstein A. *Theory of Brownian Movement* (trans. by Fürth R, Cowper AD, 1956). New York: Dover Publications, 1905.)

Figure 1.3 Overview of the human circulation, highlighting the relative roles of diffusion and convection in O_2 transport.

relies on **diffusion** to transport O_2 across the short distance between gas and blood in the lungs; but the absorbed O_2 is then washed rapidly along in a stream of pumped fluid, covering a large distance in seconds ($\sim 3\,\mathrm{cm\ s^{-1}}$). This form of transport is called bulk flow or **convective transport**, and its energy source is the contraction of the heart. Convective transport carries O_2 a metre or more from the lungs to the smallest blood vessels of the human extremities in $\sim 30\,\mathrm{s}$, whereas diffusion would take more than five years! Nevertheless, diffusion takes over as the dominant transport process for the final 10–$20\,\mu\mathrm{m}$ from blood to cell.

1.2 Functions of the cardiovascular system

- The primary function of the cardiovascular system (CVS) is the **rapid convective transport** of oxygen, glucose, amino acids, fatty acids, vitamins, drugs and water to the tissues; and the rapid washout of metabolic waste products from the tissues (carbon dioxide, urea, creatinine).
- The CVS is also a **control system**. It distributes hormones to the tissues, and secretes bioactive agents itself (natriuretic peptides, renin, nitric oxide, endothelin, prostaglandins).
- The CVS is crucial for **body temperature regulation**, because it transports heat from deep organs to the skin surface and regulates heat loss from the skin.
- In **reproduction** the CVS provides the hydraulic mechanism for genital erection.

1.3 The circulation of blood

The heart consists of two synchronous, muscular pumps, the right and left ventricles (Figure 1.4). Each pump is filled from a contractile reservoir, the right or left atrium. The right ventricle pumps deoxygenated blood through the pulmonary trunk to the lungs (Figure 1.5). Four pulmonary veins return oxygenated blood from the lungs to the left side of the heart, completing the short, low pressure **pulmonary circulation**. The left ventricle pumps an equal volume of oxygenated blood to the tissues of the body. The tissues extract some of the oxygen, and the partly deoxygenated blood returns via two great veins, the superior vena cava and inferior vena cava, to the right atrium. This completes the long, high pressure **systemic circulation**. One-way valves in the heart and veins ensure that blood follows the circular pathway described above, as first demonstrated by the London physician, **William Harvey**. Harvey's originality and groundbreaking introduction of experimentation into physiology and medicine disproved the earlier ebb-and-flow dogma of the previous 1000 years. His elegant work

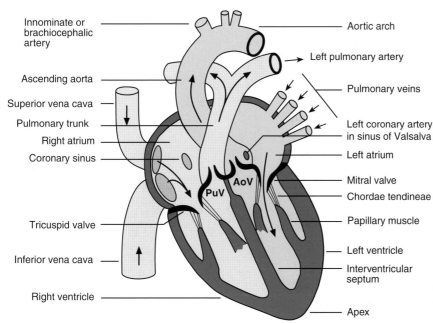

Figure 1.4 Structure of the mammalian heart. Pink indicates oxygenated blood; grey is deoxygenated blood. AoV, aortic valve; PuV, pulmonary valve.

is delightfully described in his book *De Motu Cordis* (Concerning the Motion of the Heart, 1628).

The right heart perfuses the pulmonary circulation

Venous blood enters the right atrium from the superior and inferior vena cava, and flows on through the tricuspid valve into the right ventricle. The ventricle is composed mainly of cardiac muscle, and fills with blood while the muscle is relaxed. Cardiac relaxation is called **diastole** (pronounced dia-stol-i). Contraction then follows (**systole** – pronounced sis-tol-i). Systole

pumps some of the ventricular blood into the pulmonary trunk at a low pressure. The trunk divides into the right and left pulmonary arteries, which supply each lung. Progressive branching leads to tiny blood vessels, called capillaries, in the walls of the minute air sacs of the lungs (alveoli). Here gases are exchanged by diffusion. Inhaled oxygen diffuses into the blood, raising its oxygen content from ~150 ml/litre (mixed venous blood, resting human) to ~195 ml/litre. At the same time, carbon dioxide diffuses out of the blood into the alveolar gas and is exhaled. The oxygenated blood returns through the pulmonary veins and passes through the left atrium into the left ventricle.

Figure 1.5 'Plumbing' of the human circulation. The systemic and pulmonary circulations are in series. The circulation to most systemic organs is in parallel (brain, myocardium, limbs, etc.), but the liver and renal tubules have an 'in series' or portal blood supply. Bronchial venous blood drains anomalously into the left atrium, slightly desaturating it. Red, oxygenated blood; black, deoxygenated blood. RA, LA, RV, LV, right and left atrium/ventricle, respectively.

The left heart perfuses the systemic circulation

The left ventricle contracts at the same time as the right ventricle and ejects the same volume of blood, but at a much higher pressure. The blood flows through the aorta, which gives off the major, named branches shown in Figure 1.6. Repeated arterial branching leads, ultimately, to millions of microscopic, thin-walled capillaries (Figure 1.7). Here the ultimate function of the cardiovascular system is fulfilled; dissolved gases, glucose and other metabolites diffuse between the capillary blood and the cells of the body. The deoxygenated blood returns through a convergent system of veins that, broadly speaking, accompany the named arteries and drain into the superior and inferior venae cavae (Figure 1.8).

1.4 Cardiac output and its distribution

Cardiac output is defined as the volume of blood ejected by one ventricle in one minute. Cardiac output therefore equals **stroke volume** (the volume ejected per contraction) multiplied by **heart rate** (the number of contractions per minute). In a resting adult the stroke volume is typically 70–80 ml and the heart rate is 60–75 beats per minute. Resting cardiac output is thus $\sim 75\,\text{ml} \times 70\,\text{min}^{-1}$,

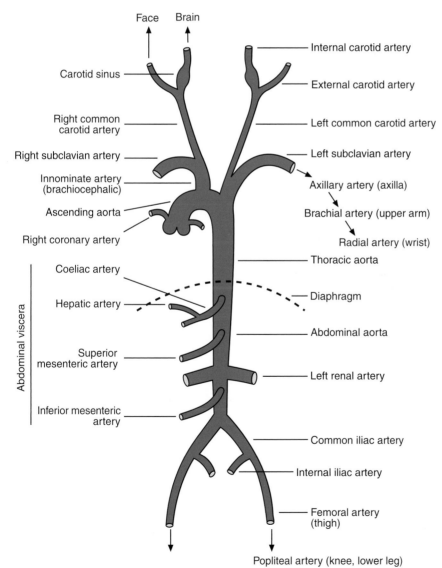

Figure 1.6 Simplified anatomy of human arterial system. Paired, thoracic intercostal arteries are not shown.

Wall/lumen	
2 mm/25 mm	Aorta
1 mm/4 mm	Muscular conduit artery
30 μm/30 μm	Arteriole
0.5 μm/6 μm	Capillary
3 μm/30 μm	Venule
0.5 mm/5 mm	Vein
1.5 mm/30 mm	Vena cava

Figure 1.7 Different types of blood vessel, seen in cross section and *en face*. The thickness of the wall relative to lumen is greatest in arterioles, though the ratio varies with vascular tone. The large-vessel dimensions apply to humans. (Sources as for Table 1.3.)

or ~5 litres min^{-1}. The output can increase greatly in response to increased peripheral oxygen demand, rising four- to five-fold during strenuous human exercise. How this increase is brought about, via autonomic nerves and physical distension, is described in Chapters 3–6.

Cardiac output is distributed in proportion to metabolic and functional demand

As a rough rule, the left ventricular output is distributed to the tissues of the body in proportion to their metabolic rate. For example, skeletal muscle accounts for ~20% of human O_2 consumption at rest and receives ~20% of the cardiac output (Figure 1.9). This egalitarian principle is overridden, however, in the kidneys, because their excretory function requires a high blood flow. The kidneys account for only 6% of human O_2 consumption, yet they receive 20% of the cardiac output, in order to generate an adequate excretion of water and urea. Since the renal blood flow is so enormous, some other tissues must receive less than their 'fair' share of the cardiac output; and, surprisingly, cardiac muscle (myocardium) is one of them. To compensate for its relative underperfusion, the myocardium extracts an unusually high proportion of the O_2 in arterial coronary blood, namely 65–75%. The norm for most tissues is only ~25%.

The distribution of the cardiac output between tissues is actively adjusted to match changing demands. For example, during exercise the fraction of the output that goes to skeletal muscle can be increased to ~80%. This is brought about by the **vasodilatation** (reversible widening) of tiny arterial vessels in the exercising muscle, called arterioles (Figure 1.7). Vasodilatation allows blood to flow more easily into the active muscle.

1.5 Introducing 'hydraulics': flow, pressure and resistance

Gradients of pressure drive the flow

What drives blood along a blood vessel? The chief factor is the gradient of blood pressure. Ventricular ejection raises aortic blood pressure to ~100 mmHg above atmospheric pressure. Pressure in the great veins, however, is close to atmospheric pressure. There is thus a large pressure difference driving blood from artery to vein. The usual cardiovascular units of pressure are 'mmHg above atmospheric pressure', because human blood pressure was, until recently, measured using a mercury column, with atmospheric pressure as the reference or zero level (see Appendix 2, 'Pressure').

Arterial pressure is **pulsatile**, because the heart ejects blood intermittently (systole), with rests in-between (diastole). During diastole the systemic arterial pressure decays from a peak of ~120 mmHg to a trough of ~80 mmHg; and pulmonary artery pressure decays from 25 mmHg to 10 mmHg (Figure 1.10). This is conventionally written as 120/80 mmHg and 25/10 mmHg, respectively.

A simple law links flow, pressure and conductance

Although arterial pressure and flow pulsate, many aspects of the circulation are best understood by using **average levels**. To get at the basic rule governing flow, let us consider a steady, non-pulsatile flow of water or plasma along a long rigid tube, driven by a constant pressure head. Under these conditions, flow $\dot{Q}$ is proportional to the pressure drop between the inlet (pressure P_1) and outlet (pressure P_2):

$$\dot{Q} \propto (P_1 - P_2) \qquad (1.2)$$

(Flow is often represented by a dotted Q in physiology, because Q stands for quantity of fluid and the

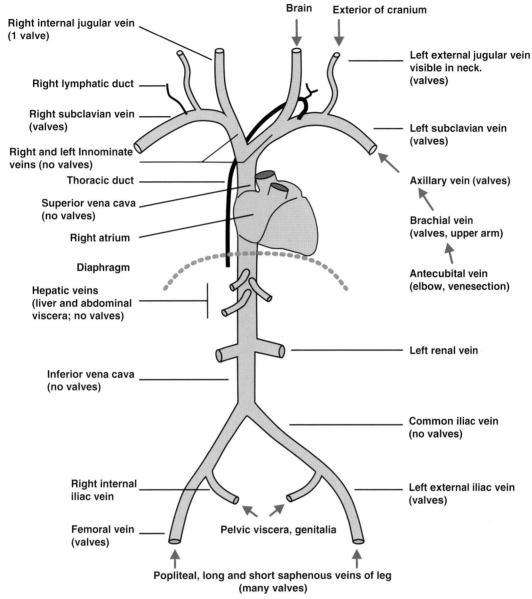

Figure 1.8 Simplified anatomy of human venous system. Valves occur in limb veins but not central veins. The drainage of the main lymphatic vessels, the thoracic duct and right lymphatic duct, into the neck veins, is shown. The lymphatic system develops as an outgrowth of the venous system during embryogenesis.

dot denotes rate of passage in Newton's original calculus notation.) Flow is, by definition, the **volume transferred per unit time**. Flow is thus a rate of transport, and the common expression 'rate of flow' is both tautologous and dimensionally incorrect!

If we insert a proportionality factor, K, into the above relation, we obtain a basic **law of flow** that tells us how much flow is generated by a given pressure difference:

$$\dot{Q} = K(P_1 - P_2) \qquad (1.3)$$

The proportionality factor K is called the **hydraulic conductance** of the tube. It is a measure of the ease of flow, and depends on tube width. The wider the tube, the greater the conductance and the bigger the flow generated by a given pressure gradient. Thus a large artery has a bigger conductance and carries a bigger flow than a narrow arteriole.

Resistance is the opposition to flow

Instead of considering the ease of flow (conductance), it is often more convenient to quantify the

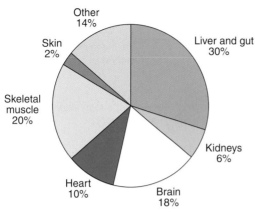

Oxygen consumption (rest)

- Other 14%
- Liver and gut 30%
- Skin 2%
- Skeletal muscle 20%
- Kidneys 6%
- Heart 10%
- Brain 18%

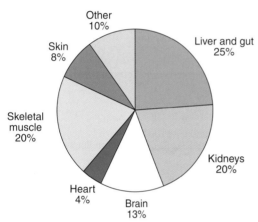

Cardiac output distribution (rest)

- Other 10%
- Liver and gut 25%
- Skin 8%
- Skeletal muscle 20%
- Kidneys 20%
- Heart 4%
- Brain 13%

Figure 1.9 Comparison of oxygen usage and cardiac output distribution in humans at rest. (Data from Wade OL, Bishop JM. *Cardiac Output and Regional Flow*. Oxford: Blackwell, 1962.)

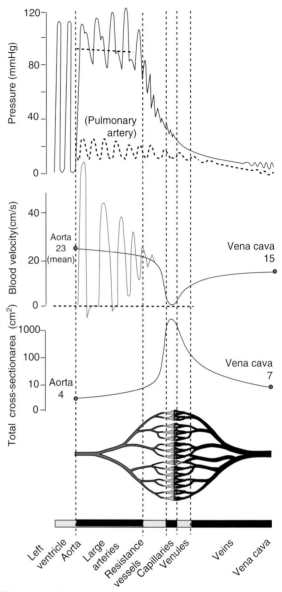

Figure 1.10 Pressure and blood velocity in systemic circulation of a resting human. (*Top trace*) The drop in mean pressure across the main arteries (dashed line) is only ~2 mmHg. The large pressure drop across the terminal arteries and arterioles (diameter 30–500 μm) shows that they are the main resistance vessels. Low pulmonary pressure profile is also shown. (*Middle trace*) Pulsation of blood velocity (red line) and change in mean velocity across circulation (black line). The same blood flow passes each vertical dashed line per minute, namely the cardiac output. Mean velocity is blood flow divided by the cross-sectional area of the vascular bed (see text). (*Bottom trace*) Increase in total cross-sectional area of the circulation in microvessels.

difficulty that blood experiences in passing through a vessel – the vessel's opposition to flow, or 'hydraulic resistance'. The hydraulic resistance of a tube is simply the inverse of its conductance (ease of flow); resistance R is $1/K$. Thus we can rewrite the above basic law of flow as:

$$\dot{Q} = \frac{(P_1 - P_2)}{R} \qquad (1.4)$$

This is called **Darcy's law of flow**. (As an aide-memoire, note its similarity to Ohm's law, i.e. flow of electrical current = voltage difference/electrical resistance.) Darcy's law tells us that $R = (P_1 - P_2)/\dot{Q}$, so **resistance is the difference in mean pressure needed to drive one unit of flow in the steady state**, and its units are mmHg per ml/min. The bigger the resistance, the bigger the difference in pressure needed to drive a given flow.

Resistance is low in wide vessels, such as the named arteries and veins, and is high in narrow vessels such as arterioles. Thus arteries need only a small pressure drop to drive the cardiac output though them, whereas the arterioles need a much bigger pressure drop (Figure 1.10). **The drop in pressure across a given class of vessel is thus an index of its resistance**. In this way we know that, in a resting human, the named large arteries account for only 2% of the total resistance of the systemic circulation; the smallest arteries and the arterioles ~60%; the capillaries ~20%; and the venous system ~15%.

The resistances of tubes in series summate

When two tubes are joined in series (end to end), the resistances add up. Consequently, although the resistance of the aorta is low, the resistance of the systemic circulation is high, due to the additional high resistances of the narrow arterioles and capillaries. (Linkage in parallel is considered in Chapter 8.) The total resistance of the human systemic circulation is ~0.02 mmHg min ml^{-1}. The resistance of the pulmonary circulation is only 1/7th as much, 0.003 mmHg min ml^{-1}, because pulmonary vessels are shorter and wider than their systemic counterparts. Consequently, a low pulmonary arterial pressure suffices to drive the cardiac output through the lungs.

Active contraction/relaxation of arterioles adjusts peripheral resistance and local blood flow

Darcy's law of flow helps us to understand how the blood flow to a peripheral organ or tissue is regulated – for example, how it is increased to an exercising muscle or a secreting gland. Equation 1.4 shows that there are only two ways to raise the blood flow – either the driving pressure must be raised or the vascular resistance reduced. Arterial blood pressure is generally kept within a narrow range by nervous reflexes, so it is normally **changes in vascular resistance that regulate local blood flow**. For example, when we salivate, the blood flow to the salivary gland increases ten-fold, because the vascular resistance of the gland is reduced to one-tenth of its former value through arteriolar vasodilatation; the arterial pressure driving the flow is unchanged. Changes in vascular resistance are brought about by the contraction and relaxation of the narrow, terminal branches of the arterial system, so we must next consider the structure of blood vessels.

1.6 Blood vessel structure

The aorta gives rise to named conduit arteries (Figure 1.6). These branch repeatedly to form tiny arteries of diameter 0.1–0.5 mm, which branch into even narrower vessels of very high resistance, the arterioles (Figure 1.7). Arterioles branch into a vast number of fine, thin-walled capillaries. Capillaries converge to form venules, which converge into small veins, which converge into large, named veins (Figure 1.8).

Branching slows down the blood

Capillary numbers are colossal; the capillaries of an adult human would girdle the earth if laid end-to-end (40 000 km). The total cross-sectional area of the vascular system at a given branch level is the number of vessels n times the cross-sectional area of an individual vessel, πr^2. As blood traverses the arterial tree, the increase in n through branching outweighs the reduction in vessel size, πr^2. Consequently, the **total cross-sectional area of the circulation increases from aorta to capillary bed** (Table 1.2 and Figure 1.10). It then falls as venous vessels converge.

The broadening of the circulation with branching is important, because it slows down the blood, just as the current in a river slows down when the river banks widen. The **blood velocity** (cm/s) at a particular branch level equals the total **flow** (cm^3/s), namely the cardiac output, divided by the total **cross-sectional area** of the branches (cm^2): velocity = flow/area. Consequently, capillary blood

Table 1.2 Comparison of number and size of different types of blood vessels, in dog mesentery[a]

Vessel	Number	Length (mm)	Diameter (mm)	Total cross-sectional area (mm²)	Volume (% of total)
Main artery	1	60	3	7	2.5
Arterioles and smallest arteries	1 380 000	1.5–2	0.024–0.031	739	8.1
Capillaries	47 300 000	0.4	0.008	2378[b]	5.7
Venules	2 100 000	1.0	0.026	1151	6.9
Small veins	180 000	1–14	0.075–0.28	1019	21.3[c]
Large veins	61	39–60	1.5–6	174	46.7[c]

[a]In the mesentery, unlike most tissues, microvessels are easy to see and therefore quantify.
[b]Capillaries have the largest cross-sectional area and therefore slowest flow.
[c]Veins contain most of the circulating blood volume.
(After Scleier J. *Archiv Gesamte Physiologie*. 1918; **173**: 172.)

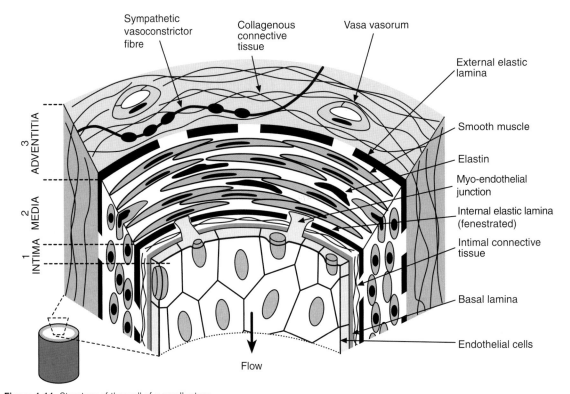

Figure 1.11 Structure of the wall of a small artery.

velocity is ~1/200th of arterial blood velocity, due to the vast increase in cross-sectional area (Figure 1.10). The slow blood velocity in systemic and pulmonary capillaries is important, because it gives the red cells **sufficient time to exchange oxygen and carbon dioxide**.

The vascular wall has three layers

The wall of all blood vessels, except capillaries, consists of three layers (Figure 1.11): the tunica intima (innermost coat), tunica media (middle coat) and tunica adventitia (outer coat).

The **intima** is a sheet of flattened endothelial cells resting on a thin layer of connective tissue. The endothelial layer is the main barrier to the escape of plasma. It also secretes many vasoactive chemicals, including the antithrombotic vasodilator, nitric oxide.

The **media** supplies mechanical strength and contractile power. It consists of spindle-shaped, smooth muscle cells, arranged helically, embedded in a matrix of elastin and collagen fibres. Two sheets of elastin, called the internal and external elastic lamina, mark the boundaries of the media. Intimal endothelial cells send processes through the internal elastic lamina in places, to make contact with smooth muscle cells. These myo-endothelial junctions transmit signals from the intima to the media.

The **adventitia** is a connective tissue sheath with no distinct outer border. Its role is to tether the vessel loosely to the surrounding tissue. The adventitia of most vessels contains **sympathetic fibre terminals**. Each terminal has numerous bead-like swellings ('varicosities') that release a vasoconstrictor agent, noradrenaline, which regulates local resistance and blood flow. In large arteries and veins the adventitia also contains small blood vessels, called **vasa vasorum** (literally 'vessels of vessels'), which nourish the thick media. In limb veins, the adventitia contains **nociceptive nerve fibres**, which mediate the pain of thrombophlebitis.

Blood vessels develop from endothelium in the embryo

The cardiovascular system is the first organ system to form in the embryo, because it is needed to deliver O_2 and nutrients to the developing tissues. Embryonic blood vessels formation, or **vasculogenesis**, is controlled by signalling molecules. Vasculogenesis begins when mesodermal precursor cells express a receptor for **vascular endothelial growth factor** (VEGF-A). Embryos lacking VEGF-A, or its receptor VEGFR-2, fail to form blood vessels and die. Vasculogenesis starts at two sites, one in the yolk sac and one in the embryo proper. In the yolk sac, VEGFR-2-positive cells develop into islands of endothelium, which enclose blood precursor cells (haemangioblasts). The islands then fuse to form a primary capillary plexus. In the embryo itself, VEGFR-2 cells form endothelial tubes that develop into the heart (Section 2.1), dorsal aorta and primary (cardinal) vein. The primary vessels then develop connections with the capillary plexus. After this the system remodels, under genetic and haemodynamic influences, to form arteries, capillaries and veins. Smooth muscle cells differentiate under the influence of transforming growth factor-β, and are recruited to blood vessels by an endothelial secretion, platelet-derived growth factor. Endothelial membrane proteins called **ephrins** determine which tubes become arteries, as opposed to veins.

Endothelial cell proliferation and VEGF also play a key role in the growth of new blood vessels in children and adults – for example, in wound healing and cancer. This is called **angiogenesis** (cf. vasculogenesis); see Chapter 9. The inhibition of angiogenesis in cancers is now a therapeutic target, because a cancer cannot grow to a large size without a growing blood supply.

1.7 Functional classes of vessel

The mature circulation has evolved along sound economic principles, namely that each vessel must fulfil at least one extra role besides conducting blood. On this basis the following major classes of vessel are recognized:

- elastic arteries
- conduit and feed (muscular) arteries
- resistance vessels
- exchange vessels
- capacitance vessels.

In each class of vessel the structure of the wall is specially adapted to its role, as follows.

Elastic arteries accommodate the stroke volume and smooth the flow

The heart ejects blood only during systole. Therefore, if arteries were completely rigid, there would be no peripheral blood flow during diastole. This potential problem is circumvented by the distensibility of the largest arteries, caused by an abundance of elastin (Table 1.3). The extracellular protein **elastin** is six times more extensible than rubber. The distensibility conferred by elastin enables the aorta, iliac arteries and pulmonary trunk (diameter 1–2 cm in humans) to act as temporary blood storage vessels; they expand by ~10% during each heartbeat to accommodate the ejected blood. The stretched elastin also stores mechanical energy. During diastole, the stored mechanical energy (tension) maintains the arterial blood pressure, which drives the blood through the resistance vessels. Thus, despite the fact that the heart ejects blood only intermittently, arterial blood pressure does not fall below ~80 mmHg, and blood flows continuously through the peripheral tissues (Figure 1.10).

Collagen is the other major extracellular protein of elastic arteries. Collagen fibrils are ~100 times less distensible than elastin. They form a partly slack network in the media and prevent overdistension if blood pressure rises. The elastic artery wall is thus a composite material, similar in many respects to a car tyre – the rubber/elastin allows expansion up to a

Table 1.3 Composition of the blood vessel wall (%)

	Endothelium	Smooth muscle	Elastin tissue	Collagen
Elastic artery	5	25	40	27
Arteriole	10	60	10	20
Capillary	95	0	0	5 (basal lamina)
Venule	20	20	0	60

(After Caro CG, Pedley TJ, Schroter RC, Seed WA. *The Mechanics of the Circulation.* Oxford: Oxford University Press, 1978; and Burton AC. *Physiology and Biophysics of the Circulation.* Chicago, IL: Year Book Medical Publishers, 1972.)

certain volume, beyond which increasing tension in inelastic fibres prevents overexpansion. As elastin fragments with age, the stiffer collagen increasingly dominates the properties of elastic vessels – a process called '**arteriosclerosis**' (Chapter 18).

Conduit arteries and feed arteries deliver blood to the organs

Medium-size conduit arteries include the brachial, radial, femoral, cerebral and coronary arteries (diameter 0.1–1.0 cm in humans). Their tunica media contains more smooth muscle and is thicker, relative to the lumen, than in elastic arteries (Figure 1.7). The thick wall prevents collapse at sharp bends such as the elbow and knee. The primary role of these **conduit or conducting arteries** is to conduct the flow from the elastic arteries to smaller arteries that feed the resistance vessels (**feed arteries**).

Conduit and feed arteries have a rich sympathetic innervation and can change their diameter actively. **Dilatation** facilitates the local increase in blood flow to skeletal muscle during exercise. **Contraction** reduces peripheral blood flow – spectacularly so in diving mammals. **Vasospasm** is an intense sustained contraction of conduit arteries. This can be life-saving in accidents, as demonstrated by a motor-cycle crash victim brought into Accident and Emergency with one leg severed at the knee. The popliteal artery was torn in half, but was scarcely bleeding, because shed blood platelets had triggered vasospasm. This prevented the patient from bleeding to death. Less beneficial is the cerebral artery vasospasm evoked by cerebral haemorrhage, which can cause a stroke; and the vasospasm of diseased coronary arteries, which can cause cardiac angina at rest (variant angina).

Pressure falls sharply across resistance vessels (terminal arteries and arterioles)

From the small feed arteries, blood enters narrow terminal arteries (diameter 100–500 μm) and the final branches of the arterial tree, the arterioles (diameter 10–100 μm). These vessels dominate the resistance of the entire circulation, as shown by **the pressure profile of the circulation** (Figure 1.10). Mean blood pressure falls very little along the elastic and conduit arteries (~2 mmHg from aorta to radial artery), because their wide diameter creates little resistance to flow. (The odd 'peaking' of the pressure wave in peripheral arteries is explained in Chapter 8.) **The major fall in blood pressure occurs across the terminal arteries and arterioles.** From the law of flow (eqn 1.4), we see there is only one possible explanation for a large pressure drop; these vessels must offer a large resistance to flow; resistance = pressure drop per unit flow. The terminal arteries and arterioles are therefore called **resistance vessels**.

The **proximal resistance vessels**, namely the terminal arteries, are richly innervated by sympathetic vasoconstrictor nerve fibres, and the muscular wall is thick, relative to the lumen (Figure 1.7). The **distal resistance vessels**, namely the terminal arterioles, are poorly innervated, and the media comprises just one to three layers of smooth muscle cells. Some workers define an arteriole as a vessel with just one layer of muscle, while others define it as an arterial vessel of diameter <100 μm. The terminal arteries and arterioles have a high resistance because the lumen is narrow and the number of vessels is relatively low (Table 1.2).

Resistance vessels act as 'taps' regulating local blood flow and capillary perfusion

Since the resistance vessels dominate the net resistance to blood flow, they act as the taps of the circulation – that is to say, they can turn local blood flow up or down to match local demand. When the resistance vessels dilate (**vasodilatation**), resistance to flow falls, so local blood flow increases. Conversely, **vasoconstriction** raises local resistance and reduces the local blood flow. The terminal arterioles also adjust the number of capillaries perfused with blood. This task used to be attributed to imaginary 'precapillary sphincters', but it is now generally accepted that true sphincters rarely exist in blood vessels.

Exchange vessels transfer O_2 and nutrients to the tissue

The exchange of oxygen, CO_2, metabolites and fluid between blood and tissue occurs chiefly in the capillaries. **Capillaries** are tiny (diameter 4–7 μm) and very numerous, so most cells lie within 10–20 μm of the nearest capillary. The capillary wall comprises a single layer of endothelial cells 0.5 μm thick, with no media or adventitia. The extreme thinness facilitates the rapid passage of solutes. Some O_2 exchange also occurs through the walls of the arterioles, upstream of the capillaries; and some fluid exchange occurs downstream, in the **postcapillary or pericytic venule** (microscopic venule that lacks a complete smooth muscle coat; diameter 15–50 μm). Strictly speaking, therefore, the term **exchange vessel** includes capillaries and microvessels immediately upstream and downstream.

Although capillaries are very narrow, the capillary bed as a whole has a surprisingly low resistance to flow, and the pressure drop across it is only ~20 mmHg (Figure 1.10). The low resistance is due to multiple factors: the very large numbers of capillaries running in parallel (Table 1.2), their shortness (~1 mm), and a special kind of flow called bolus flow (Chapter 8). The large cross-sectional area of the capillary bed slows the blood velocity to 0.5–1 mm/s (Figure 1.10). As a result, the '**transit time**' for a red cell to traverse a systemic capillary is ~0.5–2 s. This allows the red cell sufficient time to unload O_2 and take up CO_2 from the tissue.

Arteriovenous anastomoses regulate heat exchange

A few tissues, notably the skin and nasal mucosa, possess wide shunt vessels of diameter 20–130 μm that connect arterioles directly to venules, bypassing the capillaries. These shunts are called arteriovenous anastomoses (singular, anastomosis). Their thick muscular walls are richly innervated by sympathetic vasoconstrictor fibres. In the skin they are involved in the control of body temperature, and in the nasal mucosa they help to warm the inspired air. Arteriovenous anastomoses are not common in other tissues.

Capacitance vessels are venous vessels that act as blood reservoirs

Venules (diameter 50–200 μm) and veins differ chiefly in size and number. The thin wall comprises an intima, a thin media of smooth muscle and collagen, and the adventitia. In limb veins the intima has

semilunar valves at intervals, as described by Harvey's teacher, the gloriously named Hieronymus Fabricius ab Aquapendente, at Padua University in 1603. The semilunar valves prevent the backflow of venous blood in the limbs under the drag of gravity (Figure 8.26). By contrast, the large central veins and the veins of the head and neck lack functional valves.

Venules and small veins are more numerous than the corresponding arterioles and arteries (Table 1.2), so their net resistance is low. Consequently, a pressure drop of only 10–15 mmHg is sufficient to drive the cardiac output from the venules to the right atrium.

Because of their large number and size, veins and venules contain about two-thirds of the circulating blood at any one instant, and are therefore called 'capacitance vessels' (Figure 1.12). The volume of blood in this venous reservoir is variable, partly because the thin venous wall is easily distended/collapsed, and partly because many veins are innervated by sympathetic vasoconstrictor fibres. At times of physiological stress an increase in sympathetic fibre activity causes the capacitance vessels to contract, displacing blood into the heart and arteries to help maintain arterial pressure.

1.8 The plumbing of the circulation

'In parallel' versus 'in series' circulations

The systemic circulation is divided into specialized, individual circuits, each supplying a specialized tissue or organ (brain, heart wall, kidneys, intestine, etc.). The arterial supply to each organ usually comes from the aorta, so that each organ is supplied directly with arterialized blood. This form of plumbing is called an **in parallel** arrangement (Figure 1.5). In a few organs, however, the main blood supply is the venous outflow from another organ upstream. The two organs are thus connected **in series**, not in parallel. This type of arrangement is also called a **portal system**, and it has certain advantages and disadvantages, as follows.

Portal circulations provide a direct delivery service

The **liver** has the largest portal system in the body. Around 72% of the liver's blood supply comes from the portal vein, which contains deoxygenated, venous blood from the intestine and spleen (Figure 1.5). The portal vein enters the liver at the

Blood volume distribution

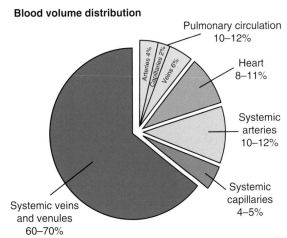

Figure 1.12 Approximate distribution of 5.5 litres blood in a supine, resting man. On standing, the percentage of blood in the lungs falls by about one-third, as does the volume in the heart, while the volume in peripheral veins increases (Adapted from Folkow B, Neil E. *Circulation*. London: Oxford University Press, 1971, by permission.)

'porta hepatis' (gateway of the liver), from which the term 'portal system' originates. In addition, the liver receives about a quarter of its blood flow via the hepatic artery; so its circuitry is partly in parallel, as well as in series. Portal systems have the advantage that they transport valuable substances directly from one site to another. For example, the portal vein transports the products of digestion directly from the intestine to the liver, for immediate metabolic processing and/or storage.

Portal systems also exist in the **kidney**, where effluent blood from the glomerulus supplies the tubules; and in the **brain**, where a portal vein carries releasing hormones from the hypothalamus to the anterior pituitary gland.

A portal system has one obvious drawback, however – the downstream tissue receives partially deoxygenated blood under a reduced pressure head. As a result the downstream tissue is vulnerable to damage during episodes of hypotension (low arterial pressure). For example, renal tubular damage is a relatively common complication of severe hypotension.

1.9 Control systems

The heart and blood vessels continually adjust their contractile state to meet the varying demands of daily life, such as standing, exercise, salivation, stress, etc. Such changes are brought about by nervous and endocrine reflexes, and are co-ordinated by the brain. One of the most important cardiovascular reflexes is the **arterial baroreceptor reflex**, which stabilizes arterial blood pressure and thus maintains the pressure driving blood to the brain. The reflex is initiated by stretch receptors, called baroreceptors, in the walls of major arteries. The baroreceptors sense changes in blood pressure and relay the information to the brainstem. This elicits reflex changes in the activity of autonomic nerves controlling the heart and blood vessels. The resulting changes in cardiac output, peripheral resistance and venous capacitance help restore arterial blood pressure to normal.

Where should we go from here? In a system as complex as the cardiovascular system there is a danger of not seeing the wood for the trees, but the above outline should help avoid this. In Chapters 2–14 (cardiac electricity, haemodynamics, etc.) we bump into the trees and even peep under the bark. In Chapters 15–18, we stand back again, to gain a broader perspective of how the system as a whole responds to physiological and medical challenges.

SUMMARY

- The beating of the heart generates a rapid, convective transport of O_2, nutrients, waste products, hormones and heat around the body. The branching vascular tree conveys O_2 to within 10–$20\,\mu m$ of most cells; the short final distance is covered by diffusion. Since diffusive transport time increases as the square of distance, tissues die in the absence of convective transport (e.g. myocardial infarction).

- The right ventricle is filled via the right atrium and pumps deoxygenated blood at low pressure (mean $\sim 15\,mmHg$) through the low-resistance pulmonary circulation for oxygenation. The left ventricle is filled via the left atrium and pumps oxygenated blood at high pressure (mean $\sim 90\,mmHg$) through the high-resistance systemic circulation.

- Human resting cardiac output is $\sim 5\,l\,min^{-1}$. Output equals heart rate (60–70 beats min^{-1}) times stroke volume (70–$80\,ml$). The distribution to individual tissues is controlled by the local resistance vessels. Blood flow is generally allocated to a tissue in proportion to its metabolic activity, but the kidneys receive a disproportionate 20% of the cardiac output to satisfy their excretory role.

- Blood flow $\dot{Q}$ is driven by the pressure drop from artery to vein, $P_A - P_V$. Darcy's law of flow states $\dot{Q} = (P_A - P_V)/R$, where R is resistance to flow. Resistance is located chiefly in the tiny terminal arteries and arterioles, as shown by the large pressure drop across them. These 'resistance vessels' can actively constrict or dilate to match local blood flow to local demand.

- Other functional categories of vessel are as follows. Elastic arteries (e.g. aorta) receive the intermittently ejected stroke volume and convert it into a continuous albeit pulsatile peripheral flow. Exchange vessels (capillaries, postcapillary venules) allow solute and water to exchange with the tissue. Capacitance vessels (venules, veins) contain about two-thirds of the circulating blood volume and act as a controlled, variable reservoir of blood.

- Except in capillaries the vascular wall comprises three layers: the tunica intima (endothelium), tunica media (vascular smooth muscle, collagen, elastin) and tunica adventitia (connective tissue, nerve fibres). The smooth muscle regulates the vessel diameter and thereby regulates local blood flow and the distribution of blood volume.

- Vascular smooth muscle is controlled by autonomic nerves, circulating hormones and local factors. Autonomic nerves and circulating hormones also regulate the rate and force of the heartbeat. In this way the brain and reflexes can control the cardiovascular system. For example, the baroreflex stabilizes arterial blood pressure.

- Most specialized circulations (coronary, cerebral, etc.) are plumbed in parallel to each other, so that each organ receives fully oxygenated blood. Portal circulations are in series with an upstream tissue and thus receive venous blood. For example, the portal vein supplies the liver with venous blood from the intestine.

Further reading

Coultas L, Chawengsaksophak K, Rossant J. Endothelial cells and VEGF in vascular development. *Nature* 2005; **438**: 937–45.

Fenger-Gron J, Mulvany MJ, Christensen KL. Mesenteric blood pressure profile of conscious, freely moving rats. *Journal of Physiology* 1995; **488**: 753–60.

Harvey W. (1628) *On the Motion of the Heart and Blood in Animals* ('*De Motu Cordis*', trans. by R. Willis). London: Prometheus Books, 1993.

Henderson JR, Daniel PM. Capillary beds and portal circulations. In: Renkin EM, Michel CC (eds). *Handbook of Physiology*, The Cardiovascular System, Vol. IV, Part 2. Bethesda, MD: The American Physiological Society, 1984: 1035–46.

Jones EAV, le Noble F, Eichmann A. What determines blood vessel structure? Genetic prespecification vs hemodynamics. *Physiology* 2006; **21**: 388–95.

Neil E. Peripheral circulation: historical aspects. In: Shepherd JT, Abboud FM (eds). *Handbook of Physiology*, Vol. III, Part 1. Bethesda, MD: American Physiological Society, 1983: 120.

Ritman EL, Lerman A. The dynamic vasa vasorum. *Cardiovascular Research* 2007; **75**: 649–58.

CHAPTER 2

The cardiac cycle

Learning objectives

After reading this chapter you should be able to:

- State the significance of the fibrotendinous ring, the four valves, papillary muscle, ventricle wall thickness and the pacemaker (2.1).
- List the four phases of the ventricular cycle and related valve positions (2.2).
- Sketch the changes in atrial and ventricular pressures over the cardiac cycle (Figure 2.5).
- Draw a ventricular pressure–volume loop, labelling each side and corner (Figure 2.6).
- Define ejection fraction and give typical values (2.3).
- Give the relative timings of diastole and systole at rest and during maximal exercise (2.4).
- State the origins of (i) the apex beat; (ii) the heart sounds; (iii) cardiac murmurs (2.5).
- Outline briefly the nature and use of echocardiography, radionuclide angiography and cardiac catheterization (2.6).

An adult human heart weighs only 250–350 g, yet it pumps out ~200 million litres of blood, via ~3 billion (3×10^9) contractions over our allotted 'three score years and ten', making the heart one of the most heavily used muscles in the body. This chapter describes the mechanical events that generate the heart's truly remarkable output.

2.1 Gross structure of the heart

The human heart is a four-chambered, hollow muscle, roughly conical in shape, ~12 cm long by 9 cm wide. It lies obliquely across the midline of the chest with the tip of the cone (the cardiac **apex**) behind the fifth left intercostal space (Figures 2.1 and 2.7). The heart is rotated around its long axis so that the right atrium and right ventricle form the anterior surface.

The four cardiac chambers are built upon a ring of fibrous fatty tissue called the **annulus fibrosus**, located at the atrioventricular junction. The atrio-ventricular plane is called the **base** of the heart, and it moves towards the apex during systole. The annulus fibrosus has three roles. First, it acts as a mechanical base for the atria and ventricles, which are attached to its upper and lower sides, respectively. Second, it defines four apertures, each containing a valve. Third, it insulates the ventricles electrically from the atria.

The cardiac chambers are lined internally by the **endocardium** (endo-, inside), comprising a thin sheet of flattened endothelial cells over connective tissue and, in places, scanty smooth muscle cells. Endothelium also lines the valve surfaces and all blood vessels. The outer surface of the heart is covered by **epicardium** (epi-, outside), a thin layer of flattened mesothelial cells over connective tissue. The entire heart is enclosed in a fibrous sac or **pericardium** (peri-, around). The narrow, mesothelium-lined space between the epicardium and pericardium contains **pericardial fluid**, which lubricates the cardiac surfaces. The lower surface of the pericardium is fused to the diaphragm.

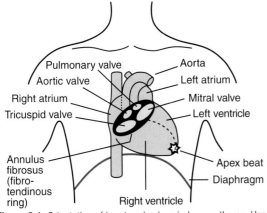

Figure 2.1 Orientation of heart and valves in human thorax. Heart lies obliquely, and is rotated so that right atrium and right ventricle form most of anterior surface. A fibrotendinous ring forms the 'base' of the heart. Tip of ventricle forms the 'apex'. Inferior surface and pericardium (not shown) rest on central tendon of diaphragm. The four valves are grouped closely in an oblique plane behind the sternum.

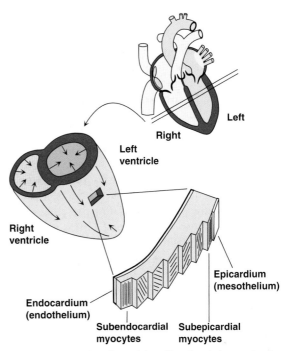

Figure 2.2 Direction of ventricle wall motion during contraction (*middle*) and orientation of muscle fibres in the ventricle wall (*bottom*). The longitudinal shortening of the left ventricle length during systole accounts for ~60% of the stroke volume and is due chiefly to the base (atrioventricular plane) descending towards the apex, rather than apex moving towards the base.

Consequently, each time the diaphragm descends during inspiration, the heart is dragged into a more vertical orientation.

Right atrium and tricuspid valve

The right atrium is the thin-walled, muscular chamber that receives the venous return from the two venae cavae and the coronary sinus. The coronary sinus is the main vein draining the heart muscle (Figure 1.4). The **pacemaker**, which is the 'sparking plug' that initiates each heartbeat, is located in the wall of the right atrium, close to the entrance of the superior vena cava.

A valve with three cusps, the tricuspid valve, connects the right atrium to the right ventricle. Each cusp is a thin, baggy flap, ~0.1 mm thick, composed of connective tissue and covered by endothelium. The free margin of each cusp is tethered by tendinous strings, the **chordae tendineae**, to an inward projection of the ventricle wall called a **papillary muscle** (Figure 1.4). The papillary muscles contract and tense the chordae tendineae during systole. This prevents the valve from inverting into the atrium as pressure builds up in the ventricle.

Right ventricle and pulmonary valve

The free wall of the human right ventricle is ~0.5 cm thick and resembles a pocket tacked around the interventricular septum (Figure 2.2). The expulsion of blood is produced partly by the free anterior wall approaching the septum, as in old-fashioned bellows, and partly by movement of the base (tricuspid valve) towards the apex. The outlet from the ventricle into the pulmonary artery is guarded by the pulmonary valve, which has three equal-sized, baggy cusps.

Left atrium and mitral valve

The left atrium receives blood from the four pulmonary veins and transmits it into the left ventricle through a bicuspid valve. The large anterior and small posterior cusps were thought to look like a bishop's mitre, hence the name mitral valve. The cusp margins are tethered by chordae tendineae to two papillary muscles in the left ventricle, which prevents eversion (Figure 1.4).

Left ventricle, apex beat and aortic valve

The left ventricle wall is about three times thicker than that of the right ventricle, because the left side has to generate higher arterial pressures. Blood is ejected by a reduction in diameter (~40% of stroke volume) and length (~60% of stroke volume).

The latter is due chiefly to the contracting muscle dragging the base (mitral plane) towards the apex, rather than apex towards base. The muscle fibres are wrapped around the chamber somewhat like a turban, i.e. their orientation changes progressively. The innermost or **subendocardial muscle fibres** are orientated longitudinally, running from the base (fibrotendinous ring) to apex (tip of left ventricle). The central fibres run circumferentially, the outermost or **subepicardial fibres** again run longitudinally, and intermediate fibres run obliquely (Figure 2.2). When the chamber contracts, it twists forwards and the apex taps against the chest wall, producing a palpable **apex beat**. This is normally felt in the fifth, left intercostal space, about 10 cm from the midline (the mid-clavicular line). Cardiac enlargement can be detected by the deviation of the apex beat from its normal location.

The root of the aorta contains a three-cusp valve. Occasionally it has only two cusps, and such valves are prone to narrowing (**stenosis**) in later life. Next to each cusp, the root of the aorta bulges out into the **sinuses of Valsalva**. The two coronary arteries originate in the sinuses, just behind the valve leaflets (Figure 1.4).

Cardiac embryogenesis and congenital cardiac abnormalities

The heart starts out as a simple endothelial tube located between the main vein and dorsal aorta. A coat of mesodermal cells differentiates into myocardial cells, which begin to contract rhythmically by day 19–20 in humans. The tube folds into an S-shape as it grows, and develops constrictions that delineate a primitive single atrium and ventricle. Each chamber is then subdivided into two. The two atria, however, remain connected by an opening, the **foramen ovale** (see Figure 4.1). This shunts most blood from the right atrium directly into the left atrium, since there is no need to perfuse the lungs for O_2 uptake *in utero*. Right atrial and ventricular blood is well oxygenated because it comes partly from the placental vein. Residual right-side blood, that has not been diverted through the foramen ovale, passes into the pulmonary trunk, from where much of it flows directly into the aorta through a connection called the **ductus arteriosus**. Thus most blood bypasses the lungs. The ductus arteriosus and foramen ovale normally close soon after birth, redirecting the entire blood flow from the right side into the lungs for oxygenation.

Due to the intricacy of cardiac development, congenital cardiac abnormalities are relatively common (~1 per 100 live births). They fall into four categories:

- defects in the ventricular septum (commonest) or atrial septum;
- persistent patent ductus arteriosus;
- aortic coarctation (narrowing of the aorta near the ductus arteriosus insertion);
- transposition of the major vessels. In Fallot's tetralogy, for example, the aortic orifice overlies the ventricular septum, and there is a ventricular septal defect, narrow pulmonary trunk and hypertrophied right ventricle.

Most of these conditions require surgical correction.

2.2 The ventricular cycle

The cycle of atrial and ventricular contraction is called the cardiac cycle (Figure 2.3). The ventricular cycle is divided into four phases, based on the positions of the inlet and outlet valves. Let us begin with the moment when both the atria and ventricles are relaxed (diastole). The timings below refer to a human cycle lasting 0.9 s, which corresponds to 67 beats/min. The information has been acquired by echocardiography (Section 2.6), cardiac catheterization (Section 2.6) and electrocardiography (Chapter 5).

Ventricular filling

Duration:	0.5 s (resting human)
Inlet valves (tricuspid, mitral):	open
Outlet valves (pulmonary, aortic):	closed

Ventricular diastole occupies nearly two-thirds of the cardiac cycle in a resting human, providing ample time to fill the ventricles. Initially the atria are likewise in diastole, so blood flows passively from the great veins through the relaxed atria and the open atrioventricular valves into the ventricles. Filling is very fast over the initial 0.15 s (Figure 2.4, ventricle blood volume plot). This **initial rapid-filling phase** displays a curious feature, namely ventricular pressure falls initially, despite blood volume increasing. The explanation is that the relaxing ventricle is recoiling elastically from its deformed end-systolic shape, and is thus sucking blood into its chamber in early diastole.

As the ventricle reaches its inherent, relaxed volume, the rate of filling slows down (**diastasis**).

Figure 2.3 Changes in valves, atrial and ventricular volumes during the cardiac cycle. For clarity, the apex is drawn here as if shifted towards the atrioventricular plane (base) during systole, but imaging shows that much of the longitudinal shortening is due to the base being pulled down towards the apex.

Further filling is driven by the venous pressure, which distends the ventricle and causes ventricular pressure to rise gradually.

In the final third of the filling phase **atrial contraction** pumps extra blood into the ventricle. In young adults atrial systole boosts the ventricular filling by 10–20% at rest, but the proportion increases with age, reaching 46% by 80 years. The atrial boost becomes more important during exercise, especially in the young, because the raised heart rate leaves less time for passive ventricular filling.

The volume of blood in a ventricle at the end of its filling phase is called the **end-diastolic volume** (EDV). The EDV is typically ~120 ml in a standing man (Figure 2.4), and ~150 ml supine. The corresponding **end-diastolic pressure** (EDP) is just a few mmHg. EDP is a little higher on the left side than on the right (Table 2.1), because the thicker left ventricle wall requires a higher pressure to distend it. Since pressures are higher in the left atrium than right atrium, congenital defects in the atrial septum in neonates usually result in a left-to-right flow of blood. Such defects do not, therefore, deoxygenate the arterial blood or cause 'blue baby' syndrome.

Isovolumetric contraction

Duration:	0.05 s
Inlet valves:	closed
Outlet valves:	closed

Atrial systole is followed by ventricular systole. This lasts 0.35 s and is divided into a brief isovolumetric phase and a longer ejection phase. As soon as ventricular pressure rises just above atrial pressure, the atrioventricular valves are closed by the reversed pressure gradient. Backflow during closure is minimal because vortices approximate the valve cusps during the late filling phase (Figure 2.3, top). Since the ventricle has temporarily become a closed chamber, the tension of its contracting wall causes the pressure of the trapped blood to rise rapidly. The maximum rate of rise of pressure, dP/dt_{max}, is often used as an index of cardiac contractility (Figure 2.4).

Ejection

Duration:	0.3 s
Inlet valves:	closed
Outlet valves:	open

When ventricular pressure exceeds arterial pressure, the outflow valves are pushed open and ejection begins. Three-quarters of the stroke volume is ejected in the first half of the ejection phase – the **rapid ejection phase** (~0.15 s). Since the blood is ejected faster than it can drain away through the peripheral vessels, most of the stroke volume is accommodated temporarily in the distended elastic arteries. This drives the arterial pressure up to its maximum or 'systolic' level. During ejection, the

Figure 2.4 Changes in pressure, volume and flow in aorta, left ventricle and left atrium during human cardiac cycle (subject upright). Right side (not shown) has similar patterns but lower pressures. *Jugular venous pulse* in neck and right atrial wave are similar to the left atrial wave shown here. EDV, end-diastolic volume; ESV, end-systolic volume; SV, stroke volume. Second heart sound splits into aortic (A) and pulmonary (P) components. (After Noble MIM. *Circulation Research* 1968; **23**: 663–70.)

Table 2.1 Mean pressures during the human cardiac cycle, in mmHg[a]

	Right	Left
Atrium	3	8
Ventricle		
End of diastole	4	9
Peak of systole	25	120

[a]Adult, at rest, supine.

cusps of the open aortic valve lie close to the entrances to the coronary arteries, but do not block them because vortices behind the cusps cause them to 'float' between midstream and the aorta wall. The vortices are due to out-pouchings of the root of the aorta, the **sinuses of Valsalva** (Figure 1.4).

Later in systole, the ejection rate slows down (Figure 2.4, aortic velocity trace). Since the rate at which aortic blood is draining away into the peripheral circulation now exceeds ventricular ejection, pressure begins to fall. Although the ventricular pressure soon falls 2–3 mmHg below arterial pressure (Figure 2.4, top trace), the outward momentum of the blood prevents immediate closure of the aortic valve. However, the reversed pressure gradient gradually decelerates the outflow (Figure 2.4, velocity curve), until finally a brief backflow closes the outflow valve. Backflow is normally less than 5% of the stroke volume, though this figure increases greatly if the aortic valve is leaky (aortic incompetence). Valve closure creates a notch in the arterial pressure trace called the **incisura**. For the rest of the cycle, the arterial pressure declines gradually as blood drains away into the periphery.

Only two-thirds of the end-diastolic blood volume is ejected in a resting human. The ejected volume, or **stroke volume**, is 70–80 ml and the residual or **end-systolic volume** is ~50 ml. The proportion ejected, or **ejection fraction**, is the stroke volume divided by end-diastolic volume, and averages 0.67 at rest. The end-systolic volume serves as a reserve that can be drawn on to raise the stroke volume and ejection fraction during exercise.

Isovolumetric relaxation

Duration:	0.08 s
Inlet valves:	closed
Outlet valves:	closed

When the aortic and pulmonary valves close, each ventricle becomes, briefly, a closed chamber, and the elastic recoil of the deformed, relaxing myocardium

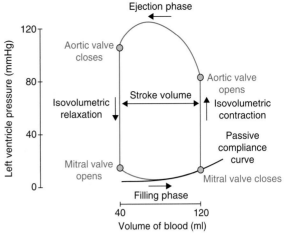

Figure 2.5 Pressure–volume loop for human left ventricle (subject resting, upright).

causes the ventricular blood pressure to fall rapidly. When pressure falls just below atrial pressure, the pressure difference pushes open the atrioventricular valves, which terminates the isovolumetric relaxation phase. Blood floods in from the atria (which have themselves been filling up during ventricular systole), and the next cycle begins.

The ventricular pressure–volume loop

A plot of ventricular blood pressure against ventricular blood volume creates a roughly rectangular, closed loop (Figure 2.5), which proves very useful when discussing left ventricular performance (Chapter 5). The bottom left corner of the loop represents the opening of the mitral valve. Moving anticlockwise with time, the bottom line shows the progressive filling of the ventricle in diastole. In the initial rapid-filling phase the pressure is falling due to the suction exerted by the elastic recoil of the ventricle. In the later, slow-filling phase (diastasis), the line coincides with the passive pressure–volume relation of the relaxed ventricle, or **compliance curve**.

At the onset of systole the mitral valve closes (bottom right corner) and isovolumetric contraction raises the ventricular pressure (the vertical right side of the loop). When ventricular pressure reaches arterial blood pressure, the aortic valve opens (top right corner). Volume then decreases as ejection occurs (top line, direction right to left). At the end of systole, the aortic valve closes (top left corner) and the ensuing isovolumetric relaxation (vertical left side) leads to mitral opening and repetition of the cycle. Note that each corner of the loop represent a valve opening or closing, and each side represents one phase of the ventricular cycle. The width of the loop is the stroke volume and its area represents the work done per beat.

The atria refill with blood during ventricular systole, so we must consider next the atrial cycle.

2.3 The atrial cycle and jugular venous pressure waves

The jugular veins in the neck are in open communication with the right atrium. Consequently, the atrial pressure cycle creates a visible jugular venous pulse, which is readily seen in a slim, recumbent human (Figure 8.27). Inspection of the jugular pulse is part of the standard clinical examination of the cardiovascular system. Pressure recordings in the jugular vein or atrium reveal two main pressure waves per cardiac cycle, the A and V waves, and a third, smaller wave, the C wave (Figures 2.5 and 8.27). There are also two sharp falls in pressure, called the X and Y descents.

The **A wave** is the increase in pressure caused by atrial systole, the 'A' referring to atrial. Atrial systole produces a slight reflux of blood through the valve-less venous entrance. This reverses the flow in the venae cavae briefly, and raises central venous pressure to its maximum point in the cardiac cycle, typically 3–5 mmHg. Backflow is small, even though there are no veno-atrial valves, because the incoming venous blood has considerable inertia.

The next event, the atrial **C wave**, is caused by the bulging of the cusps of the tricuspid or mitral valve into the atrium as the valves close. Since the jugular veins are some distance from the atria, the venous C wave occurs slightly later. The jugular C wave is also caused partly by the systolic expansion of the adjacent carotid artery, hence the nomenclature 'C', for carotid.

After the C wave the pressure falls sharply – the **X descent**. The X descent is caused by atrial relaxation and by the downwards movement of the base of the ventricle (annulus fibrosus) as the ventricle contracts (Figure 2.2). The downward movement of the base stretches the atria, sucking blood into them, so venous inflow reaches its peak velocity at this point (Figure 8.27).

As the atria fill, atrial pressure rises, creating the **V wave;** 'V' refers to the concomitant ventricular systole. Finally, the atrioventricular valves open and the atrial blood drains rapidly into the ventricles, producing a sharp drop in pressure, the **Y descent**.

Since the right atrial pressure cycle is mirrored in the internal and external jugular veins of the neck, a physician can assess the central venous pressure cycle simply by inspecting the neck of a recumbent subject. What the eye particularly notices are two sudden venous collapses, corresponding to the X and Y descents. Certain cardiac diseases produce characteristic abnormalities of the jugular venous pulse. **Tricuspid incompetence**, for example, produces exaggerated V waves in the neck, because ventricular systole forces blood back through the leaky valve into the right atrium and neck veins.

2.4 Altered phase durations when heart rate increases

The timings given above refer to a resting human. During strenuous exercise the heart rate can reach 180–200 beats per minute, and the entire cardiac cycle lasts only about one-third of a second (180 beats/min). Consequently, each phase of the cycle must be shortened. The various phases do not, however, shorten to an equal degree (Figure 2.6). Ventricular systole shortens moderately, to ~0.2 s, leaving a mere 0.13 s for diastole and ventricular refilling. The early rapid-filling phase remains important; diastasis is greatly curtailed, and atrial systole contributes more than at rest. Even so, 0.13 s is close to the minimum time for adequate refilling of the human ventricle. Further increases in heart rate, such as the **pathological tachycardia** of Wolff–Parkinson–White syndrome (>250 beats/min), actually cause the cardiac output to decline, because the diastolic interval is too brief to refill the ventricle adequately. **Diastolic refilling time thus sets a limit to the maximum useful heart rate**.

Figure 2.6 Effect of heart rate on the diastolic period available for filling. d, diastole; s, systole. Diastole is curtailed more than systole as heart rate increases. (Courtesy of Professor Horst Seller, University of Heidelberg.)

2.5 Heart sounds and valve abnormalities

Heart sounds are of great value to clinicians in assessing valve function.

The normal heart sounds

When a cardiac valve closes, the cusps balloon back as they check the momentum of the refluxing blood. The sudden tensing of the cusps sets up a brief vibration, rather as a sail slaps audibly when filled by a sudden gust of wind. The vibration of the valve is transmitted through the tissues to the chest wall and can be heard through a stethoscope. With healthy valves only closure is audible; opening is silent, as with a well-oiled door.

Two heart sounds are easily heard per beat – the first and second heart sounds. They are usually represented as lubb-dupp followed by a pause, roughly in waltz time; the first heart sound (lubb) is the one immediately after the pause. (Lubb-dupp should not be taken too seriously, however, since only English-speaking hearts go lubb-dupp. German ones go duhp-teup and Turkish ones rrup-ta!) The heart sounds can be recorded through a microphone placed on the precordium (skin over the heart) and printed out as a **phonocardiogram** (Figure 2.4). **The first heart sound** is a vibration of ~100 cycles/s (100 Hz), caused by the near-simultaneous closure of the tricuspid and mitral valves. The **second heart sound**, of similar frequency, is caused by the closure of the aortic and pulmonary valves.

The second sound is sometimes audibly split into an initial aortic component and a fractionally delayed pulmonary component (**split second sound**). A first sound followed by a split second sound can be imitated as 'lubb-terrupp'. Splitting is most pronounced during inspiration, for two reasons: (i) inspiration lowers intrathoracic pressure, which increases right ventricular filling which prolongs the right ventricular ejection time and delays pulmonary valve closure; (ii) inspiration also expands the lung blood vessels, which transiently reduces the return of pulmonary blood to the left ventricle. This reduces the left ventricular stroke volume, shortens left ventricular ejection time, and thus hastens aortic valve closure. Splitting of the second sound is caused, therefore, by equal and opposite movements of the aortic and pulmonary components.

Two further faint rumbles can be detected by phonocardiography, but they are of low frequency and difficult for the untrained ear to detect. The

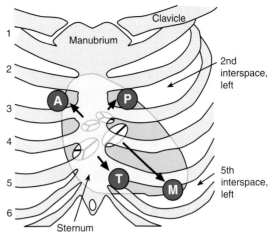

Figure 2.7 Location of cardiac valves and auscultation areas. A, aortic valve area; P, pulmonary valve area; T, tricuspid area; M, mitral area.

third heart sound, common in young people, is caused by the rush of blood into the relaxing ventricles during early diastole. The **fourth heart sound** occurs just before the first sound and is caused by atrial systole.

Each valve has a separate auscultation (listening) area

All four heart valves lie close together under the sternum (Figure 2.7). Fortunately, each valve is best heard over a distinct, well-separated auscultation area, which is located over the chamber fed by the valve. The **mitral valve** is best heard in the mid-clavicular line of the fourth–fifth left intercostal space; the **tricuspid valve** in the fifth interspace at the left sternal edge; the **aortic valve** in the second interspace at the right sternal edge; and the **pulmonary valve** in the second interspace at the left sternal edge.

Valve abnormalities cause cardiac murmurs

Valve abnormalities fall into two classes: incompetence and stenosis. **Valvular incompetence** is a failure of the valve to seal properly. This allows blood to regurgitate through the valve. **Valvular stenosis** is a narrowing of the open valve. As a result, an abnormally high pressure gradient is needed to drive blood through the open valve.

In **aortic valve stenosis**, systolic pressure in the left ventricle is raised, because a large pressure gradient is required to force blood through the narrowed valve (Figure 2.8, top). Also the aortic pressure, which feeds the coronary arteries, is reduced.

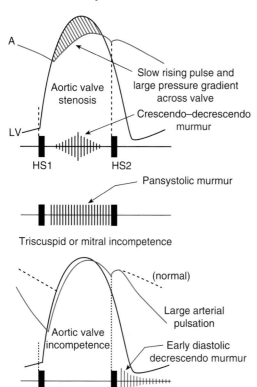

Figure 2.8 Three cardiac murmurs caused by valve pathology. (*Top*) Aortic valve stenosis creates a large pressure gradient between aorta (A) and left ventricle (LV) during ejection (hatched zone). The slow-rising arterial pulse is associated with a crescendo–decrescendo ejection murmur. (*Middle*) In tricuspid or mitral incompetence, regurgitation from ventricle to atrium during systole creates a pansystolic murmur. (*Bottom*) In aortic valve incompetence, diastolic leakage from the aorta to left ventricle causes a characteristic wide pulse pressure (systolic minus diastolic) and an early diastolic, decrescendo murmur as the pressure head decays. Pressure and time axes as in Figure 2.4.

The combination of increased ventricular work and reduced coronary O_2 supply can cause angina during exercise. (Angina is reversible cardiac pain that arises when the myocardial O_2 demand exceeds coronary O_2 supply.) Clinical case 5 at the end of this book describes a patient with this condition.

Blood flows through a stenosed or incompetent valve as a turbulent jet, which creates a high-frequency vibration. The vibration can be heard through the stethoscope and is called a **murmur**. Since there are four valves and two pathologies, there are eight basic valve murmurs. Three common examples are illustrated in Figure 2.8. **Aortic valve stenosis** is characterized by a systolic, **crescendo-decrescendo murmur** (one that rises and falls as ejection waxes and wanes), loudest over the aortic area (Figure 2.8, top). In **mitral incompetence**, blood regurgitates into the left atrium during ventricular systole. This creates a **pansystolic murmur** (one that extends throughout systole), loudest over the mitral area (Figure 2.8, middle). The sound may be represented roughly as 'lu-shshshsh-tupp'. By contrast, **aortic valve incompetence** produces an early, **diastolic decrescendo murmur** (one that dies away), sounding roughly like 'lubb-dubbshsh' (Figure 2.8, bottom). Additional noises (clicks and snaps) can also occur.

Murmurs can arise from other causes besides valve disease. Hypochondriac readers should note that a **benign systolic murmur** is common in young people, caused by turbulence in the ventricular outflow tract. Benign systolic murmurs are common during pregnancy, strenuous exercise and anaemia (Section 8.2). Ventricular septal defects too can cause murmurs.

2.6 Clinical assessment of the cardiac cycle

The human cardiac cycle is assessed at the bedside by examining five physical signs, namely:

- the arterial pulse (to assess heart rate and force)
- systolic and diastolic arterial blood pressure
- the jugular venous pulse
- the apex beat
- the heart sounds.

If pathology is suspected, more specialized investigations may be undertaken, as follows.

Electrocardiography

The electrocardiogram (ECG) is a cutaneous recording of cardiac electrical events, described fully in Chapter 5. Here we will simply note the relation of the ECG waves to the cardiac cycle (Figure 2.4). The ECG **P wave** is produced by electrical activation of the atria, so it marks the onset of atrial contraction. The **QRS complex** is produced by electrical activation of the ventricles, so it is followed almost immediately by the onset of ventricular contraction and the first heart sound. The **T wave** is produced by the electrical recharging of the ventricles. Since this marks the onset of diastole, the T wave is closely followed by the second heart sound.

Non-invasive imaging: echocardiography and MRI

Echocardiography is a non-invasive tool that records the motion of the heart walls and valves.

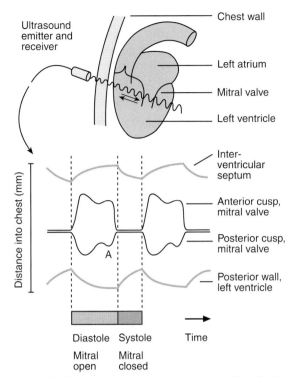

Figure 2.9 M-mode echocardiogram showing motion of mitral valve cusps and walls of the left ventricle. Note fast filling phase in early ventricular diastole and fast ejection phase in early systole. Atrial systole (A) increases cusp separation in late ventricular diastole.

Table 2.2 Echocardiography results for a normal human left ventricle

Wall or septum thickness	0.7–1.1 cm
End-diastolic internal diameter	3.5–5.6 cm
End-systolic internal diameter	1.9–4.0 cm
Ejection fraction (estimated from cube of diameter change)	62–85%
Aortic valve orifice	1.6–2.6 cm

Values from Swanton RH. *Cardiology.* Oxford: Blackwell Science, 1998.

Additional information is extracted from the frequency of the reflected ultrasound, which is altered by the moving blood cells (**Doppler shift).** From the Doppler shift, a colour-coded map of blood flow through a valve and chamber can be constructed. This provides a non-invasive, semi-quantitative measure of regurgitation across leaky valves.

Magnetic resonance imaging (MRI) is a further, non-invasive technique now available in some centres to image the cardiac chambers and walls.

Cardiac catheterization

This is a powerful but invasive investigative technique. Under local anaesthesia a fine catheter is threaded through the antecubital vein in the crook of the elbow and advanced, under X-ray guidance, through the right atrium into the right ventricle or pulmonary artery. Similarly, a catheter introduced through the femoral artery can access the aorta, coronary arteries and left ventricle. The cardiac catheter can then be put to a number of uses, as follows.

Cardiac angiography

A radio-opaque contrast medium is injected through the catheter and its progress through the cardiac chambers is recorded by X-ray cinematography. This displays the movement of the heart wall and any valvular regurgitation. It also reveals atheromatous obstructions in the coronary arteries.

Radionuclide angiography

A gamma-ray emitting isotope, technetium, is injected into a central vein. The ensuing gamma emission from the heart is recorded by a gamma camera over the precordium. Images of the heart are computed in diastole and systole, and the ejection fraction is calculated from the change in counts per ejection.

Intracardiac pressure measurement

Chamber pressures can be measured by an external pressure transducer connected to the cardiac

A beam of ultra-high frequency sound is directed across the heart from a precordial emitter, namely a piezoelectric crystal emitting 1000 brief pulses of ultrasound per second (Figure 2.9). Between each microsecond pulse, there is a millisecond 'listening' interval, during which sound reflected by the chamber walls and valve cusps is collected. The reflected sound is computer-processed to build up a picture of cardiac structure and motion as follows.

In **motion mode** (M-mode) the positions of anatomical features are plotted against time. This gives a linear display of the motion of the heart walls and valve leaflets, as in Figures 2.9 and 6.24.

In **two-dimensional mode** (2-D mode) an anatomical image of a slice through the heart is displayed at successive instants in time. This produces a moving image of the valve leaflets and heart wall, and reveals pathologies such as valve lesions, abnormal wall motions (e.g. infarcts) and hypertrophic cardiomyopathy (pathological wall thickening). Also, ejection fraction and cardiac contractility can be estimated from the change in left ventricular dimensions over the cycle (Table 2.2).

catheter, or by a miniature transducer mounted in the catheter tip. A reduced pressure difference across a closed valve is the gold standard test for valvular incompetence. Conversely, an elevated pressure gradient across an open valve indicates stenosis (Figure 2.8, top). A pulmonary artery catheter can be wedged in the pulmonary arterioles to record 'pulmonary wedge pressure', which is used as an estimate of capillary pressure in the lungs.

Intracardiac pacing

This is a therapeutic rather than diagnostic application of cardiac catheterization. To replace a defective atrial pacemaker, a wire catheter is wedged in the ventricle and used to stimulate each heartbeat from an external electrical device.

Measurement of cardiac output by thermal dilution

This application of cardiac catheterization is described in Section 7.2.

SUMMARY

- The four muscular chambers of the mammalian heart are based on a fibrotendinous ring (**annulus fibrosus**) with four apertures, each occupied by a valve. The ring isolates the atria electrically from the ventricles.

- The ventricular cycle comprises **four phases** of unequal duration, with the right and left sides essentially in synchrony.

- In the **filling phase** the ventricle is in diastole. The arterial outlet valves (aortic and pulmonary) are closed. The atrioventricular inlet valves (tricuspid and mitral) are open. Initial rapid, passive filling is aided by the elastic recoil of the ventricles. Filling then slows (diastasis). Late filling is boosted by **atrial systole**, especially in exercise and the elderly.

- In the **isovolumetric contraction phase** the onset of ventricular systole raises ventricular pressure, which closes the atrioventricular valves and creates the **first heart sound**. Pressure in the closed chamber rises rapidly, and this short phase is quickly terminated by the opening of the arterial outlet valves.

- During the ensuing **ejection phase**, two-thirds of the ventricular blood (the **ejection fraction**) is expelled in resting subjects, and more during exercise.

- As the ejection wanes and pressures fall, a slight backflow closes the aortic and pulmonary valves. The resulting **second heart sound** is split during inspiration. In the ensuing **isovolumetric relaxation phase**, the ventricular pressure falls rapidly until below atrial pressure. The atrioventricular valves then open and the cycle repeats.

- The **ventricular pressure–volume loop** is roughly rectangular. Each corner represents a valve action, each side a phase. The width equals stroke volume. The area equals stroke work.

- The right atrial cycle is reflected in the jugular veins, visible in the neck during recumbency. The **A wave** (atrial systole) and **C wave** (closure of tricuspid valve) are followed by the **X descent** (atrial diastole). Pressure rises again as venous return continues (**V wave**), then falls as the opening of the tricuspid valve dumps the atrial contents into the ventricle (**Y descent**).

- **Phase durations** depend on heart rate. Ventricular diastole occupies two-thirds of the cycle at rest but only one-third at high heart rates. The fall in filling interval limits the maximum useful human heart rate to $180–200\,\text{min}^{-1}$.

- **Abnormalities of the human cardiac cycle** may be detected at the bedside by inspecting the jugular venous pulse, measuring arterial blood pressure and pulse rate, palpating the apex beat and auscultating the heart sounds. Characteristic **murmurs** are caused by valve stenosis or incompetence. Further investigations include electrocardiography, echocardiography, radionuclide angiography and diagnostic cardiac catheterization.

Further reading

Benavidez O, Goldblatt A, Lilly LS. Heart sounds and murmurs. In: Lilly LS (ed.). *Pathophysiology of Heart Disease*, 3rd edn. Baltimore, MD: Williams & Wilkins, 2003.

Burkhoff D, Mirsky I, Suga H. Assessment of systolic and diastolic ventricular properties via pressure–volume analysis: a guide for clinical, translational and basic researchers. *American Journal of Physiology* 2005; **289**: H501–12.

Carlsson M, Ugander M, Mosen H, Buhre T, Arheden H. Atrioventricular plane displacement is the major contributor to left ventricular pumping in healthy adults, athletes and patients with dilated cardiomyopathy. *American Journal of Physiology* 2007; **292**: H1452–9.

Chung CS, Karamanoglu M, Kovacs SJ. Duration of diastole and its phases as a function of heart rate during supine bicycle exercise. *American Journal of Physiology* 2004; **287**: H2003–8.

Horesh S, Pendse S, Come, PC. Diagnostic imaging and catheterisation techniques. In: Lilly LS (ed.). *Pathophysiology of Heart Disease*, 3rd edn. Baltimore, MD: Williams & Wilkins, 2003.

Nishikawa Y, Roberts JP, Tan P, Klopfenstein CE, Klopfenstein HS. Effect of dynamic exercise on left atrial function in conscious dogs. *Journal of Physiology* 1994; **481**: 457–68.

Udelson JE, Bacharach SL, Cannon RO, Bonow RO. Minimum left ventricular pressure during beta-adrenergic stimulation in human subjects: evidence of elastic recoil and diastolic 'suction' in the normal heart. *Circulation* 1990; **82**: 1174–82.

CHAPTER 3

The cardiac myocyte: excitation and contraction

Learning objectives

After reading this chapter you should be able to:

- Outline the ultrastructure and functions of the sarcomere, sarcoplasmic reticulum, transverse tubules and gap junctions (3.1).
- Explain how Ca^{2+}-actin–myosin interactions produce contraction (3.2).
- Sketch a ventricular action potential, label the various phases and name the ion channels responsible for each (3.3, 3.5).
- Explain the link between the action potential plateau and contractility (3.6).
- Describe the myocyte Ca^{2+} cycle and the factors affecting Ca^{2+} store size (3.7).
- State the effect of diastolic length on contractile force (3.8).
- Outline the effect of the following agents on contractile force: catecholamines; calcium channel blockers; phosphodiesterase inhibitors; digoxin (3.7, 3.8).
- Draw and explain a delayed afterdepolarization (3.9).

Each heartbeat is triggered by an electrical system within the heart wall called the **pacemaker–conduction system**. This is composed of modified muscle fibres, not nerves. The pacemaker initiates an electrical discharge, which is conducted from one muscle fibre to the next by local electrical currents. When the electrical stimulus reaches the **contractile muscle cells** that make up the bulk of the heart (cardiac myocytes), they fire off an **action potential**, which raises the intracellular calcium ion concentration. The **Ca^{2+} ions** then activate the myocyte's contractile machinery, comprising **actin and myosin filaments**. The cardiac action potential lasts almost as long as the contraction, unlike the situation in skeletal muscle. Moreover, the cardiac myocytes are coupled together electrically, so every single one contracts during each heartbeat. This means that contractile force cannot be boosted by recruiting additional muscle fibres, as in skeletal muscle. Instead, contractile force is regulated by adjusting the intracellular Ca^{2+} level and the stretch of the fibres in diastole.

Although the heart wall comprises mainly muscle fibres, two other important cell types are present. Intermingled **fibroblasts** secrete collagen and other extracellular matrix polymers, which determine the stiffness of the wall and its elastic recoil from contraction during early diastole. **Endothelial cells** line the internal chambers to create a non-thrombogenic surface. The muscle fibres themselves fall into two categories, as indicated above. The great majority, the cardiac myocytes, do mechanical, contractile work, and are quiescent until stimulated by the second type of muscle fibre, the pacemaker–conduction system. This chapter describes the electrical and contractile properties of the workhorse cardiac myocytes, while Chapter 4 describes the specialized pacemaker–conduction system.

3.1 Ultrastructure of a cardiac myocyte

The human cardiac myocyte is a roughly cylindrical cell, 10–20 μm wide × 50–100 μm long. Some cardiac myocytes are branched, and all possess a single, central nucleus.

Junctions provide mechanical and electrical connection

Adjacent myocytes are attached end-to-end at a stepped face, the **intercalated disc**. There are two distinct types of junction within the intercalated disc: the gap junction provides electrical conduction, and the desmosome provides mechanical strength (Figure 3.1).

The **gap junction**, or nexus, is oddly named, because the adjacent myocyte membranes approach each other extremely closely, to within 2–4 nm. Gap junctions transmit ionic currents, and hence electrical excitation, from one myocyte to the next,

Figure 3.1 Schematic section of myocardium parallel to fibre axis, based on electron micrographs.

because the junction consists of hollow tubes. Six subunits of the protein connexin form a hollow tube, or **connexon**, spanning the cell membrane. Pairs of connexons from opposing myocytes unite end-to-end, so that the joined hemi-tubes create a continuous channel across the narrow intercellular gap. Ions can thus flow from the cytoplasm of one myocyte into the next. As a result, the entire muscle mass of the atria or ventricles behaves as an **electrically continuous sheet**, interrupted only by the annulus fibrosus. This ensures that all the myocytes in a given chamber contract nearly simultaneously. In myocardial ischaemia, increases in intracellular acidity and Ca^{2+} cause closure of some connexons, leading to poor electrical coupling, which facilitates arrhythmia.

Desmosomes provide mechanical strength by riveting the myocytes together. Desmosome are composed of cadherin, a transmembrane glycoprotein that spans the 25 nm-wide space between adjacent myocyte membranes. Cytoskeletal cables, called intermediate or desmin filaments, are anchored internally to the desmosomes. These cables run through the myocyte and give it tensile strength.

The fundamental contractile unit is called a sarcomere

The myocyte is packed with long, contractile bundles ~1 μm wide, called myofibrils. Each myofibril is composed of numerous, basic contractile units called sarcomeres, joined end-to-end and aligned in register across the cell. The transverse alignment gives the cardiac myocyte its characteristic stripy appearance.

The resting length of a sarcomere is 1.8–2.0 μm. It comprises a set of filamentous proteins between two thin partitions, the **Z lines**, composed of the protein α-actinin (Figures 3.1 and 3.2); 'Z' is for 'zwischen', German for 'between'. Between the Z lines there are two kinds of filament: thick filaments composed of the protein myosin and thin filaments composed primarily of the protein actin. Cardiac myosin and actin are different isoforms to those found in skeletal muscle.

The **thick myosin filament** is 1.6 μm long by 11 nm wide. Multiple filaments are arranged in parallel in the central part of the sarcomere, which is called the A band due to its anisotropic appearance under polarized light. Each filament consists of ~400 myosin molecules. Each molecule resembles a golf club with a double head. The 'handle', 150 nm long, lies along the filament axis and the head protrudes from the side of the filament (Figure 3.3).

The **thin actin filament** is 1.05 μm long by 6 nm wide. Actin filaments are interposed between the myosin filaments, with one end free in the A band and the other rooted in the Z line. The actin filaments form the pale I (isotropic) band. The I band is only ~0.25 μm wide, because most of the actin filament is in the space between the myosin filaments,

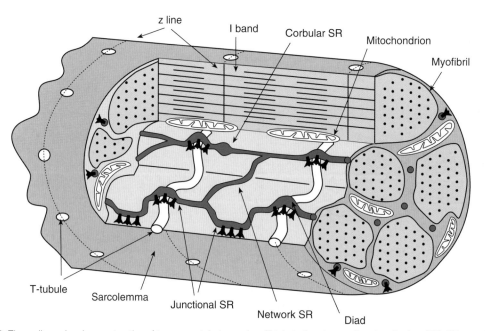

Figure 3.2 Three-dimensional reconstruction of transverse tubular system (T-tubules) and sarcoplasmic reticulum (SR). SR occupies ~5% of the cell volume. The black 'feet' are Ca^{2+}-release channels, also called ryanodine receptors (RyR).

in the A band. In other words, the actin and myosin filaments interdigitate. The filamentous actin (F-actin) is a polymer of globular actin subunits (G-actin), which are bonded side-by-side. The thin filament consists of two such F-actin strings, arranged as a two-stranded helix (Figure 3.3). The groove of the double helix contains a regulatory protein, **tropomyosin**. Also, a regulatory complex composed of **troponins** is attached to the tropomyosin and actin at regular intervals. The tropomyosin–troponin complex plays a key role in initiating contraction.

Besides the contractile filaments, the sarcomere contains spring-like filaments of **titin**, which run from Z line to Z line. Their role is to align the myosin filaments and to contribute elasticity to the heart wall, along with the extracellular collagen.

A transverse tubular system carries excitation into the interior

At each Z line the surface membrane, or **sarcolemma**, is invaginated into a set of fine transverse tubules (**T-tubules**) that run into the cell interior (Figure 3.2). The T-tubules, like the surface

Figure 3.3 Three stages of crossbridge cycle. (a) Rest. Actin binding sites (white star) are blocked by tropomyosin. (b) Ca^{2+} displaces the troponin–tropomyosin complex, exposing actin binding sites. This allows the myosin head to form a crossbridge. (c) Flexion of myosin head shifts the thin filament and Z-line towards sarcomere centre. Head then disengages and reattaches further along actin filament. Figure shows only one of numerous actin binding sites, four of ~400 myosin heads and one of the two heads per myosin molecule.

membrane, possess Na^+ and Ca^{2+} channels, so they transmit electrical excitation rapidly into the interior of the cell. This helps activate the numerous myofibrils virtually simultaneously. T-tubules are well developed in ventricular myocytes, but are scanty in atrial and Purkinje cells, and absent in the hearts of birds and lower vertebrate.

Sarcoplasmic reticulum contains a store of releasable Ca^{2+}

Within the muscle cytoplasm (sarcoplasm) there is a second set of tubes called the sarcoplasmic reticulum (SR), which is derived from endoplasmic reticulum. The SR is a closed set of anastomosing tubes, 20–60 nm wide, that course over the myofibrils. The SR also pass very close to the T-tubules and sarcolemma in places, without actually opening into them. The SR is of major importance, because it contains a store of Ca^{2+} ions, which are partially released into the sarcoplasm when the cell is excited, leading to contraction.

The SR has two functionally distinct regions, with different roles in Ca^{2+} handling, namely the junctional SR (Ca^{2+} release) and network SR (Ca^{2+} uptake) (Figure 3.2).

Junctional SR approaches to within 15 nm of the sarcolemmal surface or, more commonly, a T-tubule, forming a 'diad'. The lumen of junctional SR contains a store of Ca^{2+} ions loosely attached to a storage protein, calsequestrin. Tiny feet extend from the junctional SR towards the T-tubule or sarcolemma. Each foot is actually a gigantic protein, with a plethora of names – 'Ca^{2+} **release channel**' (describing its function), '**ryanodine receptor, RyR**' (because it binds the drug ryanodine) or **CICR channel** (calcium-induced calcium release channels, because it is activated by a rise in free Ca^{2+}).

Network SR comprises tubes that run over the myofibrils and actively take up sarcoplasmic Ca^{2+} by means of abundant **Ca^{2+}-ATPase pumps**. Pump activity is regulated by an inhibitory protein, **phospholamban**.

As indicated above, when the myocyte is excited electrically, Ca^{2+} is released from the junctional SR via the Ca^{2+} release channels, and the released Ca^{2+} activates the contractile machinery. This brings us to the question of how the contractile machinery works.

3.2 Mechanism of contraction

The contraction of the heart is brought about by the shortening of sarcomeres, as follows.

Sarcomeres shorten by a sliding filament mechanism

Sarcomere contraction is brought about by the thin actin filaments sliding into the spaces between the thick myosin filaments, as described independently by Andrew Huxley and Rolf Niedergerke, and by Hugh Huxley and Jean Hanson, in 1954. Part of their evidence was that, during a contraction, both I bands shorten, but the A band does not. The filaments are propelled past each other by the repeated making, rotation and breaking of biochemical bonds, or **crossbridges**, between the thin and thick filaments. The crossbridges, noted in electron micrographs by Hugh Huxley in 1957, are actually the heads of myosin molecules protruding from the side of the thick filament. Each head acts an **independent force generator**, and the swivelling action of hundreds of myosin heads per filament add up to a substantial force generation (Figure 3.3). The process can be likened to a rowing eight (the thick filament) moving up a river (the thin filaments) by repeatedly placing, moving and withdrawing their oar blades (myosin heads). The speed of the crossbridge cycling, and hence filament sliding, is determined by the particular isoform of myosin; the adult human ventricle contains 97% slow-sliding β-myosin and 3% fast-sliding α-myosin.

Ca^{2+} initiates shortening via the troponin–tropomyosin complex

Each actin subunit has a binding site for a myosin head, but the binding sites are blocked at rest by the ribbon-like tropomyosin molecule. Tropomyosin is a 42 nm-long protein that lies in the groove of the F-actin double helix, and it overlies seven G-actin subunits. Each tropomyosin has a troponin complex attached to one end, composed of three units. Troponin C is a Ca^{2+}-binding protein; troponin I is inhibitory; and troponin T binds the complex to tropomyosin.

Exposure of the myosin-binding sites on actin is brought about by a sudden rise in the concentration of free Ca^{2+} ions in the sarcoplasm, brought about mainly by Ca^{2+} release from the SR store. Some of the Ca^{2+} binds to the troponin C. This causes a change in molecular configuration that shifts the tropomyosin–troponin complex deeper into the F-actin groove, thereby exposing the myosin-binding sites of the F-actin. The myosin head can now bind to the actin, forming a crossbridge, and contraction ensues.

Force and movement are generated by a change in the angle of the attached myosin head, which advances the filament by 5–10 nm. After this, the head disengages and the process repeats itself at a new actin site further along the thin filament. This process occurs in hundreds of myosin heads all along the filament, though not synchronously. Thus, to pursue the rowing analogy, the thick filament rows itself into the space between the thin filaments.

The number of crossbridges determines contractile force

In skeletal muscle, excitation raises the sarcoplasmic Ca^{2+} concentration so high (10 μM), that troponin C is saturated and crossbridge formation is maximal. Every twitch of an individual skeletal muscle fibre therefore occurs at full power. In the heart operating at resting outputs, this is not so. The Ca^{2+} concentration during excitation reaches only 0.5–2 μM, which activates only a fraction of the potential crossbridge sites. Consequently, the contraction is **submaximal**, typically around 40% maximal. Anything that increases the intracellular Ca^{2+} level, such as adrenaline, will therefore cause more crossbridges to form and increase the force of the heartbeat. In cardiac muscle, **the force of the contraction is proportional to the number of crossbridges formed**, and thus **depends on sarcoplasmic Ca^{2+} concentration during excitation**.

ATP energizes the myosin head

Energy for the rowing movement of the myosin heads is supplied by adenosine triphosphate, ATP. ATP binds to an ATPase site on the myosin head at the end of stage (c) of Figure 3.3. Energy is released immediately from the ATP by hydrolysis to adenosine diphosphate (ADP) and inorganic phosphate. The released energy activates the myosin head by cocking it back into a high energy 'firing' angle, as in stage (a) of Figure 3.3. 'Firing', i.e. the power stroke in the sequence (b)–(c), is powered by the energy inherent in the cocked position.

Contractile performance is tightly linked to O_2 supply

Each crossbridge cycle breaks down one ATP molecule, so a continuous supply of ATP is needed for contraction. Consequently, cardiac myocytes have an exceptionally high mitochondrial density. The mitochondria occupy 30–35% of the cell volume, forming rows between the myofibrils. ATP is manufactured in the mitochondria by oxidative phosphorylation, for which O_2 is obligatory. Cardiac performance is therefore heavily dependent on the supply of O_2 by the **coronary arteries**. The partial pressure of oxygen in arterial blood (P_{O_2}, 100 mmHg) is much higher than in the myocyte (5–20 mmHg), so a large gradient drives the diffusion of O_2 into the myocyte. Moreover, myocyte sarcoplasm contains **myoglobin**, an O_2-binding protein, at ~3.4 g/l. The myoglobin is ~50% saturated at a P_{O_2} of 5 mmHg, and therefore holds a small store of O_2. It also facilitates the rapid diffusion of O_2 through the sarcoplasm.

The release of the SR Ca^{2+} store, which activates the contractile machinery, is itself triggered by an action potential. So we must next consider the electrical properties of the cardiac myocyte.

3.3 Resting membrane potential

The potential difference between the interior and exterior of a myocyte can be measured by driving a fine, sharp-tipped microelectrode into the sarcoplasm (Figure 3.4). A **microelectrode** is a glass tube that has been heated, drawn out to a very fine point, filled with a conducting solution, and connected to an amplifier and voltmeter. The other lead of the voltmeter is connected to an extracellular electrode. The **intracellular potential** of the resting cardiac myocyte is −80 mV to −90 mV, i.e. 80–90 mV lower than the extracellular fluid. In atrial and ventricular cells the resting potential is stable (Figure 3.4), whereas in pacemaker cells and many conduction fibres (Purkinje fibres) it is unstable, and drifts towards zero with time – a complication we will defer to Chapter 4.

Membrane potentials are the result of differences in ion concentration across the cell membrane and the presence of ion-conducting channels in the membrane. The ion channels have been characterized by **patch clamping**, in which a tiny patch of cell membrane is sucked onto the end of a micropipette and the electrical current through the channels in the patch is recorded (Figure 4.3). By applying different ions, potentials and blocking agents to the patch, specific ion channels can be identified. Cardiac myocytes express three classes of cation-conducting channel, namely K^+-, Na^+- and Ca^{2+}-selective channels, with many subtypes in each group. Channel selectivity is not absolute; for example, a 'potassium channel' has a K^+/Na^+ permeability ratio of ~100/1. Most of these channels can flip repeatedly between open and closed states, and the probability that one state predominates depends on the membrane potential and other factors.

Potassium ions generate the resting membrane potential

The resting potential is the result of a high intracellular K^+ concentration (140 mM) relative to extracellular K^+ (4 mM), in combination with open, K^+-permeable channels in the resting cell membrane. The membrane also has Na^+ and Ca^{2+} channels, but these are mostly closed at negative potentials. By contrast, a specific type of K^+ channel, the inward rectifier channel (K_{ir}), is partly in the

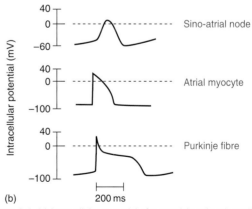

Figure 3.4 (a) Intracellular potential of a ventricle subendocardial myocyte during an action potential. Resting potential −80 mV. Ion equilibrium potentials marked for comparison. Top inset shows measurement of potential. (b) Different forms of cardiac action potential. SA node and some Purkinje fibres have unstable resting potentials. The atrial potential is triangular in many species, as shown here, but has a spike-and-plateau form in humans.

open state at negative potentials. (Mammals have a bewildering variety of K^+ channels, with 7 genes for inward rectifiers, 12 genes for voltage-activated K^+ channels (see below) and 5 genes for Ca^{2+}-activated K^+ channels.) Since intracellular K^+ concentration is ~35 times higher than extracellular K^+ concentration (Table 3.1), K^+ tends to diffuse out of the cell through the K_{ir} channels, creating a resting outward current of K^+ ion, i_{Kir} (or i_{K1}). The negative intracellular ions, mainly organic phosphates and charged proteins, cannot accompany the K^+ ions, because the cell membrane is impermeable to them (Figure 3.5). Consequently, the outward diffusion of K^+ ions quickly creates a tiny separation of charge, which leaves the cell interior negative with respect to the exterior. The electrical charge on a single ion is very large (see Faraday's constant, Appendix 2), so just one excess negative intracellular ion per 10^{15} ion pairs is enough to generate the resting potential of $-80\,mV$. This minute imbalance is far too tiny to be detected by chemical analysis.

Table 3.1 Concentration of ions in myocardial cells

	Intracellular (mM)	Extracellular (mM)	Nernst equilibrium potential (mV)
K^+	140	4	-94
Na^+	10	140	$+70$
Ca^{2+}	0.0001^a	1.2^c	$+124$
Cl^-	30	120	-37^b
pH	7.0–7.1	7.4	–

^{a}In resting myocyte.
^{b}At $-80\,mV$ resting potential there is Cl^- efflux through Cl^- channels. During an action potential, e.g. $+20\,mV$, there is Cl^- influx through Cl^- channels.
^{c}The total Ca^{2+} concentration in plasma is about double this, but only 1.2 mM is in ionic form.

The Nernst equation predicts the K^+ equilibrium potential

If the intracellular potential were big enough (namely $-94\,mV$), the negative intracellular potential attracting positive K^+ ions into the cell would exactly offset the tendency of K^+ to diffuse out of the cell down the concentration gradient. There would then be no net movement of K^+ out of the cell. The electrical potential at which this equilibrium would occur is called the potassium equilibrium potential, E_K. This **electrical potential** is, by definition, equal in magnitude to the outward-driving effect of the concentration gradient, or **chemical potential**. The chemical potential depends on the ion concentration outside (C_o) and inside the cell (C_i). The relation between the electrical equilibrium potential of **any** ionic species X (E_x) and the concentration ratio is given by the **Nernst equation**:

$$E_x = (RT/zF)\log_e(C_o/C_i) \qquad (3.1a)$$

where R is the gas constant (Appendix 2), T is absolute temperature, z is ion valency and F is Faraday's constant. More simply, for a cation at human body temperature (310°K, 37°C), the equilibrium potential in millivolts works out to be:

$$E_x = (61.5/z)\log_{10}(C_o/C_i) \qquad (3.1b)$$

Since the ratio C_o/C_i for potassium is 1:35 and the valency is +1, the K^+ equilibrium potential is $-94\,mV$. Microelectrode measurements show that the resting membrane potential is close to E_K but never quite equals it (Figure 3.6). We will see why in the next section.

Figure 3.5 Ion gradients and currents across resting membrane (i, inside; o, outside). 'A$^-$' inside cell refers to impermeant intracellular anions, mainly phosphate and charged amino acids. Straight arrows show concentration gradients for ions permeating the resting sarcolemma; i_{Kir}, outward background current of K^+; i_b, inward background current (mainly Na$^+$). Reflected arrows indicate ions unable to penetrate the resting membrane. Surface pump and Na$^+$–Ca^{2+} exchanger shown at the top.

External potassium conc. (mM)

Figure 3.6 Effect of extracellular K^+ on resting membrane potential of myocyte (circles) or Purkinje fibre (dotted line). Solid line is Nernst equilibrium potential E_K. Deviation from E_K is due to inward background current i_b. Increasing deviation in hypokalaemia is due to a fall in potassium conductance g_K and reduced outward current carried by $3Na^+$–$2K^+$ pump. (Adapted from Noble D. *The Initiation of the Heart Beat*. Oxford: Clarendon Press, 1979.)

The Nernst equation has important clinical implications, because extracellular K^+ concentration can rise excessively in some conditions, e.g. renal failure, or locally in cardiac ischaemia. The Nernst equation tells us that this will reduce the resting membrane potential, i.e. make it less negative (Figure 3.6). This can trigger a fatal cardiac arrhythmia.

A Na^+ background current creates non-equilibrium conditions

In reality the resting membrane potential is never quite as big as the K^+ equilibrium potential (Figure 3.6). This is due to a small, resting inward current of positive charge, mainly Na^+ ions, called the **inward background current**, i_b. Although the permeability of the resting membrane to Na^+ is only 1/10th to 1/100th of its permeability to K^+, both the electrical and chemical gradient for Na^+ are directed into the cell (Table 3.1). The sum of the two gradients, the **electrochemical gradient**, drives a small inward current of Na^+ into the cell (Figure 3.5). As a result, the resting potential is typically 10–20 mV more positive than the potassium equilibrium potential.

Since the resting potential is not quite negative enough to halt completely the outward diffusion of K^+ ions, there is a continuous trickle of K^+ out of the resting myocyte, creating an **outward background current** i_{Kir}. The outward current i_{Kir}, along with another small outward current generated by the Na^+–K^+ pump (see below), is equal and opposite to the inward current i_b. Thus the resting membrane potential remains stable despite a continuous slow exchange of K^+ for Na^+.

Membrane potential depends on the ratio of ionic permeabilities

We can use a basic law of electricity, Ohm's law, to understand how the relative permeability of the membrane to K^+ and Na^+ affects the membrane potential. **Ohm's law** states that current i is proportional to potential difference ΔV and electrical conductance g (1/resistance). In other words, $i = g \cdot \Delta V$. The conductance of the cell membrane to a particular ion is proportional to its permeability to that ion (Appendix 2). The potential difference ΔV that drives the outward background current of K^+ ions (i_{Kir}) is the difference between the actual membrane potential V_m and the potassium equilibrium potential E_K. Ohm's law thus tells us that the outward background current is:

$$i_{Kir} = g_K (V_m - E_K) \quad (3.2)$$

where g_K is membrane potassium conductance. By similar reasoning, the inward background current of sodium ions i_b is:

$$i_b = g_{Na} (V_m - E_{Na}) \quad (3.3)$$

where E_{Na} is the sodium equilibrium potential, about $+70$ mV. If the resting potential is stable, the inward and outward currents must be equal and opposite; so the right hand sides of (3.2) and (3.3) are equal, neglecting other minor currents. Combining the two expressions, we get an equation describing the resting potential, called **the conductance equation**:

$$V_m = \frac{E_K + E_{Na} \cdot g_{Na}/g_K}{1 + g_{Na}/g_K} \quad (3.4)$$

The conductance equation is a simple version of a more complex expression that incorporates chloride currents too (the Goldman constant field equation, Appendix 2); but it is ideal for our present purpose, because it highlights the importance of the **sodium to potassium conductance ratio** g_{Na}/g_K in setting the membrane potential. The conductance equation tells us that the resting potential is a potassium equilibrium potential (E_K, -94 mV) that has been reduced by a small fraction of the sodium equilibrium potential (E_{Na}, $+70$ mV). The fraction is typically 1/10th, because the ratio g_{Na}/g_K is 1:10. The conductance equation therefore predicts that the resting potential should be (-94 mV $+ 7$ mV)/1.1, which is -79 mV. This is very close to the measured potential in resting cardiac myocytes. The conductance equation also tells us that if g_{Na} becomes bigger than g_K, as happens during an action potential (see below), the membrane potential will become positive – the characteristic feature of an action potential.

Current–voltage relationships for ion channels are commonly non-linear

One problem in applying Ohm's law to ion channels is that the conductance g of an ion channel, unlike that of a copper wire, often changes with the potential. Consequently, the current–voltage relation is non-linear. An Ohmic expression such as (3.2) or (3.3) tells us the current at a given conductance and potential, but does not tell us the shape of the current–voltage relation. The K^+ channel chiefly responsible for the resting potential, **the inward rectifier K^+ channel** K_{ir}, is a good example. Its conductance falls when the membrane is depolarized (loses charge), so less K^+ leaks out during the action potential (Figure 3.8). This is called inward rectification, and is important because it **conserves intracellular K^+ during the very long cardiac action potential**. The fall in channel permeability upon depolarization is caused by positively charged magnesium ions and polyamines, which are drawn into the inner mouth of the channel and obstruct it.

3.4 Role of pumps and exchangers

A Na^+–K^+ pump preserves the intracellular ion levels

The myocyte is a chemical battery, but the chemical that powers the battery, K^+, is slowly but continuously leaking out of the cell. Unchecked, the concentrations of K^+ and Na^+ would eventually equilibrate across the cell membrane, leaving the battery flat. This is prevented by active pumps in the sarcolemmal membrane, which preserve the chemical composition of the interior.

The **sodium–potassium pump** is an ATPase that uses metabolic energy to pump Na^+ ions out of the cell and, simultaneously, K^+ ions into the cell (Figure 3.5). Three Na^+ ions are expelled from the cell for every two K^+ ions pumped in. The pump therefore generates a net outflow of positive charge, and is said to be 'electrogenic'. The contribution of the pump current to the resting potential is a minor one, however, since blocking the pump with

ouabain reduces the myocyte potential by only 2–4 mV. The pump rate is increased by a rise in intracellular Na^+ concentration or extracellular K^+.

The operation of several ion exchangers depends on the Na^+ gradient set up by the Na^+–K^+ pump. The **Na^+–Ca^{2+} exchanger** is of major importance (next section). The **Na^+–H^+ exchanger** regulates intracellular pH by transporting protons out of the cell, in exchange for a flow of Na^+ into the cell down the gradient established by the Na^+–K^+ pump. The Na^+–H^+ exchanger is particularly important in myocardial ischaemia (Section 3.10 and Figure 6.22).

Calcium transporters regulate diastolic Ca^{2+} and the Ca^{2+} store

During diastole the myocyte expels the Ca^{2+} ions that entered from the extracellular fluid during the preceding action potential (see below). The main Ca^{2+} transporter in the surface membrane (sarcolemma) is the **sodium–calcium exchanger**. This transmembrane protein is particularly abundant in sarcolemma close to junctional SR. The exchanger operates in '**forward mode**' over most of the cardiac cycle, allowing three extracellular Na^+ ions into the cell in exchange for the expulsion of one intracellular Ca^{2+} ion (Figure 3.5). The entry of the excess Na^+ ions creates a small inward current. The exchanger is not powered by ATP but is driven by the inward-directed Na^+ concentration gradient, rather as a waterwheel is turned by a water gradient. Calcium expulsion thus depends, indirectly, on the active Na^+–K^+ pump, which creates the Na^+ gradient – a crucial point for understanding the cardiac drug digoxin (Section 3.7).

Since the forward mode carries a net positive charge into the cell, it is also promoted by negative intracellular potentials. The exchanger is reversible, however, and can be driven briefly into **reverse mode** (Ca^{2+} entry, Na^+ expulsion) when the intracellular potential is positive (peak of action potential), especially if intracellular Na^+ is high, as during treatment with the drug digoxin.

The $3Na^+$–$1Ca^{2+}$ exchanger accounts for around three-quarters of Ca^{2+} expulsion from cardiac myocytes. The other quarter is pumped out by a relatively small number of ATP-powered, sarcolemmal **calcium pumps**. Calcium pumps are more abundant in the network SR, where they build up the Ca^{2+} store. The active and passive Ca^{2+} transporters together reduce cytosolic Ca^{2+} concentration to an extremely low level in resting myocytes, namely 10^{-7} M (0.1 μM).

3.5 Cardiac action potentials

The cardiac action potential has five phases

An action potential is an abrupt reversal of the membrane potential to a positive value (Figures 3.4 and 3.7). The myocyte action potential is triggered by an action potential in the conduction system or an adjacent myocyte. The neighbouring action potential creates a current that reduces the negative resting potential (Section 4.3). When the membrane potential reaches a **threshold** of −60 mV to −65 mV, the electrical conductance of the sarcolemma suddenly increases (Figure 3.7, middle), due to the opening of Na$^+$ channels (Figure 3.8). This allows a sudden, inward current of Na$^+$ ions (Figure 3.7, bottom). The resulting influx of positive charge causes the cell to **depolarize** extremely quickly, and flip to a positive potential of +20 mV−+30 mV, called the **overshoot**. This is called phase 0 of the cardiac action potential (Figure 3.7, top).

In most myocytes the membrane then begins to repolarize (phase 1). This early repolarization is only partial, however. When the membrane potential reaches 0 to −20 mV, it becomes relatively stable for a remarkably long period, 200–400 ms. This is called the **plateau**, or phase 2. As a result of the plateau, myocardial action potentials last ∼100 times longer than nerve or skeletal muscle action potentials (1–4 ms). The combination of a marked phase 1 and phase 2 gives the action potential a characteristic spike-and-plateau appearance in the human atrium, ventricular subepicardial (outer) muscle and Purkinje conduction fibres (Figure 3.4b, bottom). Subendocardial myocytes, however, lack a marked phase 1 (Figure 3.4a). Finally, the membrane **repolarizes** (phase 3), though at only 1/1000th of the rate of depolarization. Phase 4 is the resting potential.

Figure 3.7 Phases of cardiac action potential (a), changes in net electrical conductance of membrane (b), and net electrical current across membrane, with inward current downwards (c). The changes represent the sum of the individual K$^+$, Na$^+$ and Ca^{2+} changes shown in Figure 3.8. This particular myocyte is a Purkinje cell, with an unstable resting potential and relatively negative plateau potential. (Wiedmann's seminal observation of 1956, redrawn from Noble D. *The Initiation of the Heartbeat*. Oxford: Clarendon Press, 1979, by permission.)

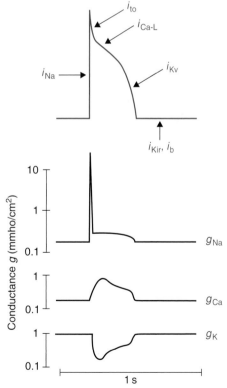

Figure 3.8 Myocyte action potential, ionic currents responsible, and changes in membrane conductances to individual ions, which together account for the net membrane conductance changes in Figure 3.7b. (Based on Noble D. The surprising heart. *Journal of Physiology* 1984; **353**: 1–50, with permission from Wiley-Blackwell.)

The **shape of the cardiac action potential** differs between sites, and also between species (Figures 3.4 and 3.7–3.11). Atrial potentials last only 150 ms and are triangular in many non-human species (Figure 3.4, middle). Ventricular potentials last longer (400 ms) and are more rectangular, due to a distinct plateau at $+30$ mV to 0 mV (Figure 3.8). The phase 1 repolarization spike is well developed in subepicardial myocytes but not in subendocardial myocytes, so the subendocardial action potential lasts longer – a point that is important for understanding the ECG T wave (Section 5.5). Purkinje cells have the longest action potentials of all (up to 450 ms), with a pronounced phase 1 spike and a low plateau potential, at around -20 mV (Figure 3.7).

The myocardial action potential is generated by a sequence of changes in sarcolemmal permeability to Na^+, Ca^{2+} and K^+, which allows ionic currents to flow down their electrochemical gradients, as described next.

Fast Na⁺ channels cause rapid depolarization (phase 0)

Depolarization and overshoot are caused by an extremely rapid increase in sarcolemmal permeability to Na^+ ions. **Fast sodium channels** open (activate) beyond their threshold of -60 to -65 mV, raising the net membrane conductance abruptly by $\sim$100-fold (Figure 3.7). This allows a rapid influx of Na^+ ions, the **first inward current**, i_{Na}, down the electrochemical gradient (Figure 3.8). The inward current drives the potential towards the Nernst equilibrium potential for sodium, E_{Na}, which is $+70$ mV (Table 3.1). However, the potential never quite reaches E_{Na}, because there is still a small outward current of K^+ ions. The situation at the **overshoot** is essentially a mirror image of that at rest, and the same equation (3.4) applies. Equation 3.4 predicts an overshoot membrane potential of $+55$ mV for a Na:K conductance ratio of 10:1.

The fast Na^+ channel is said to be **voltage-dependent**, because it opens at a critical, threshold potential; and **time-dependent**, because its open state is of short duration. Due to the time dependency, Na^+ channels **inactivate** automatically, and the overshoot is very brief. The molecular basis of these properties is explained in Section 3.6.

Transiently open K⁺ channels cause early repolarization (phase 1)

In myocytes with a marked phase 1, such as subepicardial myocytes and Purkinje fibres, the membrane next undergoes a rapid but incomplete repolarization, due to a **transient outward current**, i_{to} (Figure 3.8). The current is carried mainly by voltage-gated K^+ channels, which open transiently in response to depolarization, then quickly inactivate (Figure 3.10). Also, an influx of chloride ions through chloride channels contributes to i_{to}.

Partial repolarization by i_{to} has two roles: it enhances the electrochemical gradient for Ca^{2+} entry in the next phase and it **influences action potential duration**. For example, subepicardial myocytes express more transient outward K^+ channels than subendocardial myocytes, so the subepicardial action potential is shorter. Conversely, in failing hearts, the K^+ channel expression is reduced, so the action potential is prolonged.

L-type Ca²⁺ channels cause the early plateau (phase 2)

The cardiac action potential next displays its unique feature, a plateau lasting 200–400 ms. The first part of the plateau is generated by a small but long-lasting inward current of Ca^{2+} ions, i_{Ca}. The Ca^{2+} current is the second inward current of the action potential (i_{Na} being the first), and it prevents the myocyte from repolarizing rapidly, as would a nerve axon or skeletal muscle fibre. The existence of two different inward currents, i_{Na} and i_{Ca}, can be demonstrated using tetrodotoxin, a dangerous poison from the Japanese puffer fish; this blocks fast Na^+ channels and abolishes the initial spike of the action potential, but not the plateau phase (Figure 3.9). Figure 3.9 also shows that the plateau current i_{Ca} is increased by adrenaline – a point we will return to later.

The inward Ca^{2+} current is driven by the electrochemical gradient, and is carried by channels

Figure 3.9 Effect of adrenaline and tetrodotoxin (TTX) on action potential of calf Purkinje fibre. The control recording (C) shows a normal Purkinje action potential. Adrenaline enhanced the plateau calcium current. Tetrodotoxin abolished the initial spike depolarization, because it blocks the fast Na^+ channels. The residual action potential resembles that of the SA node (see Figure 3.4). (After Carmeliet E, Vereeke J. *Pfluger's Archiv* 1969; **313**: 303–15, with kind permission from Springer Science and Business Media.)

called long-opening or **L-type Ca^{2+} channels**. These are particularly abundant in the T-tubules. L-type Ca^{2+} channels are voltage-gated channels that are rapidly activated by depolarization (though not as rapidly as fast Na$^+$ channels) – so current i_{Ca} has already reached 40% of its peak during phase 1. The current peaks at 2–7 ms, then continues to flow at a declining rate for a long time, because long-opening Ca^{2+} channels inactivate slowly. Figure 3.8 shows the increase in Ca^{2+} conductance and its prolonged, slow decay. The latter explains the decaying net membrane conductance during the plateau in Figure 3.7b. The L-type Ca^{2+} channels can be partially inhibited by calcium channel blockers, such as verapamil and diltiazem.

The total conductance of the activated Ca^{2+} channels is much lower than that of the fast Na$^+$ channels, so i_{Ca} is a much smaller current. But it is just the right size to counterbalance, very nearly, the repolarizing effect of the small outward K$^+$ current that flows throughout the action potential. In this way, the membrane potential is held close to 0 mV for hundreds of milliseconds.

The **outward K$^+$ current i_{Kir} is reduced during the plateau**, because the membrane K$^+$ conductance falls upon depolarization (Figures 3.8 and 3.10). This is the phenomenon of **inward rectification**, described earlier. Inward rectification is caused by the obstruction of the inner mouth of K$_{ir}$ channels by intracellular magnesium ions and polyamines during depolarization. Inward rectification is a helpful economy measure, because it minimizes the number of K$^+$ and Ca^{2+} ions that are exchanged during the exceptionally long cardiac action potential, and thus reduces the energy cost incurred by an action potential.

Na$^+$–Ca^{2+} exchange maintains the late plateau

If Na$^+$ ions are removed from the fluid bathing an isolated myocyte, the plateau becomes shorter. This shows that the late part of the plateau, when more and more L-type Ca^{2+} channels are closing, is maintained by an inward current of Na$^+$ ions. The plateau Na$^+$ current is carried by the Na$^+$–Ca^{2+} exchanger (Figure 3.5), not Na$^+$ channels. The exchanger creates a net inward current, because it lets three Na$^+$ ions into the cell for every Ca^{2+} expelled. Moreover, the exchanger current increases during the plateau phase, due to the rise in sarcoplasm Ca^{2+} concentration. The exchanger current is most marked when the plateau is at a relatively negative potential (e.g. Purkinje fibres, Figures 3.4b bottom and 3.7 – cf. ventricular

myocyte, Figure 3.4a), because the exchanger, being electrogenic, is affected by membrane potential as well as ion concentrations. Indeed, during the positive overshoot phase of the action potential the exchanger may even briefly go into reverse mode, helping to move Ca^{2+} into the cell (Appendix 2).

Slow potassium channel opening causes repolarization (phase 3)

As the plateau progresses, the depressed net potassium conductance begins to rise (Figure 3.8). This is due to the gradual opening of voltage-activated K$^+$ channels, called **delayed rectifier or slow K$^+$ channels** (K$_V$, K$_S$). Unlike the voltage-activated Na$^+$ and Ca^{2+} channels, delayed rectifier channels activate very slowly (Figure 3.10). As they do so, the outward K$^+$ current i_{Kv} gradually increases, until it outweighs the small, late-plateau inward current, and thereby initiates repolarization. As repolarization proceeds, the **inward rectifier** conductance is restored, and contributes to the final stage of repolarization (Figure 3.10).

The magnitude of the inward K$^+$ current affects the **duration of the plateau**. When the heart rate is increased by sympathetic stimulation, channel phosphorylation increases the repolarizing K$^+$ current i_{Kv}, which induces early repolarization and thus shortens the plateau – a necessary step to allow more action potentials per minute

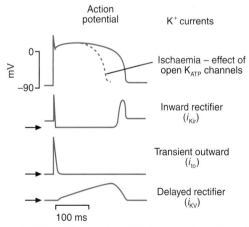

Figure 3.10 Three K$^+$ currents contributing to cardiac action potential. Arrows mark zero current. Dashed line shows effect of acute ischaemia; increased open probability of K$_{ATP}$ channels shortens the action potential. Hypoxic shortening is abolished by the K$_{ATP}$ blocker glibenclamide, and by knockout of the pore-forming Kir6.2 protein in mice. (Adapted from Sanguinetti MC, Keating MT. *News in Physiological Sciences*, 1997; **12**: 152–7, with permission from the American Physiological Society.)

(Section 4.5). Action potential duration also alters in pathological conditions, shortening in hypoxia (Figure 3.10, top) and lengthening in chronic heart disease. A variant of the delayed rectifier protein gene *KCNQ1* impairs channel function, prolongs the plateau and causes a long QT interval in the ECG. This form of **long QT syndrome** underlies some cases of sudden cardiac death in apparently healthy, young individuals. Long QT syndromes can also result from mutations of other channel proteins, such as the sodium channel gene *SCN5A*.

Refractory period and its relation to contraction period

The myocyte is electrically inexcitable (refractory) throughout its prolonged depolarization. This is called the **absolute refractory period** (Figure 3.11). By the time repolarization reaches $-50\,mV$, many but not all of the fast Na^+ channels have reset from the inactivated state to a closed but activatable state. (The difference between 'inactivated' and 'closed' is explained in Section 3.6.) Consequently, the cell begins to regain some degree of electrical excitability at this point. A larger-than-normal excitatory stimulus is necessary, however, due to the substantial number of Na^+ channels still inactivated. The period between $-50\,mV$ and full repolarization is therefore called the **relative refractory period**. After this, the myocyte regains its normal ease of electrical excitation.

Myocyte contraction starts about $10\,ms$ or so after phase 0 and lasts 200–250 ms overall (Figure 3.11). Contraction therefore peaks near the end of the absolute refractory period, and the myocyte is into the relaxation phase by the end of the relative refractory period. Tension development is thus completed before the cardiac myocyte becomes re-excitable. This is important, because it limits the contractile behaviour of the heart to repeated **single twitches**. In skeletal muscle, by contrast, the very brief action potentials follow each other so quickly that one twitch fuses with the next one to generate a sustained contraction. This cannot happen in the heart, because the refractory period lasts as long as tension development. This seems an excellent arrangement, because a sustained myocardial contraction would quickly prove fatal!

A relatively small quantity of ions is exchanged per action potential

The numerous ionic currents described above are all small, even the Na^+ current. Consequently, **the change in intracellular ion concentration caused by a single action potential is tiny**. Students often assume, wrongly, that the 'rush' of Na^+ ions into the cell must raise the intracellular Na^+ concentration substantially – but this is mistaking speed for quantity. Around 40 million Na^+ ions enter a myocyte during depolarization. Since a myocyte contains about 200 000 million Na^+ ions, Na^+ concentration rises by a mere 0.02%. The change is even smaller for K^+, a fall of 0.001% (Appendix 2, 'Quantity of ions'). The Na^+–K^+ and Na^+–Ca^{2+} transporters are therefore able to restore the chemical composition of the sarcoplasm without excessive expenditure of metabolic energy.

The main ionic currents are summarized in Table 3.2. The numerous subtypes of channel are summarized in more detail, for reference purposes, in Table 4.2.

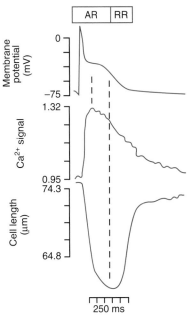

Figure 3.11 Relation between electrical, chemical and mechanical events in a single myocyte (rat). The myocyte was loaded with a fluorescent dye to measure free sarcoplasmic Ca^{2+} concentration. Note the sequence of the peaks – first electrical, then chemical, then mechanical. AR, absolute refractory period to $-50\,mV$ repolarization; RR, relative refractory period from $-50\,mV$ to full repolarization. Rat myocytes have an unusually negative plateau potential. (Records from Spurgeon *et al. American Journal of Physiology* 1990; **258**: H574–86.)

Table 3.2 Chief ionic currents in cardiac work cell. For a more detailed subdivision, see Table 4.2

Current	Ion	Direction[a]	Function	Blockers
$i_{K, total}$	K^+	Outward	1 Generates resting membrane potential 2 Repolarization	Ba^{2+} Tetraethyl ammonium
i_b	Na^+ (mostly)	Inward	Inward background current makes resting potential smaller than E_K	–
i_{Na}	Na^+	Inward	Fast depolarization, to help propagate excitation.	Tetrodotoxin, lidocaine, procaine, quinidine
i_{Ca}	Ca^{2+}	Inward	1 Excitation–contraction coupling 2 Plateau maintenance	Mn^{2+}, Nifedipine, amlodipine, verapamil
$i_{Na–Ca}$	$3Na^+$ in $1 Ca^{2+}$ out	Net inward current (forward mode of Na–Ca exchanger)	Sustains late plateau. Expels intracellular Ca^{2+}. Arrhythmogenic afterdepolarization in ischaemic Ca^{2+} overload	–

[a] 'Inward' means a flow of positive charge from the extracellular to the intracellular compartment.

CONCEPT BOX 3.1

Cardiac potentials are generated by ionic gradients and sequential activation of ion channels

- The resting potential, −80 mV, is created by the tendency of intracellular K^+ to diffuse out of the myocyte through open, K^+-selective channels, leaving behind a slight excess of intracellular negative charge.
- The resting potential approaches the Nernst equilibrium potential for K^+, modified by a small, inward background current of Na^+.
- At the start of an action potential, voltage-gated Na^+ channels admit a brief influx of positive ions into the cell, depolarizing it.
- The overshoot of the action potential (+30 mV) approaches a Nernst equilibrium potential for Na^+, modified by a small outward background current of K^+.
- The activation of long-opening Ca^{2+} channels then allows an influx of Ca^{2+} (i_{Ca}). This nearly counterbalances the outward K^+ current and generates a long plateau at around zero potential, lasting 200–400 ms.
- The plateau is terminated by an increasing efflux of K^+ ions through slowly activating, delayed rectifier K^+ channels. The K^+ efflux repolarizes the cell. Large K^+ currents shorten the plateau and small K^+ currents lengthen it.

3.6 Advanced aspects: structure–function relations of ion channels

Although the molecular structure of ion channels is complex, a broad outline helps us to understand certain key properties, such as the time-dependent inactivation of Na^+ channels. Moreover, the genetic mutation of certain channel proteins underlies cardiac disorders, such as long QT syndromes.

All ion channels are formed by transmembrane proteins arranged in a ring around a central, aqueous pore (Figure 3.12). In K^+ channels, four individual proteins, called α subunits, make up the ring; in Na^+ and Ca^+ channels, four α-like domains of a single protein make up the ring. The simplest cardiac channel is the inward rectifier channel (K_{ir}), where each α subunit has two hydrophobic transmembrane helices. This probably evolved into the voltage-sensitive K^+ channels, with six transmembrane helices per α subunit. This in turn probably evolved into Na^+ and Ca^{2+} channels, where four α-like units are strung together as a single molecule.

Inward rectifier K^+ channel family (Figure 3.12, top). This family includes K_{ir} and some related channels that we will meet later (K_{ATP}, K_{ACh}). Mutation studies indicate that the K^+ selectivity of the central pore is conferred by a specific amino acid motif, glycine–tyrosine–glycine, in an intramembrane loop lining the pore (P or H5 loop). There are no voltage-sensitive loops. However, depolarization reduces K_{ir} conductance (inward rectification), because intracellular magnesium ions and polyamines impede the inner mouth of the channel when current is flowing outwards.

Voltage-gated K^+ channel family, K_v. Two members of this family are particularly important for cardiac function.

(a) Delayed rectifier (slow) channel, K_s. Each α subunit is formed by protein KCNQ1, which has six hydrophobic transmembrane loops, S1–S6 (Figure 3.12, middle). Mutation studies show that

Figure 3.12 Ion channel topography. The inward rectifier channel (K_{ir}), with two transmembrane helices per α subunit, probably evolved into voltage-sensitive K^+ channels, with six transmembrane helices, which evolved into Na^+ and Ca^{2+} channels. In each case a hollow channel is created by four proteins, called α subunits (K^+ and TRP channels), or by four α-like domains of a single protein (Na^+ and Ca^+ channels). Each α subunit/domain has a P loop (red line) that dips into the lipid membrane to line the pore and determine its ion selectivity. The positively charged, arginine-rich S4 loop is the voltage sensor. S4 is uncharged in TRP channels (see Table 12.2). Phosphorylation of sites on intracellular loops by protein kinases can regulate channel activity, e.g. Ca^{2+} channel phosphorylation by cAMP-activated protein kinase A promotes the open state, following adrenergic stimulation. The Ca^{2+} channel is broadly similar to the Na^+ channel, but its slow, inactivation gate may be the intracellular loop linking domains I and II.

positively charged arginine and lysine residues in the S4 loops act as a voltage sensor, making this a voltage-activated channel. Inactivation is brought about by a ball-on-chain (the last 20 amino acids of the intracellular N-terminal), which slowly blocks the intracellular opening following depolarization. Mutations of KCNQ1 impair channel function, leading to delayed repolarization and sudden death in young individuals (long QT syndrome). The channel also has two regulatory β subunits (protein KCNE1).

Transient outward K^+ channel, K_{to}. This has a similar structure to K_S but is composed of different proteins, $K_V4.3$ and KChIP2. It has a faster activation and inactivation than K_S. $K_V4.3$ expression is reduced in failing hearts, leading to prolonged action potentials.

Voltage-gated Na^+ channel. The cardiac fast Na^+ channel, $Na_V1.5$, is one of eight types of voltage-dependent Na^+ channel in the genome. It is formed by a large, single protein of ~2000 amino acids, which loops back and forth across the cell

Figure 3.13 Activation–inactivation cycle of voltage-sensitive Na^+ channel. Outward displacement of the charged S4 loops by depolarization opens the activation gate (S6 loops). The slower, inactivation gate is a hinged lid, formed by the intracellular loop linking molecular domains III and IV. Enzymatic cleavage of this loop abolishes inactivation. As long as the inactivation gate is closed, the myocyte is incapable of re-excitation (refractory).

membrane to form four near-identical groups called domains I–IV (Figure 3.12, bottom). Each domain has six hydrophobic transmembrane loops, S1–S6, as in K_v channels. Positively charged arginine and lysine residues in S4 again act as the voltage sensor, and amino acids in the pore-lining P loop confer Na^+ selectivity. The anti-arrhythmia drugs lidocaine, procaine and quinidine inhibit Na^+ channels by plugging the pore.

The excitation–inactivation cycle of the Na^+ channel is due to the operation of two 'gates', which are parts of the polypeptide chain (Figure 3.13). The m or **activation gate** (probably S_6 loops) is closed at resting potentials, blocking the pore. A second, intracellular gate, the h or **inactivation gate**, is open at resting potential. The inactivation gate is a hinged lid over the channel entrance, formed by the positively charged intracellular loop linking domains III and IV. A channel in this configuration is closed but excitable ('deactivated'). When the membrane is depolarized to threshold potential, an outward shift in the positively charged, voltage-sensitive S_4 loops opens the activation gate, allowing Na^+ passage. At the same time, however, the inactivation gate begins to close; but since the inactivation gate moves more slowly than the activation gate, there is a millisecond or so when the channel is open, before the inactivation gate closes. This is the instant in which the brief first inward current i_{Na} flows. Once the second gate has closed, the channel is inactivated. It cannot be re-excited until it has been re-set to the closed-but-activatable

starting configuration (Figure 3.13, bottom). This requires repolarization to beyond $-70\,mV$.

Voltage-gated L-type Ca^{2+} channel

The cardiac L-type Ca^{2+} channel comprises a single, pore-forming protein, $Ca_V1.2$ (the $\alpha1$ subunit), and several regulatory subunits. Like the Na^+ channel, $Ca_V1.2$ has four domains, each with six transmembrane segments, including a charged S4 voltage sensor. Ca^{2+} selectivity is attributed to glutamate residues in the pore-lining P loop. As with Na^+ channels, time-dependent inactivation is brought about by an intracellular lid docking process; but the lid may be the intracellular loop linking domains I and II. Closure of the inactivation gate is enhanced by intracellular Ca^{2+} via a binding protein, calmodulin (Ca^{2+}-dependent inactivation). Consequently, the rise in intracellular Ca^{2+} during the action potential helps to terminate opening. Adrenergic stimulation leads to the phosphorylation of the C-terminus domain by protein kinase A, increasing the duration of the open state.

3.7 Physiological and pathological changes in action potential

As noted earlier, differences in transient outward K^+ channel expression result in a gradient of action potential duration across the ventricle wall. The action potential can also be regulated physiologically, and can be by altered by disease, as described next.

Catecholamines boost the plateau current and contractile force

The contractile force of a cardiac myocyte is proportional to the size of the plateau current, i_{Ca}, which can be increased by circulating **adrenaline** and by **noradrenaline** from cardiac sympathetic fibres. The increased current creates a dome-shaped plateau (Figure 3.9) and leads to a bigger free Ca^{2+} transient and contractile force. This is called the **inotropic** (strengthening) action of catecholamines. The biochemical steps that lead to the rise in i_{Ca} are described in Section 4.5, and the way in which i_{Ca} influences the size of the cytosol Ca^{2+} transient is described in Section 3.8. **L-type calcium channel blockers**, such as verapamil and nifedipine, have the opposite effect; they attenuate i_{Ca} and thus weaken the heartbeat.

Acute ischaemia shortens the action potential, via K_{ATP} channels

During a coronary artery thrombosis, the acute myocardial hypoxia reduces the plateau duration (Figure 3.10, top). This is due to the activation of a specialized form of K_{ir} channel, the K_{ATP} channel (Figure 3.12, top right). At a normal intracellular ATP concentration of ~5 mM, the open probability of K_{ATP} channels is low; but the open probability increases as ATP concentration falls, and as ADP, adenosine and H^+ concentration rise in hypoxic cells. The increased K^+ conductance induces early repolarization. This shortens the plateau, which in turn truncates calcium entry. This may be helpful, in that it reduces the work of the Ca^{2+} pumps/exchangers, and thus reduces oxygen demand during hypoxia.

Chronic heart disease prolongs the action potential

Whereas acute hypoxia shortens the action potential, chronic cardiac failure, ventricular hypertrophy and chronic infarction lengthen it, by reducing the K^+ channel expression, especially the transient outward K^+ channel. The reduced K^+ current leads to delayed repolarization, a prolonged plateau and a high frequency of arrhythmias. The importance of the timing of repolarization is vividly demonstrated by **long Q–T syndrome**, which can be caused by a genetic abnormality of the delayed rectifier protein KCNQ1. The prolonged plateau leads to Ca^{2+} overload and afterdepolarization (Section 3.10), which in turn can trigger arrhythmia and sudden death in an otherwise healthy, young individual.

3.8 Excitation–contraction coupling and the Ca^{2+} cycle

Extracellular Ca^{2+} and intracellular Ca^{2+} are both essential for cardiac contraction. The need for extracellular Ca^{2+} was discovered by the London physiologist **Sidney Ringer** in 1883, and, as with many seminal discoveries, chance played a part. It was the job of Ringer's assistant to prepare solutions of sodium and potassium chloride, which maintained the beating of an isolated frog heart for many hours. But when Ringer himself made up the 'same' solution, using distilled water, the heart quickly weakened and failed. Ringer discovered that his assistant had been using the 'hard' London tap water, and that the Ca^{2+} in the water was essential to cardiac contraction. Indeed, if the extracellular Ca^{2+} around an isolated myocyte is quickly washed away, the very next beat fails. The reason is that the entry of extracellular Ca^{2+} into the subsarcolemmal space during the early phase of i_{Ca} is necessary to trigger the release of the SR Ca^{2+} store (calcium-induced calcium release), which then initiates crossbridge formation.

A sarcoplasmic Ca^{2+} transient initiates contraction

The arrival of an action potential triggers a sharp rise in sarcoplasmic free Ca^{2+}, from 0.1 µM to ~0.5–2 µM. Some of the Ca^{2+} binds to troponin C to activate contraction (Figure 3.3). To prove that sarcoplasmic Ca^{2+} causes contraction, Fabiato and Fabiato performed a classic experiment in 1975, in which the sarcolemma was stripped from the myocyte, so that intracellular Ca^{2+} could be equilibrated with a known Ca^{2+} concentration in the bathing fluid. These 'skinned' cells were found to relax at 0.1 µM Ca^{2+}, contract moderately at 1 µM Ca^{2+} and contract maximally at >10 µM Ca^{2+}. The correlation between contractile force and sarcoplasmic [Ca^{2+}] was later confirmed in non-skinned myocytes, using intracellular, Ca^{2+}-sensitive fluorescent dyes; the fluorescent signal begins to rise immediately after depolarization, and is quickly followed by contraction (Figure 3.11). Intact myocytes are more sensitive to Ca^{2+} than are skinned ones, and the free Ca^{2+} during a normal, submaximal twitch is probably ~0.55–0.75 µM.

How does the action potential induce an order-of-magnitude increase in sarcoplasmic Ca^{2+} concentration? As Figure 3.14 shows, the Ca^{2+} come from two sources: the main source is the sarcoplasmic

Figure 3.14 The calcium cycle during systole (left) and diastole (right). A T-tubule L-type Ca^{2+} channel and adjacent cluster of $\sim$10 Ca^{2+}-release channels (only two shown here) form a functional unit. SR, sarcoplasmic reticulum; CICR, calcium-induced calcium release.

reticulum store ($\sim$75–90%) and the plateau current i_{Ca} supplements it ($\sim$10–25%).

Calcium-induced calcium release from SR is the main source of the Ca^{2+} transient

Junctional SR contains a concentrated store of Ca^{2+} ($\sim$1 mM), and is studded with Ca^{2+}-release channels (or ryanodine receptors, RyR). Each release channel is a giant protein of molecular mass 2.3 million dalton. The protein forms a 'foot' with a T-shaped tube through its centre, through which Ca^{2+} is presumably released. The foot terminates only nanometres from the sarcolemma of a T-tubule or cell surface, and is thus extremely close to the L-type Ca^{2+} channels (Figure 3.14). In junctional regions there is typically one L-type Ca^{2+} channel for every ten Ca^{2+}-release channels. The Ca^{2+}-release channels are activated by a rise in free Ca^{2+} concentration in their local, subsarcolemmal environment, brought about by the opening of the adjacent L-type Ca^{2+} channel. This is called **calcium-induced calcium release** (CICR).

During diastole the free intracellular Ca^{2+} concentration is so low that the release channels are closed, except for occasional random discharges,

which can be seen as local **calcium sparks** in myocytes loaded with Ca^{2+}-sensitive fluorescent dye. Each spark represents a cluster of release channels, and most occur close to T-tubules, though some occur under the surface sarcolemma. When an action potential arrives, the sarcolemmal current i_{Ca} quickly raises the Ca^{2+} concentration in the subsarcolemmal space (Figure 3.14). This is called **trigger calcium**. The trigger calcium from a single L-type channel probably activates a cluster of 6–20 release channels. Since this happens all over the cell, there is a near-synchronous firing of thousands of Ca^{2+} sparks ($\sim$10 000 per cell), which releases a substantial fraction of the SR store, typically $\sim$50%. This raises the sarcoplasmic Ca^{2+} concentration roughly ten-fold over $\sim$50 ms, from $\sim$0.1 μM to a peak of $\sim$1 μM. The released Ca^{2+} diffuses rapidly into the sarcomere, and the cell begins to contract (Figure 3.11).

SR Ca^{2+} release is graded, not all-or-none

A potential problem with CICR is that positive feedback (Ca^{2+} release causing more Ca^{2+} release) could, in principle, cause an ungraded discharge of the entire SR store. This does not happen in practice; studies show unequivocally that a small i_{Ca} causes a small Ca^{2+} transient and weak contraction, while a large i_{Ca} causes a large Ca^{2+} transient and strong contraction. This is probably because the activation of release channels requires a **highly localized, very large rise** in subsarcolemmal Ca^{2+} concentration, mediated by an immediately adjacent L-type Ca^{2+} channel; a lesser, diffuse rise in cytosolic Ca^{2+} is not sufficient to activate the release channels. Consequently, one cluster does not generally trigger others. Activation within a given cluster may possibly be all-or-none, due to positive feedback (the cluster bomb model), but **the number of clusters activated is proportional to the size of i_{Ca}.** The greater the number and duration of L-type Ca^{2+} channel opening events, the greater is the recruitment of subsarcolemmal release clusters and the greater the fraction of the SR store released.

The release channels activate rapidly, then inactivate slowly, over ~30–100 ms (mechanism unknown). Inactivation is followed by a slow recovery of the channel's resting ability to respond to Ca^{2+}. This is part of the process of restitution, the return of the system to its original resting state.

Restitution: pumps in the network SR restock the store

The Ca^{2+}-ATPase pumps of the network SR are stimulated by the systolic rise in sarcoplasmic Ca^{2+}, and pump 75–90% of the raised Ca^{2+} back into the SR interior. The other 10–25% is expelled by the sarcolemmal $Na^+–Ca^{2+}$ exchanger (Figure 3.14). Since sarcolemmal expulsion normally equals Ca^{2+} entry during the action potential (as i_{Ca}), the cell Ca^{2+} content is unchanged in diastole. As the sarcoplasm Ca^{2+} concentration falls, Ca^{2+} dissociates from the troponin–tropomyosin complex and the muscle relaxes. Calcium uptake by the network SR is followed by restocking of the calsequestrin stores in the junctional SR. The process of **restitution**, that is to say the restocking of the store and restoration of release channel excitability, is normally completed well before the next excitation.

The SR Ca^{2+} pumps are regulated by an inhibitory protein, **phospholamban**. The braking effect of phospholamban on the pump is reduced by adrenaline and noradrenaline. Consequently, adrenaline and noradrenaline increase the rate of myocardial relaxation (**lusitropic action**), as well as increasing the contractile force via an increase in i_{Ca} (**inotropic action**), as described next.

β_1-adrenergic stimulation increases the Ca^{2+} transient and contractility

As well as providing the trigger Ca^{2+}, the current i_{Ca} continues through the early plateau phase and accounts for ~10–25% of the rise in sarcoplasmic Ca^{2+} concentration. Consequently, the force of contraction correlates with the amplitude and duration of i_{Ca}. **Adrenaline** and **noradrenaline** increase i_{Ca}, via the signal transduction pathway shown in Figure 4.9. This increases the size of the free Ca^{2+} transient, and hence contractile force, through two mechanisms. First, the increase in trigger i_{Ca} in the subsarcolemmal space recruits more clusters of release channels, releasing a greater **fraction** of the Ca^{2+} store. Second, the raised i_{Ca} during the plateau increases the amount of Ca^{2+} available for subsequent uptake into the SR store, leading to an increase in the **size** of the Ca^{2+} store over several beats. This focuses our attention on the important question, 'What governs the size of the calcium store?'

Factors governing size of SR calcium store

The amount of Ca^{2+} in the SR store depends on the balance between the influx of extracellular Ca^{2+} during the plateau and its expulsion during diastole. Consequently, Ca^{2+} store size depends on:

1 extracellular Ca^{2+} concentration, which is normally very stable;
2 the size of the plateau current, which is increased by the β_1-adrenoceptor ligands, noradrenaline and adrenaline, and reduced by Ca^{2+}-channel blockers;
3 heart rate, which affects the duration of systole (extracellular Ca^{2+} influx) relative to diastole (Ca^{2+} expulsion). Store size and contractile force generally increase with heart rate, as described under 'Bowditch effect' (Section 6.11).

The size of the SR store can also be raised by pharmacological agents, such as **digoxin**, a drug used to treat chronic heart failure (next section). **Caffeine** at very high concentrations *in vitro* activates Ca^{2+}-release channels, leading to a sustained contraction called a contracture. At therapeutic, lower levels, however, caffeine improves contractility by inhibiting phosphodiesterase, as does **milrinone**, a drug used to treat acute cardiac failure. The **phosphodiesterases** are a group of enzymes that degrade cyclic adenosine monophosphate (cAMP), which is

Figure 3.15 In 1785, William Withering reported that a folklore remedy based on an infusion of foxglove leaves (*Digitalis*) was beneficial for 'dropsy' (cardiac failure). The bicentennial experiment shown here confirms that foxglove extract increases contractile force and intracellular Ca^{2+} concentration in ferret papillary muscle. Light emission from the aequorin-injected muscle (*top trace*) was used to measure systolic free Ca^{2+} concentration; aequorin, a jellyfish protein, emits blue light in the presence of free Ca^{2+}. (From Allen DG, Eisner DA, Smith GL, Wray S. *Journal of Physiology* 1985; **365**: 55P, with permission from Wiley-Blackwell.)

the intracellular messenger mediating the effect of adrenaline and noradrenaline (Figure 4.9). Caffeine and milrinone elevate cAMP and thus mimic the contractility enhancing action of adrenaline and noradrenaline. **Ischaemic heart disease** can cause overloading of the SR store, leading to arrhythmia (Section 3.10).

Digoxin increases the systolic Ca^{2+} transient

Digoxin, a cardiac glycoside produced by foxgloves, has been used for over two centuries to treat chronic cardiac failure. It enhances myocardial contractile force by increasing the size of the systolic Ca^{2+} transient (Figure 3.15). Its pharmacological target is actually the sarcolemmal Na^+–K^+ pump, which it inhibits by $\sim$25%. This raises the subsarcolemmal Na^+ concentration. Since the transmembrane Na^+ gradient drives the Na^+–Ca^{2+} exchanger, Ca^{2+} expulsion is slowed, the Ca^{2+} store builds up and cardiac contractility improves. However, the toxic dose of digoxin is only a little higher than the therapeutic dose; at toxic doses, excessive accumulation of intracellular Ca^{2+} causes store overload. This is a potent trigger for afterdepolarization and arrhythmia; so digoxin over-dosage can trigger arrhythmia (Section 3.10).

3.9 Regulation of contractile force

The degree of activation of the contractile machinery is continually adjusted by physiological mechanisms during our daily lives (Chapter 6). When we are at rest, only about 40% of the potential actin–myosin crossbridges are activated during systole, so the heartbeat is gentle. During exercise or stress, the number of crossbridges is increased, so the heart beats harder, i.e. with increased force. There are two, fundamentally different ways of increasing crossbridge formation.

1 The **systolic Ca^{2+} transient** can be increased, as described above. This is normally brought about by noradrenaline released locally from

---

Contractile force is proportional to crossbridge activation

- A crossbridge is a myosin head that extends from the thick myosin filament to a binding site on the thin actin filament. Flexion of the head generates contraction.
- Contractile force is increased by increasing the number of crossbridges.
- Crossbridge formation is induced by a rise in sarcoplasmic free Ca^{2+} concentration.
- The free Ca^{2+} transient is due chiefly to the partial discharge of the sarcoplasmic reticulum (SR) store of Ca^{2+}. Store discharge is triggered by the arrival of extracellular Ca^{2+} as current i_{Ca} at the start of an action potential (calcium-induced calcium release).
- During a quiet heartbeat the free Ca^{2+} transient is only big enough to activate a fraction of the potential crossbridges.
- Sympathetic stimulation increases i_{Ca} and stored Ca^{2+}, leading to bigger free Ca^{2+} transients, more crossbridge formation and increased contractile force.
- Stretching the cell increases its sensitivity to Ca^{2+}, and therefore increases crossbridge formation and contractile force.

CONCEPT BOX 3.2

cardiac sympathetic fibres, and also circulating adrenaline from the adrenal gland.

2 **Stretching the myocyte** in diastole provides a second, fundamentally different way of increasing crossbridge formation. In normal life the myocardium becomes more stretched whenever diastolic filling increases, for example every time we lie down. Stretch increases the **sensitivity to Ca^{2+}**, rather than the size of the Ca^{2+} transient. This is the basis of the fundamental **Starling law of the heart** or **length–tension relation** described in Chapter 6. An account of its underlying mechanism is deferred to that chapter.

3.10 Store overload, afterdepolarization and arrhythmia

Coronary artery disease causes cardiac ischaemia, which often triggers an arrhythmia, such as a fatal ventricular fibrillation (Chapter 5). The primary pro-arrhythmogenic change is often the **overloading of the SR calcium store**. The store becomes overloaded through two main mechanisms:

1 Ischaemia raises intracellular Na^+ concentration, partly because the energy supply for the Na^+–K^+ pump is reduced, and partly because intracellular acidosis stimulates the sarcolemmal Na^+–H^+ exchanger. A raised intracellular Na^+ concentration reduces the forward mode turnover of the Na^+–Ca^{2+} exchanger, leading to intracellular Ca^{2+} accumulation (Figure 6.22).

2 Cardiac ischaemia reflexly increases cardiac sympathetic nerve activity, raising noradrenaline and adrenaline levels. This activates myocardial β-adrenoceptors, which, via intracellular cAMP (Figure 4.9), boost the plateau Ca^{2+} current, i_{Ca}. High sympathetic activity in ischaemic hearts thus promote store overload and arrhythmia (see below). Conversely, it is difficult to induce ventricular fibrillation by regional ischaemia in a chronically denervated heart. Phosphodiesterase inhibitors can have similar arrhythmogenic effects to high sympathetic activity, because they too raise intracellular cAMP and hence i_{Ca}.

The overloaded Ca^{2+} store is prone to spontaneous, **partial discharge during early diastole –** possibly exacerbated by increased leakiness of the

Figure 3.16 Partial discharge of overloaded internal Ca^{2+} store in diastole (*lower trace*) stimulates the electrogenic $3Na^+$–$1Ca^{2+}$ exchanger, causing a net inflow of positive charge (Na^+) and a delayed afterdepolarization (DAD, *upper trace*). If the DAD reaches threshold, it triggers a premature action potential (*dashed line*). *Dotted line* shows effect of replacing external Na^+ by Li^+, to inhibit the Na–Ca exchanger; the shortening of the plateau shows that exchanger current normally contributes to the late plateau; also the DAD is abolished. (Based on Benardeau *et al. American Journal of Physiology* 1996; **271**: H1151–61, with permission from the American Physiological Society.)

Ca^{2+}-release channels (RyR) due to β-adrenoceptor-driven phosphorylation. The diastolic rise in sarcoplasmic Ca^{2+} stimulates Ca^{2+} expulsion by the sarcolemmal $3Na^+$–$1Ca^{2+}$ exchanger. Since this entails a net inward flow of positive charge, it causes a depolarization after the action potential (Figure 3.16). If the afterdepolarization reaches threshold, a premature action potential follows and may trigger an arrhythmia. The afterdepolarization may occur after the cell has fully repolarized (**delayed afterdepolarization, DAD**) or during its repolarization phase (**early afterdepolarization, EAD**). Delayed afterdepolarizations probably trigger most of the arrhythmias associated with acute cardiac ischaemia, chronic cardiac failure, digoxin toxicity and phosphodiesterase inhibitors.

Since an increased calcium current, i_{Ca}, contributes to the above chain of events, the risk of sudden death from arrhythmia after myocardial infarction can be reduced by L-type Ca^{2+} channel blockers (verapamil, diltiazem) and β-adrenoceptor blockers (propranolol, atenolol, metoprolol).

SUMMARY

- The myocyte **resting potential**, $-80\,mV$, approximates to a K^+ equilibrium potential, modified by a small inward background current of Na^+ ions. The ATP-powered $3Na^+$–$2K^+$ pump maintains the intracellular ion concentrations and contributes 2–4 mV to the potential.

- Contraction is initiated by an **action potential**. Voltage-dependent Na^+ channel conducts a rapid inward current of Na^+, i_{Na}, which depolarizes the myocyte (spike of action potential, phase 0). The Na^+ channels rapidly inactivate, and a transient outward K^+ current i_{to} causes an early partial repolarization (phase 1). A second inward current, mainly of extracellular Ca^{2+} ions (i_{Ca}), maintains a prolonged depolarization, the **plateau**, lasting 200–400 ms (phase 2). An inward Na^+ current through the $3Na^+$–$1Ca^{2+}$ exchanger maintains the late plateau. Contraction begins during the plateau, and the cell is absolutely refractory to re-excitation.

- **Repolarization** by outward K^+ currents i_{Kv} and i_{Kir} terminates the plateau (phase 3). During tachycardia and hypoxia, increased K^+ currents shorten the plateau; in chronic heart disease, reduced K^+ currents lengthen it.

- Immediately after depolarization, extracellular 'trigger' Ca^{2+} passes through L-type Ca^{2+} channels into the subsarcolemmal space (early i_{Ca}). This activates clusters of Ca^{2+}-release channels (ryanodine receptors) in the junctional sarcoplasmic reticulum (**calcium-induced calcium release**). The release of around half the SR Ca^{2+} store transiently raises sarcoplasmic free Ca^{2+} to $\sim 1\,\mu M$.

- Ca^{2+} binds to the troponin–tropomyosin complex on actin filaments, leading to the exposure of myosin-binding sites. Myosin heads then form **crossbridges**, extending from the thick myosin filaments to the thin actin filaments. The myosin heads swivel, rowing the thick myosin filaments into the spaces between the thin actin filaments. This generates tension and shortening. Recocking of the myosin heads consumes ATP, so mitochondrial density is high and normal contractility requires a high O_2 supply via the coronary arteries.

- **Contractile force**, typically $\sim 40\%$ maximal at rest, depends on the fraction of the potential crossbridges activated. This is regulated by two factors.

- Stretch of the sarcomere in diastole increases the **sensitivity** of the contractile machinery to Ca^{2+}, which leads to more crossbridge activation and contractile force (the length–tension relation).

- The **size** of the systolic Ca^{2+} transient determines the number of crossbridges activated at a given length. Adrenaline and noradrenaline increase i_{Ca}, which increases the store size and also supplies more trigger Ca^{2+}, releasing a greater fraction of the store. This leads to bigger Ca^{2+} transients and hence stronger contractions.

- In **ischaemia** the SR Ca^{2+} store becomes overloaded, especially when β-adrenoceptor stimulation by catecholamines is high. Spontaneous partial discharge of the overloaded store in diastole evokes afterdepolarization, due to the increased $3Na^+$–$1Ca^{2+}$ exchanger current. This can trigger premature action potentials and arrhythmia.

Further reading

Reviews and chapters

Aidley DJ The contractile mechanism of muscle. In *The Physiology of Excitable Cells*, 4th edn. Cambridge: Cambridge University Press, 1998: 336–71.

Bers DM. Calcium cycling and signaling in cardiac myocytes. *Annual Review of Physiology* 2008; **70**: 23–49.

Blaustein MP, Lederer WJ. Sodium/calcium exchange: its physiological implications. *Physiological Reviews* 1999; **79**: 764–854.

Boyett MR, Harrison SM, Janvier NC, McMorn SO, Owen JM, Shui Z. A list of vertebrate cardiac ionic currents – nomenclature, properties, function and cloned equivalents. *Cardiovascular Research* 1996; **32**: 455–81.

Brady AJ. Mechanical properties of isolated cardiac myocytes. *Physiological Reviews* 1991; **71**: 413–42.

Brette F, Orchard C. Resurgence of cardiac T-tubule research. *Physiology* 2007; **22**: 167–73.

Hiraoka M, Furukawa, T. Functional modulation of cardiac ATP-sensitive K1 channels. *News in Physiological Sciences* 1998; **13**: 131–7.

Jespersen T, Grunnet M, Olesen S-P. The KCNQ1 potassium channel: from gene to physiological function. *Physiology* 2005; **20**: 408–16.

Jongsma HJ, Gros D. The cardiac connection (gap junction). *News in Physiological Sciences* 1991; **6**: 34–40.

Kjeldsen K, Norgaard A, Gheorghiade M. Myocardial Na, K-ATPase: the molecular basis for the hemodynamic effect of digoxin therapy in congestive heart failure. *Cardiovascular Research* 2002; **55**: 710–13.

Roden DM, Balser JR, George AL, Anderson ME. Cardiac ion channels. *Annual Reviews of Physiology* 2002; **64**: 431–475.

Solaro RJ, Rarick HM. Troponin and tropomyosin; proteins that switch on and tune in the activity of the cardiac myofilaments. *Circulation Research* 1998; **83**: 471–80.

Venetucci LA, Trafford AW, O'Neill SC, Eisner DA. The sarcoplasmic reticulum and arrhythmogenic calcium release. *Cardiovascular Research* 2008; **77**: 285–92.

Research papers

See www.hodderplus.com/cardiovascularphysiology for a full list of Research papers for this chapter.

CHAPTER 4

Initiation and nervous control of the heartbeat

Learning objectives

After reading this chapter you should be able to:

- Sketch the anatomy of the cardiac excitation–conduction system and state the role of each component (4.1).
- Explain 'dominance' (4.1) and the emergence of a slower pacemaker in heart block.
- Draw the sino-atrial node potential over one cardiac cycle and state the ionic basis of each phase (4.2).
- Explain how depolarization propagates through the myocardium (4.3).
- State the chronotropic actions of (i) sympathetic and (ii) parasympathetic nerves, and the underlying mechanisms (4.5, 4.6).
- Explain the inotropic and lusitropic effects of sympathetic stimulation (4.5).
- Describe the deleterious effect of hyperkalaemia (4.7).
- State the actions of (i) β-blockers and (ii) Ca^{2+}-channel blockers on the heart (4.8).

If the heart is excised from a cold-blooded animal and placed in a suitable solution of electrolytes, it will continues to beat for a long period. This simple experiment shows that the heartbeat is initiated from within the heart itself. Unlike skeletal muscle, extrinsic nerves are not necessary to initiate contraction. The heartbeat is initiated by an intrinsic electrical system composed of modified myocytes, not nerves. These specialized myocytes are organized into (i) the sino-atrial node (pacemaker), a group of cells that discharge spontaneously at regular intervals to initiate the heartbeat; and (ii) cells that conduct the electrical impulse across the annulus fibrosus into the ventricle wall, triggering ventricular systole. Although pacemaker activity does not depend on extrinsic nerves, the frequency of pacemaker firing can be modified by autonomic nerves; sympathetic activity increases it, parasympathetic activity decreases it. Sympathetic fibres also regulate the contractile force, and therefore the

stroke volume. Thus both components of the cardiac output, namely heart rate and stroke volume, are under central nervous control.

4.1 Organization of pacemaker–conduction system

The sino-atrial node initiates the heartbeat

The sino-atrial node (SA node, pacemaker) is a strip of myocytes roughly 20 mm long and 4 mm wide in man, located on the posterior wall of the right atrium close to the superior vena cava (Figure 4.1). The mammalian sino-atrial node is so called because it evolved from the sinus venosus, an antechamber to the right atrium in lower vertebrates. The node is made up of small myocytes that have scanty myofibrils and an unstable membrane potential. Human nodal cells fire an action potential spontaneously about once every second at rest. This excites the adjacent atrial myocytes. The action potential is then conducted from myocyte to myocyte, creating a wave of depolarization that sweeps across both atria. The wave travels at ~1 m/s and initiates atrial systole.

The atrioventricular node delays ventricular excitation

The electrical impulse quickly reaches the atrioventricular node (AV node), a small mass of cells and connective tissue in the lower, posterior region of the atrial septum. The AV node is the start of the only electrical connection across the annulus fibrosus, which otherwise insulates the atria from the ventricles (Section 2.1). The impulse is delayed in the node for ~0.1 s at resting heart rates. The delay is generated by the complex local circuitry and the small diameter of the nodal cells, 2–3 μm, which reduces the conduction velocity to ~0.05 m/s. The delaying role of the AV node is important, because it allows time for the atria to contract before the ventricles.

The bundle of His and its branches excite the ventricles

The role of the ventricular conduction system is to excite the entire ventricular wall as near simultaneously as possible. A bundle of fast-conducting muscle fibres, the **bundle of His**, conveys the electrical impulse from the AV node through the annulus fibrosus into the fibrous upper part of the interventricular septum. Here the bundle turns and runs forwards along the crest of the main, muscular part of the septum (Figure 4.1). The bundle gives off a

left bundle branch, which comprises two sets of fibres, one anterior and one posterior. These course down the left side of the muscular septum and supply the left ventricle. The remaining bundle, the **right bundle branch**, runs down the right side of the interventricular septum and supplies the right ventricle.

The bundle fibres are wide, fast-conducting myocytes arranged in a regular, end-to-end fashion. They terminate in an extensive network of large fibres in the subendocardium, described by the Hungarian histologist Purkinje in 1845. **Purkinje fibres** are the widest cells in the heart (diameter 40–80 μm), and consequently have the highest conduction velocity (3–5 m/s). Their role is to distribute the electrical impulse rapidly to the subendocardial myocytes. From here the impulse passes from myocyte to myocyte at ~0.5–1 m/s in a generally outward, epicardial direction, until the whole wall has been excited. This takes ~90 ms.

The fastest pacemaker dominates a hierarchy of slower, latent pacemakers

There are other potential pacemakers in the heart besides the SA node, but they have slower intrinsic frequencies of firing. The SA node normally determines the heart rate simply because its cells have the fastest frequency of firing, and therefore excite the heart before other, slower pacemakers have reached their firing threshold. If the SA node is destroyed, myocytes in the AV node or atrium take over as the new pacemaker, because they have the next highest rate of firing. The bundle of His too can pacemake, but only at ~40 beats/min. Purkinje cells have an even slower pacemaking frequency, ~15 beats/min,

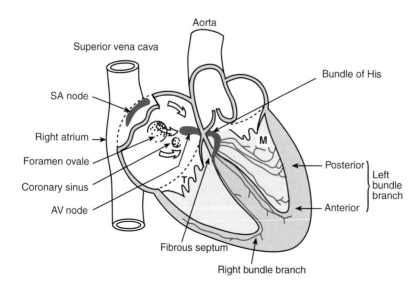

Aorta

Superior vena cava

Bundle of His

SA node

Right atrium

Foramen ovale

Coronary sinus

AV node

M

Posterior
Anterior
} Left bundle branch

T

Fibrous septum

Right bundle branch

Figure 4.1 The cardiac conduction system. The posterior fibres of the left bundle branch are seen *en face*, running just inside the septum, then curling round in the left ventricular subendocardium. Broad arrows show conduction through atrial muscle. Note the proximity of the valves (T, tricuspid; M, mitral) to the bundle of His; valve lesions can affect the main bundle. The foramen ovale is the remnant of the fetal connection between right and left sides. The coronary sinus is the outlet of the main coronary vein.

which is too slow to maintain an adequate cardiac output. There is thus a **gradient of intrinsic pacemaker frequencies along the cardiac electrical system**. The slower, lower centres are normally excited by the SA node before they have time to fire spontaneously. This is called **dominance**.

The emergence of a slow, distal pacemaker can be seen in the pathological condition of **heart block**. In heart block the bundle of His fails to transmit excitation through the annulus fibrosus, so the SA node can no longer dominate the ventricle. Pacemaker cells in the bundle then take over, driving the ventricles at ~40 beats/min (Figure 5.4e). This is too slow for many daily activities, and such patients usually benefit from the insertion of an artificial pacemaker.

4.2 Electrical activity of pacemaker

Pacemaker potential decay determines heart rate

The membrane potential of SA node cells is small and unstable. The initial potential is only −50 to −70 mV, because nodal cells express few inward rectifier K^+ channels (K_{ir}), the channels responsible for the big, stable resting potential in atrial and ventricular myocytes. The pacemaker cell does, however, express voltage-dependent, delayed rectifier K^+ channels, K_v (Table 4.1), and K^+ efflux through these channels generates the starting potential of around −60 mV.

The membrane potential then decays spontaneously with time (Figure 4.2). This slowly declining potential is called the **pacemaker potential**. When the pacemaker potential reaches a threshold of −40 to −55 mV, it triggers an action potential, which sparks off the next heartbeat. The rate of decay of the pacemaker potential, i.e. its slope, is important, because it determines the time interval needed to reach threshold, and thus the interval between heartbeats. The steeper the slope, the sooner the threshold is reached and the shorter the interval between the heartbeats. Thus a steeply decaying pacemaker potential causes a high heart rate.

Multiple ionic currents cause the potential to decay

The decay of the pacemaker potential is brought about by several, different inward currents, and also by a decay of the outward current, as follows:

1 The delayed rectifier, voltage-activated K^+ channels, K_V, inactivate slowly with time at negative potentials, due to the ball-and-chain mechanism shown in Figure 3.12. This is why membrane electrical conductance declines during phase 4 in Figure 3.7. Consequently, the polarizing (negative-making) **outward current i_K decays with time**. The decay in outward K^+ current allows inward, depolarizing currents to become increasingly dominant (Figure 4.2). The inward currents are as follows:

2 A small, inward current of Na^+ ions slowly depolarizes the cell. The current may be partly the inward background current i_b, described in Chapter 3. In addition, many SA node cells possess a specialized pacemaker current called the **'funny' current**, i_f. Current i_f is only active at

Table 4.1 Main ionic currents in nodal pacemaker cells

Current	Ion	Direction	Function	Channel inhibitor
(i_{Na})	(Na^+)	−	Voltage-operated Na^+ channels are largely absent/inactivated in nodal cells	−
i_f and i_b^*	Na^+	Inward	Supply inward depolarizing current during initial part of pacemaker potential	Cs^+ and ivabradine block i_f
$i_{Na\text{-}Ca}^\dagger$	Na^+	Inward	Imporant contribution to later part of pacemaker depolarization	
i_{Ca}	Ca^{2+}	Inward	1. Contributes to last third of pacemaker potential 2. Generates slow-rising action potential	Mn^{2+}, verapamil, nifedipine
i_{Kv}	K^+	Outward	Delayed rectifier, voltage-operated channel 1. Supplies decaying current during pacemaker potential 2. Supplies repolarization current	Ba^{2+}

*i_f is funny current; i_b is background current.
†Net inward current produced by the expulsion of one intracellular Ca^{2+} in exchange for three extracellular Na^+ ions.

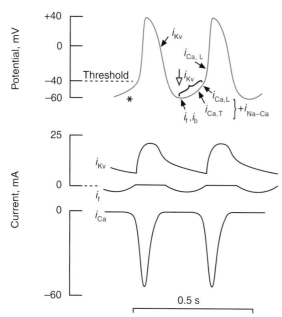

Figure 4.2 Ionic basis of pacemaker potential and action potential in sino-atrial cell. Slope of pacemaker potential (asterisk) determines time to reach threshold, and hence heart rate. Inward currents downwards, outward currents upwards. i_{Kv}, potassium current; i_f, 'funny' Na$^+$ current; i_b, background Na$^+$ current; $i_{Ca,T}$, Transient Ca^{2+} channel current; $i_{Ca,L}$, Long-lasting Ca^{2+} channel current; i_{Na-Ca}, inward current due to 3Na$^+$–1Ca^{2+} exchanger. (Based on Petit-Jacques J *et al. News in Physiological Sciences* 1994; **9**: 77–9, with permission from the American Physiological Society; and Noble D. In: Zipes DP, Jalife J (eds). *Cardiac Physiology from Cell to Bedside*. Philadelphia, PA: WB Saunders, 1995: 305–13.)

potentials negative to about −50 mV, and it is funny-peculiar in the sense that the channel is activated by hyperpolarization – whereas most voltage-sensitive channels are activated by depolarization (e.g. K$_V$ and Ca^{2+} channels). Although the i_f channel is non-selective between Na$^+$ and K$^+$, the i_f current is carried chiefly by Na$^+$ ions, because the electrochemical gradient favours Na$^+$ influx at negative membrane potentials. Caesium ions block i_f and slow the rate of pacemaker depolarization, as does a recently introduced i_f blocker, **ivabradine**. These agents do not stop the pacemaker decay completely, however, indicating the existence of additional pacemaking currents.

3 The **3Na$^+$–1Ca^{2+} exchanger** generates a net inward Na$^+$ current, i_{Na-Ca}, that contributes substantially to pacemaker depolarization. Blocking this current can abolish the late part of the decay of the pacemaker potential.

4 As the membrane potential decays below −55 mV or so, an **inward current of Ca^{2+}**

ions begins to contribute to depolarization. The SA node expresses voltage-sensitive Ca^{2+} channels of a type called transient or **T-type**. T-type channels have an increased probability of being in the open state beyond −55 mV (Figure 4.3, left). As the potential declines further, voltage-sensitive **L-type** Ca^{2+} channels also begin to open. L-type channels activate at more depolarized (**L**ower) potentials than the T-type (Figure 4.3, right). Thus an increasing Ca^{2+} influx accelerates the depolarization rate in the late stages of the pacemaker potential, triggering the action potential and next heartbeat.

Node action potentials are small, sluggish and Ca^{2+}-based

Node action potentials are small in amplitude and slow-rising, similiar to the tetrodotoxin-blocked myocyte of Figure 3.9. This is because the nodal cell has few functional fast Na$^+$ channels. The action potential in both the SA and AV node is generated solely by an inward Ca^{2+} current (Table 4.1). Therefore, calcium-channel inhibitors, such as verapamil, reduce the size of the nodal action potential, as well as pacemaker decay rate. Repolarization is brought about by an outward K$^+$ current through delayed rectifier K$^+$ channels, K$_V$ (Figure 3.10). These voltage-gated channels activate very slowly during depolarization (time constant 300–400 ms), so they open gradually during the action potential. Upon repolarization they begin to inactivate slowly, thus contributing to the next pacemaker cycle.

4.3 Transmission of excitation

Propagating currents spread the excitation

The spread of excitation through the atria, conduction system and ventricles is brought about by local electrical currents that act ahead of the action potential (Figure 4.4). In the active, depolarized region the membrane interior is positively charged, while in the resting zone ahead it is negative. The two regions are connected by an internal, electrically conductive pathway, namely the sarcoplasm and **gap junctions** (Figure 3.1). Positive charge therefore flows intracellularly into the resting membrane region, depolarizing it. Externally the converse applies; the extracellular fluid is a conducting medium, so positive charge flows from the outside of the resting membrane to the active

Figure 4.3 Cardiac Ca^{2+} currents recorded by patch clamp. A tiny patch of membrane is sealed to the glass micropipette by suction to record single channel activity (*top left*). The patch can be ruptured mechanically or chemically, to record net current through all the ion channels in the cell ('perforated patch' or 'whole cell' mode, *top right*). Depolarization beyond −55 mV (*top left trace*) caused a single T-type channel to flicker open sporadically (*middle left*), admitting *T*iny pulses of current. This soon ceases, so the average current passed by hundreds of T-type channels is *T*ransient (*bottom left*). When the membrane is depolarized further (*top right trace*), a single, higher threshold L-type Ca^{2+} channel opens sporadically, admitting *L*arger pulses of current, for longer (*middle right*). The average current passed by hundreds of such channels is thus *L*ong-lasting (*bottom right*) and inactivates only slowly. (Redrawn from Nilius B *et al. Nature* 1985; **316**: 443–6, with permission from Macmillan Publishers Ltd.)

region, reducing the charge on the outside of the resting membrane. This process is in fact the **passive discharge of a capacitor**, namely the lipid membrane. When the resting membrane potential reaches threshold, an action potential is triggered, setting up fresh local currents to excite the next region and so on. Since the membrane to the rear is in its **refractory period**, excitation proceeds unidirectionally.

The safety margin for propagation; conduction rate depends on fibre diameter and local current magnitude

The conduction of excitation is fastest in the widest cells, the Purkinje fibres. A **wide diameter** confers a low axial electrical resistance, which enables the local circuits in Figure 4.4 to reach out a greater distance ahead of the active region. Conduction rate also depends on the magnitude and rate of rise of

Figure 4.4 Excitation is transmitted through the conduction system and myocardium by local currents acting ahead of the action potential. Internal current flows through the sarcoplasm and gap junctions of the intercalated disc. External current flows through the extracellular fluid. The currents discharge the membrane ahead, triggering its action potential.

the action potential. Conduction is fast in myocytes with large, rapid-rising action potentials, such as ventricular myocytes, because these potentials generate **big propagating currents**, and big currents can extend well ahead of the active region. Action potential depolarization rate, i.e. the steepness of the phase 0, Na^+-mediated spike (500 volts/s), is particularly important for the generation of big propagating currents and the reliable propagation of excitation. During ischaemia and hyperkalaemia, the deterioration in ventricular action potential size and phase 0 depolarization rate can impair conduction, contributing to ventricular arrhythmia (Section 4.7). Nodal cells, which have small, slow-rising action potentials, generate small propagating currents and have a **poor safety margin for conduction**; so conduction is slow and easily blocked in nodal tissue.

4.4 Regulation of the heart rate

The human heart beats 50–100 times per minute at rest and a little slower in endurance-trained athletes. In other mammals the heart rate is proportional to $1/mass^{0.25}$: for example, the shrew's heart rate is 600/min and the elephant's is 25/min! The heart rate is modulated by sympathetic and parasympathetic autonomic nerves innervating the pacemaker and AV node.

Sympathetic fibres innervate the whole heart

The short, preganglionic cardiac sympathetic fibres leave the spinal cord at segments T1–T5 and synapse

in the paravertebral sympathetic ganglia (Figure 4.5). The much longer postganglionic fibres run along the surface of the great vessels to reach the heart. Unlike parasympathetic fibres, the sympathetic fibres richly innervate the ventricular muscle, as well as the atria and pacemaker–conduction system. The pacemaker is innervated chiefly by fibres from the right paravertebral ganglia, and the ventricles by fibres from the left paravertebral ganglia.

Parasympathetic fibres have a more restricted distribution

Cardiac parasympathetic fibres originate in the vagal motor nuclei of the brainstem, and the very long, preganglionic fibres travel in the right and left vagus nerves (Figure 4.5). The right fibres generally innervate the pacemaker and the left the AV node, but there is considerable anatomical variation. The long preganglionic fibres synapse with the postganglionic parasympathetic neurons within the myocardium, mostly around the SA and AV nodes. Short postganglionic fibres innervate the nodes. The ventricles receive only a sparse parasympathetic innervation.

Autonomic fibres continuously modify the intrinsic pacemaker rate

Both the sympathetic and parasympathetic fibres are tonically (continuously) active, so the pacemaker firing rate is continuously influenced by them, even at rest. Increased sympathetic activity speeds up the heart rate (**tachycardia**) (Figure 4.6). Increased parasympathetic activity slows it down (**bradycardia**) (Figure 4.7). Although both autonomic systems are tonically active, the **parasympathetic, inhibitory effect predominates at rest**. This follows from the finding that the intrinsic heart rate is ~105 beats/min in young humans after parasympathetic blockade by atropine and sympathetic blockade by propranolol. Physiological changes in heart rate are usually brought about by **reciprocal changes in sympathetic and parasympathetic activity**. For example, the tachycardia of exercise is brought about by increased sympathetic activity and reduced parasympathetic activity.

Parasympathetic regulation acts faster than sympathetic regulation

The tachycardia elicited by sympathetic stimulation is relatively sluggish in onset and decays relatively slowly when stimulation ceases (Figure 4.6). By contrast, the bradycardia elicited by parasympathetic stimulation

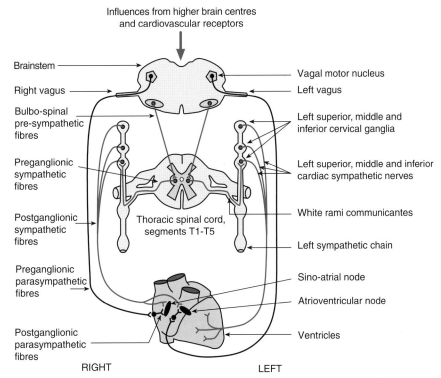

Figure 4.5 Innervation of heart by sympathetic fibres (red) and vagal parasympathetic fibres (black). The sympathetic outflow arises from the intermediolateral horns of the thoracic spinal cord segments T1–T5.

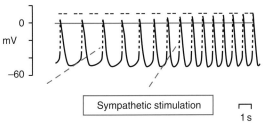

Sympathetic stimulation

1 s

Figure 4.6 Effect of continuous sympathetic stimulation (box) on pacemaker potential. Note the relatively sluggish onset of tachycardia. The dashed, red gradients highlight the increased slope of the pacemaker potential. The upper double-dashed line draws attention to the increase in action potential size, caused by the increased inward Ca^{2+} current induced by noradrenaline-activated β-adrenoceptors. (From Hutter OF, Trautwein W. *Journal of General Physiology* 1956; **39**: 715–33, with permission from the Rockefeller University Press.)

has a very short latency and resolves more quickly when fibre activity ceases (Figure 4.7). Consequently, changes in parasympathetic activity account for rapid changes in heart rate, such as the slowing of the heart during each expiration (sinus arrhythmia) and fainting. The fast 'on' effect is brought about by a hyperpolarizing pathway activated by acetylcholine (see later). The fast 'off' effect is due to the rapid removal of acetylcholine by the enzyme cholinesterase.

Temperature too affects heart rate

The pacemaker rate is influenced by temperature. A **fever** causes the heart rate to increase by ~10 beats/min per degree Centigrade. Conversely, cooling can be used to slow the heart during open heart surgery.

4.5 Effects of sympathetic stimulation

Sympathetic stimulation increases heart rate, contractility and relaxation rate

The arrival of an action potential in a sympathetic postganglionic terminal triggers the release of the neuroeffector **noradrenaline** ('norepinephrine' in the American literature); for details, see Section 14.1. Noradrenaline binds to $β_1$-adrenoceptors on the cardiac cell membrane. Cardiac myocytes also express α- and $β_2$-adrenoceptors, but $β_1$-receptors outnumber $β_2$ by around four to one in humans. The circulating hormone **adrenaline** (epinephrine), which is secreted by the adrenal medulla in response to sympathetic stimulation, likewise activates cardiac $β_1$-adrenoceptors. Adrenaline and noradrenaline are known collectively as the

Vagal stimulation, 10 impulses/second

0 mV

Threshold

-62 mV

Slope of pacemaker potential

Reduced slope

Hyper-polarization

1 second

Figure 4.7 Changes in the SA node pace-maker potential and attendant bradycardia caused by stimulation of vagal cardiac parasympathetic fibres (guinea pig). Note the brisk hyperpolarization of the resting membrane and the sustained slope reduction (dashed red line), which increase the time needed to reach threshold. (After Bolter CP, Wallace DJ. and Hirst GDS (2001). *Autonomic Neuroscience: Basic and Clinical* **94**, 93–101, with permission from Elsevier.)

CONCEPT BOX 4.1

Rate of decay of pacemaker potential determines heart rate

- The negative potential of a pacemaker cell decays with time (becomes less negative), due to inward currents of Na^+ and Ca^{2+} and a fall in K^+ conductance.
- The rate of decay (slope) determines how long it takes the pacemaker to reach the threshold for an action potential, which triggers the next heartbeat. Decay rate thus determines the interval between heartbeats (heart rate).
- Sympathetic stimulation increases the decay rate, so threshold is reached more quickly and the number of beats per minute increases.
- Parasympathetic stimulation reduces the decay rate, so it takes longer to reach threshold and the heart rate falls.
- Parasympathetic stimulation also rapidly hyperpolarizes the pacemaker cells, by activating acetylcholine-sensitive K^+ channels. This increases the time needed to decay to threshold, slowing the heart rate abruptly.

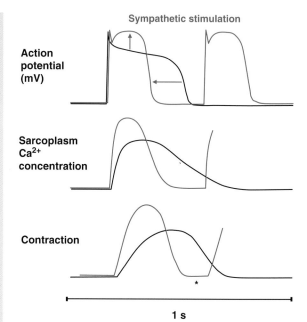

Sympathetic stimulation

Action potential (mV)

Sarcoplasm Ca^{2+} concentration

Contraction

1 s

Figure 4.8 Effect of sympathetic stimulation on a ventricular myocyte. Heart rate approximately doubled in this illustration. (*Top pair of traces*) Membrane potential before (black) and after (red) sympathetic stimulation. Vertical arrow highlights increased inward Ca^{2+} current during the plateau, producing domed appearance. Horizontal arrow highlights shortening of action potential by increased outward, repolarizing K+ current. (*Middle traces*) Increased sarcoplasmic Ca^{2+} transient and faster removal. (*Bottom traces*) The contraction is stronger, of shorter duration, and relaxation is more rapid. Despite this, the diastolic period for refilling is severely curtailed (asterisk).

catecholamines. Activation of β_1-receptors leads, over several beats, to:

- an increase in heart rate (the **chronotropic effect**, Figure 4.6)
- increased AV node conduction velocity (the **dromotropic effect**)
- shortening of the myocyte action potential (Figure 4.8)
- increased contractile force (the **inotropic effect**, Figures 4.8 and 6.18)
- increased rate of relaxation (the **lusitropic effect**, Figures 4.8 and 6.18).

The action of noradrenaline is terminated partly by diffusion into the bloodstream, which washes it away; and partly by reuptake into the sympathetic nerves. Since these processes are relatively slow, the recovery from sympathetic stimulation is slow.

The intracellular pathways that lead to the above dramatic changes in cardiac performance are as follows.

β_1-adrenoceptors activate the cAMP–PKA pathway

Activated β_1-receptors trigger a biochemical cascade that amplifies the signal and leads to multiple changes in ion channel and pump activity (Figure 4.9). Each receptor catalyses the dissociation of many molecules of an intramembrane G protein,

Figure 4.9 Signal transduction pathways activated by sympathetic transmitter noradrenaline and parasympathetic transmitter acetylcholine, in a myocardial or pacemaker cell. Aden. cyclase, adenylate or adenylyl cyclase; PLB, phospholamban; G_s, stimulatory guanosine triphosphate (GTP)-binding protein; G_i, inhibitory GTP-binding protein. Each G protein is a heterotrimer of α, β and γ subunits. On activation it dissociates into an α and a $\beta\gamma$ subunit (*lower panel*). The α_s subunit activates adenylate cyclase. The α_i subunit inhibits adenylate cyclase. The $\beta\gamma_i$ subunit activates K_{ACh} (K_G) channels.

G_s ('s' for stimulatory). This trimeric (three part) protein dissociates into α_s and $\beta\gamma$ subunits. The α_s subunit diffuses within the membrane and activates a membrane-bound enzyme, **adenylate (or adenylyl) cyclase**, which catalyses the conversion of numerous ATP molecules into the intracellular messenger **cyclic adenosine monophosphate (cAMP)**. Due to the substantial amplification along the pathway, the activation of a single adrenoceptor generates a large number of intracellular messenger molecules. The cAMP has the following actions:

- cAMP interacts directly with **pacemaker i_f channels** to increase their open-state probability. The rise in current i_f accelerates the rate of pacemaker potential decay and contributes to the chronotropic effect.
- cAMP activates the intracellular enzyme **protein kinase A (PKA)**. PKA catalyses the phosphorylation of **L-type Ca^{2+} channels**, which increases their open-state probability and duration. In atrial and ventricular myocytes, the

resulting increase in plateau Ca^{2+} current creates a 'spike and dome' action potential, and contributes to the inotropic effect (Figure 4.8). In SA node myocytes the increase in Ca^{2+} current accelerates the pacemaker potential decay and thus contributes to the chronotropic effect.

- PKA phosphorylates the slow, **delayed rectifier K^+ channels**. The resulting increase in the repolarizing outward current i_{Kv} contributes to the shortening of the ventricular action potential (Figure 4.8). Shortening also occurs, however, during purely electrical pacing (cf. sympathetic stimulation), because the intracellular Na^+ and Ca^{2+} concentrations rise when action potential frequency is increased. These ionic changes affect several currents influencing action potential duration. The reduction in action potential duration allows more excitations to fit into each minute, a necessary, permissive step when heart rate increases.
- PKA phosphorylates **phospholamban**, reducing its inhibitory effect on the Ca^{2+}-ATPase

pump of the network SR. This 'disinhibition' increases the Ca^{2+} affinity of the pump, and thus boosts Ca^{2+} transfer from sarcoplasm into SR. This accounts for most of the lusitropic (relaxation-speeding) effect. Beta-adrenergic stimulation may also phosphorylate the **Ca^{2+} release channels** (RyR), so that a bigger fraction of the raised Ca^{2+} store is released per excitation.

The above biochemical transduction pathway is relatively long and slow, so the 'on' response to sympathetic stimulation is slow (Figure 4.6). As well as the classic PKA pathway, long-term β-adrenergic stimulation may activate another kinase, **Ca^{2+}/ calmodulin-dependent kinase II** (CaMK II). This phosphorylates phospholamban at a different site, and maintains the inotropic effect of β-adrenergic stimulation. To return the cell to its baseline state, the various phosphorylated proteins are dephosphorylated by the **phosphatases** PP1 and PP2A. Many of these regulatory enzymes – PKA, CaMK II, PP1 and PP2A – are organized into massive regulatory protein complexes around their subcellular targets (phospholamban, RyR, etc.).

The $β_1$ receptor itself is subject to continual turnover. While occupied by a catecholamine molecule, the receptor can be phosphorylated by a receptor kinase. This uncouples the receptor from the G_s–adenylate cyclase system and leads to its internalization (downregulation). Fresh $β_1$-receptors are normally inserted into the membrane to maintain the appropriate receptive level. The balance between removal and replacement go awry, however, in heart failure (Chapter 18).

The above intracellular events enhance cardiac performance as follows.

The chronotropic and dromotropic effects

1 **The rate of decay of the pacemaker potential is increased**, so the threshold is reached sooner and the heart rate increases (Figure 4.6). The increased decay rate is caused by increases in the depolarizing currents i_f, i_{Ca-L} and i_{Na-Ca}, aided by an increased rate of deactivation of the delayed rectifier K^+ channel, reducing i_{Kv}. For the heart to function effectively at a higher pacing rate, the cardiac cycle too must be shortened. Sympathetic stimulation brings this about as follows.

2 **Conduction through the AV node is speeded up** by the activated nodal $β_1$-receptors (dromotropic effect). This reduces the time lag between SA node firing and ventricular contraction and shortens the ECG PR interval.

3 **The action potential of atrial and ventricular myocytes is shortened**, due to early repolarization (Figures 4.8 and 4.9). Without this change the long plateau would limit the maximum possible heart rate. This change shortens the QT interval of the ECG.

The inotropic effect is due to an increased Ca^{2+} transient

Over the course of several beats, the raised plateau Ca^{2+} current i_{Ca-L} (Figures 3.9, 4.6 and 4.8), in conjunction with the increased Ca^{2+} affinity of the SR pumps, increases the size of the SR store. The **enlarged Ca^{2+} store** and **increased trigger Ca^{2+}** (increased i_{Ca-L}) generate a bigger systolic-free Ca^{2+} transient (Figure 4.8). This activates more crossbridges and thus increases the force of atrial and ventricular systole.

The lusitropic effect is due mainly to faster Ca^{2+} reuptake by the SR

The **duration of contraction falls** and **relaxation rate increases** (Figure 4.8). This shortens the ejection and isovolumetric relaxation phases of the cardiac cycle, and thereby **minimizes the reduction in diastolic interval** (Figure 2.6). This is essential, since the heart needs sufficient time to refill. The lusitropic effect is brought about chiefly by the accelerated removal of sarcoplasmic Ca^{2+} by the network SR pumps. Studies of genetically engineered, phospholamban knock-out mice show that 85% of the lusitropy is due to pump stimulation by phosphorylated phospholamban. The rest is due to the phosphorylation of thin filament troponin I, which speeds up the crossbridge cycling and thus allows faster relaxation.

cAMP-raising drugs mimic sympathetic stimulation

Intracellular cAMP concentration depends not only on the rate of production by adenylate cyclase but also on the rate of degradation by **phosphodiesterase**. Agents that inhibit phosphodiesterase, such as **caffeine**, **theophylline** and **milrinone**, raise intracellular cAMP. They therefore mimic the effects of $β_1$-agonists, i.e. they increase the heart rate and contractility. However, despite their beneficial cardiodynamic effects these drugs increase the mortality rate in patients with heart failure.

4.6 Effects of parasympathetic stimulation

The parasympathetic neurotransmitter is acetylcholine

The arrival of an action potential in a parasympathetic postganglionic terminal triggers the release of the acetylcholine. Acetylcholine, discovered by Otto Loewi in 1921, was the first neurotransmitter to be identified. Loewi sampled fluid from a frog heart during vagal stimulation and found that the fluid caused bradycardia when applied to an isolated frog heart. Acetylcholine binds to and activates **muscarinic M_2-receptors** on the myocyte membrane. The acetylcholine is quickly removed from the junctional region, however, by the enzyme **cholinesterase**. Consequently, the heart rate picks up briskly when vagal activity is reduced.

Vagal parasympathetic fibres are tonically active, and the tonic activity is increased by endurance training, causing bradycardia in athletes. The amount of acetylcholine released from the terminal can be enhanced by a pathway involving neural nitric oxide synthase, which likewise is enhanced by training.

Acetylcholine slows the pacemaker potential

Vagal stimulation produces bradycardia through two electrophysiological actions (Figure 4.7). The chief effect is to reduce the rate at which the pacemaker potential decays. In addition, the membrane is rapidly hyperpolarized, i.e. made more negative. As a result of these two effects, the potential takes longer to reach the threshold and the heart rate decreases. Of the two effects, the reduction in slope is the more important over long periods, because it can be elicited by a lower concentration of acetylcholine and is better sustained. The chronic bradycardia of a trained athlete is an example of this effect.

M_2-receptors inhibit adenylate cyclase and activate K_{ACh} channels

Acetylcholine reduces the pacemaker slope by reducing both the Na^+ current i_f and the L-type Ca^{2+} current i_{Ca-L}. The mechanism is the reverse of that triggered by β_1-adrenoceptors. The M_2-receptor activates an inhibitory trimeric G protein, G_i, causing it to dissociate into α_i and $\beta\gamma_i$ subunits. The α_i subunit inhibits adenylate cyclase (Figure 4.9, upper panel), leading to a fall in cAMP and reduced protein kinase A activity. These changes in turn reduce the activity of i_f and L-type Ca^{2+} channels.

Acetylcholine-induced hyperpolarization is mediated by the $\beta\gamma_i$ subunit of the dissociated G_i protein (Figure 4.9, bottom). The $\beta\gamma_i$ subunit rapidly activates a specialized form of inward rectifier K^+ channel, the K_G or K_{ACh} **channel**. The resulting increase in outward K^+ current shifts the membrane potential closer to the Nernst equilibrium potential for K^+, $-94\,mV$ (eqn 3.1), causing hyperpolarization. The shortness of the M_2–$G\beta\gamma_i$–K_G linkage accounts for the rapidity with which vagal stimulation slows the heart.

Physiological roles

Examples of vagal bradycardia in man include:

- slowing of the heart during expiration (sinus arrhythmia, Figure 5.4a)
- the low heart rate of a trained athlete
- slowing of the heart during a dive (Chapter 17)
- transient arrest of the heart at the onset of fainting (vasovagal attack, Chapter 18).

An extreme example of vagal bradycardia has given rise to the everyday expression, 'playing possum'. To fool a predator, the possum feigns death by collapsing and developing a profound bradycardia:

Quoth Fox to Brer Possum
'You're due in my antrum'.
Old possum smiled; he had a hunch
His flaccid apnoee-a
And bradycardee-a
Would leave Fox in no mood for lunch.

4.7 Dangers of altered ionic environment

Since cardiac function depends on ionic gradients, any severe disturbances of extracellular ion concentration will obviously be 'A Bad Thing' for the heart. As Ringer showed, **hypocalcaemia** reduces myocardial contractility. Conversely, extreme **hypercalcaemia** arrests the heart in systole.

Hyperkalaemia can cause arrhythmia

The plasma K^+ concentration in a resting human is normally maintained at 3.5–5.5 mM by means of renal excretion and cellular uptake by the Na^+–K^+ pump. Renal K^+ excretion is regulated by the angiotensin–aldosterone system (Chapter 14), while the cellular pump is stimulated by a rise in extracellular K^+ concentration. Clinical hyperkalaemia can arise from reduced renal excretion (renal failure, angiotensin inhibitors, spironolactone) or the escape of intracellular K^+ following acidosis, tissue breakdown, crushing injury, outdated blood transfusion and haemolysis (e.g. fresh-water drowning). Hyperkalaemia weakens the heartbeat and can lead to arrhythmia. A hyperkalaemia of >7 mM in a resting human can be a medical emergency, since a rapid increase to >7.5 mM can arrest the heart in diastole (**asystole**). Indeed, for cardiac transplant surgery the donor heart is deliberately perfused with **cardioplegic solution** containing 20 mM K^+, to arrest the heart. An arrested heart needs less O_2, so is better able to survive until transplantation.

Hyperkalaemia reduces the Nernst K^+ equilibrium potential and therefore the resting membrane potential (Figure 3.6). This in turn diminishes the action potential, because the low resting potential prevents many Na^+ channel from resetting from the inactivated state to the closed-but-activatable state (Figure 3.13, top right). At a resting potential of -70 mV about half the inactivation gates are closed, while at -50 mV most are closed. As a result the action potential begins to lose its sharp phase 0, and is eventually reduced to a sluggish rise of small amplitude dependent on i_{Ca-L} (Figure 4.10). Since small, slow-rising action potentials generate less propagating current, electrical transmission is slower and less secure than normal. This can lead to heart block (Figure 5.4) or a pathological ventricular tachycardia/fibrillation. The raised extracellular K^+ also stimulates the electrogenic $3Na^+-2K^+$ pump and enhances the activity of K^+ channels K_{ir} and $K_{v(r)}$, causing early repolarization. The attendant ECG changes include a wide QRS complex (due to slow electrical propagation in the ventricle) and a tall, peaked T wave (due presumably to enhanced repolarizing K^+ current).

Some of the above changes also occur in **ischaemic myocardium**, because ischaemia causes a local increase in myocardial interstitial K^+

Figure 4.10 Effect of hyperkalaemia on the membrane potential of a Purkinje fibre (see text). The spike to the left of each action potential marks stimulation by an external impulse some distance away. Note the increasing conduction time, reduced resting potential, reduced action potential size and slowed rate of rise. (After Myerburg RJ, Lazzara R. In: Fisch E (ed.). *Complex Electrocardiography.* Philadelphia, PA: Davis, 1973.)

concentration (Figure 6.22). Treatment of the hyperkalaemia is by correction of the cause and, in an emergency, intravenous insulin and glucose, which causes a widespread cellular uptake of K^+.

Remarkably, and despite the above catalogue of horrors, the plasma K^+ concentration in a normal human can double to 8 mM in severe exercise without evident harm. The K^+ is released by the exercising skeletal muscle. It appears that the large increase in adrenaline and noradrenaline during exercise protects the myocardium against the hyperkalaemia – probably by boosting the action potential current i_{Ca-L}.

Hypokalaemia too can cause arrhythmia

Hypokalaemia is an extracellular K^+ concentration below 3 mM. Clinical hypokalaemia arises mainly from increased renal excretion (caused usually by K^+-losing thiazide diuretics) or severe diarrhoea and vomiting. The low extracellular K^+ reduces the activity of the electrogenic $3Na^+-2K^+$ pump and potassium channels K_{ir} and $K_{v(r)}$, thereby reducing the repolarizing currents. This prolongs the plateau duration and phase 3 repolarization, particularly in the K_v-rich subepicardial myocytes. As explained in Section 5.5, an upright T wave in the ECG depends on the fact that the subepicardial action potential is normally shorter than the subendocardial action potential. Prolongation of the subepicardial action potentials thus leads to flattened or inverted T waves, and sometimes a late wave called a **U wave**. Although these electrophysiological changes predispose to arrhythmia, hypokalaemic arrhythmia is seen mainly in patients with pre-existing cardiac disease.

H^+ and ischaemia weaken the heartbeat

Intracellular H^+ ions compete with Ca^{2+} for the troponin C binding site. Consequently, intracellular acidosis weakens the contraction. Intracellular pH is normally held at 7.1–7.2 by membrane transporters, namely the Na^+-H^+ exchanger and $Na^+-HCO_3^-$ importer. These can be overwhelmed, however, in ischaemia, leading to intracellular acidosis and weak contractions (Section 6.12).

4.8 Pharmacological manipulation of cardiac currents

Beta-blockers. The tonic, stimulatory effect of sympathetic activity can be reduced by non-selective β-adrenoceptor blockers (propranolol, oxprenolol) and specific β_1-adrenoceptor blockers (atenolol,

Table 4.2 Cardiac ion channels: advanced aspects. To paraphrase Professor Noble in *The Surprising Heart*, the description of ionic currents in the preceding text 'may already have exhausted the reader, but it certainly does not exhaust the mechanisms that have been found'. This table lists, for advanced students and reference purposes, the main ionic currents, component proteins and genes (in brackets) of the pore-forming α subunit. Regulatory β and other subunits are not listed. ***First-year students should not attempt to memorize these details!***

Channel and current	Properties and activators	Inhibitor	Roles
Potassium conducting channels			
(a) based on Kir protein; not voltage gated			
Inward rectifier channel Kir – current i_{K1} or i_{Kir} – heterotetramer* of Kir2.1 (*KCNJ2*) and Kir2.2 (*KCNJ12*)	Open at negative potentials. Little K^+ efflux at positive potentials because internal aperture blocked by Mg^{2+} and polyamines	Ba^{2+}	Supplies outward current for resting potential of myocytes and late phase of repolarization, from $-20\,mV$ to $-80\,mV$. Few in SA node, hence small resting potential
Muscarinic G-protein activated K_G, K_{Ach} – current $i_{K\text{-}Ach}$ – hetero-tetramer of Kir3.1 (*KCNJ3*) and Kir3.4 (*KCNJ5*)	Activated by ACh and adenosine receptors through release of $G_{\beta\gamma}$. Some spontaneous opening	Ba^{2+} partially. Pertussis toxin blocks the G_i protein	In SA node, ACh and adenosine receptors slow heart rate via hyperpolarizing effect of K_G channels. In SA node, K_G contributes to background K^+ current
ATP-sensitive K channel K_{ATP}, K_{NDP} – current $i_{K\text{-}ATP}$ – octamer of 4 Kir6.2 surrounded by 4 SUR2	Opened by low ATP ($<0.1\,mM$), raised nucleoside diphosphate (ADP), adenosine, H^+, nicorandil, cromakalim, pinacidil, diazoxide	Glibenclamide	Abundant. In ischaemia, $\uparrow$ opening terminates ventricle action potential early, reducing contractile force
(b) based on Kv protein; voltage gated			
Delayed rectifier, voltage-activated Kv: subtypes Ks, Kr – current $i_{Kv} = i_{Ks} + i_{Kr}$ – Ks gene *KvLQT1* (*KCNQ1*); Kr gene *HERG* (*KCNH2*)	Activates slowly on depolarization beyond $-40\,mV$, then inactivates slowly (i_{Ks}) or rapidly (i_{Kr}). Shortens action potential. Ks is enhanced by β-adrenergic stimulation	Ba^{2+} TEA[a] 4AP[b]	Slow inactivation causes decaying g_K of pacemaker potential. Terminates action potential by supplying initial repolarization current down to $-20\,mV$. $\uparrow$ by β-adrenergic stimulation to shorten myocyte action potential. *KCNQ1* mutation causes ~50% cases of long QT syndrome; *HERG* less often
Transient outward – current i_{to} – Kv4.3 (*KCND3*)	Activated by depolarization. More in subepicardial than subendocardial myocytes	4AP	Causes phase 1 repolarization, shortening the subepicardial action potential. Shortens action potentials in rat and mouse to allow high heart rates. $\downarrow$ in heart failure, causing prolonged action potentials.
Sodium conducting channels			
Fast-inactivating Na channel, Na_V – current i_{Na} – cardiac isoform is $Na_V1.5$ (*SCN5A*)	Open state is voltage- and time-dependent	Tetrodotoxin. Local anaesthetics	Depolarization spike of action potential in ventricles, atria Scarce in SA node, so no spike here *SCN5A* mutations are a rare cause of long QT syndrome ($<5\%$ cases)
Hyperpolarization-activated – 'funny' current i_f – tetramer of HCN1–4	Opens slowly at potentials negative to $-45, -60\,mV$. **H**yperpolarization-activated **c**yclic **n**ucleotide-gated, hence 'HCN' protein	Cs^+, ivabradine	Contributes to pacemaker depolarization; Cs^+ slows pacemaker depolarization by 10–40% Activity increased by cAMP during β-adrenergic stimulation; reduced by acetylcholine M2 receptors
Background – current i_b	Passive background current		Attenuates the resting membrane potential
(Na–Ca exchanger, NCX) – current i_{Na_Ca}, i_{NCX}	Not a channel but transfers 3 Na^+ into cell for each Ca^{2+} expelled (forward mode). Activated by intracellular Ca^{2+}	Li^+, Cd^{2+}, La^{3+}	1. Forward mode supplies net inward current in late plateau 2. Brief reverse mode after Na^+ spike may contribute to early Ca^{2+} influx 3. Can generate DADs
(Na–K pump) – current i_{NaK}	Not a channel, but transfers 3 Na^+ out of cell for every 2 K^+ in, generating a small net outward current	Digoxin, ouabain	Minor outward current, contributing 2–4 mV to resting membrane potential

(Continued)

Table 4.2 (Continued)

Channel and current	Properties and activators	Inhibitor	Roles
Calcium conducting channels			
L-type Ca channel – current i_{Ca-L} – protein $Ca_v1.2$, $\alpha1C$ (*CACN1AC*)	Voltage-operated; activated by depolarization. '*L*'ong-lasting activation. Inactivation is time-dependent and Ca^{2+}-dependent	Cd^{2+} Ni^{2+} Verapamil	1. Supplies trigger Ca^{2+} for CICR 2. Carries most of the early plateau current 3. Generates SA and AV node action potentials 4. C-terminus phosphorylation following β-adrenergic stimulation mediates increased Ca^{2+} influx and contractility
T-type Ca channel – current i_{Ca-T} – $Ca_v3.1$–3.3, $\alpha1H$ (*CACNA1H*)	Activates at more negative potentials than L-type, e.g. $-55\,mV$. '*T*'ransient activation state	Ni^{2+} Insensitive to verapamil or β agonists	Contributes to pacemaker depolarizing current
Chloride conducting channels			
cAMP-dependent – current $i_{Cl(AMP)}$	Activated by cAMP and therefore β_1 agonists		Contributes to phase 1 repolarization after β_1 activation, from +ve potentials down to E_{Cl} of $-40\,mV$ (Table 3.1)
Ca^{2+} dependent – current $i_{Cl(Ca)}$	Activated by cytosol Ca^{2+}	DIDS	E_{Cl} is $-40\,mV$, so contributes to phase 1 repolarization, pacemaker depolarization and DADs
Swelling activated	Stretch-activated, opened by osmotic swelling of cell		Regulates cell volume.
Stretch-activated channels (SAC)			
Non-specific cation conducting – TRP protein family	Activated by stretch	Gd^{3+}	Mechanoelectric feedback.
K^+-selective SAC – protein TREK-1	Activated by stretch		Mechanoelectric feedback
Cl^--selective SAC	See under *Chloride*		See under *Chloride*

[a]TEA, tetraethylammonium.
[b]4AP, 4-aminopyridine.
*'Heterotetramer' means composed of four subunits which are not all identical.

metoprolol). These agents attenuate the cardiac Ca^{2+} currents and SR pump, leading to a fall in heart rate, contractile force and cardiac output. This is beneficial in the treatment of hypertension (Section 18.4) and angina (ischaemic heart pain when cardiac work exceeds the capacity of diseased coronary arteries to deliver O_2 – Section 15.1).

Ca^{2+}-channel blockers. Verapamil and diltiazem partially inhibit L-type Ca^{2+} channels, reducing the plateau current i_{Ca-L}. This shortens the action potential and has a negative inotropic (weakening) effect. Verapamil has a greater effect on the heart than nifedipine and is used to reduce cardiac work and hence O_2 demand in angina patients. Verapamil also slows AV node conduction, so it can suppress arrhythmias that depend on a 'circus', re-entry mechanism (Section 5.8).

K^+-channel openers. The metabolically sensitive K_{ATP} channel, which we met in Section 3.6, can be activated by cromakalim, pinacidil, minoxidil and nicorandil. K_{ATP} activation causes hyperpolarization. The main therapeutic effect is the relaxation of peripheral blood vessels, which helps to relieve angina.

Adenosine is sometimes given intravenously to terminate **supraventricular tachycardia**, a pathologically high heart rate driven by an abnormal atrial pacemaker. Adenosine acts on purinergic A_1 receptors to activate nodal K^+ channels, leading to hyperpolarization. This reduces the heart rate and slows AV node conduction.

Na^+-channel blockers. Procainamide, lignocaine and quinidine are used as anti-arrhythmic drugs.

'Funny' channel blocker. The recently introduced drug ivabradine blocks the pacemaker current i_f, thus reducing the rate of pacemaker depolarization. The attendant slowing of the heart rate reduces myocardial O_2 demand, so ivabradine is used to treat angina.

4.9 Mechano-electrical feedback

A sharp thump on the chest will sometimes restart an arrested heart, or correct a pathological tachycardia. Therefore, mechanical stimuli can affect cardiac electrical activity. Mechanical stretch can activate stretch-activated ion channels (SACs), which transmit an inward, depolarizing cation current. The following effects are attributed to SACs (Table 4.2).

1 **The Bainbridge 'reflex'.** Bainbridge discovered in 1915 that the rapid infusion of a large volume of saline into the venous system causes a transient tachycardia (Section 16.3). The tachycardia may be due in part to the activation of SACs in the pacemaker cells. The effect is of little physiological importance.

2 **Catheter-induced arrhythmia.** Mechanical stimulation of the wall of the atrium or ventricle during cardiac catheterization can trigger extra systoles and other arrhythmias. Gadolinium ions, Gd^{3+}, block SACs and prevent stretch-induced arrhythmias.

3 Atrial myocytes secrete the hormone **atrial natriuretic peptide** in response to stretch (Section 14.9). This response is presumably mediated by SACs.

SUMMARY

- The sino-atrial node (pacemaker) initiates atrial contraction. The atrioventricular node delays the transmission of excitation to the ventricle, so that atrial contraction precedes ventricular contraction. The bundle of His and Purkinje system distribute the electrical impulse rapidly throughout the ventricular muscle mass.

- The membrane potential of a pacemaker cell decays with time (the pacemaker potential). The decay is caused by multiple inward currents (Na^+ currents i_f, i_b; exchanger current i_{Na-Ca}; Ca^{2+} currents i_{Ca-T}, i_{Ca-L}) combined with a decaying K^+ permeability. The decay rate determines the time needed to reach threshold and fire an action potential that initiates the next heartbeat. Heart rate is thus controlled by the slope of the decaying pacemaker potential. The nodal action potential is small, sluggish and generated solely by L-type Ca^{2+} channels.

- Sympathetic fibre terminals release noradrenaline, which activates cardiac β_1-adrenoreceptors. In the SA node the β_1-activation accelerates the decay of the pacemaker potential and thus increases heart rate (chronotropic effect). The increased decay rate is due to increases in the depolarizing pacemaker currents i_f and i_{Ca-L}, and an accelerated decay in K^+ permeability.

- Activation of β_1-adrenoceptors on atrial and ventricular myocytes increases the open probability of L-type Ca^{2+} channels, leading to a bigger plateau current, Ca^{2+} store and trigger Ca^{2+}, and thus a bigger Ca^{2+} transient and stronger contraction (inotropic effect). Ca^{2+} reuptake by the SR pumps is enhanced, so systole is shortened and relaxation speeded up (lusitropic effect). The effects of β_1-activation are mediated through the G_s-adenylate cyclase–cAMP–protein kinase A cascade.

- Parasympathetic vagal fibres release acetylcholine, which activates muscarinic M_2-receptors. This activates G_i protein, which inhibits the adenylate cyclase–cAMP–PKA pathway. The inhibition of PKA reduces the inward pacemaker currents i_f and i_{Ca-L}, and thus slows pacemaker depolarization and heart rate. Muscarinic receptors also hyperpolarize pacemaker cells by activating K_{ACh} channels. This produces an abrupt fall in heart rate, e.g. on expiration or fainting.

- Electrical activity can be altered by ionic environment and drugs. Hyperkalaemia depolarizes the myocytes, leading to conduction impairment and arrhythmias. Beta-blockers such as propanolol, and Ca^{2+}-channel blockers such as verapamil, reduce the plateau current i_{Ca}, which reduces contractile force and heart rate. Since this reduces myocardial O_2 demand, these drugs are beneficial in ischaemic heart disease.

Further reading

Reviews and chapters

Accili EA, Proenza C, Baruscotti M, DiFrancesco D. From funny current to HCN channel: 20 years of excitation. *News in Physiological Science* 2002; **17**: 32–7.

Eisner DA, Dibb KM, Trafford AW. The mechanism and significance of the slow changes of ventricular action potential duration following a change of heart rate. *Experimental Physiology* 2009; **94**: 520–8.

Kurachi Y, Ishii M. Cell signal control of the G protein-gated potassium channel and its subcellular location. *Journal of Physiology* 2004; **554**: 285–94.

Mangoni ME, Nargeot J. Genesis and regulation of the heart automaticity. *Physiological Reviews* 2008; **88**: 919–82.

Sanguinetti MC, Keating, MT. Role of delayed rectifier potassium channels in cardiac repolarization and arrhythmias. *News in Physiological Sciences* 1997; **12**: 152–7.

Simmerman HKB, Jones LR. Phospholamban: protein structure, mechanisms of action and role in cardiac function. *Physiology Reviews* 1998; **78**: 921–47.

White E. Length-dependent mechanisms in single cardiac cells (mechano-electric aspects). *Experimental Physiology* 1996; **81**: 885–97.

Zipes DP, Jalife J. *Cardiac Electrophysiology from Cell to Bedside*, 4th edn. Philadelphia, PA: WB Saunders, 2004.

Research papers

See www.hodderplus.com/cardiovascularphysiology for a full list of Research papers for this chapter.

CHAPTER 5

Electrocardiography and arrhythmias

Learning objectives

After reading this chapter you should be able to:

- Draw, label and scale a typical ECG trace, stating the chosen lead (5.1).
- State the origin of the P, QRS and T waves, and the PR and ST intervals (5.2).
- Explain what a cardiac dipole is (5.4).
- Sketch out how the cardiac dipole changes with time in the frontal plane during ventricular depolarization (5.5).
- Explain why different leads record different QRS patterns during the same systole (5.6).
- Give the meaning, mechanism and significance of:
  - sinus arrhythmia
  - ectopic beat
  - heart block
  - pathological tachycardia
  - atrial fibrillation
  - ventricular fibrillation.
- State the roles of afterdepolarization, vulnerable period and re-entry circuits in arrhythmogenesis (5.8, 3.9).
- Outline the ECG changes caused by ischaemic heart disease.

5.1 Principle of electrocardiography

The electrocardiogram (ECG) is a recording of potential changes at the skin surface that result from the depolarization and repolarization of heart muscle. The method was developed in the early twentieth century by Willem Einthoven in Leiden, who invented the string galvanometer, and Augustus Waller in London, whose demonstration to the Royal Society in 1909 provoked protests in Parliament (Figure 5.1). As explained earlier (Figure 4.4), the spread of cardiac excitation creates currents in the extracellular fluid. The currents generate small potential differences across the body surface, of around 1 mV, and these can be recorded by a sensitive voltmeter connected to metal electrodes on the skin surface. The potential difference is recorded on a strip of moving paper or computer screen to produce the familiar ECG trace. The paper speed is standardized at 0.2 s per large division (25 mm/s).

The magnitude of the skin potential difference depends on the size of the extracellular current, which in turn depends on the **mass of myocardium** that is activated. Consequently, the surface ECG detects the activity of atrial and ventricular muscle, but fails to detect the pacemaker–conduction system. The activity of the latter can, however, be recorded via a cardiac catheter.

Figure 5.1 Electrocardiogram demonstrated to the Royal Society by Waller's pet bulldog, Jimmie, in 1909; Waller is just behind Jimmie. Jimmie has his front and hind paws in pots of normal saline connected to a galvanometer. (From the *Illustrated London News*, 22 May 1909.)

The Times newspaper, July 9, 1909, reported that Mr Ellis Griffith (MP for Anglesey) questioned the Secretary of State in Parliament over Waller's 'public experiment' on a dog with 'a leather strap with sharp nails secured around the neck, his feet being immersed in glass jars containing salts connected by wires with galvanometers'. Had the Cruelty to Animals Act (1876) been contravened?

Mr Gladstone: 'I understand the dog stood for some time in water to which sodium chloride had been added or in other words a little common salt. If my honourable friend has ever paddled in the sea he will understand the sensation. (Laughter) The dog – a finely developed bulldog – was neither tied nor muzzled. He wore a leather collar ornamented with brass studs. Had the experiment been painful the pain would no doubt have been immediately felt by those nearest the dog.' (Laughter)

Mr MacNeill (Donegal South): 'Will the right honourable gentleman inform the person who furnished him with his jokes that there are members in this House who regard these experiments on dogs with abhorrence?' (Hear)

Mr Gladstone: 'I certainly shall not. The jokes, poor as they are, are mine own.' (Laughter and cheers)

(From Waller AD. *Physiology the Servant of Medicine*. London: Hodder and Stoughton, 1910.)

5.2 Relation of ECG waves to cardiac action potentials

The human ECG shows three main deflections per cardiac cycle (Figure 5.2). The P wave is caused by atrial depolarization; the QRS complex by ventricular depolarization and the T wave by ventricular repolarization. The trace returns to the baseline, or 'isoelectric state', during the PR interval and the ST segment. The lettering has no particular meaning; letters were simply allotted sequentially by Einthoven. The ECG waves are

Figure 5.2 Human ECG, Leads I–III. Lead II (60°) has the largest P, R and T waves. Lead I (0°) has a smaller R wave than Lead III, so this subject's electrical axis is between 60° and 90° (see Section 5.7). Ordinate divisions, 0.1 mV; time marks, 1/30th second. Thick baseline is an interference artefact of early string galvanometers, cf. Figure 5.4a. (From Sir Thomas Lewis's classic monograph *The Mechanism and Graphic Registration of the Human Heart*. London: Shaw and Sons, 1920.)

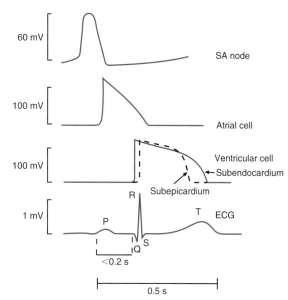

Figure 5.3 Timing of ECG waves compared with intracellular recordings of cardiac action potentials. Subepicardial myocytes (dashed trace) have ~3 times more repolarizing i_{to} K$^+$ channels than subendocardial myocytes, so they repolarize first. This causes the T wave to be upright (Section 5.5).

aligned with the underlying cardiac action potentials in Figure 5.3, and with the other events of the cardiac cycle in Figure 2.4.

P wave marks atrial excitation

The first ECG wave, the small, broad P wave, coincides with the upstrokes of thousands of right and left atrial action potentials, spread over ~0.08 s. The P wave thus marks atrial depolarization. Atrial contraction occurs during the PR interval.

PR interval marks AV node delay

The interval between the start of the P wave and the start of the QRS complex is called the PR interval, even when it is strictly speaking a P–Q interval. The PR interval represents the time taken for excitation to spread across both atria, then through the AV node and His–Purkinje system into the ventricle. Much of the PR interval represents the delay in transmission through the AV node, which allows atrial systole to precede ventricular systole. The PR interval should not exceed 0.2 s. Longer intervals indicate a defect in the conduction pathway called **heart block** (Figure 5.4c).

The ECG is isoelectric for much of the PR interval, despite the potential difference between the depolarized atria and polarized ventricles. This is because the insulating annulus fibrosus breaks

the electrical circuit shown in Figure 4.4; consequently, no detectable extracellular current is flowing.

Atrial repolarization does not register on the ECG, because it is asynchronous and slow (Figure 5.3), and therefore does not generate sufficient extracellular current to be detected. It is often stated, incorrectly, that atrial repolarization is not seen because it is obscured by the QRS complex – a classic example of a 'factoid', i.e. something that is persistently taught, eminently plausible, tenaciously believed, but demonstrably false! The ECG of patients with third-degree heart block, where P waves are not followed by an 'obscuring' QRS wave, show clearly that atrial repolarization simply does not register on the ECG (Figure 5.4e).

QRS complex marks ventricular excitation

The rapid depolarization of a large mass of ventricular muscle produces a large deflection, the QRS complex (Figure 5.3). The Q wave is an initial downward spike, the R wave is an upward spike and the S wave is a second downward spike. All three components are not necessarily present in every record – the complex may be just RS (e.g. Figure 5.2, Lead I) or just QR. The complex normally lasts ≤0.1 s. Wider QRS complexes indicate either a ventricular ectopic beat (Figure 5.4b) or a block in

Figure 5.4 A cornucopia of arrhythmias. (a) Sinus arrhythmia in a healthy 19-year-old medical student. (b) The first example of an extrasystole (ventricular ectopic, asterisk) recorded by Einthoven (CP, compensatory pause). The upper trace, the radial pulse, shows that the patient experiences a missed heartbeat. (c–e) Progressive stages of heart block. (c) First-degree block, with prolonged PR interval. (d) Second-degree block; no QRS after every third P. (e) Third-degree block. QRS unrelated to P. (f) Atrial fibrillation with 'f' waves. (g) Ventricular fibrillation triggered during the vulnerable period (late T wave of second beat), in an ischaemic heart showing ST segment depression and T wave inversion. (Records c–f are from Lewis' classic book, *The Mechanism and Graphic Registration of the Heart Beat.* London: Shaw and Sons, 1920.)

one of the bundle branches. In bundle branch block, the R wave has a characteristic 'M'-shaped notch, due to the staggered activation of the ventricle. The first heart sound follows just after the QRS complex (Figure 2.4).

ST segment is displaced in ischaemic heart disease

The ST segment extends from the end of the QRS wave to the start of the T wave. It coincides with the plateau of the ventricular action potential and rapid ventricular ejection. Since the ventricle is uniformly depolarized, no extracellular current is flowing and the ST segment is isoelectric. In ischaemic heart disease, however, the ST segment can be depressed (angina) or elevated (transmural infarct shortly after a heart attack), due to injury currents (Section 5.9).

T wave marks repolarization

Ventricular repolarization is slower and less synchronous than depolarization, so it generates a broad, asymmetrical wave, the T wave (Figure 5.3). The second heart sound follows closely after the T wave. Both the T wave and R wave are upright in most ECG recordings, despite the fact that repolarization is the electrical opposite of depolarization. The explanation of this oddity is deferred to Section 5.5, because it depends on the concept of 'cardiac dipole' (Section 5.4). Myocardial ischaemia can cause **T wave inversion**, as in the first beat of Figure 5.4g and Figure 5.11, right.

5.3 Standard ECG leads

To understand the QRS complex we have to consider three things:

(i) the anatomical location of the recording electrodes relative to the heart;
(ii) the concept of an electrical dipole; and
(iii) the change in dipole orientation as depolarization spreads across the ventricles.

Let us deal first with the positioning of the recording electrodes. The most basic ECG is recorded using three **limb electrodes**, one on each arm and one on the left leg (Figure 5.5). Wrists and ankles are usually used, but the exact position makes no difference to the recording; the limb simply serves as a tube of conducting electrolyte solution (the extracellular fluid) connected to the torso.

There are three bipolar limb leads

Pairs of limb electrodes can be connected across a voltmeter in three different combinations, called the bipolar limb leads. When the left arm is connected to the positive terminal of the voltmeter and right arm to the negative terminal, this is a called a Lead I recording. If the potential on the left side of the

Figure 5.5 Electrode positions to record a 12-lead ECG. The bipolar limb leads (I, II and III) and unipolar limb leads (aVL, aVR and aVF) record in the frontal plane. Precordial chest leads V1–V6 record in a transverse plane. For explanation of unipolar limb leads, see text. Typical records on right. Red arrows show direction of biggest potential difference during ventricular excitation (main dipole), in the frontal and transverse planes.

body is more positive than on the right during cardiac excitation, Lead I records a positive potential. The three bipolar combinations are as follows.

Left arm (+) to Right arm (−) = LEAD I (angle of view 0°)

Left leg (+) to Right arm (−) = LEAD II (angle of view 60°)

Left leg (+) to Left arm (−) = LEAD III (angle of view 120°).

Because each limb serves as an electrical conductor connected to the trunk, the limb electrodes in effect record from each shoulder and the pelvis. They thus form a sensing triangle around the heart, called **Einthoven's triangle** (Figure 5.5). Each lead views the heart from a different angle in the frontal plane. Lead I, forming the top of Einthoven's triangle, is horizontal, and this angle is taken as zero. Lead II is at roughly 60° to Lead I and Lead III at roughly 120°.

There are three unipolar limb leads

A cunning ruse provides three additional viewing angles from the same limb electrodes. The trick is to feed the signal from two electrodes simultaneously

into the negative terminal of the voltmeter, thereby producing an averaged signal located roughly in mid-chest. When the signal from the foot is connected to the other terminal, the angle of view is from the pelvis to mid-chest, ~90° to the horizontal (Figure 5.5). This is called unipolar limb Lead aVF (**a**ugmented **V**oltage from **F**oot). The three unipolar limb leads are:

Left arm to + terminal = aVL (angle of view −30°)

Right arm to + terminal = aVR (angle of view −150°)

Foot to + terminal = aVF (angle of view +90°).

Lead aVR looks into the inside of the ventricles, so it records negative rather than positive waves (Figure 5.5). Lead aVF records the inferior surface of the heart. Since aVF is at a right angle to I, it is useful for working out the cardiac electrical axis, as explained later.

There are six unipolar precordial leads

In clinical practice, an additional six electrodes, V1–V6, are placed across the chest for connection to the positive terminal of the voltmeter. All three limb leads are connected to the negative terminal to create a mid-chest reference point. The six precordial leads encircle the heart and 'look' transversely across the chest. This is useful, because the wave of excitation travels in three dimensions, not just the frontal plane recorded through limb leads. Leads V1–V2 lie over the fourth intercostal space, immediately right and left of the sternum, respectively; they record right ventricle activity best. V3 is between V2 and V4. V4 is placed over the fifth intercostal space in the mid-clavicular line. V3–V4 record interventricular septal activity best. V5–V6 are at the same level in the anterior axillary and mid-axillary line, respectively, and record the left ventricular activity best.

The ECG records an upward deflection when the positive pole of a potential difference is directed towards the left arm (Lead I) or left leg (Leads II and III), or a unipolar/precordial lead. We must therefore consider next the polarity of the heart during excitation.

5.4 The cardiac dipole

Two clouds of charge can be represented by two poles

At any instant during the spread of excitation through the ventricle there is a resting zone, with a diffuse cloud of positive extracellular charges, and an excited zone, with a diffuse cloud of negative extracellular charges (Figure 5.6a). Just as a diffuse mass can be represented by a centre of gravity, so a diffuse charge can be represented as a single charge at its electrical centre, or pole. Thus, during the spread of excitation the ventricles can be represented by one negative pole and one positive pole, i.e. by an electrical dipole. The size of the attendant ECG deflection depends not only on the **magnitude** of the dipole but also on its **orientation** relative to the recording lead, as follows.

Detection depends on the angle of the recording leads

A dipole is surrounded by positive and negative potential fields, which grow weaker with increasing distance, like the fields around a magnet (Figure 5.6b). When the leads of a voltmeter are aligned with the two poles, the difference between the positive and negative potential fields is recorded optimally, whereas leads at right angles to the dipole detect no potential difference (Figure 5.6b). The potential difference recorded by the ECG voltmeter thus depends on the orientation of the recording electrodes relative to the dipole. You can get a sense of this effect by viewing a ruler face-on, then slowly rotating it through 180°. The visible length changes from maximum to zero and back to maximum as the angle of view changes.

The dipole can be resolved into vectorial components

The dipole is a **vector** quantity. That is to say, it possesses direction as well as magnitude, just like a

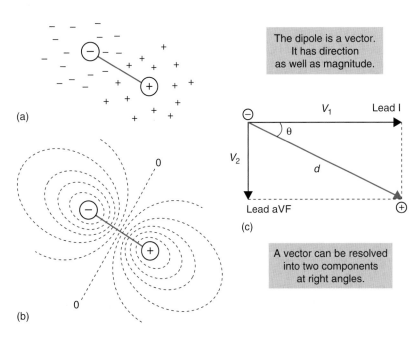

The dipole is a vector. It has direction as well as magnitude.

A vector can be resolved into two components at right angles.

Figure 5.6 Properties of an electrical dipole. (a) Two diffuse groups of opposite charge can be represented by a dipole, i.e. two points of opposite charge, like the terminals of a battery. (b) Equipotential lines around a dipole. The zero potential runs across the middle of the dipole. (c) Resolution of dipole vector (red arrow) into two components at right angles. The length of the red arrow represents vector magnitude d. The voltage difference V_1 detected by Lead I depends on angle θ ($V_1 = d$ cosine θ). If V_1 and V_2 are drawn the same lengths as the R waves in Leads I and aVF, respectively, the electrical axis of the heart equals θ.

mechanical force. The symbol for a vector is an arrow whose length represents the size of the vector and whose direction represents the angle of the vector. Just as with a force vector, the electrical vector can be resolved into two components at right angles, and the ECG registers **the magnitude of the component aligned with the recording leads** (Figure 5.6c). But this raises another question: in which direction does the cardiac dipole point?

5.5 The excitation sequence

Both the magnitude and orientation of the cardiac dipole change continuously as excitation spreads through the ventricles. For simplicity we will consider only changes in the frontal plane here; but since the ventricles are three-dimensional bodies lying in an oblique, rotated position, the dipole size and direction change in the transverse plane too.

The ventricular dipole swings anticlockwise in the frontal plane during depolarization

The first part of the ventricles to depolarize is the left side of the interventricular septum, which is activated by the left bundle branches (Figure 5.7). The dipole magnitude is small, because only a small mass of muscle has been activated; and the dipole angle is ~120° to the horizontal, i.e. pointing down and rightwards. Next, the remaining septum and most of the subendocardium depolarize, while the subepicardium is still polarized. Since the bulky left ventricle predominates, the dipole magnitude is large and the dipole angle is ~60°, i.e. pointing down and leftwards. The last region to be excited by the advancing wave of depolarization is the base of the ventricles, close to the annulus fibrosus. The bulky left ventricle again predominates, creating a small dipole pointing headwards. The sequence of ventricular activation thus causes the cardiac vector to rotate anticlockwise in the frontal plane, and to wax and wane in size as it rotates. This entire sequence takes ~90 ms.

Repolarization occurs in reverse, creating an upright T wave

We now have the information needed to answer a puzzle raised earlier – why is the T wave upright? This seems odd on first acquaintance, since repolarization is the electrical opposite of depolarization. The explanation is that the myocytes repolarize in reverse order to depolarization. In other words, the subepicardium repolarizes before the subendocardium (Figure 5.8). This is because the outer ventricular myocytes have shorter action potentials than the inner myocytes, due to their higher density of transient outward K^+ channels (Figure 5.3). Repolarization begins, therefore, in the subepicardium and spreads towards the subendocardium, whereas depolarization does the reverse. As a result, the same polarity develops transiently across the heart during repolarization as during depolarization (Figure 5.8). This is why the T wave is upright.

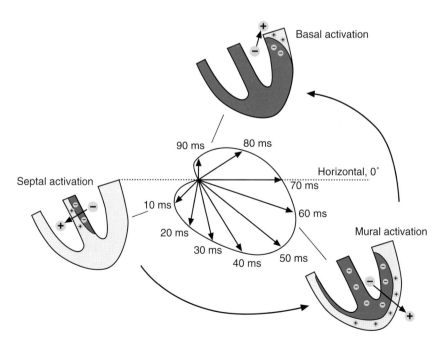

Figure 5.7 Changes in size and angle of cardiac dipole (straight arrows) with time during ventricular excitation. Charges refer to extracellular fluid, not intracellular. Grey areas are myocytes at resting potential, so they carry a positive extracellular charge. Red areas are depolarized myocytes with negative extracellular charge. Cardiac dipole rotates anticlockwise and waxes and wanes over ~90 ms. Electrical axis here is ~40° below the horizontal.

Figure 5.8 Depolarization/repolarization state of ventricles at three points in time, namely partial depolarization (red zone, R wave, *top*), full depolarization (ST segment, *middle*) and partial repolarization (grey zone, T wave, *bottom*). Signs refer to extracellular charge. Arrows show direction of advance of wave front. Since myocytes repolarize in reverse order to depolarization, the dipoles are in the same direction. Consequently, the T wave is upright.

5.6 Why the QRS complex is complex

Knowing the orientation of the ECG leads and dipole, we are now in a position to understand why the QRS complex has negative as well as positive waves; and why the same heartbeat generates differently shaped QRS complexes in different leads (Figure 5.5). To work through an example, let's consider the dipole at three instants – the beginning, middle and end of ventricular excitation – as detected by bipolar limb leads I–III. In the individual shown in Figure 5.9, the small initial dipole at ~120° is directed obliquely away from Lead I. Resolving the vector, we find there is small component directed at 180°. Since the positive pole points away from Lead I (0°), Lead I records a small, negative deflection, i.e. a Q wave (point 'a' in Figure 5.9). At the same instant, however, Lead III (120°) detects the full dipole (120°), so it records a positive deflection, i.e. the start of an R wave.

By 50 ms, the dipole has grown to its maximum size and swung anticlockwise to ~40°. The dipole

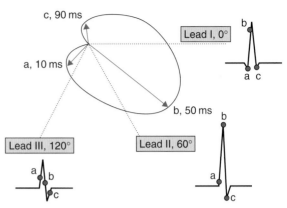

Figure 5.9 Illustration of how the changing magnitude and direction of the dipole (red arrows) creates different QRS complexes in different frontal leads. The dipole is shown at three instants in time: a, b and c. The vectorial component recorded by Leads I, II and III at each instant is marked by a red dot on the corresponding ECG trace.

now has a large vectorial component directed at Lead I (0°), which therefore records a substantial upward deflection – a large R wave (point 'b', Figure 5.9). Lead II (60°) is almost exactly aligned with the dipole, so **Lead II usually registers the biggest R wave**. Lead III (120°) is almost at right angles to the dipole, and so Lead III records little potential difference.

By 90 ms the dipole has dwindled in magnitude and, in the illustrated case, swung round to about −100°, creating a small, downward deflection in each limb lead, i.e. an S wave. Thus the same wave of ventricular excitation produced a QRS complex in Lead I, a very large RS complex in Lead II and a small RS complex in Lead III. Using similar reasoning, the reader should now be able to work out why the **P wave, QRS complex and T wave are all inverted in Lead aVR** (Figure 5.5); and why the Q wave generated by the initial depolarization of the interventricular septum is best seen in aVL.

The precordial (chest) leads record the dipole in the transverse plane. In this plane, the maximum dipole points towards the left axilla (Figure 5.5, bottom right, red arrow); so the R wave increases in height from V2 to V3 and peaks in axillary leads V4–V5. Since the maximum dipole points away from V1, the main wave of the QRS complex is downwards in V1.

Confusingly for students, not all ECG traces are identical to those in Figures 5.5 and 5.9. This is because the orientation of the cardiac dipole varies between individuals. For example, the subject of Figure 5.2 had the biggest R wave in Lead II, as expected; but Lead III showed a bigger R wave than Lead I. This indicates a more vertically orientated electrical axis, and brings us to the issue of the electrical axis of the heart.

5.7 Electrical axis of the heart

The direction of the largest dipole in the frontal plane is called the electrical axis of the heart. In Figures 5.5 and 5.9 the electrical axis is ~40° below the horizontal. The electrical axis can be worked out numerically by comparing the height of the R wave in Leads I and aVF, using the method shown in Figure 5.6c. In a busy clinic, a quick estimate can be made as follows: (i) Compare the size of the R wave in Leads I–III. If the largest R wave is in Lead II, the electrical axis is closer to 60° than to 0° or 120°. (ii) Look for the lead with the smallest QRS complex, with R and S waves of nearly equal height. This lead must be roughly at right angles to the electrical axis (e.g. Lead I in Figure 5.2).

The electrical axis has a very wide, normal range, from −30° to +110°. The axis depends partly on an individual's anatomy; the heart and electrical axis are more vertical in a tall, thin person than in a short, broad-chested individual. The axis also becomes more vertical during each inspiration, because the descending diaphragm tugs on the pericardium and drags down the apex. The electrical axis depends too on the relative thickness of the right and left ventricle walls. Hypertrophy of the left ventricle due to a cardiomyopathy shifts the electrical axis to the left (**left axis deviation**). Hypertrophy of the right ventricle due to pulmonary disease produces **right axis deviation**.

5.8 Arrhythmia and arrhythmic mechanisms

The ECG is invaluable for the diagnosis of irregular rhythms (arrhythmia, dysrhythmia), myocardial ischaemia (Section 5.9) and ventricular hypertrophy. Arrhythmias range from the benign, perfectly normal sinus arrhythmia, to pathological but relatively harmless 'palpitations' and serious, life-threatening fibrillation. The arrhythmia of heart block is caused by a failure of the conduction system; but most other pathological arrhythmias are triggered by a **delayed afterdepolarization**, which results from the discharge of an overloaded SR Ca^{2+} store (Figure 3.16). After the triggering event, a continuous arrhythmia is usually sustained by a **re-entry (circus) mechanism** (see below).

The depolarizing ventricle forms an electrical dipole

- During the 90 ms that it takes depolarization to spread through the ventricles, the excited region carries a cloud of negative extracellular charges (the negative pole) and the resting region a cloud of positive extracellular charges (the positive pole). A dipole thus forms across the heart.
- The dipole is biggest midway through excitation, because roughly half the wall is negative and half positive.
- The direction of the biggest dipole is called the electrical axis of the heart. It is typically 0–90° below the horizontal, in the frontal plane.
- An ECG lead detects the part of the dipole directed towards itself. Lead II, aligned at 60° to the horizontal, is roughly in line with the biggest dipole, so it usually has the biggest R wave.
- The dipole waxes and wanes, and swings anticlockwise, as excitation sweeps through the ventricles. The changes in dipole size and orientation generate the Q, R and S waves.

Sinus arrhythmia

Sinus arrhythmia is the normal, regular, physiological slowing of the heart during expiration and speeding up during inspiration. Sinus arrhythmia is especially marked in children and young adults; in the medical student of Figure 5.4a, for example, the heart rate oscillated between $52\,min^{-1}$ during expiration and $92\,min^{-1}$ during inspiration. The inspiratory tachycardia partially compensates for a fall in left ventricular stroke volume during inspiration. The latter is due to a fall in left ventricle filling as inspiration expands the pulmonary vascular bed.

Sinus arrhythmia is brought about by an increase in vagal parasympathetic activity during expiration, followed by a decrease during inspiration. This phasic change in vagal activity persists even when breathing is paralysed, showing that it is driven primarily by a central (cf. reflex) mechanism, namely an input from the respiration centre to the vagal motor nuclei in the brainstem (Figure 16.17).

Ventricular ectopic beats

Aberrant myocytes may occasionally fire before the SA node, triggering a premature beat, also known as an ectopic beat or extra systole (Figure 5.4b). If the trigger site lies in the ventricle, the resulting QRS wave is broad and ill-synchronized, because excitation was not disseminated along the normal, rapid His–Purkinje pathway. The contraction is ill co-ordinated and fails to eject blood normally, as shown by the blood pressure trace in Figure 5.4b. The subsequent, normal excitation wave from the SA node finds the ventricular myocytes still in their **refractory period**, so no contraction is elicited. This results in a long interval before the next normal beat, called a **compensatory pause**. The patient often notices this delay, commenting that 'My heart keeps missing a beat'.

Occasional ectopic beats are not uncommon in normal individuals, and are common after a heart attack. The ectopic beat is probably triggered by a **delayed afterdepolarization** (DAD). The DAD is the result of a discharge of the SR Ca^{2+} store in early diastole, which increases the net inward exchanger current, i_{Na-Ca} (Figure 3.16). DADs are most likely to occur in ischaemic heart disease, or when the SR Ca^{2+} store is overloaded due to the action of digoxin, catecholamines, caffeine (strong coffee) and other phosphodiesterase inhibitors.

Heart block

The AV node, bundle of His or a bundle branch may begin to fail to transmit electrical excitation properly, due to fibrosis of the adjacent atrioventricular valves or ischaemic heart disease. Three degrees of main bundle block are recognized. **First-degree heart block** is a lengthening of the PR interval to >0.2 s (e.g. 0.45 s in Figure 5.4c). This is caused by a slowing of conduction between the AV node and ventricle. **Second-degree heart block** is an intermittent failure of excitation to pass from the atria to the ventricles. In Figure 5.4d, for example, there are only three QRS complexes for four P waves; the PR interval lengthens with each beat, until a point is reached where transmission fails completely (the Wenkebach phenomenon). Transmission fails at every third P wave in Figure 5.4d, and the sequence then repeats. In **third-degree or complete heart block**, the transmission fails completely, so the atria and ventricles beat independently, at different rates. In Figure 5.4e, the atria (P waves) are beating at 72 min^{-1}, driven by the SA node. The ventricles are beating at 30 min^{-1}, driven by a latent pacemaker in the bundle of His or Purkinje system that has escaped from dominance by the SA node. Complete heart block can occur intermittently, causing **Stokes–Adams attacks** (sudden, temporary loss of consciousness). Such patients are treated by artificial pacemaker implantation.

Re-entry (circus) mechanisms sustain pathological tachycardias

Sometimes an abnormal conduction pathway develops, often in ischaemia, such that the wave of excitation travels in a never-ending circle (**circus**, Figure 5.10). Myocytes emerging from their refractory period then find themselves re-excited prematurely by the return of the local excitation

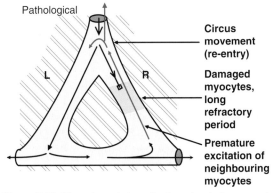

Figure 5.10 Circus (re-entry) mechanism of arrhythmogenesis. (*Top and middle*) Normal spread of excitation around non-conducting obstacles such as a blood vessel or connective tissue. (*Bottom*) Pathology, such as ischaemia or chronic heart failure, causes a long refractory period in the fibres on the right (R), and also slow conductions. As a normal excitation arrives at R, it finds the myocytes refractory from the previous impulse, so it propagates no further. By the time the slowly propagating wave has spread down L, then retrogradely up R, myocytes at R are no longer refractory. They conduct the impulse back up to the junction with L, which is re-excited (re-entry), setting up a self-perpetuating loop or 'circus'.

wave (**re-entry**). A slow rate of wave propagation favours re-entry, because it allows time for the myocytes to regain excitability after their refractory period. Slow propagation is often the result of local ischaemia, which reduces the resting potential and thereby prevents some fast Na^+ channels from recovering from the inactivated state (Figure 3.13). The resulting impairment of the action potential upstroke reduces the propagating currents, which slows conduction (Figure 4.10).

Re-entry probably sustains fibrillation (see below) after a triggering DAD, and also sustains many pathological tachycardias. The unforgettably named **Wolff–Parkinson–White syndrome** comprises episodes of paroxysmal tachycardia (palpitations) at >200 beats/min, resulting from an anatomically definable re-entry pathway, the accessory bundle of Kent. This is an extra electrical connection across the annulus fibrosus, additional to the bundle of His. Under certain circumstances the ventricular depolarization wave passes up the bundle of Kent to re-excite the atria, thus producing a self-perpetuating circus pathway and tachycardia. The sensation of palpitations is frightening, and the truncated diastolic filling interval reduces the cardiac output, leading to light-headedness and even collapse. Treatment is by the destruction of the bundle of Kent.

The aim of pharmacological therapy for re-entry dysrhythmias is to disrupt the timing of re-entry, using a Ca^{2+} channel inhibitor (**verapamil**), K^+ channel activator (**adenosine**, Section 4.8) or Na^+ channel inhibitor (**procainamide**, **quinidine**). Also, a pathological tachycardia can sometimes be halted by applied physiology. **Massage of the carotid sinuses**, a reflexogenic area just below the angle of the jaw (Figure 16.2), elicits a reflex increase in vagal parasympathetic drive to the heart. This slows the pacemaker and reduces the conduction velocity through the AV node, which terminates some tachycardias.

Atrial fibrillation

Fibrillation is an uncoordinated, repetitive excitation of myocytes, resulting in a writhing movement of the chamber wall, with no effective ejection of blood. Fibrillation is probably sustained by multiple, local re-entry circuits within the wall. Atrial fibrillation is not uncommon in the elderly, and is compatible with a sedentary life. Excitation is transmitted sporadically through the AV node to the ventricles, resulting in a characteristic, easily diagnosed radial pulse of **irregularly irregular** rhythm and variable amplitude (Figure 5.4f, upper trace). Small, irregular 'f' waves replace the P wave in the ECG. The main danger is that an organized blood clot or **thrombus** may form in a stagnant region of the atrium and then embolize, i.e. float away downstream, with serious consequences for the tissue in which it lodges.

Ventricular fibrillation

Fibrillation of the ventricle wall is a fatal sequel to anaesthetic overdose, electrocution and, most commonly, myocardial ischaemia. In Figure 5.4g the first two beats show abnormalities characteristic of chronic myocardial ischaemia, namely ST segment depression and T wave inversion. After the second sinus beat a ventricular ectopic arises during the second half of the T wave, a period called the **vulnerable period**. An ectopic during the vulnerable period is particularly prone to trigger fibrillation, because some myocytes have repolarized but others are still in their refractory period; consequently, multiple local circus pathways are readily triggered. This creates numerous rapid, uncoordinated electrical

---

Afterdepolarization and re-entry cause arrhythmias

- In an ischaemic heart the overloaded SR calcium store may discharge in early diastole. This increases Ca^{2+} expulsion by the $3Na^+$–$1Ca^{2+}$ exchanger. The net positive charge (Na^+) transferred into the cell by the exchanger causes an afterdepolarization.
- A delayed afterdepolarization (DAD) can reach threshold, triggering an action potential and poorly co-ordinated ectopic beat (extra systole).
- In the latter half of the T wave ('vulnerable period'), ectopic activation readily triggers re-entry-based arrhythmias, such as ventricular fibrillation.
- During the vulnerable period local circus pathways can develop, because some myocytes have repolarized while others have not. An ectopic excitation propagating slowly through a circus pathway will re-excite myocytes emerging from their refractory period (re-entry). This re-excites the circus pathway – a self-perpetuating process.
- Ischaemia slows myocardial conduction, due to inactivation of some Na^+ channels. Slow conduction allows the return of circus excitation after the refractory period, and thus favours re-entry-based arrhythmias. Re-entry underlies fibrillation.

CONCEPT BOX 5.2

waves and an ineffective rippling motion of the ventricle wall (fibrillation). With no cardiac output, death follows within minutes. 'Cardioversion' by a DC electric shock to the chest wall sometimes succeeds in restoring sinus rhythm.

5.9 ECG in ischaemic heart disease

Coronary artery disease is a common cause of local ventricular ischaemia, which manifests itself as a displacement of the ST segment above/below the isoelectric baseline. ST segment displacement is caused by a fall in resting potential and action potential magnitude in ischaemic myocytes. This creates a potential difference between the ischaemic myocytes and surrounding healthy myocytes, which causes **injury current** to flow during normally isoelectric periods. This shifts the level of the ST segment and/or ECG baseline. Exercise-induced **angina** causes ST segment depression, as explained in Figure 5.11a. The change is reversible with rest (Figure 15.7). By contrast, a **transmural infarct**, i.e. damage to the full thickness of a segment of wall, initially elevates the ST segment – the first definitive ECG change after a heart attack (Figure 5.11b). A few days later pathological Q waves and T wave inversion develop.

(a) Angina ECG ST

(b) Transmural infarct; early and late ECG

Figure 5.11 Effect of myocardial ischaemia on ventricle extracellular charge distribution and ECG. (a) ST segment depression during an angina attack. The potential difference between normal myocytes and ischaemic myocytes (usually subendocardial) creates a dipole and injury current during the ST interval (cf. normally uniform depolarization, Figure 5.8 middle) and a reversed one during the T–P interval. This depresses the ST segment relative to the baseline. The ECG reverts to normal when the angina is relieved by rest. A partial thickness, subendocardial infarct can likewise cause ST depression, but this is not relieved by rest. (b) Full thickness (transmural) infarct, caused by coronary artery thrombosis. (*Upper schematic*) Ventricle during ST interval, a few hours after infarction. The potential difference between the ischaemic and normal myocytes during ST creates a dipole and injury current, which causes ST elevation in leads facing the infarct, e.g. V1–6 for anterior infarcts, aVF and III for an inferior infarct. (*Lower schematic*) Ventricle during spread of excitation, several days later. As ischaemic cells die (necrosis), they become electrically silent, so ST elevation dwindles and is replaced by pathological Q waves and T wave inversion. Pathological Q waves are deep Q waves (>2 mm, 0.2 mV) in leads not normally showing them, persisting for years. These features are caused by the altered dipole during excitation; cf. Figure 5.7. The infarcted myocardium acts as an 'electrical window' for leads facing it. A partial thickness subendocardial infarct does not generate pathological Q waves.

SUMMARY

- The 12-lead electrocardiogram is a recording of small potential differences ($\sim$1mV) in the frontal plane (three bipolar limb leads and three unipolar limb leads) and transverse plane (six precordial leads).

- The P wave is caused by atrial depolarization, the QRS complex by ventricular depolarization and the T wave by ventricular repolarization.

- The PR interval is a delay caused chiefly by slow transmission through the atrioventricular node. It should not exceed 0.2 s in humans. The delay allows atrial systole to precede ventricular systole.

- The isoelectric ST segment corresponds to the plateau of the ventricular action potential. It is displaced by injury currents during angina or after a heart attack (infarct).

- The T wave is upright in most leads, because repolarization occurs in reverse sequence to depolarization, due to the short action potentials of subepicardial myocytes.

- At any instant during the spread of ventricular excitation, negative and positive extracellular charges create an electrical dipole.

- The QRS complex differs between leads, because each lead detects the dipole from a different angle. Lead I (left arm–right arm) is horizontal (0°). Lead II (left leg–right arm) is at 60° and Lead III (left leg–left arm) at 120° in the frontal plane. These three leads form Einthoven's triangle.

- The component Q (down), R (up) and S (second down wave) result from changes in the dipole over <0.1 s. Excitation spreads first into the left interventricular septum, then out through the subendocardium to the subepicardium and base. The resulting dipole, which is dominated by the left ventricle, rotates anticlockwise in the frontal plane, waxing and waning as it does so.

- The angle of the largest dipole in the frontal plane, usually 0–90°, is called the electrical axis of the heart.

- The ECG is used to diagnose cardiac ischaemia (angina, infarcts) and arrhythmia. Pathological arrhythmia can be caused by conduction impairment (heart block), afterdepolarization resulting from SR Ca^{2+} store discharge (extra-systole, or trigger for fibrillation) and re-entry circuits (pathological tachycardia, fibrillation). Afterdepolarization during the vulnerable period (late T wave) may trigger multiple re-entry circuits, causing fatal ventricular fibrillation.

Further reading

Carmeliet E. Cardiac ionic currents and acute ischemia: from channels to arrhythmias. *Physiological Reviews* 1999; **79**: 917–1017.

Jalife J. Ventricular fibrillation: mechanisms of initiation and maintenance. *Annual Review of Physiology* 2000; **62**: 25–50.

Rowlands DJ. The electrocardiogram. In: Warrell DA, Cox TM, Firth JD, Benz EJ (eds). *Oxford Textbook of Medicine*, 4th edn. Oxford: Oxford University Press, 2005.

Volk T, Nguyen TH-D, Schultz J-H, Faulhaber J, Ehmke H. Regional alterations of repolarizing K$^+$ currents among the left ventricular free wall of rats with ascending aortic stenosis. (Epicardial versus endocardial potentials and T wave.) *Journal of Physiology* 2001; **530**: 443–55.

Waldo AL, Wit AL. Mechanisms of cardiac arrhythmias. *Lancet* 1993; **341**: 1189–93.

Zipes DP, Jalife J (eds) (2004) *Cardiac Electrophysiology: From Cell to Bedside*, 4th edn. Philadelphia, PA: W.B. Saunders, 2004.

CHAPTER 6

Control of stroke volume and cardiac output

Learning objectives

After reading this chapter you should be able to:

- Sketch the length–tension relation and give its probable mechanism (6.2, 6.3).
- State Starling's law of the heart and its importance for stroke volume regulation (6.4).
- Draw a ventricular function (Starling) curve and define stroke work (6.4, 6.5).
- List the chief factors influencing central venous pressure (6.6).
- State the roles of the Frank–Starling mechanism in man (6.7).
- Use Laplace's law to explain why cardiac distension is harmful in heart failure (6.8).
- State the direct and secondary effects of arterial pressure on stroke volume (6.9).
- Define contractility and draw a graph to show how altered contractility affects the Starling curve (6.10).
- List the effects of sympathetic stimulation on cardiac performance (6.10).
- Draw a ventricular pressure–volume loop and sketch the effect of (i) increased filling pressure (preload); (ii) increased contractility; (iii) increased arterial pressure (afterload); and (iv) exercise (6.5, 6.10).
- Name two important inotropic hormones and two classes of inotropic drug (6.11).
- Outline the negative inotropic and arrhythmogenic effects of myocardial ischaemia (6.12).
- Outline the co-ordinated cardiac response to exercise (6.13).
- Explain the tight link between myocardial performance and coronary blood flow (6.14).

6.1 Overview

In a resting adult each ventricle pumps out 4–7 litres of blood per minute – the cardiac output. The **cardiac index**, which relates resting output to body size, is 3 l/min per square metre of body surface area ($\sim 1.8\,m^2$ for a 70-kg adult). The cardiac output is not fixed, however, but is continually adjusted to meet changes in demand. For example, the cardiac output is reduced by $\sim 10\%$ during sleep, and is increased by 20–30% during excitement, stress or a heavy meal. It rises by up to 40% during pregnancy and four- to six-fold during hard exercise, though less than this in ischaemic hearts (Table 6.1). These changes are brought about by changes in both heart rate and stroke volume. The control of **heart rate** by autonomic nerves was described in Chapter 4. In this chapter we focus initially on the control of stroke volume, followed by the co-ordinated regulation of stroke volume, heart rate and peripheral vascular tone when cardiac output is raised.

Stroke volume is influenced by two opposing factors, namely the **energy of contraction** of the ventricles and the **aortic pressure** that has to be overcome before any blood can be expelled (Figure 6.1). A highly energetic contraction produces a large stroke volume. A high arterial pressure, on the other hand, opposes ejection and reduces the stroke volume, unless there are compensatory changes.

The **energy of contraction** can be raised by two mechanisms. (i) Stretching the myocardium in diastole by raising the end-diastolic pressure enhances the contractile energy. This is called **Starling's law of the heart**. (ii) The strength of contraction at a given degree of stretch can be increased by sympathetic nerves and circulating adrenaline. This is called an increase in **contractility**.

Arterial pressure depresses stroke volume, because ejection cannot begin until ventricular pressure exceeds aortic pressure. If arterial pressure is high, much of the contractile energy of the heartbeat is needed to raise ventricular blood pressure during the isovolumetric contraction phase, so less energy remains for the ejection phase.

Stroke volume thus depends on the interplay of three factors:

- diastolic stretch, which depends on venous filling pressure;
- contractility, which is regulated by sympathetic fibres and hormones and is reduced by cardiac disease;
- arterial pressure, which opposes ejection.

This chapter describes first the effect of diastolic stretch (Sections 6.2–6.8), then arterial pressure (Section 6.9) and then contractility (Sections 6.10–6.12).

6.2 Contractile properties of isolated myocardium

Isolated strips of myocardium, such as an isolated papillary muscle, have been studied as an aid to understanding the behaviour of the more complex, intact heart. These studies *in vitro* have demonstrated the importance of 'preload' and 'afterload' in contractile performance, as follows.

Preload enhances contractile force; the isometric length–tension relation

A relaxed strip of myocardium can be stretched to a set length by hanging a weight from it, called the **preload** (Figure 6.2). If the ends of the muscle are

Table 6.1 Output of adult human heart in litres/min (mean and standard deviation)

	Rest	Exercise[a]
Normal adult	6.0 (1.3)	17.5 (6.0)
Coronary artery disease	5.7 (1.5)[b]	11.3 (4.3)

[a]The output of the diseased heart became inadequate during exercise at 85% of maximum heart rate or to onset of angina.
[b]The output of the diseased heart was within the normal range at rest.
After Rerych SK, Scholz PM, Newman GE *et al. Annals of Surgery* 1978; **187**: 449–58.

Figure labels: Filling pressure (preload): Starling's law of the heart; Stroke volume; Arterial pressure opposing ejection (afterload); Total peripheral resistence; Energy of contraction; Contractility: – sympathetic nerves – circulating agents

Figure 6.1 Factors that regulate stroke volume. Total peripheral resistance, which arises mainly in the arterioles and terminal arteries, is represented here by the narrow tube in series with the aorta.

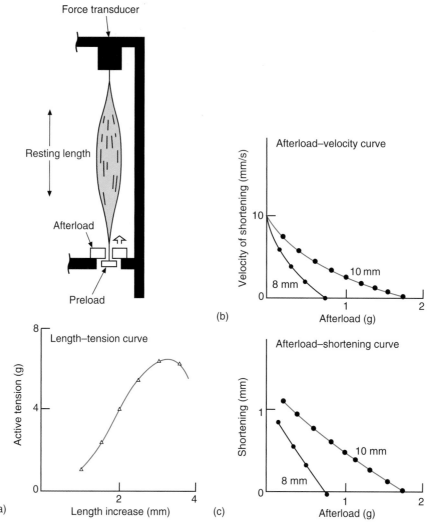

Figure 6.2 Contractile behaviour of isolated cat papillary muscle. Preload weight sets resting length. If preload is clamped, shortening is prevented and the electrically stimulated contraction is isometric. Graph (a) shows effect of resting length on isometric contractile force. If the muscle is allowed to shorten, it lifts a constant weight, the afterload, and the contraction is isotonic (b and c). Isotonic contractions starting from 10-mm resting length (high preload) are stronger than from 8-mm resting length (low preload). (After Sonnenblick EH. *American Journal of Physiology* 1962; **202**: 931–9, with permission from the American Physiological Society.)

then anchored to rigid points and the muscle is stimulated electrically, it develops active tension (force) but cannot shorten. This is called an **isometric contraction** (iso-, same; -metric, length). Remarkably, the greater the initial stretch, the greater the contractile force on stimulation (Figures 6.2a and 6.3). This important effect is called the **length–tension relation**. Translating this to the intact ventricle, the stretch of the muscle fibres is set not by a weight but by the **diastolic filling pressure**; the ensuing **isovolumetric contraction** is roughly equivalent to an isometric contraction; and the increase in contractile energy with stretch is called **Starling's law of the heart** (Section 6.4).

Afterload impairs shortening; the isotonic afterload–shortening relation

To study shortening, as opposed to tension development, one end of the isolated myocardial strip is left free to move upon stimulation; but as it begins its contraction, it lifts a constant weight, the **afterload** (Figure 6.2, left). This compels the muscle to shorten while exerting a fixed, known force – a mode of contraction called **isotonic contraction** (iso-, same; -tonic, force). If the afterload is increased, both the rate and degree of shortening decrease, unsurprisingly (Figure 6.2b,c). This is called the **afterload–shortening relation**. If the starting length is increased by raising the preload, however, the speed and degree

Figure 6.3 Effect of resting sarcomere length on contractile force in 'skinned' myocardium. The sarcolemma has been permeabilized by a detergent, then exposed to a near-physiological systolic Ca^{2+} concentration (8.9 μM), or a saturating one that causes maximal contracture (50 μM). The lower but steeper curve is similar to intact cardiac muscle. Sketches at top show how stretch reduces interference by myosin heads (red) that are pulling in the 'wrong' direction beyond the sarcomere mid-point. (Adapted from Kentish JC, ter Keurs HEDJ, Ricciardi L, Bucx JJJ, Noble MIM. *Circulation Research* 1986; **58**: 755–68, by permission.)

6.3 Mechanisms underlying the length–tension relation

Stretching the sarcomere increases contractile energy

When the myocardium is stretched by a preload, every sarcomere in the myocyte is lengthened, as shown by laser diffraction measurements. A plot of contractile force versus relaxed sarcomere length forms a curve. Maximum force is attained at a sarcomere length of 2.2–2.3 μm (Figure 6.3), and stretch beyond this point reduces contractile force; but such lengths are probably never reached *in vivo*, because myocytes become very stiff above 2.3 μm. In intact hearts at normal end-diastolic pressure, the sarcomere length is ~1.8–2.0 μm, so **myocytes normally operate on the ascending part of the length–tension curve**.

Stretch can raise contractile force without raising intracellular Ca^{2+}

The reader may have come away from Chapters 3 and 4 with the impression that a stronger heartbeat must always be due to a rise in intracellular Ca^{2+}; but this is not so. Figure 6.4 shows the effect of diastolic stretch on twitch force and sarcoplasmic Ca^{2+} transient. Stretch causes an **immediate force increase** with no increase in the systolic Ca^{2+} transient − unlike the Ca^{2+}-mediated effect of catecholamines (Sections 3.8 and 4.5). If the stretch is maintained, there is a further, slow increase in force over ~5 min, which is due to increased Ca^{2+} transients. The immediate force increase accounts for 60% of the eventual response, and is the basis of the length–tension relation. The subsequent Ca^{2+}-mediated **slow force response** underlies the **Anrep effect** in intact hearts (Section 6.9).

Stretch reduces filament overlap and raises Ca^{2+} sensitivity

How is the immediate force increase achieved? Two mechanisms contribute to it, namely changes in actin–myosin filament overlap and increased sensitivity to Ca^{2+}. The latter mechanism is the more important one in cardiac muscle, unlike skeletal muscle.

Filament overlap and interference. When the sarcomere is less than 2.0 μm long, the actin filaments (1 μm long) extend across the mid-line into the 'wrong' half of the sarcomere (Figure 6.3, top left). Consequently, a fraction of the myosin crossbridges

of shortening increase, because stretch increases the contractile force (Figure 6.2b,c, red curves).

The moment when an isolated strip begins to pick up the afterload corresponds, in an intact heart, to the moment when the tensing ventricle opens the outlet valve by slightly exceeding arterial pressure. Therefore, **arterial pressure** determines afterload *in vivo*; the **ejection phase** is roughly equivalent to isotonic shortening; and the cardiac **pump-function curve** (Section 6.9) is roughly equivalent to the afterload–shortening relation. The qualifier 'roughly' is used because the afterload is not constant in a contracting heart; it waxes and wanes as arterial pressure peaks and falls. This form of contraction is called **auxotonic**. The afterload–shortening relation is important clinically, because it underlies the use of arterial pressure-reducing drugs to improve the output of failing hearts.

are pulling in the opposite direction to the majority, reducing the net tension generated. Moreover, in sarcomeres less than 1.6 μm long, the myosin filament hits the Z lines. Stretch between 1.6 and 2 μm reduces these interference problems and thus increases the net contractile force. This explanation is clearly incomplete, however, because it applies equally to skeletal muscle, yet the **cardiac muscle is much more sensitive to stretch than skeletal muscle**, i.e. the length–tension curve is much steeper for cardiac than skeletal muscle (Figure 6.5). An additional, more important mechanism must therefore operate in cardiac muscle.

Increased sensitivity to Ca^{2+}. If all possible crossbridges at a given sarcomere length are activated *in vitro*, by raising intracellular Ca^{2+} to supra-normal levels, there is still a length–tension relation, but it is less steep than normal (Figure 6.3, upper curve). The relation now resembles that for skeletal muscle, and is explained by the filament interference effect (above). At a more physiological Ca^{2+} level (Figure 6.3, lower curve), the active tension is lower, because only a fraction of the potential crossbridges is activated; but

the force increases much more steeply with stretch, approaching closer and closer to the line for full activation. This experiment shows that **stretch increases the fraction of crossbridges activated by a given Ca^{2+} level**. Stretch thus increases the sensitivity of the contractile machinery to Ca^{2+}. This has been confirmed by plotting contractile force against Ca^{2+} concentration at two different sarcomere lengths; stretch shifts the curve to the left (Figure 6.6). In other words, a stretched myocyte needs less Ca^{2+} to produce a given contractile force.

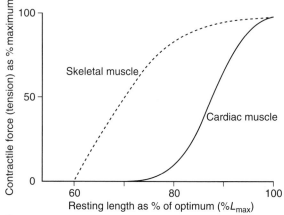

Figure 6.5 Length–tension relation of cardiac muscle compared with skeletal muscle. Cardiac muscle has a much steeper curve than skeletal muscle at physiological lengths (80–100%, L_{max}), even though the filament overlap is the same. This is because stretch increases the Ca^{2+} sensitivity of cardiac myocytes. (Adapted from Fuchs F, Smith SS. *News in Physiological Science* 2001; **16**: 5–10, with permission from the American Physiological Society.)

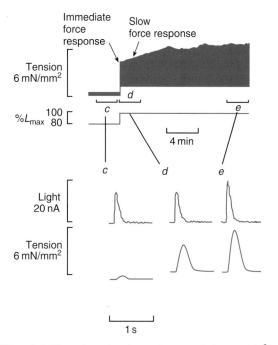

Figure 6.4 Effect of stretch on isometric contractile force and Ca^{2+} transients in isolated papillary muscle. The muscle was stretched from 80% of optimum length (L_{max}) to 100%. Note immediate, large increase in force at *d*, then a smaller, slow force response. Light signal from the Ca^{2+}-sensitive protein, aequorin, shows that the big initial response, *d*, does not require an increased Ca^{2+} transient, whereas the slow force response at *e* does (Anrep effect). (After Allen DG, Nichols CG, Smith GL. *Journal of Physiology* 1988; **406**: 359–70, with permission from Wiley-Blackwell.)

Figure 6.6 Contractile tension developed by chemically permeabilized rat ventricular muscle in response to bathing solution Ca^{2+} concentration, at two different resting sarcomere lengths. The Ca^{2+} concentration needed to generate a 50% maximum contraction, [Ca]$_{50\%}$, was reduced by stretch, i.e. Ca^{2+} sensitivity was increased by stretch (From Hibberd MG, Jewell BR. *Journal of Physiology* 1982; **329**: 527–40, with permission from Wiley-Blackwell.)

The cause of length-dependent Ca²⁺ sensitivity remains controversial

The mechanism underlying length-dependent Ca^{2+} sensitivity is still not fully established, but the **lattice spacing hypothesis** holds sway at present. In a myocyte of fixed volume, any increase in length is associated with a fall in diameter. This reduces the side-to-side separation of the actin and myosin filaments, which may allow crossbridges to form more readily. In support of this hypothesis, reducing the myocyte diameter by immersing it in a hyperosmotic solution increases its contractile force. The magnitude of this effect, however, may be too small to explain fully the physiological Ca^{2+} sensitization. We have to conclude that the mechanism is still not fully understood.

Having defined the properties of isolated cardiac muscle, we can now turn to the intact organ, and consider how stretch affects ventricular performance.

6.4 The Frank–Starling law of the heart

The isovolumetric contracting heart; Frank's experiment

The isometric length–tension relation of Figure 6.5 operates in intact hearts too, as shown by the German physiologist Otto Frank in 1895. Frank ligated the aorta of a frog heart, so that each contraction was purely isovolumetric, similar to an isometric contraction. When the ventricle wall was stretched in diastole, by increasing the diastolic fluid volume (preload), a greater pressure was generated by the systolic contractions (Figure 6.7a).

Therefore, **the energy of contraction of the intact heart increases as a function of diastolic distension** (Figure 6.7b, red curve). We will see later that this isovolumetric contraction curve sets an upper limit to ventricular pressure–volume loops (Section 6.5).

The ejecting heart; Starling's experiment

A more physiological situation, namely ventricular ejection, was studied by Ernest Starling and his co-workers in London in the early twentieth century. In their classic experiment the isolated heart and lungs of a dog were perfused with warm oxygenated blood from a venous reservoir (Figure 6.8). The height of the reservoir controlled the central venous pressure (CVP). CVP is the pressure at the entrance to the right atrium, and it is important because it determines the right ventricular end-diastolic pressure (RVEDP) and hence the stretch of the resting chambers. In other words, **the CVP determines the preload experienced by right ventricular muscle**. Similarly, pulmonary vein pressure governs left ventricle end-diastolic pressure and preload. A useful term encompassing these various pressures is **filling pressure**.

Since aortic pressure influences afterload, Starling kept it constant by means of a variable resistance. The combined stroke volume of the two ventricles was recorded by a bell cardiometer. Being isolated and denervated, the heart–lung preparation was free from any extrinsic nervous or hormonal influences, so any response was a property of the heart itself. The chief findings were as follows.

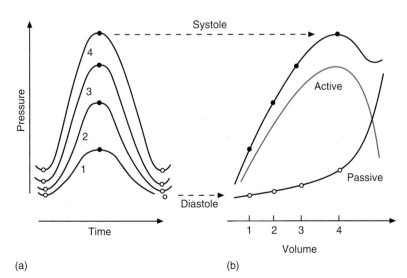

(a)

(b)

Figure 6.7 Pressure generated by isovolumetric contraction frog ventricle (aorta ligated), over a range of diastolic volumes. (a) The 'active' pressure generated between diastole (open circles) and systole (closed circles) increased as ventricular volume was raised from 1 to 4 (arbitrary units). (b) Effect of volume on pressure. Bottom curve is the passive compliance curve, showing effect of volume on diastolic pressure of relaxed ventricle. Note the increasing stiffness (upswing) as the ventricle is distended. Top curve shows corresponding systolic pressures. Red curve shows pressure generated actively, i.e. systolic pressure minus diastolic pressure. (After Otto Frank's seminal experiment of 1895.)

Figure 6.8 Starling's isolated dog heart–lung preparation. The height of the venous reservoir and the screw-clamp control central venous pressure (CVP). CVP and arterial pressure (AP) were measured by the manometers. AP was held constant by a variable resistance equal to total peripheral resistance (TPR). Ventricular volume was measured by a Henderson bell cardiometer – an inverted glass bell attached to the atrioventricular groove by a rubber diaphragm. Beat-by-beat volume changes were recorded on a rotating smoked drum. (After Knowlton FP, Starling EH. *Journal of Physiology* 1912; **44**: 206–19.)

Raising central venous pressure increases stroke volume

When CVP is raised, the RVEDP and ventricular volume increase. This stretches the right ventricle fibres. As a result, the ventricle develops a greater contractile energy and ejects a greater stroke volume. The left ventricle quickly follows suit, because the increased right ventricular output raises the pressure in the pulmonary circulation. This increases the filling pressure and distension of the left ventricle, raising contractile energy in the left heart. Thus a rise in CVP increases the output of both ventricles (Figure 6.9).

The human ventricular function curve reaches a plateau

A plot of stroke volume versus filling pressure is called a ventricular function curve or Starling curve (Figure 6.10). At filling pressures between zero (atmospheric) and 10 mmHg the stroke volume increases as a curvilinear function of pressure. This is called the **ascending limb**. Above 10 mmHg, the human ventricle reaches a **plateau** (Figure 6.10b). To put this into an everyday context, a standing or sitting human has a left ventricular end–diastolic pressure (LVEDP) of 4–5 mmHg, and is thus on the ascending limb of the Starling curve. A supine human has a higher LVEDP, 8–9 mmHg, due to the redistribution of blood from the lower body, and the heart is close to the plateau of the Starling curve.

In the isolated dog hearts studied by Starling, the stroke volume declined when the CVP was raised

Figure 6.9 Beat-by-beat recording of ventricular volume in the isolated heart–lung preparation. Note the inverted volume scale (ml): diastolic volume is at the bottom, systolic volume at the top. Stroke volume is top-to-bottom distance. Raising central venous pressure (VP) from 9 cmH$_2$O (period A) to 15 cmH$_2$O (period B) distends the ventricles in both diastole and systole, and increases stroke volume by 64%. The later, modest reduction in ventricular distension with no fall in stroke volume indicates a small rise in contractility (the Anrep effect). (From the original smoked-drum recordings of Patterson SW, Piper H, Starling EH. *Journal of Physiology* 1914; **48**: 465–511, by permission.)

above 25 mmHg. This produced a **descending limb** on the ventricular function curve (Figure 6.10a). It is unlikely, however, that human hearts ever reach such extreme filling pressures. The stroke volume declines

(a)

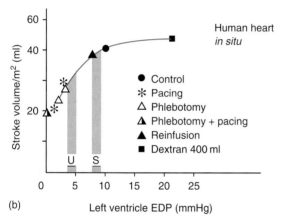

(b)

Figure 6.10 Ventricular function curves of dog (a) and human (b). (a) Effect of filling pressure on stroke volume of isolated dog heart pumping against a constant arterial pressure. Solid line shows Starling's results for effect of left atrial pressure on left ventricular (LV) stroke volume. Dashed line shows effect of central venous pressure on right ventricular (RV) stroke volume. (b) Human ventricular function curve. LV end-diastolic pressure (LVEDP) was varied *in vivo* by phlebotomy (venous bleeding) and other manoeuvres. Stroke volume is expressed per unit body surface area (stroke index). Grey bands mark normal human LVEDP when supine (S) and upright (U). Human stroke volume reaches a plateau at filling pressures above ~10 mmHg. (After Parker JD, Case RB. *Circulation* 1979; **60**: 4–12, by permission.)

in over-distended hearts for two reasons. One is that the atrioventricular valves begin to leak. The other is that the reduced curvature of the wall impairs the conversion of wall tension into blood pressure (Laplace's law, see later).

Ventricular function curves appear in a bewildering variety of guises. Any plot whose ordinate (y-axis) is a measure of contractile energy and whose abscissa (x-axis) is an index of resting fibre

length is called a ventricular function curve. The abscissa is often CVP, because human CVP is easily measured through a catheter; but other indices include RVEDP, LVEDP and echocardiograph ventricle diameter. For the ordinate, stroke volume is a reasonable index of contractile energy if mean arterial pressure is constant, as in Starling's heart–lung preparation. However, it obviously takes more energy to raise a given stroke volume to a high pressure than a low pressure; so stroke volume × mean arterial pressure, or **stroke work**, is a better measure of contractile energy (Section 6.5).

The 'law of the heart'

The results in Figure 6.10 prove that **the greater the stretch of the ventricle in diastole, the greater the stroke work achieved in systole**. As Patterson, Piper and Starling concluded in 1914, 'The energy of contraction of a cardiac muscle fibre, like that of a skeletal muscle fibre, is proportional to the initial fibre length at rest'. This statement is now honoured as **Starling's law of the heart**, or the **Frank–Starling mechanism** – though, as so often in science, Starling's definitive studies actually built on evidence from many previous workers, including that of the great German physiologist Ludwig in 1856. The physiological and pathophysiological roles of Starling's law in humans are described in Section 6.7. But first we need to consider the concept of stroke work a little more fully.

6.5 Stroke work and the pressure–volume loop

Stroke work depends on stroke volume and arterial pressure

The energy expended by the myocardium in systole is converted partly into heat and partly into useful mechanical work. The latter takes the form of an increase in the pressure and volume of blood in the arteries. To calculate how much useful work is achieved, we must first define work and pressure. Work (W) is force (F) times distance moved (L): $W = F \times L$. For example, 1 joule of work is 1 newton of force moved 1 metre. Pressure (P) is force per unit area (A): $P = F / A$. From the latter definitions, we see that the active force F exerted by a contracting ventricle equals the rise in pressure ΔP times the wall area A. If the wall then contracts over a distance L, the volume ΔV displaced into the aorta is $L \times A$, as illustrated by the top manikin in

Figure 6.11. So, applying our definition of work, the work per stroke W is given by:

$$W = F \times L = \Delta P \times A \times L$$
$$= \Delta P \times \Delta V$$

In other words, the stroke work equals the systolic increase in ventricular blood pressure multiplied by the stroke volume.

Stroke work is the area inside the pressure–volume loop

The ventricle pressure–volume loop, introduced in Section 2.2, is a useful, graphical way of depicting stroke work, which we will use later to illustrate changes in cardiac performance. Each side of the roughly rectangular loop represents one phase of the cardiac cycle, and each corner represents the opening or closing of a valve (Figure 2.5). The width of the loop is the stroke volume and its height is the systolic increase in pressure. Since stroke work is stroke volume $\times$ pressure increase, **stroke work equals the area inside the ventricular pressure–volume loop** (Figure 6.11). During the isovolumetric contraction phase B–C the ventricle is 'working' in the everyday sense (it is consuming O_2 and generating force) but no blood is entering the aorta, so the ventricle is accomplishing no external work. This phase is like a man trying to push over a house; he consumes a lot of O_2, but achieves no external work! At point C the aortic valve opens, because diastolic arterial pressure has been reached. The ejection phase C–D is loosely equivalent to an isotonic contraction, or more strictly an auxotonic contraction, and this is the phase during which mechanical work is accomplished.

The pressure–volume loop is confined inside active and passive boundary curves

The loop is constrained by two boundaries (Figure 6.11b). The lower boundary is the **passive compliance curve** of the ventricle, which shows the end-diastolic pressure at increasing end-diastolic volumes. Every contraction starts from this line. This 'compliance curve' is not linear, because the ventricle is relatively stretchy (compliant) at low pressures and stiff at high pressures – rather like a bicycle tyre. Thus changes in CVP in the physiological range, 0–10 mmHg, evoke bigger changes in filling than do changes above ~10 mmHg.

The upper boundary is set by the **isovolumetric pressure relation**, i.e. the systolic pressure that would be generated if ejection were prevented,

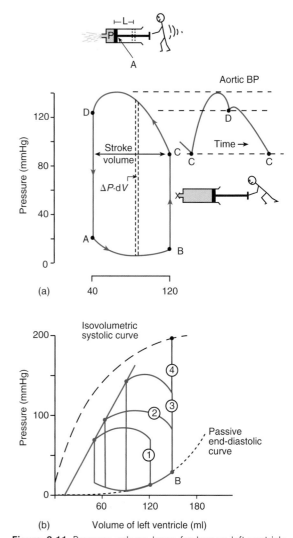

Figure 6.11 Pressure–volume loops for human left ventricle. (a) Relation to aortic pressure wave. A, mitral valve opens; AB, filling phase; B, mitral valve closes at onset of systole; BC, isovolumetric contraction; C, aortic valve opens; CD, ejection phase; D, aortic valve closes; DA, isovolumetric relaxation. Stroke work is sum of all $\Delta P \cdot dV$ strips inside the loop, i.e. total loop area. Sketches illustrate high energy expenditure and O_2 consumption by the myocardial manikin during isovolumetric contraction, achieving no external work, followed by lower energy cost of ejection. The subject is probably middle aged/elderly, since aortic pressure was 130/85 mmHg. (b) Set of pressure–volume loops for a constant contractility. Lower boundary is passive pressure–volume curve of relaxed ventricle (compliance curve). Upper boundary is systolic pressure of a purely isovolumetric contraction at increasing end-diastolic volumes (Frank–Starling mechanism). Loop 1 is basal. Raising end-diastolic volume to B increases stroke volume (loop 2), due to Starling's law. Note that end-systolic volume increases too. Raising peripheral resistance increases arterial pressure but reduces stroke volume (loop 3), due to the 'pump function' effect (Figure 6.15). A purely isovolumetric contraction (loop 4) reaches the upper boundary line. A line joining the end-systolic points is almost straight (diagonal red line). Its slope, the end-systolic elastance, is an index of contractility. (Based in part on Burkhoff D, Mirsky I, Suga H *American Journal of Physiology* 2005; **289**: H501–12.)

as in Frank's experiment (Figure 6.7). This curve has an ascending limb and plateau, due to the Frank–Starling mechanism; the greater the end-diastolic volume, the greater the contractile energy, and hence the greater the isovolumetric pressure generation. In an ejecting heart the systolic pressure never reaches the isovolumetric boundary curve, because some of the contractile energy is used to eject the blood.

Figure 6.11b illustrates how preload and after-load alter the loop within its boundaries. Loop 1 represents a human left ventricle ejecting a stroke volume of 70 ml at a low pressure. Loop 2 shows the effect of increasing the **preload**. The end-diastolic volume and pressure have been raised, e.g. by lying down, so corner B has moved up the passive compliance curve (lower boundary). The increased stretch raises the contractile energy via the Frank–Starling mechanism, so the stroke volume and loop area (stroke work) increase. Note that the Frank–Starling mechanism involves the ventricle getting bigger both at end-diastole (side BC) and at end-systole (side DA).

Loop 3 shows the deleterious effect of increasing the **afterload**, e.g. by raising arterial blood pressure with a vasoconstrictor drug. In our example, loop 3 starts from the same end-diastolic stretch as loop 2; but more energy is consumed in raising the ventricle pressure to a high enough level to open the aortic valve, leaving less energy available for ejection. As a result the stroke volume declines. If ejection were prevented totally, as in line 4, the ventricle would generate maximum systolic pressure and touch the upper boundary; but stroke volume and useful work would be zero, so the loop has no width.

The top left corner of the loop shows the myocardium at the instant of greatest shortening, i.e. end-systole. When a set of pressure–volume loops is plotted as in Figure 6.11b, the end-systolic points fall on a nearly straight line, the **end-systolic pressure–volume relation**. The slope of this line, called the end-systolic elastance, has been used as a measure of ventricular **contractility** (Section 6.10). For example, adrenaline, which increases ventricular contractility, steepens the end-systolic pressure–volume line.

6.6 Central venous pressure and cardiac filling

Any event that changes the central venous pressure (CVP), such as a blood transfusion or a haemorrhage, changes the stroke volume via the Frank–Starling mechanism. The CVP depends partly on the total volume of blood in the circulation and partly on the distribution of blood between the central and peripheral veins. Volume distribution is affected by five main factors: gravity (posture), peripheral venous tone, the skeletal muscle pump, the pumping action of the heart and breathing pattern.

Low blood volume reduces filling pressure

About two-thirds of the entire blood volume is in the venous system (Figure 1.12). Consequently, a fall in blood volume (hypovolaemia), resulting from a **haemorrhage** or **dehydration**, lowers the CVP. This reduces the stroke volume via the Frank–Starling mechanism, and can cause hypotension in patients with severe hypovolaemia. Conversely, a blood transfusion raises CVP and thereby improves the stroke volume and arterial blood pressure after a haemorrhage.

Gravity: standing reduces CVP

In a standing human the drag of gravity redistributes ~500 ml of blood from the thorax into the veins of the lower limbs. This **venous pooling** reduces the CVP. As a result, human stroke volume is reduced in the standing or sitting position. Conversely, lying down redistributes venous blood from the lower body to the thorax, raising the CVP and stroke volume (Figure 6.10b).

Sympathetic nerves regulate peripheral venous tone

The veins of the skin, kidneys and splanchnic (gastrointestinal) system are innervated by sympathetic venoconstrictor fibres, and peripheral venoconstriction shifts blood into the central veins (Figures 14.5 and 14.14). The central nervous system can thus regulate cardiac filling pressure to some degree. Peripheral venoconstriction occurs during exercise, stress, deep respiration, haemorrhage and shock, and contributes significantly to the raised filling pressure of heart failure. Conversely, cutaneous venodilatation in a hot climate (for temperature regulation) coincidentally reduces CVP and stroke volume – hence the greater propensity of humans to dizziness and fainting in hot weather.

The venous muscle pump boosts CVP in exercise

During rhythmic exercise, skeletal muscle contraction repeatedly compresses the deep veins of the limbs. Since the limb veins have semilunar valves, the compression displaces the blood centrally

(Figure 8.26). This raises the CVP and stroke volume moderately during dynamic exercise. Conversely, soldiers standing at attention for long periods in hot weather have an inactive muscle pump, leading to an embarrassing tendency to faint on parade. The combination of gravitational venous pooling, heat-induced venodilatation and lack of muscle pump activity reduces the CVP and stroke volume, leading to cerebral hypoperfusion and fainting.

An increase in cardiac pumping reduces filling pressure

The heart is a pump; that is to say, it removes blood from the venous system and transfers it into the arterial system. It is easy to forget that pumping not only increases the volume and pressure of blood in the arterial system but also **reduces the volume and pressure of blood in the central veins** (Figure 6.12). Stimulation of the cardiac output, for example by the sympathetic system, speeds up the transfer of blood from the central veins to the arteries, so the central venous filling pressure and preload tend to fall, while the arterial pressure and afterload rise. Both changes have an adverse effect on the stroke volume unless compensatory changes are brought into play, as they often are (Section 6.13). Conversely, **if cardiac output is suddenly reduced by acute cardiac failure, e.g. a heart attack, the filling pressure rises**. This rise is exacerbated by a reflex sympathetic peripheral venoconstriction, as noted above.

Respiration and coughing affect cardiac extramural pressure and output

Ventricular filling in diastole depends not only on the internal blood pressure but also on the external pressure on the heart. The true filling pressure is the difference between the internal and external pressures, or **transmural pressure** (trans-, across; mural, wall). The external pressure on the heart is the subatmospheric intrathoracic pressure, namely $-5\,cmH_2O$ at end-expiration and $-10\,cmH_2O$ at end-inspiration. Since intrathoracic pressure becomes more negative during inspiration, and at the same time intra-abdominal pressure becomes more positive (due to the descent of the diaphragm), inspiration boosts the filling of the thoracic venae cavae and right ventricle (Figure 8.27, top). Consequently, **inspiration raises right ventricular stroke volume**. At the same time,

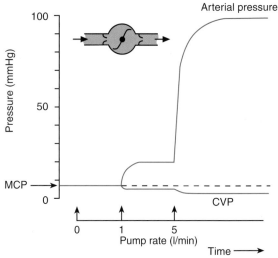

Figure 6.12 Effect of a pump on input and output pressure. At zero pumping rate, the central venous pressure (CVP) and arterial pressure equalize (mean circulatory pressure, MCP). When the pump starts, it removes fluid from the input line, so it reduces input pressure, CVP, as well as raising output pressure (arterial pressure). CVP changes less than arterial pressure, because venous compliance (volume accommodated per unit pressure change) is greater than arterial compliance. (Based in part on Berne RM, Levy MN. *Cardiovascular Physiology*. St Louis, MO: Mosby, 1997, with permission from Elsevier.)

however, the expansion of the lungs during inspiration increases the pulmonary blood pool, which temporarily reduces the return of blood to the left ventricle. So **inspiration reduces left ventricular stroke volume**. The reduction in left ventricular output is partly offset by sinus arrhythmia, the tachycardia associated with inspiration (Section 5.8); but left ventricular output nevertheless falls during inspiration. Expiration reverses these effects. As a result, breathing causes synchronous oscillations in arterial pressure, called **Traube–Hering waves**.

Coughing, and other forms of forced expiration, such as the Valsalva manoeuvre (Section 17.2), raises intrathoracic pressure to positive values; up to 400 mmHg has been recorded during coughing! This reduces or even reverses the ventricular transmural pressure in diastole. The resulting fall in ventricular filling and cardiac output contributes to the dizziness associated with a severe bout of coughing.

Disorders of the pericardium impair filling

Cardiac extramural pressure can also be raised by diseases of the pericardium, the fibrous, fluid-filled sac that encloses the heart. **Pericardial effusions** and **constrictive pericarditis** both raise the pressure around the heart. This impairs ventricular filling and can reduce the cardiac output severely, requiring surgical intervention.

6.7 Operation of Starling's law in humans

The single most important role of the Frank–Starling mechanism is to **balance the outputs of the right and left ventricles** (see below). It also contributes to the **increased stroke volume of exercise** (Section 17.3); mediates **postural hypotension** (fall in cardiac output and blood pressure on standing, Section 17.1); mediates **hypovolaemic hypotension** following a haemorrhage or dehydration (Section 18.2); and accounts for the **fall in stroke volume during forced expiration** (Valsalva manoeuvre, Section 17.2).

The Frank–Starling mechanism equalizes right and left ventricular outputs

It is essential that right ventricular output equals left ventricular output over any period longer than a few beats. Imagine a right ventricular output that is merely 1% greater than left ventricular output. The pulmonary blood volume, normally 0.6 litres, would increase with each heart beat and reach 2 litres within half an hour, causing catastrophic pulmonary congestion and oedema. In heavy exercise, with outputs around 25 l/min, catastrophic congestion would build up within minutes. Conversely, a sustained excess of left ventricular output would quickly drain the pulmonary vessels dry.

The Frank–Starling mechanism prevents such catastrophes by equalizing the two outputs. If right ventricular output begins to exceed left ventricular output, the increase in pulmonary blood volume raises the pressure in the pulmonary veins, which increases the filling of the left ventricle. By Starling's law this raises the left ventricular output until balance is restored. The opposite happens if left ventricular output transiently exceeds right output. The two outputs are thus automatically equalized in the long term.

Imbalances do occur, but they are transient. On standing up, the right output is less than left output for a few beats, due to venous pooling. Also, as noted above, the different effects of respiration on right and left outputs cause a regular, alternating imbalance, synchronous with the respiratory cycle.

CVP, not 'venous return', is the true regulator of stroke volume

Students (and some professionals!) sometimes get into an awful muddle by trying to explain the control of cardiac output in terms of 'venous return' rather than filling pressure. 'Venous return' is the flow of blood into the right atrium. When the circulation is in a steady state, the venous return equals the cardiac output, because the circulation is a closed system of tubes; any inequality can only be transient. Under steady-state conditions, the **venous return is simply the cardiac output observed in veins**, rather than arteries. The popular notion that venous return 'controls' the cardiac output is an unhelpful, literally circular viewpoint, because venous return **depends** on the cardiac output. Imagine a plot of cardiac output as a function of venous return; it would be a straight line of slope 1.0! By contrast, CVP is an **independent** variable; it can be adjusted independently of cardiac output, for example by changes in venoconstrictor tone or blood volume. CVP is thus an independent determinant of the stroke volume, unlike venous return.

The Guyton cross-plot highlights the role of CVP

The pivotal role of CVP is illustrated by an ingenious cross-plot devised by the American physiologist Arthur Guyton (Figure 6.13). The '**cardiac output curve**' on the Guyton plot represents the positive effect of CVP on stroke volume, via Starling's law. The other line, the '**venous return curve**', shows a negative effect of CVP on venous return, as defined by Darcy's law of hydraulics (Section 1.5). That is to say, a rise in CVP reduces the pressure gradient driving blood from the capillaries to the central veins, and thus tends to reduce venous flow. The venous return curve reaches zero at ~7 mmHg CVP, because 7 mmHg is the **mean circulatory pressure** – the pressure of blood when all flow has stopped in the circulation and pressures have equalized. In the steady state *in vivo*, **the cardiac output and venous return must be equal**, and this happens at only one point on the plot, namely where the two curves cross. The stable intersection occurs at a CVP that generates an identical cardiac output and venous return.

The Starling curve is depressed in heart failure

Guyton's cross-plot provides insights into many pathophysiological states, including cardiac failure

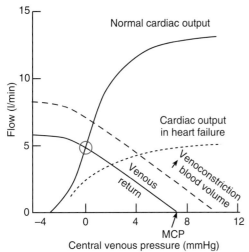

Figure 6.13 Guyton's graphical analysis of the circulation. The cardiac output curve reflects the increase in ventricular output as CVP increases (Starling's law). The 'venous return curve' shows the fall in blood flow from the capillaries into the central veins as CVP rises (Darcy's law of flow). At zero venous return (circulatory arrest), CVP equals the mean circulatory pressure, MCP. Cardiac output must equal venous return in the steady state, so where the two lines cross is the steady state (open circle). Heart failure depresses the output curve (reduced contractility, short dashes) but raises the venous return curve (long dashes), because MCP is increased by venoconstriction and increased plasma volume. The new steady state, where the dashed lines cross, occurs at a raised CVP but almost normal cardiac output. Hypovolaemia shifts the venous return curve downwards (not shown). Increased contractility (exercise) shifts the output curve upwards (not shown). (After Guyton AC, Jones CE, Coleman TG. *Circulatory Physiology: Cardiac Output and its Regulation.* Philadelphia, PA: WB Saunders, 1973, with permission from Elsevier.)

(Figure 6.13). In cardiac failure, the output curve (Starling curve) is depressed by a fall in contractility. At the same time, there is a rise in mean circulatory pressure, due to sympathetic peripheral venoconstriction and renal fluid retention. This displaces the venous return curve upwards. The new steady state for the failing heart occurs at the new intersection. The failing output is, surprisingly, only slightly below normal, because the CVP has increased. These are the characteristic features of moderate ventricular failure (Chapter 18).

6.8 Laplace's law and swollen hearts

Radius links wall tension and pressure

The radius of the ventricle determines how effectively the active wall tension raises blood pressure. This consideration is particularly important in failing hearts, which become very swollen and have an abnormally large radius. The degree of curvature of any hollow chamber (heart, football, soap-bubble) links the wall tension to the internal pressure, as pointed out by a French mathematician, the Marquis de Laplace, in 1806 – in a treatise on celestial mechanics! Laplace's law states that, for a hollow sphere, the internal pressure P is proportional to the wall tension T and is inversely proportional to the internal radius r:

$$P = \frac{2T}{r} \qquad (6.1)$$

(A simple proof for a cylinder appears in Figure 8.17. The factor '2' in the sphere formula results from the fact that a sphere has two planes of curvature, compared with one for a cylinder.) **Tension** is a force, equal to wall stress (S) times wall thickness (w). **Wall stress** is defined as force per unit cross-sectional area of wall, so Laplace's law can also be written as:

$$P = \frac{2Sw}{r} \qquad (6.2)$$

The involvement of radius is readily understood by considering the curvature of the wall (Figure 6.14). As radius increases, curvature decreases. Consequently, a smaller component of the wall tension is angled towards the cavity, generating less pressure. The curvature of the ventricle wall thus determines how effectively the active wall tension is converted into intraventricular pressure.

Laplace's law affects cardiac performance in several ways, as follows.

The Laplace effect facilitates late ejection

Wall stress equals the afterload against which the myocytes must shorten during ejection (Figure 6.2). Laplace's law tells us that the afterload S is not simply the ejection pressure (a common but loose assumption) but is ejection pressure $P \times$ radius/$2w$ (eqn 6.2). In other words, **afterload depends on chamber radius, as well as arterial pressure**. The bigger the radius, the bigger the afterload, for a given arterial pressure. Since the radius of the chamber falls as ejection proceeds, afterload falls too, facilitating the late phase of ejection; in other words, ejection gets easier as it proceeds. The decreasing chamber radius likewise contributes to the peaking of aortic pressure after ejection has been under way for a little while (Figure 2.4).

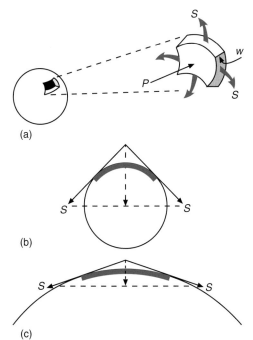

Ventricular 'preload' and 'afterload'

- Preload is the wall stress S (force applied to unit cross-sectional area) in resting myocardium. It can be adjusted *in vitro* by suspending a weight from a muscle strip.
- In the intact ventricle, the preload (diastolic wall stress) depends on the end-diastolic pressure P, chamber radius r and wall thickness w (Laplace's law); $S = Pr/2w$. The end-diastolic pressure itself is often referred to, inaccurately, as the preload.
- Afterload is the force per unit cross-sectional area (stress) that opposes the shortening of an isotonically contracting muscle strip. It can be adjusted *in vitro* by making a muscle pick up a weight as it begins to shorten.
- In the intact ventricle, the afterload (systolic wall stress) depends on arterial pressure, chamber radius and wall thickness (Laplace's law). Arterial pressure itself is often referred to, inaccurately, as the afterload.

Figure 6.14 Effect of curvature of a hollow sphere on the conversion of wall stress S into internal pressure P (Laplace's law). (a) Hollow sphere with an 'exploded' segment, showing the two circumferential wall stresses. Stress is force per unit cross-sectional area, of thickness w. The wall stress in the ejecting heart equals the afterload on the myocytes. (b) Cross section showing how the wall stresses (tangential arrows) give rise to an inwardly directed stress equal and opposite to the pressure. The thick red line represents a muscle segment exerting tension. Arrow length is proportional to stress magnitude. (c) Increasing the radius reduces the curvature, and therefore the inward component of the wall stress; so pressure falls (Laplace's law).

Ventricular distension has advantages and disadvantages

The Laplace effect and the Frank–Starling mechanism clearly have opposite effects on ventricular performance. Distension of the ventricle raises its force of contraction, due to Starling's law; but distension also reduces the pressure generated by a given contractile force, due to Laplace's law. Fortunately, in a healthy heart the gain in contractile energy resulting from moderate distension (Starling's law) greatly outweighs the fall in pressure-generating efficiency (Laplace's law). This is not so, however, in the grossly dilated, failing heart (Section 6.14 and below).

The dilated, failing heart operates at low mechanical efficiency

The failing heart is often grossly dilated (Figure 18.12), making the Laplace effect the dominant one. An increase in radius in an already swollen heart causes little to no increase in contractile force, because the ventricle is on the plateau of the Starling curve; but the increase in radius impairs the generation of systolic pressure and hence ejection (Laplace's law). **Reduction of cardiac distension is an important therapeutic goal in heart failure**, because it improves the conversion of contractile force into intraventricular pressure. Distension is usually reduced by lowering the cardiac filling pressure, using diuretics to reduce plasma volume.

Summary of Starling and Laplace laws in man

Few summaries of the operation of Starling's law in man could be more memorable than Professor Alan Burton's rhyme, 'What goes in, must come out':

The great Dr. Starling, in his Law of the Heart
Said the output was greater if, right at the start,
The cardiac fibres were stretched a bit more,
So their force of contraction would be more
   than before.
Thus the larger the volume in diastole,
The greater the output was likely to be.

If the right heart keeps pumping more blood
   than the left,
The lung circuit's congested; the systemic bereft.

Since no-one is healthy with pulmo-congestion,
The Law of Doc Starling's a splendid
   suggestion.
The balance of outputs is made automatic
And blood–volume partition becomes
   steady–static.

When Guardsmen stand still and blood pools in
   their feet
Frank–Starling mechanics no longer seem neat.
The shift in blood volume impairs C–V–P,
Which shortens the fibres in diastole.
Contractions grow weaker and stroke volume
   drops,
Depressing blood pressure; so down the Guard
   flops.

But when the heart reaches a much larger size,
This leads to heart failure, and often demise.
The relevant law is not Starling's, alas,
But the classical law of Lecompte de Laplace.
Your patient is dying in decompensation,
So reduce his blood volume or call his relation.

(From *Physiology and Biophysics of the Circulation*.
Chicago, IL: Year Book Medical Publishers, 1972,
by courtesy of the publishers. With apologies to
Alan Burton's spirit for the addition of verse 3.)

6.9 Multiple effects of arterial pressure on the heart

Arterial blood pressure affects cardiac output
through several, opposing mechanisms. Overall, a
high arterial pressure has an adverse effect, depressing the output in the short term and leading to ventricular hypertrophy and eventually cardiac failure
in the long term.

Increasing the afterload reduces stroke volume; the pump function curve

It will be recalled that the greater the afterload on a
strip of myocardium *in vitro*, the less it shortens
(Figure 6.2c). In the intact heart the afterload is
often increased by a rise in arterial pressure and this
reduces shortening during systole. Thus **a rise in
arterial blood pressure impairs stroke volume**,
as in Figure 6.11b, loop 3. **Pulmonary embolism**
provides a clinically important example. If a large
venous thrombus becomes detached, often from a
deep leg vein, it is swept along (embolizes) through
the right heart and into the pulmonary arterial tree,
where it jams in a branch. This raises pulmonary

vascular resistance, pulmonary arterial pressure and
right ventricular afterload. The increased afterload
causes a sharp fall in right ventricular output and
the patient may collapse.

The deleterious effect of arterial pressure on
stroke volume is shown graphically by the **pump
function curve** (Figure 6.15). For any pump operating at a fixed power, be it the heart or a laboratory
roller pump, the maximum stroke volume occurs at
zero outflow pressure. As the pressure opposing outflow is raised, the stroke volume declines (point W
to point 1, Figure 6.15). Maximum pressure is generated at zero stroke volume, as in loop 4 of Figure
6.11b. If the energy of the pump is increased, for
example through the Frank–Starling mechanism,
the pump function curve is shifted upwards (e.g.
from point 1 to point 2, Figure 6.15). If the contractile energy is reduced by heart failure, the pump
function curve is shifted downwards (point W to
point 3).

Since the resistance of the peripheral circulation
is a major determinant of mean arterial pressure, it
also affects stroke volume. This is put to practical use

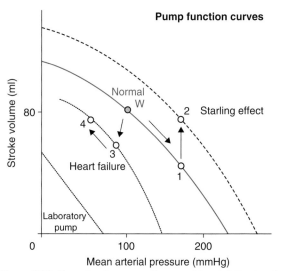

Figure 6.15 Pump function curves for normal heart, failing heart
and laboratory roller pump. W, normal work point. Raising the
peripheral resistance raises pressure but depresses stroke volume
(point 1), if end-diastolic volume is held constant (as in loop 3,
Figure 6.11). Ventricular distension can restore the stroke volume
by shifting the pump function curve to a higher energy level
(point 2) – the Frank–Starling mechanism. Impaired contractility
(heart failure) shifts the curve to a lower energy level (point 3). The
stroke volume of a failing heart can be improved by pressure-reducing
drugs (point 4). (Based on concepts from Elzinga G, Westerhof N.
Circulation Research 1979; **32**: 178–86; and Nichols WW,
O'Rourke MF. *McDonald's Blood Flow in Arteries*, 5th edn. London:
Arnold, 2005.)

in the treatment of heart failure; **the stroke volume of a failing heart can be improved by lowering the peripheral resistance**, using vasodilator drugs. The fall in peripheral resistance reduces arterial pressure, which reduces ventricular afterload and enhances stroke volume (as in point 4, Figure 6.15, or loop 3 to loop 2, Figure 6.11b).

A raised arterial pressure evokes conflicting secondary effects

1 **Compensation through the Frank–Starling mechanism**. If arterial pressure is raised acutely, ejection is at first reduced, as above (point 1, Figure 6.15). Then, as returning blood begins to accumulate in the left ventricle, the end-diastolic volume expands over a few beats (Figure 6.16). This raises the contractile energy of the ventricle through the Frank–Starling mechanism. As a result the pump function curve is shifted to a higher level and the stroke volume improves, though at the expense of cardiac dilatation (point 2, Figure 6.15).

2 **Compensation through the Anrep response**. Over the next 5–10 min there is a further adaptation (Figure 6.16). The contractility of the ventricle increases, and this enables the ventricle to maintain the stroke volume from a lower, near-normal end-diastolic volume. This is called the Anrep response, and it is equivalent to the **slow force response** in isolated myocardium (Figure 6.4). It arises from at least three mechanisms. (i) Inotropic (strengthening) agents are produced within the myocardium, namely myocardial angiotensin II and endothelin 1. These act in an autocrine/paracrine fashion to increase the myocyte Ca^{2+} store and Ca^{2+} transient. (ii) Activation of the Na^+–H^+ exchanger raises the intracellular Na^+, which slows the expulsion of Ca^{2+} by the Na^+–Ca^{2+} exchanger. (iii) Stretch-activated channels increase the entry of extracellular Ca^{2+}, boosting the Ca^{2+} store.

3 **Depression of output by the baroreflex**. In an intact animal, as opposed to an isolated heart, an acute rise in arterial pressure also triggers a neurophysiological reflex, the baroreceptor reflex (Chapter 16). This reduces cardiac sympathetic nerve activity, which reduces ventricular contractility, stroke volume and heart rate in order to return the arterial pressure to normal (Figure 6.17).

The **overall effect** of an acute rise in arterial pressure on stroke volume thus depends on the interplay between two negative influences (increased afterload and the baroreflex) and two compensatory changes (the Starling and Anrep effects) (see Figure 6.17). In general, the depressor influences predominate, i.e. a high vascular resistance usually depresses the stroke volume, as in the case of pulmonary embolism described earlier.

Chronic hypertension causes concentric ventricular hypertrophy

In patients with clinical hypertension, the long-standing (chronic) elevation of the arterial pressure has additional, slow effects on the heart. The left ventricle gradually undergoes concentric hypertrophy; that is to say, the wall grows thicker without any increase in chamber size. This contrasts with the response in endurance-trained athletes, where chamber size increases. The hypertrophy is driven by local growth factors, such as angiotensin II and endothelin. These trigger a kinase pathway, the MAP kinase cascade, that activates nuclear transcription factors, which in turn activate hypertrophy genes. Hypertrophy helps the ventricle cope with the persistent, high afterload, at least for a while. In the long term, however, the overloaded ventricle often goes into failure. This is one of several reasons why clinical hypertension should always be treated, despite being asymptomatic.

Figure 6.16 Three effects of raising peripheral resistance and arterial pressure (middle trace, *B.P.*) on stroke volume (excursion of upper trace) and ventricular end-diastolic volume (EDV, lower border of upper trace), in the Starling heart–lung preparation. Volume record is inverted as in Figure 6.9; time scale same. White arrowhead marks immediate reduction in stroke volume on raising arterial pressure, due to the **pump function relation**. As returning blood accumulates in the heart, venous pressure (*V.P.*) and EDV increase, restoring stroke volume (**length–tension or Frank–Starling relation**). Thereafter, around *C*, contractility increases gradually, as shown by a fall in EDV with no reduction in stroke volume (the **Anrep effect**). (From Patterson SW, Piper H, Starling EH. *Journal of Physiology* 1914; **48**: 465–511, by permission.)

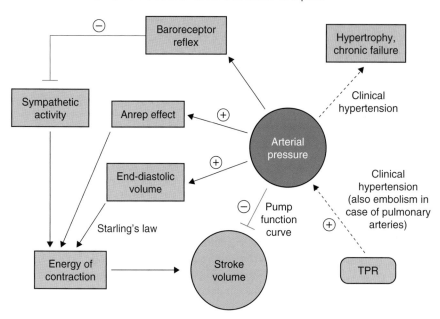

Figure 6.17 An acute rise in arterial pressure, resulting from a rise in total peripheral resistance (TPR), affects stroke volume through two negative and two positive mechanisms. TPR may be increased acutely by sympathetic vasomotor activity, or chronically by clinical hypertension. Chronic hypertension introduces additional factors: ventricular hypertrophy and eventual failure. On the right side, pulmonary resistance may be increased acutely by pulmonary embolism, raising pulmonary arterial pressure.

6.10 Sympathetic regulation of contractility

The meaning of contractility

Up to this point the chapter has focused on changes in contractile energy brought about by changes in resting fibre length (intrinsic regulation). Contractile energy is also regulated, however, by neurohumoral factors (extrinsic regulation). **A change in contractile energy that is caused by neurohumoral factors, not altered fibre length, is called a change in contractility**. The term 'contractility' thus specifically excludes changes brought about by the Frank–Starling mechanism. The most important inotropic (strengthening), neurohumoral agent, physiologically, is the sympathetic neurotransmitter noradrenaline. Other inotropic agents include circulating adrenaline, angiotensin II, extracellular Ca^{2+} ions, inotropic drugs and reduced beat interval.

Sympathetic stimulation produces a stronger, briefer beat

Cardiac sympathetic nerve activity increases during exercise, orthostasis (standing up), stress and haemorrhage. The left cardiac sympathetic fibres innervate the atrial and ventricular myocardium, and the right fibres innervate the pacemaker–conduction system (Figure 4.5). The sympathetic terminal varicosities release noradrenaline, which activates

Contractility

- Contractility is the force of contraction achieved from a given initial fibre length.
- Contractile force can be increased either by increased contractility and/or by increasing the resting fibre length through end-diastolic stretch (the Frank–Starling mechanism).
- Positive inotropic agents are factors that increase contractility. They include the sympathetic neurotransmitter noradrenaline, circulating adrenaline, β_1-agonist drugs, phosphodiesterase inhibitors, digoxin and reduced beat interval.
- Negative inotropes include acute myocardial ischaemia (acting through intracellular acidosis), chronic cardiac failure, anaesthetics, parasympathetic fibre activity (a minor effect), β_1-receptor antagonists and Ca^{2+} channel blockers.

myocyte β_1-adrenoceptors. The receptors activate the G_s–α_s–adenylate cyclase–cAMP–protein kinase A– phosphorylation cascade shown in Figure 4.9. The ensuing rise in extracellular Ca^{2+} current, i_{Ca}, increases the sarcoplasmic reticulum (SR) Ca^{2+} store and also boosts the amount of trigger Ca^{2+} at the start of each contraction. As a result, the magnitude of the **cytosolic free Ca^{2+} transient increases**, causing more crossbridge formation and force development (Figure 4.8). At the same time the Ca^{2+} uptake pumps of the SR are stimulated

Figure 6.18 Effect of sympathetic stimulation or noradrenaline on cardiac performance. (a) Left ventricular pressure climbs faster (dP/dt_{max}), systolic pressure increases, systole shortens, relaxation is quicker and end-diastolic pressure (EDP) falls. (b) Combined stroke volume recorded by a cardiometer at a constant, paced heart rate. The left cardiac sympathetic nerves were stimulated continuously from point A. The increased ejection fraction reduced right atrial pressure and ventricular volumes. However, the Frank–Starling mechanism, operating at reduced end-diastolic volume, attenuated the increase in stroke volume. The enhanced contractility is evident from the fact that stroke volume increased slightly despite the much reduced end-diastolic volume. At B the filling pressure was artificially restored to its previous level, allowing the effect of contractility on stroke volume to emerge fully. Vertical bar represents size of control stroke volume. (Adapted from Linden RJ. *Anaesthesia* 1968; **23**: 566–84, with permission from Wiley-Blackwell.)

through the phosphorylation of phospholamban, and the increased rate of removal of sarcoplasmic Ca^{2+} by the pumps **shortens the Ca^{2+} transient** and hence the duration of systole. Sympathetic stimulation thus causes a shorter, more forceful contraction of the individual myocytes, with the following effects on ventricular performance (additional to **tachycardia**, Figure 4.6):

- **Ventricular pressure** climbs more rapidly in systole and reaches a higher level, because the elastic arteries receive an increased volume of blood in a shorter time (Figure 6.18a). The maximum rate of pressure increase, dP/dt_{max}, has been used as an index of contractility, although it is also increased by the Frank–Starling mechanism (Figures 6.2b and 6.7).
- **Ejection fraction** rises above two-thirds, which is the resting fraction. This is a popular clinical measure of contractility, because it is readily estimated by echocardiography.
- **Diastolic volume** falls, because the ejection fraction has increased. Note that a rise in contractility makes the ventricle **smaller in both diastole and systole** (Figure 6.18b), whereas the Frank–Starling mechanism makes the ventricle bigger in both diastole and systole.
- **Stroke volume** increases. In an isolated preparation the increase is attenuated by the concomitant fall in end-diastolic volume (which

reduces the Frank–Starling effect) and increase in arterial pressure (the afterload effect). The full increase in stroke volume is only achieved when these adverse changes are prevented or minimized by reflex changes in the peripheral circulation, as happens in intact animals. During exercise, for example, peripheral vascular adjustments minimize the fall in end-diastolic volume and rise in arterial pressure, thus allowing an optimal increase in stroke volume.

- The **duration of systole** shortens (Figure 6.18a). This prevents excessive shortening of the diastolic filling time as the heart rate increases. Increased contraction velocity enables the stroke volume to be ejected during the shortened systole.

The net effect of sympathetic nerve stimulation, therefore, is to increase the arterial pressure, stroke volume, ejection fraction and heart rate, and to reduce the ejection time, end-diastolic pressure and ventricle size.

Graded sympathetic activity generates a family of ventricular function curves

Since sympathetic stimulation increases the contractile energy produced at a given end-diastolic volume, it shifts the entire Starling curve upwards

Figure 6.19 Family of ventricular function curves (Starling curves) generated by graded sympathetic stimulation of dog heart. Sympathetic activity in range $0-4 \, s^{-1}$ increased contractility in a graded fashion. Arrows to red points show how enhanced contractility reduces filling pressure, as well as raising stroke volume. (From Sarnoff SJ, Mitchell JH. *Handbook of Physiology Cardiovascular System*, Vol. 1. Baltimore, MD: American Physiological Society, 1962: 489–532, by permission.)

(Figure 6.19). Sarnoff showed in the 1960s that the shift is graded and proportional to the level of sympathetic activity. The heart therefore operates not on a single Starling curve but on an entire family of curves. Stroke volume can be altered by moving along a curve (i.e. by changing contractile energy through the Frank–Starling mechanism) or by moving from one curve to a higher or lower one (i.e. by changing the contractility). A combination of both changes is common *in vivo*. For example, during upright exercise increased filling pressure shifts the ventricles along a Starling curve, and increased ventricular contractility shifts the curve upwards.

Sympathetic stimulation widens the pressure–volume loop and shifts it leftwards

Sympathetic stimulation raises the upper limit of the pressure–volume loop, i.e. the isovolumetric systolic pressure line. Peak pressure (loop height), stroke volume (loop width) and stroke work (loop area) all increase, within the confines of the raised boundary (Figure 6.20a, loop 2). Cardiac sympathetic stimulation alone also shifts the loop to the left, because it reduces end-diastolic volume (unless compensatory mechanisms are brought into play); so the Frank–Starling mechanism attenuates the increase in stroke volume. In an intact animal, however, the end-diastolic volume is prevented from

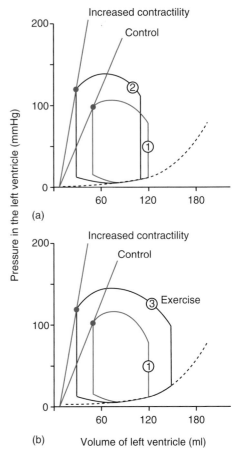

Figure 6.20 Effect of increased left ventricular contractility on human pressure–volume loop. The slope of the straight line through each end-systolic point, the end-systolic elastance, is an index of contractility, as in Figure 6.11b. (a) Loop 1 is basal state. Loop 2 shows effect of increased contractility *per se*. Ejection fraction is increased, so end-diastolic volume falls. Loop area (stroke work) is increased. (b) During exercise (loop 3), contractility is raised by sympathetic activity and in addition end-diastolic volume is raised by peripheral venoconstriction and the skeletal muscle pump. The increase in stroke volume is now greater.

falling, or even raised, by peripheral venoconstriction and the muscle pump, e.g. during upright exercise. Consequently, the loop widens in both directions, resulting in a bigger increase in stroke volume and stroke work (Figure 6.20b, loop 3).

6.11 Other positive inotropic influences

Adrenaline and other β-agonists

The human adrenal medulla secretes adrenaline and noradrenaline in the ratio of approximately 4:1. Adrenaline activates cardiac β_1-adrenoceptors and therefore has the same direct effects on the heart as noradrenaline. The plasma concentrations of both substances increase ~20 times in maximal exercise. Even so, the cardiac response to exercise is normally dominated by the powerful cardiac sympathetic nerves.

β-agonist drugs, such as **isoprenaline, dopamine** (a precursor of adrenaline) and the synthetic analogue **dobutamine**, have similar inotropic and chronotropic effects. β-agonists can be used to support an acutely failing heart for a short period.

Broad-spectrum phosphodiesterase inhibitors, such as **caffeine** and **theophylline**, and selective phosphodiesterase type III inhibitors such as **milrinone**, raise intracellular cAMP and thus mimic the effects of β-agonists (Figure 4.9). This action of caffeine probably accounts for the tendency of strong coffee to cause palpitations in some subjects.

Angiotensin II

The circulating concentration of the hormone angiotensin II increases during exercise and heart failure (Section 14.8). Much of its positive inotropic effect results from neuromodulation; angiotensin AT_1 receptors on central neurons and sympathetic ganglia increase sympathetic activity, while AT_1 receptors on sympathetic nerve terminals facilitate noradrenaline release (Figure 14.2). Angiotensin also acts directly on cardiac myocyte receptors to enhance i_{Ca}.

Other circulating inotropes

The hormones thyroxine (Section 14.5), insulin, glucagon and corticosteroids all have a long-term, positive inotropic effect. The inotropic drug **digoxin** inhibits the sarcolemmal Na^+–K^+ pump by ~25%, leading to a rise in intracellular Ca^{2+} (Section 3.7).

Beat interval influences on contractile force

The American physiologist Bowditch reported in 1871 that shortening the interval between the heartbeats causes a gradual increase in contractile force. If the frequency of electrical stimulation is suddenly raised, there is a single weaker beat, then the beats grow progressively stronger in a 'staircase' pattern, until a new steady state is reached. Conversely, if the beat interval is increased (reduced frequency), there is one stronger beat, then the contractions become weaker (Figure 6.21a). The Bowditch staircase effect, or interval–tension relation, occurs in amphibia and some mammals, including man; but it is blunted or even reversed in failing hearts.

Figure 6.21 Effect of beat interval on contractility. (a) Twitches of an isolated rat ventricular myocyte stimulated at 1, 0.2 and 2 beats/s. Intracellular Ca^{2+} was monitored by the fluorescent dye Fura-2. (b) In a patient with heart failure a premature systole (beat A) is feeble, and beat B after the compensatory pause is stronger than usual (**post-extrasystolic potentiation**). ((a) From Frampton JE, Orchard CH, Boyett MR. *Journal of Physiology* 1991; **437**: 351–75, by permission; (b) from Voss A, Baier V, Schumann A *et al. Journal of Physiology* 2002; **538**: 271–78, with permission from Wiley-Blackwell.)

The increase in contractility with heart rate is caused by an increase in the SR Ca^{2+} store, leading to bigger systolic Ca^{2+} transients (Figure 6.21a). The store is increased by (i) the reduced diastolic period for Ca^{2+} expulsion and (ii) a rise in intracellular $[Na^+]$, caused by the increased action potential frequency. The rise in intracellular Na^+ slows Ca^{2+} expulsion by the Na^+–Ca^{2+} exchanger. Although the Bowditch rate effect is an interesting phenomenon, it contributes only a little to the increased contractility of exercise. The latter is due chiefly to increased β_1-adrenoceptor activation.

After an interval reduction, the first beat is weaker rather than stronger, unlike all the subsequent beats. Similarly, a **premature ectopic beat** in a patient produces a weak beat, even when excitation follows the normal conduction pathway

(Figure 6.21b, beat A). The premature beat is weak because the SR Ca^{2+}-release channels recover relatively slowly from their inactivated state, so they are partially refractory during a premature beat.

After a premature ectopic beat there is a compensatory pause, and the next beat is stronger than normal (Figure 6.21b, beat B). This is called **post-extrasystolic potentiation**. The patient may feel the post-extrasystolic potentiation and complain 'My heart gives a jump, Doctor'. The increased filling time occasioned by the compensatory pause raises the end-diastolic volume and thus contributes to post-extrasystolic potentiation in a patient. However, post-extrasystolic potentiation also occurs in isolated myocardium, where it is attributed to the increased filling of the SR Ca^{2+} store during the prolonged beat interval.

6.12 Negative inotropism, ischaemia and arrhythmia

Negative inotropic influences are factors that reduce myocardial contractility. Aside from parasympathetic activity, negative inotropic effects are usually non-physiological, and often a component of cardiac disease. They include:

- parasympathetic (vagal) activity and cholinergic agonists;
- β-blocker drugs, such as propranolol, oxprenolol and atenolol (Section 4.8)
- calcium-channel blockers, such as verapamil (Section 4.8)
- hyperkalaemia (Section 4.7)
- barbiturates and many general anaesthetics
- acidosis and hypoxia, often the result of ischaemic heart disease
- chronic cardiac failure (Section 18.5).

Parasympathetic fibres have only a weak effect on ventricular contractility

Vagal parasympathetic fibres innervate the pacemaker–conduction system and atrial myocardium (Figure 4.5). They markedly reduce heart rate, but have relatively little effect on ventricular contractility. The human ventricles receive only a scanty parasympathetic innervation, and even maximal vagal stimulation reduces ventricular contraction by only 15–38%. Interestingly, there is a concomitant fall in noradrenaline in the coronary venous blood, because some parasympathetic fibres terminate close to sympathetic fibres and inhibit the sympathetic terminals. Conversely, sympathetic fibres release not only noradrenaline but also neuropeptide Y and galanin, which inhibit acetylcholine release from vagal fibres. In the SA node, this **cross-inhibition** facilitates an increase in heart rate.

Ischaemia impairs contractility and causes arrhythmia

Ischaemia is an inadequate tissue oxygenation, resulting usually from an inadequate blood flow. In the heart, atheromatous narrowing of one or more coronary arteries is usually responsible (Figure 15.6). The reduced blood supply causes local hypoxia, leading to anaerobic glycolysis and intracellular lactic acidosis (Section 6.14). These metabolic changes impair contractility and cardiac output, especially during exercise, so exercise capacity is reduced (Table 6.1). Cardiac ischaemia also causes chest pain (angina/heart attack), and can precipitate an arrhythmia. The ECG shows the characteristic changes illustrated in Figure 5.11. The multiple effects of ischaemia are described in a little more detail below, and are summarized in Figure 6.22.

Impaired contractility. The fall in mitochondrial oxidative metabolism leads to a fall in the creatine phosphate energy reserve, a rise in inorganic phosphate and ADP, and eventually a fall in ATP. Pyruvate oxidation is diverted into lactic acid formation, causing intracellular acidosis. **Acidosis has a strongly negative inotropic effect** (Figure 6.23), probably because H^+ ions compete with Ca^{2+} for the troponin C binding sites. The rise in inorganic phosphate likewise impairs contractility, though less strongly. A reduction in the open-state probability of SR Ca^{2+}-release channels further impairs contractility.

Arrhythmia. The ischaemic heart is prone to impaired electrical conduction and arrhythmia. These changes are the result of multiple mechanisms, as follows (Figure 6.22):

- Resting membrane potential decreases, because interstitial $[K^+]$ increases as the Na^+–K^+ ATPase runs down.
- Action potential size (phase 0) and duration (phase 2) are reduced. Phase 0 is impaired because the low resting membrane potential traps some of the Na^+ channels in the inactivated state (Figure 3.13, top right). Phase 2 duration is reduced by K_{ATP} channel activation (Figure 3.10).
- Connexon conductivity is reduced, impairing the electrical coupling between cells. Ventricular

Figure 6.22 Summary of the multiple mechanisms by which acute ischaemia impairs contractility and causes arrhythmia. Acute myocardial ischaemia is usually caused by coronary artery disease. For chronic heart failure, see Section 18.5.

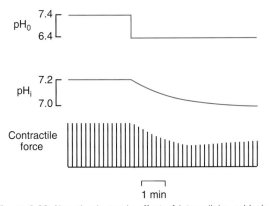

Figure 6.23 Negative inotropic effect of intracellular acidosis. Intracellular pH, pH_i, was changed by adding extracellular acid (pH_o). Reduction of pH_i by only 0.2 units halves the contractility. (Based on Hongo K, White E, Orchard CH. *Experimental Physiology* 1995; **80**: 701–12, with permission from Wiley-Blackwell; and Bountra C, Vaughan-Jones RD. *Journal of Physiology* 1989; **418**: 163–87, with permission from Wiley-Blackwell.)

fibrillation is especially likely to arise at moderate levels of uncoupling, because a mix of slow conduction and blocked conduction favours circus formation (Figure 5.10).

- Intracellular [Na^+] increases, because Na^+–K^+ ATPase activity declines and intracellular acidosis stimulates the Na^+–H^+ exchanger (Figure 3.14). The rise in [Na^+]$_i$ reduces the Na^+ gradient that drives Ca^{2+} expulsion by the Na^+–Ca^{2+} exchanger. Consequently, acidosis causes intracellular Ca^{2+} accumulation.
- The SR Ca^{2+} store becomes overloaded, partly for the above reason and partly because there is an increase in extracellular Ca^{2+} influx i_{Ca}, due to a reflex increase in sympathetic activity.

The overloaded Ca^{2+} store may discharge spontaneously in early diastole, stimulating the $3Na^+$–$1Ca^{2+}$ exchanger to generate an afterdepolarization, which may trigger an ectopic beat (Figure 3.16). Re-entry circuits may then develop, because the reduced action potential size and reduced connexon conductivity slow conduction, and the abnormalities are not uniformly distributed (Figure 5.10). Thus, an **ectopic** triggered by an **afterdepolarization** during the **vulnerable period** (late T wave, when some myocytes are repolarized and others not) can initiate a **re-entrant arrhythmia** such as fibrillation (Figure 5.4g).

The paradox of myocardial ischaemia–reperfusion injury

An adequate O_2 supply is essential for a healthy myocardium. Yet, paradoxically, the reperfusion of ischaemic myocardium with oxygenated blood increases the amount of cell damage. Two factors cause the damage. (1) Re-oxygenation enables the Na^+–K^+ ATPase pump to restore the Na^+ gradient, which drives the sarcolemmal Na^+–H^+ exchanger. The latter quickly corrects the intracellular acidosis and thereby restores contractility; but if the intracellular Ca^{2+} overload has not yet been corrected, the restored contractility results in a severe, sustained **contracture**. Contracture can damage the cytoskeleton, disrupt cell membranes and cause **necrosis** (cell death). (2) The myocytes are also damaged by the formation of toxic **oxygen-derived free radicals**, as described in Section 13.9. The oxygen-derived free radicals damage the sarcolemma, leading to arrhythmia.

The Na^+–H^+ exchange inhibitor, amiloride, greatly reduces reperfusion injury in experimental animals. It prolongs the duration of the intracellular acidosis and depressed contractility. This gives the myocyte sufficient time to restore its normal, low free Ca^{2+} concentration and avoid contracture.

Myocardial stunning and ischaemic preconditioning

If the coronary blood flow remains low after a coronary thrombosis, myocardial contractility remains low (**hibernation**). If the coronary flow is then restored, and the ischaemia was not too severe, there may be little cellular necrosis yet cardiac performance remains depressed for days. This is called **myocardial stunning**. 'Stunning' is decreased contractile function despite normal Ca^{2+} transients, normal energetic status and restored perfusion. It is caused by troponin I degradation, which reduces the thin filament responsiveness to Ca^{2+}.

In animal experiments, prior exposure to sublethal ischaemia has a protective effect, in that there is less cardiac damage during a second episode of ischaemia. This is called **ischaemic preconditioning**. The protection lasts up to 3 days. Ischaemic preconditioning is thought to be mediated by the release of certain chemicals (adenosine, nitric oxide and others) that activate intracellular kinase cascades (protein kinase C and others). These promote the transcription of cardioprotective genes (inducible nitric oxide synthase, cyclooxygenase 2 and others), which increases the production of the cardioprotective agents nitric oxide and prostaglandins.

6.13 Co-ordinated control of cardiac output

An uncoordinated stimulus is relatively ineffective

To achieve an effective regulation of cardiac output in humans, as opposed to isolated hearts, the cardiac changes must be co-ordinated with changes in the arterial and venous systems. It is illuminating to see how ineffective an uncoordinated change in a single cardiac factor can be. The relatively trivial change in stroke volume upon sympathetic stimulations of an isolated heart provides one example (Figure 6.18b). Another example is the relatively small increase in cardiac output when the pacing frequency is raised in a patient with an artificial pacemaker; there is remarkably little increase in cardiac output at paced rates above $100\,min^{-1}$, and output actually declines at high pacing rates, due to the reduced diastolic filling time. Thus, changes in a single cardiac variable are relatively ineffective. Co-ordinated, cooperative changes in both cardiac and vascular function are required for cardiac output to increase effectively. This is well illustrated by the response to exercise.

Exercise involves co-ordinated cardiac and vascular changes

Human cardiac output increases by ~6 l/min for every extra litre of O_2 consumed per minute. The increased output is brought about by increases in heart rate and stroke volume. Tachycardia is generally the major factor; the human heart rate increases in proportion to O_2 consumption, to a maximum 180–200 beats/min. Studies using echocardiography and aortic Doppler flowmetry show that the contribution of increased stroke volume depends on posture, exercise intensity and age. During upright exercise the stroke volume can increase by 50–100% (Table 6.2 and Figure 6.24). In the supine position, however, stroke volume is already high at rest, so it increases relatively less during exercise. The co-ordinated cardiac and peripheral changes that underlie the increase output are as follows.

1 Cardiac sympathetic stimulation and reduced vagal activity **raise the heart rate** and **shorten systole**. The **reduced diastolic filling interval** is offset by a sympathetic-mediated rise in **atrial contractility**, which enhances the atrial contribution to ventricular filling.

2 Cardiac sympathetic stimulation, and to a lesser degree circulating adrenaline, increase ventricular contractility. This **raises stroke volume** and ejection fraction, by **reducing end-systolic volume** (Figure 6.24).

3 Sympathetic vasomotor nerves cause **venoconstriction** in the splanchnic circulation, and the **skeletal muscle pump** compresses limb veins. The resulting transfer of blood into the central veins prevents the **CVP** from falling, which is otherwise an effect of increased cardiac pumping (Figure 6.12). The CVP can increase by a mmHg or so during exercise in the upright position, **raising end-diastolic volume** (Figure 6.24). As a result, the **Frank–Starling mechanism** contributes to the increase in stroke volume. This contribution is most marked during sudden, intense, upright exercise and in the elderly.

4 **Vasodilatation** in the exercising skeletal muscle reduces the peripheral vascular resistance, and thus prevents arterial pressure from rising excessively as the cardiac output increases. In this way, the stroke volume is not restrained by a big increase in afterload.

The increased cardiac output of exercise thus involves a co-ordinated interaction between changes within the heart (rate, contractility) and vascular changes that adjust the CVP (preload) and vascular resistance (afterload).

Transplanted and artificially paced hearts respond to exercise

Cardiac transplantation necessarily entails cutting the autonomic nerves to the heart (denervation). Rather surprisingly, exercise performance is only moderately impaired. Indeed, racing greyhounds with denervated hearts experienced only a 5% reduction in track speed (Figure 17.7). This is due to a **redundancy of cardiac control**

Table 6.2 Typical cardiac response to upright exercise in a non-athlete

	Rest	Hard exercise[a]
Oxygen consumption (l/min)	0.25	3.0
Cardiac output (l/min)	4.8	21.6
Heart rate (beats/min)	60.0	180.0
Stroke volume (ml)	80.0	120.0
End-diastolic volume (ml)	120.0	140.0
End-systolic residual volume (ml)	40.0	20.0
Ejection fraction	0.67	0.86
Cycle time (s)	1.0	0.33
Duration of systole (s)	0.35	0.2
Duration of diastole (s)	0.65	0.13

[a]Exercise intensity; ~85% of maximum increase in heart rate.
After Rerych SK, Scholz PM, Newman GE *et al. Annals of Surgery* 1978; **187**: 449–58.

mechanisms. Although the denervated heart does not show the usual, immediate tachycardia at the start of exercise, the stroke volume increases rapidly, because the CVP increases (effect of leg muscle pump), raising preload; and the arterial pressure dips (effect of muscle resistance vessel dilatation), reducing afterload. Moreover, the heart rate and contractility increase over the next 1–2 min, due to increases in circulating adrenaline and angiotensin II. Greyhound track performance only deteriorates substantially if the heart is denervated and the adrenergic back-up is blocked by a β-antagonist (Figure 17.7).

Like the denervated greyhound, a patient with a transplanted heart or artificial pacemaker benefits from the redundancy of cardiac control systems. Even at a fixed pacing rate, exercise increases the stroke volume, due to the skeletal muscle pump, peripheral vasodilatation and adrenaline-enhanced contractility. This may not make for Olympic records, but it enables thousands of people to walk in the park, do the shopping and generally lead a full life.

6.14 Cardiac energetics and metabolism

Ventricular systole adds potential energy and kinetic energy to arterial blood

Part of the energy expended in ventricular systole is 'useful', in the sense that it accomplishes mechanical work on the arterial system; the rest is dissipated as heat. The useful, mechanical work takes the form of an increase in the pressure of the ejected blood

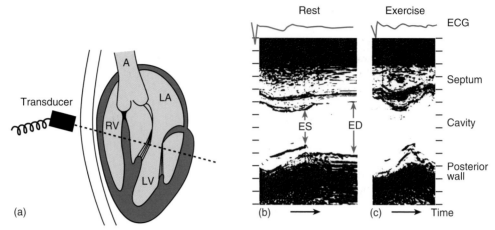

Figure 6.24 Effect of exercise on ventricular dimensions and contraction. (a) Ultrasound beam directed across ventricle (saggital section). (b) and (c) M-mode echocardiograms of human left ventricle during rest (b) and upright exercise (c). The end-diastolic dimension (ED) increased by 2 mm on average. End-systolic dimension (ES) fell by 5 mm. The ED–ES difference, an index of stroke volume, increased by 24%. (From Amon KW, Crawford MH. *Journal of Clinical Ultrasound* 1979; **7**: 373–76.)

(potential energy) and an increase in its velocity (kinetic energy).

Pressure work (stroke work) predominates. As explained in Section 6.5, the work done by the ventricle in pressurizing and shifting the stroke volume into the arteries is called the stroke work. Stroke work equals stroke volume ΔV multiplied by the mean increase in pressure ΔP. Stroke work is therefore the area inside the ventricle pressure–volume loop, $\Delta V \cdot \Delta P$ (Figure 6.11). If the left ventricle raises the blood's pressure by 100 mmHg ($1.33 \times 10^4 \, \text{N/m}^2$) and adds 75 cm^3 of this blood to the arterial system ($0.75 \times 10^{-4} \, \text{m}^3$), it performs $\sim 1 \, \text{N} \cdot \text{m}$ of work (1 joule). The arterial system gains 1 joule of potential energy.

Kinetic work is low in a resting human. The ventricle also imparts velocity to the ejected blood, i.e. it adds **kinetic energy** KE. Kinetic energy, the energy of motion, is proportional to velocity squared (v^2) and moving mass m. Total ventricular work W equals the pressure work plus the kinetic work, i.e.

$$W = \Delta V \Delta P + KE = \Delta V \Delta P + mv^2/2.$$

Under resting conditions $\sim 0.08 \, \text{kg}$ (80 ml) of blood is ejected at a mean velocity of 0.5 m/s during systole, so the kinetic energy imparted by either ventricle is $0.01 \, \text{kg m}^2\text{s}^{-2}$, or 0.01 joules. This is only 1% of the left ventricular stroke work and $\sim 5\%$ of right ventricular stroke work (stroke work being lower on the right side due to the low ejection pressure).

Kinetic work increases substantially during exercise. During heavy exercise the ejection velocity of each ventricle increases around five-fold, to $\sim 2.5 \, \text{m/s}$. Pressure and stroke volume, by contrast, increase only moderately. As a result, kinetic energy accounts for 14% of left ventricular work and 50% of right ventricular work during heavy exercise.

Cardiac power. Power is rate of working, so cardiac power equals ventricular work $\times$ heart rate. Cardiac power ranges from ~ 1.2 joules/s (1.2 watts) at rest to ~ 8 watts in heavy exercise. The latter is about an eighth of the power of a traditional household light bulb.

Emotional stress and high blood pressure increase cardiac work

A raised arterial blood pressure increases stroke work, and therefore myocardial O_2 consumption. An angry, emotional scene causes a large rise in blood pressure, so it greatly increases the myocardial O_2 demand. This is clearly something to be avoided by patients with **coronary artery insufficiency**. As the celebrated eighteenth-century anatomist John Hunter remarked in relation to his own ischaemic heart, 'My life is at the mercy of any rascal who chooses to annoy me' – and the couch on which Hunter expired after a stormy committee meeting can still be seen in the library of St George's Hospital Medical School in London.

Cardiac efficiency improves during exercise

Gross mechanical efficiency is the amount of external work achieved per unit energy expended. Cardiac efficiency is only 5–10% in a resting human, partly because the ion pumps consume about a quarter of the energy, and partly because tension generation during isovolumetric contraction consumes a lot of energy. Myocardial O_2 consumption is in fact dominated by internal work rather than external mechanical work, and correlates well with the active tension multiplied by the period for which it is maintained (the **tension–time index**). This may seem odd, until one recalls that the O_2 consumption of a tug-of-war team depends mainly on the huge tension they exert, rather than on the external work involved in shifting the opposition over a metre or so. In cardiology, the tension–time index is estimated as heart rate $\times$ systolic pressure.

During dynamic exercise, cardiac efficiency improves markedly, to $\sim$15%, because flow increases much more than arterial pressure; there is relatively little increase in the energy-expensive isovolumetric phase. This is helpful to patients with cardiac disease. By contrast, isometric exercise, such as weight lifting, is best avoided by cardiac patients, because it greatly raises arterial pressure and hence O_2 demand.

Cardiac efficiency is reduced by dilatation in heart failure

When treating heart failure, it is important to improve cardiac efficiency as much as possible. Heart failure leads to cardiac dilatation (Figure 18.12), which impairs efficiency. **Laplace's law** tells us that to maintain a normal systolic pressure P, a heart of enlarged radius r has to exert a greater contractile tension T, because $P = 2T/r$ (Section 6.8). To generate a given pressure, a dilated ventricle consumes more O_2 and has a lower mechanical efficiency than a ventricle of normal radius. Since **excessive cardiac dilatation impairs efficiency**, it must be reduced, using diuretic drugs.

Myocardial metabolism and O_2 consumption

High energy phosphate. Myocardial metabolism is normally aerobic. The immediate energy source for the myosin head is the high energy third phosphate bond of ATP, which is generated by oxidative phosphorylation in the abundant cardiac mitochondria. There is a small, back-up store of high-energy phosphate bonds in the form of **creatine phosphate**, but this is only sufficient for $\sim$15 beats. Consequently, cardiac performance depends entirely on mitochondrial ATP production increasing in proportion to myosin ATP consumption. This coupling is remarkably good; myocardial O_2 consumption increases linearly with myocardial work without any measurable change in ATP or creatine phosphate concentration – a phenomenon called the **metabolic stability paradox**. So how is mitochondrial ATP production coupled so tightly to myosin ATP consumption? The traditional answer was that Ca^{2+} not only triggers contraction but also stimulates mitochondrial oxidative phosphorylation; but it now appears that **creatine kinase** has a key role. Creatine kinase is present in the myosin filaments and in the mid-membrane space of the mitochondria, and it transfers high energy phosphate from creatine phosphate to ADP to keep up a constant cellular ATP level.

Oxygen. Cardiac myocytes have only a small reserve of O_2, bound to myoglobin, so a continuous supply of O_2 is necessary to maintain mitochondrial ATP production. In a resting human the myocardial O_2 consumption, $\sim$10 ml/min per 100 g, represents 65–75% of the O_2 delivered in the coronary arterial blood, leaving little in reserve. Consequently, during exercise the **increased myocardial O_2 demand can only be met by increased coronary blood flow**. In other words, myocardial performance is critically dependent on coronary blood flow. Since the heart, unlike skeletal muscle, cannot stop for a rest, coronary perfusion must keep pace with mitochondrial demand at all times.

Metabolic substrates. The substrates consumed by myocardium have been worked out by comparing coronary sinus (venous) and arterial plasma concentrations. Broadly speaking, **free fatty acids** normally supply 60–90% of cardiac energy. The other 10–40% is supplied by **glucose** and **lactate**. In contrast to skeletal muscle, well-oxygenated myocardium can oxidize blood lactate. This is a useful asset during hard exercise, since lactate is released into the bloodstream by the active skeletal muscle. During 25 min of cycling at moderate intensity (30–55% maximal), the glucose consumption by the human heart approximately doubles; but at higher exercise intensities the glucose consumption falls as the plasma lactate level increases. If the myocardium becomes hypoxic, however, it switches from lactate consumption to **anaerobic lactate production**, leading to intracellular acidosis and impaired contractility.

Myocardial enzymes appear in plasma after a heart attack

Lactate is normally oxidized by the heart through the enzyme **myocardial lactic dehydrogenase** (LDH), an isoform specific to the heart. When myocytes undergo ischaemic damage after a coronary thrombosis, LDH and other intracellular enzymes, such as creatine kinase and aspartate aminotransferase, escape into the circulation. Their plasma levels are a valuable laboratory test for myocardial infarction. The plasma level of troponin T too is highly specific for cardiac damage; plasma troponin T increases 2–4 h after an infarct and persists for up to a week.

SUMMARY

- Cardiac output equals heart rate × ventricular stroke volume. Stroke volume is influenced by three physiological factors: (i) diastolic stretch increases contractile force; (ii) noradrenaline and adrenaline increase contractility; (iii) arterial pressure opposes ejection.

- Ventricular diastolic stretch is determined by filling pressure, i.e. central venous pressure (CVP) on the right, pulmonary venous pressure on the left. Stretch increases the Ca^{2+} sensitivity of myocytes, and therefore contractile force and stroke work (stroke volume × pressure). This is called the length–tension relation/Frank–Starling mechanism/Starling's law of the heart.

- The Frank–Starling mechanism equalizes right and left stroke volumes and helps increase stroke volume in upright exercise and after transfusions. It reduces stroke volume during orthostasis (standing) and hypovolaemia.

- Human CVP, and therefore stroke volume, is influenced by blood volume, posture, sympathetic-mediated peripheral venous tone, the skeletal muscle pump and breathing.

- In heart failure an excessively high CVP over-distends the heart. The increased radius R impairs the conversion of active wall tension T into internal pressure P, because $T = 2P/R$ (Laplace's law). Treatment therefore aims to reduce CVP, using diuretics.

- An increase in force mediated not by stretch but by neurohumoral agents is called an increase in contractility. Ventricular contractility is raised by the sympathetic neurotransmitter noradrenaline and by circulating adrenaline. These activate the myocyte β_1-adrenoceptor – adenylate cyclase – cAMP – protein kinase A cascade. The cascade enhances the action potential Ca^{2+} current, boosts the SR Ca^{2+} store and systolic free Ca^{2+} transient, and stimulates Ca^{2+} re-uptake into the store to speed up relaxation. The result is a stronger, shorter contraction, a bigger stroke volume, ejection fraction and systolic pressure, and a reduced end-systolic volume. The pressure–volume loop becomes wider, taller and is shifted leftwards.

- Increased contractility steepens the Starling curve (stroke work versus filling pressure). The effect is graded, i.e. proportional to sympathetic activity. The heart thus operates on a 'family of ventricular function curves'.

- Other positive inotropic influences include β-agonist drugs (isoprenaline, dobutamine), phosphodiesterase inhibitors (caffeine, milrinone), Na^+–K^+ pump inhibitors (digoxin, ouabain) and increased beat frequency (Bowditch effect). Premature beats (extra systoles) are weaker than normal and the beat after the compensatory pause is stronger than normal, due to the effect of time on Ca^{2+} store restocking.

- Negative inotropic influences include myocardial ischaemia (causing hypoxia and acidosis) and chronic heart failure. Arrhythmias, a common complication, can result from the reduced membrane potentials, increased intracellular $[Na^+]$ and premature discharge of overloaded SR Ca^{2+} stores in early diastole, triggering afterdepolarization.

- An acute rise in arterial pressure increases the 'afterload' on ventricular myocytes, which reduces the stroke volume (the afterload–shortening relation, or pump function curve). Reduction of arterial pressure by vasodilator drugs is therefore used to improve stroke volume in failing hearts.

- An acute rise in arterial pressure also evokes multiple, conflicting secondary effects. The subsequent diastolic distension raises contractile force (Starling's law) and, more slowly, contractility (Anrep effect). But the baroreflex reduces sympathetic drive and contractility. Chronic hypertension evokes concentric ventricular hypertrophy and eventually heart failure.

■ During exercise, changes in the peripheral circulation and heart cooperate to raise cardiac output. Peripheral venoconstriction and the skeletal muscle pump maintain or raise the CVP (preload) and end-diastolic volume, activating the Frank–Starling mechanism. End-systolic volume is reduced by sympathetic stimulation. Stroke volume can double. Vasodilatation in active muscle minimizes the rise in arterial pressure and afterload. Sympathetic stimulation raises heart rate.

■ Myocardial performance is tightly coupled to O_2 delivery by the coronary arteries. Much of the O_2 is consumed in raising ventricular pressure. Since emotional stress raises pressure, it should be avoided by patients with coronary artery insufficiency.

Further reading

Reviews and chapters

Allen DG, Xiao XH. Role of the cardiac Na^+/H^+ exchanger during ischemia and reperfusion. *Cardiovascular Research* 2003; **57**: 934–41.

Bolli R. Preconditioning: a paradigm shift in the biology of myocardial ischemia. *American Journal of Physiology* 2007; **292**: H19–27.

Burkhoff D, Mirsky I, Suga H. Assessment of systolic and diastolic ventricular properties via pressure-volume analysis: a guide for clinical, translational and basic researchers. *American Journal of Physiology* 2005; **289**: H501–12.

Casadei B. Vagal control of myocardial contractility in humans. *Experimental Physiology* 2001; **86**: 817–23.

Cingolani HE, Perez NG, Camilion de Hurtado MC. An autocrine/paracrine mechanism triggered by myocardial stretch induces changes in contractility. *News in Physiological Science* 2001; **16**: 88–91 (Anrep effect).

Fuchs F, Smith SS. Calcium, cross-bridges, and the Frank–Starling relationship. *News in Physiological Science* 2001; **16**: 5–10.

Katz AM. Ernest Henry Starling, his predecessors, and the "Law of the Heart". *Circulation* 2002; **106**: 2986–92.

Molkentin JD, Dorn GW. Cytoplasmic signaling pathways that regulate cardiac hypertrophy. *Annual Review of Physiology* 2001; **63**: 391–426.

Piper HM. Mechanism of myocardial injury during acute reperfusion. *News in Physiological Sciences* 1997; **12**: 53–4.

Saks V, Dzeja P, Schlattner U, Vendelin M, Terzic A, Walliman T. Cardiac system bioenergetics: metabolic basis of the Frank–Starling law. *Journal of Physiology* 2006; **571**: 253–73.

Stanley WC, Recchia FA, Lopaschuk GD. Myocardial substrate metabolism in the normal and failing heart. *Physiological Reviews* 2005; **85**: 1093–129.

Research papers

See www.hodderplus.com/cardiovascularphysiology for a full list of Research papers for this chapter.

CHAPTER 7

Assessment of cardiac output and peripheral pulse

Learning objectives

After reading this chapter you should be able to:

- Define the Fick principle (cf. Fick's law of diffusion!) (7.1).
- Apply the Fick principle to estimate pulmonary blood flow from measurements of O_2 uptake (7.1).
- Draw a typical concentration or temperature versus time plot for the indicator or thermal dilution method, and explain how cardiac output is derived from it (7.2).
- Outline three modern 'high-tech' methods for estimating human stroke volume (7.3, 7.5).
- Describe the relation between the peripheral pulse and cardiac output (7.4).
- Define arterial compliance and state three major factors affecting it (7.4).

The cardiac output is the volume of blood ejected by one ventricle in one minute, and equals the stroke volume × number of beats per minute. The need to measure human cardiac output arises in many areas of research, e.g. evaluating the cardiac adaptation to physical training, and also in clinical practice e.g. to quantify the severity of cardiac disease and its response to treatment.

Cardiac output can be measured as a single entity in humans using the **Fick principle** or the **dilution method**. Alternatively, stroke volume can be measured separately by **Doppler ultrasound**, **radionuclide counting** or **echocardiography**, and the result multiplied by heart rate to give cardiac output. The heart rate is obtained by counting the radial pulse, or by ECG, or by a pulse oximeter (see later). All the above cardiac output methods require complex technology. A much simpler and more convenient estimate, albeit rather indirect, is to measure the **arterial pulse**. We will begin here with the gold standard but invasive method, the Fick principle, then move in the direction of less direct but less invasive methods. The Fick principle

has a wider, physiological importance, besides cardiac output measurement. It is a general principle describing the transport of any solute across a capillary bed, and is thus crucial to understanding a core role of the cardiovascular system – the uptake of O_2 in the lungs.

7.1 Fick's principle and pulmonary oxygen transport

Adolf Fick pointed out in 1870 that the rate at which the pulmonary capillaries take up O_2 in the lungs must equal the increase in O_2 concentration in the blood multiplied by the pulmonary blood flow. Since the pulmonary blood flow is the right ventricular output, it follows that cardiac output can be calculated from measurements of O_2 transport.

Fick's principle quantifies O_2 uptake in the lungs

As noted above, Fick's principle is more than just a method – it is basic to understanding O_2 uptake in the lungs, CO_2 elimination and many other

Figure 7.1 The Fick principle. (a) Applied to measure pulmonary blood flow ($\dot{Q}$). PA, pulmonary artery containing venous blood; PV, pulmonary vein containing arterialized blood. For other symbols, see text. (b) Applied to measure flow ($\dot{Q}$) of football supporters through a gate, based on the rate of takings (J) and the 'concentration' of money in the supporters' pockets before and after the gate. In other scenarios, each individual could be a red cell giving up CO_2 to the lungs; or a volume of plasma giving up glucose to the brain; the principle has wide application.

physiological exchanges (Figure 7.1). The amount of O_2 carried into the lungs per minute in venous blood equals pulmonary blood flow $\dot{Q}$ times venous oxygen concentration C_V:

$$\text{O}_2 \text{ in venous blood entering lungs per minute} = \dot{Q}C_V$$

Similarly, the amount of O_2 carried away from the lungs per minute in the oxygenated blood equals the pulmonary blood flow times the arterial oxygen concentration C_A:

$$\text{O}_2 \text{ in arterialized blood leaving lungs per minute} = \dot{Q}C_A$$

The amount of O_2 taken up by the blood as it passes through the lungs is the difference between the amount of O_2 entering and the amount leaving, i.e.:

$$\text{O}_2 \text{ uptake by pulmonary blood per minute} = \dot{Q}C_A - \dot{Q}C_V$$

In the steady state, the amount of O_2 taken up by the blood per minute must equal the amount of O_2

removed from the lung alveolar gas per minute, $\dot{V}_{O_2}$, so we can write:

$$\text{O}_2 \text{ removal from alveolar gas} = \text{O}_2 \text{ uptake by pulmonary blood}$$

or in symbols:

$$\dot{V}_{O_2} = \dot{Q}C_A - \dot{Q}C_V$$

Re-expressing this in terms of the O_2 arteriovenous concentration difference $C_A - C_V$:

$$\dot{V}_{O_2} = \dot{Q}(C_A - C_V) \qquad (7.1)$$

This is the **Fick equation**. It tells us that the rate of O_2 uptake from the inspired air, in ml O_2/min, equals pulmonary blood flow (in litre/min) multiplied by the arteriovenous difference in O_2 concentration (in ml O_2/litre blood).

Since the pulmonary blood flow $\dot{Q}$ is the right ventricular output, we can rearrange the Fick equation to work out the cardiac output, thus:

$$\text{Cardiac output } \dot{Q} \text{ (l/min)} = \frac{\text{Oxygen uptake rate } V_{O_2} \text{ (ml/min)}}{\text{Arterial O}_2 \text{ conc } C_A - \text{Venous O}_2 \text{ conc } C_V \text{ (ml/l)}}.$$

An example should make this clear. A resting human absorbs ~250 ml O_2 per minute from the alveolar gas ($\dot{V}_{O_2}$). Arterial blood contains 195 ml O_2 per litre and the mixed venous blood entering the lungs contains 145 ml O_2 per litre; so each litre of blood takes up 50 ml O_2 as it passes through the alveoli, i.e. ($C_A - C_V$) = 50 ml/l. To take up 250 ml O_2, 5 litres of blood are required (250/50). This amount of O_2 is taken up in 1 min. Right ventricular output at rest is therefore 5 litres/min.

Fick's method requires cardiac catheterization

Fick's method only became practicable in humans in the twentieth century, when the advent of cardiac catheterization enabled **mixed venous blood** sampling from the right ventricle/pulmonary trunk. Mixed venous blood analysis tells us the average O_2 concentration entering the lungs. Peripheral venous blood is no good for this purpose, because its O_2 concentration varies markedly between tissues, e.g. renal venous O_2 170 ml/l, coronary venous O_2 70 ml/l. The different streams of venous blood only become fully mixed in the right ventricle.

The difficult problem of sampling mixed venous blood in humans was solved by the German physician Werner Forssman, who in 1929 passed a ureteric catheter up his own arm vein into the right heart, watching its progress on an X-ray screen. This brave act founded human cardiac catheterization, won Forssman the disapproval of his head of department and, later, a Nobel prize.

The Fick method is now applied as follows. The subject's resting O_2 consumption, $\dot{V}_{O_2}$ is measured for 5–10 min by spirometry, or by collecting expired air in a Douglas bag. During this period an arterial blood sample is taken from the brachial, radial or femoral artery, and a mixed venous sample is taken from the right ventricle outflow tract/pulmonary trunk, using a cardiac catheter introduced through the antecubital (elbow) vein. The O_2 content of each blood sample is measured and the cardiac output calculated as above.

The Fick method has several limitations

Although the Fick method is the yardstick by which new methods are judged, it has its limitations. The O_2 uptake measurement takes 5–10 min to perform, so beat-by-beat changes in stroke volume cannot be resolved. Also, the method is only valid in the steady state, so a rapidly changing cardiac output cannot be measured. Being invasive, the method is inadvisable during hard exercise, because the cardiac catheter may trigger an arrhythmia in a violently beating heart. The **indirect Fick method** avoids cardiac catheterization and estimates C_V indirectly, by the analysis of re-breathed gas – an approach used recently in an orbiting space laboratory.

The Fick principle has many applications

The Fick principle is an important, general physiological principle that applies to the exchange of any material in any perfused organ – for example, glucose transport from blood to skeletal muscle or the brain (Section 10.10). The Fick principle even applies to heat exchange in a water-perfused radiator, or money turnover at the turnstile of a football ground (Figure 7.1b). In general terms, the transfer rate, J, of any substance between a flowing body and its surroundings equals the flow $\dot{Q}$ multiplied by the concentration difference between the incoming fluid, C_{in}, and the outgoing fluid, C_{out}:

$$J = \dot{Q}(C_{out} - C_{in}) \qquad (7.2)$$

The Fick principle has therefore been used to work out the rate at which an organ consumes a metabolite, such as glucose, based on measurements of local blood flow and arteriovenous concentration difference.

7.2 Indicator and thermal dilution methods

The thermal dilution method has been much used in cardiology departments, but we will first consider its parent, the indicator dilution method, which is easier to understand.

Indicator dilution method

A known mass of a foreign substance, the indicator, is injected rapidly into a central vein or the right heart. It is necessary that the indicator is confined to the bloodstream and easy to assay, such as dyes that bind to plasma albumin (Evans blue, indocyanine green), radiolabelled albumin or radiolabelled red cells. The indicator becomes diluted in the venous bloodstream, then carried through the heart and lungs and ejected into the systemic arteries (Figure 7.2a). Systemic arterial blood is sampled from the radial or femoral artery, and its indicator content is plotted against time.

For simplicity, let us first suppose that the ejected bolus of arterial blood has a uniform concentration of the indicator (Figure 7.2b). The concentration versus time plot tells us two things: the time t taken by the labelled bolus to pass a given point and the average concentration of indicator in the bolus. Concentration C is by definition the injected mass m divided by the volume of plasma in which the indicator has become distributed, V_D: in other words, $C = m/V_D$. The distribution volume of the indicator is thus:

$$V_D = m/C$$

For example, if 1 mg of indicator produced a mean plasma concentration of 1 mg/l, its volume of distribution must be 1 litre. If this volume takes t seconds to pass the sampling point, the left ventricle must be ejecting plasma at the rate V_D/t. In Figure 7.2b, the rate is 1 litre in 20 s, or 3 l/min. Thus plasma output is:

$$\text{Cardiac output (plasma)} = \frac{V_D}{t} = \frac{\text{Mass of indicator, } m}{\text{Mean concentration } C \times \text{passage time } t}.$$

The output of blood is the plasma output divided by 1 − haematocrit; the haematocrit is the fraction of the blood that is made up of red cells (0.40–0.45).

(a)

(b)

(c)

Figure 7.2 Hamilton's dye-dilution method. (a) Arterial concentration C depends on the mass of indicator injected (m) and the volume of blood in which it became diluted. (b) Idealized plot of C against time. Area $C \times t$ is 20 mg s litre^{-1} here. Height and duration depend on injection rate, but area is not affected; an increase in concentration produced by a fast injection is offset by the shorter duration of the bolus, due to a smaller distribution volume. If m is 1 mg, the cardiac output of plasma is 1 mg/20 mg s litre^{-1} = 0.05 l/s, or 3 l/min. For a haematocrit of 0.4, the cardiac output of blood is 5 l/min. (c) The grim reality – the concentration peaks and decays over time, then shows a recirculation hump. Fortunately, when C is plotted on a logarithmic scale, the early decay is linear. This allows extrapolation past the recirculation hump (asterisk). Area under the extrapolated curve is used to calculate the cardiac output. (After Asmussen E, Nielsen M. *Acta Physiologica Scandinavica* 1953; **27**: 217 with permission from Wiley-Blackwell.)

Since the denominator $C \times t$ is actually the area under the plot of concentration versus time, we can simplify the above expression to:

$$\text{Cardiac output (plasma)} = \frac{\text{Mass of indicator, } m}{\text{Area under the } C \text{ versus } t \text{ plot}}.$$

This simplification is very helpful, because in reality the arterial concentration is not constant (Figure 7.2c, cf. 7.2b) – but we can still measure the area under the curve. The concentration rises to a peak, after which it decays exponentially, because the ventricle only ejects about two-thirds of its contents per systole. The residual indicator in the ventricle is diluted by indicator-free venous blood returning during the next diastole, and the diluted blood is in turn only partially ejected in systole and so on.

After about 15 s the concentration decay curve is interrupted by a recirculation hump – the asterisk in Figure 7.2c. This is caused by blood with a high indicator content returning to the heart after one complete transit of the myocardial circulation, which is the shortest, quickest circulation in the body. To use the area equation, we need to work out the area under the curve excluding the recirculation hump. To this end, the pre-hump part of the decay curve is extrapolated underneath the recirculation hump. A semilogarithmic plot converts the exponential decay into a straight line, which can then be extrapolated under the hump to a negligible concentration (usually 1% of the peak), as in Figure 7.2c. The area under the corrected C versus t curve is used to calculate the cardiac output.

A modern, computerized version of the method is based on intravenous **lithium ion** injection. The lithium can be detected in the arterial blood by an ion-sensitive electrode. It appears that lithium loss during passage through the lungs is negligible.

Pros and cons of the indicator dilution method

The indicator dilution method agrees with the Fick method to within 5%. The dilution method has a better time resolution (30 s) than the Fick method (5–10 min). Also, it can be used in exercise, since there is no need for ventricular catheterization. The error involved in extrapolating the decay curve is, however, a drawback, and becomes a serious limitation in diseased hearts, where the initial part of the decay curve may be short and distorted.

Thermal dilution method

This variant method has been used widely in cardiac departments, owing to its greater convenience. Instead of a soluble indicator, temperature is used. A thermistor (temperature sensor) at the tip of a Swan–Ganz catheter is advanced into the pulmonary trunk/artery. A known mass of cold saline is then injected quickly into the right atrium, right ventricle or proximal pulmonary trunk. The distal thermistor records the dilution of the cold saline by the warm pulmonary bloodstream. Cardiac output is calculated as the injected amount of heat (i.e. cold) divided by the area under the temperature–time plot.

Pros and cons of thermal dilution

The major advantage of thermal dilution over indicator dilution is that it circumvents the recirculation hump problem, because the cold saline has warmed up to body temperature by the time it recirculates to the right ventricle. Heat transfer across the walls of the right ventricle and pulmonary artery can cause an overestimation of the distribution volume and hence cardiac output, but a computed correction is made for this.

7.3 Aortic flow by pulsed Doppler method

To estimate left ventricular stroke volume, pulses of ultrasound are directed down the ascending aorta from a transmitter crystal placed over the suprasternal notch (Figure 7.3, top). The moving red cells alter the frequency of the ultrasound reflected off them, and the frequency shift is proportional to the red cell velocity. This is called the Doppler shift, and is analogous to the change in pitch of a police car siren as it speeds past. The reflected ultrasound is recorded and used to compute the mean blood velocity across the aorta, millisecond by millisecond. The aortic blood velocity is plotted against time (Figure 7.3, bottom), and interpreted as follows.

Stroke distance is distance advanced along the aorta per ejection

Since distance is velocity × time, the distance that blood advances along the aorta during one systole, the **stroke distance**, equals the area under the aortic velocity–time curve. To convert stroke distance into stroke volume, the cross-sectional area of the aorta is measured by echocardiography (see Section 2.6). The area, in cm², multiplied by stroke distance in cm, gives stroke volume in cm³, less the volume drained off by the coronary arteries.

Pros and cons of Doppler method

The Doppler method is difficult to calibrate and has noise problems. But it has two enormous advantages – it is non-invasive and has an extremely high temporal resolution, recording every instant of ejection, unlike the Fick or dilution methods.

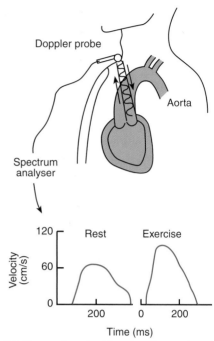

Figure 7.3 Transaortic pulsed Doppler ultrasound method. The Doppler shift in the frequency of reflected ultrasound is used to compute the mean velocity of blood across the aorta at successive moments during systole. Stroke distance is area under curve. (From Innes JA, Simon TD, Murphy K, Guz A. *Quarterly Journal of Experimental Physiology* 1988; **73**: 323–41, with permission from Wiley-Blackwell.)

7.4 Peripheral pulse and its relation to cardiac output

The oldest, cheapest, quickest and easiest way to assess human cardiac output is to palpate the radial pulse at the wrist. **Heart rate** can be counted and the **strength of the pulse** can be estimated subjectively. A strong pulse is the result of a large stroke volume, for example during exercise; and a weak pulse is the result of a low stroke volume, for example after a haemorrhage. What the finger actually detects is the expansion of the artery as pressure rises during systole. The rise in pressure, or **pulse pressure**, equals systolic pressure minus the diastolic pressure. Pulse pressure is easily quantified by sphygmomanometry (Section 8.5), and is closely related to stroke volume, as follows.

Stroke volume and pulse pressure are linked by arterial compliance

The relation between left ventricular stroke volume and systemic arterial pressure is one of the key haemodynamic relations of the circulation. It is introduced here, and is analysed in more detail in

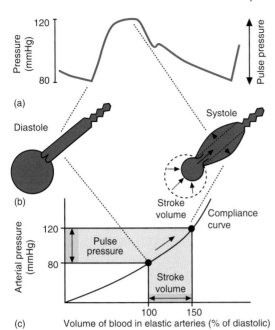

Figure 7.4 Relation between pulse pressure and stroke volume. Dotted lines link coincident points in time. (a) Aortic pressure wave. (b) Ejection of left ventricle stroke volume into elastic arteries. (c) Pressure–volume relation (compliance curves) of young human aorta. Note increase in stiffness (steeper slope) with pressure. (Based on Nichols WW, O'Rourke MF. *McDonald's Blood Flow in Arteries,* 5th edn. London: Arnold, 2005.)

Chapter 8. During ejection most of the stroke volume (70–80% at rest) is accommodated in the elastic arteries, because the ventricle ejects blood faster than it can drain away through the resistance vessels. The increase in arterial volume distends the arteries, and the arterial wall tension raises the blood pressure (Figure 7.4). The magnitude of the increase in pressure, or pulse pressure, thus depends on the **stroke volume** and the **compliance** (distensibility) of the arterial system. Compliance is defined as change in volume per unit change in pressure:

$$\text{Arterial compliance} = \frac{\text{Increase in blood volume}}{\text{Increase in arterial pressure}}. \quad (7.3)$$

Arterial compliance in a young adult is ~2 ml per mmHg at normal blood pressure. The increase in arterial blood volume during systole equals stroke volume minus the volume that drains away during the ejection period (runoff). Inserting this statement into the top line of 7.3 and rearranging, we see that the increase in arterial pressure per heart beat, the **pulse pressure**, is related to stroke volume as follows:

$$\frac{\text{Pulse}}{\text{pressure}} = \frac{\text{Stroke volume} - \text{runoff in systole}}{\text{Arterial compliance}}. \quad (7.4)$$

Changes in pulse pressure can thus serve as a guide to changes in stroke volume. In intensive care units, pulse pressure in the finger is monitored continuously, and the data are processed by a computer, based on eqn 7.4, to display a beat-by-beat estimate of stroke volume, heart rate and cardiac output.

Arterial compliance is not a fixed quantity

A significant problem when interpreting pulse pressure is that arterial compliance does not have a unique, unchanging value; its magnitude varies, as follows:

- Arterial compliance falls (stiffness increases) as pressure and volume increase; so the arterial pressure–volume plot is a steepening curve (Figure 7.4c).
- Arterial compliance is reduced by high ejection velocities, because the artery wall is a viscoelastic material, and takes time to relax (see Appendix 2). During exercise the pulse pressure increases relatively more than the stroke volume, because there is less time for viscous relaxation of the wall during a fast ejection.
- Arterial compliance declines with age, due to a degenerative stiffening of elastic arteries called **arteriosclerosis**. Consequently, pulse pressure increases with age, and this increases stroke work

---

Arterial compliance links pulse pressure and stroke volume

- Compliance is a measure of distensibility; it is the inverse of stiffness. Arterial compliance C is defined as the increase in blood volume in the arterial system, ΔV, required to produces unit increase in arterial pressure, ΔP. Thus $C = \Delta V / \Delta P$.
- Pulse pressure is the increase in pressure between diastole and systole.
- From the above definitions, pulse pressure ΔP = stroke volume (minus the runoff during ejection)/arterial compliance. Pulse pressure can thus be increased by a rise in stroke volume (e.g. exercise) or a fall in arterial compliance (e.g. ageing).
- Arterial compliance falls as pressure increases, due to the tensing of collagen in the artery wall. Consequently, a rise in mean arterial pressure also causes a rise in pulse pressure.
- Arterial compliance declines with age due to arteriosclerosis, a diffuse stiffening of the media of elastic vessels. As a result pulse pressure can double between youth and old age.

CONCEPT BOX 7.1

(Sections 8.4 and 17.7). Arteriosclerosis is the diffuse stiffening of ageing elastic arteries, due primarily to changes in the tunica media. It should not be confused with **atheroma**, which is primarily a cholesterol-related disease of the tunica intima (Table 17.4).

Pros and cons of pulse method

- The variable nature of arterial compliance can introduce some ambiguity, as can runoff during ejection, since runoff increases when peripheral resistance falls. Nevertheless, changes in pulse pressure, recorded with nothing more sophisticated than a wrist watch and sphygmomanometer cuff, offer a convenient, instant, bedside indication of changes in cardiac output in an individual from hour to hour, for example during recovery from an acute haemorrhage. At a more sophisticated level, computer models make reasonably accurate computations of acute changes in stroke volume from continuous recordings of peripheral arterial pressure. The latter can be measured continuously by an electronic, finger-volume clamp method (see Finapress, Section 8.5). This has enabled **continuous computer monitoring** of stroke volume, heart rate and cardiac output in intensive care units.

Pulse oximetry monitors pulse rate

- The heart rate can be measured using a watch and palpation of the radial artery; or a miniaturized ECG that transmits the heart rate to a wrist monitor, or a **pulse oximeter**. An oximeter is a small device that shines a light through superficial tissue, usually an ear lobe or finger, and measures the transmitted light, using a photoelectric cell. Red cells absorb some of the light, and oxyhaemoglobin absorbs a different wavelength to deoxyhaemoglobin. As the arterial system expands with each pulse, the light transmission changes. From this the pulse rate and blood oxygen saturation are computed.

7.5 Radionuclide ventriculography, echocardiography and other methods

Radionuclide ventriculography

A gamma-emitting radionuclide, usually a technetium-99 compound bound to red cells, is injected intravenously, and a precordial gamma camera records the gamma counts emanating from the ventricles. The difference between the radioactive content of the ventricles in diastole and systole is used to calculate the ejection fraction and stroke volume. The method requires, obviously, the services of a nuclear medicine department.

Quantitative echocardiography (ultrasound cardiography)

Echocardiography is non-invasive, and can measure the end-diastolic and end-systolic dimensions of the ventricle (Figures 2.9 and 6.24). The stroke volume and ejection fraction are then computed from the linear dimensions, using an assumed chamber geometry. Typical values are listed in Table 2.2. **Magnetic resonance imaging** (MRI) of the cardiac chambers can be used in a similar way.

Impedance cardiography

Chest and neck leads pass a small current through the thorax, to measure its cyclically changing electrical resistance (impedance). Aortic blood volume increases and decreases over each cardiac cycle, and since blood is a better conductor than air, the electrical impedance of the thorax oscillates likewise. Aortic stroke volume can be estimated, albeit rather indirectly, from the impedance oscillation. The method is non-invasive, but very indirect.

Electromagnetic 'flow' meter

This method is invasive, and is only used in laboratory animals for research purposes. Under general anaesthesia a miniature, semicircular magnet is surgically implanted, with its magnetic poles on either side of the blood vessel of interest, e.g. pulmonary artery. Blood is an electrical conductor, and as it cuts through the magnetic field it induces an electrical potential, which is measured. The potential is proportional to the blood velocity (cm/s), not flow. To convert mean velocity to flow, the internal diameter of the vessel is required. Being small, an electromagnetic flowmeter can be left inside a conscious animal, transmitting a signal by telemetry (radio-waves). In this way, much has been learned about the regulation of stroke volume in unfettered, conscious animals, such as dogs running on a treadmill.

SUMMARY

- The gold standard method for measuring human cardiac output is the **Fick principle**. This states that solute transfer rate = blood flow × concentration difference between incoming and outgoing blood. O_2 uptake in the lungs is measured over 5–10 min by spirometry or expired air collection. The O_2 content of mixed venous blood is measured in a blood sample taken from the right ventricle by cardiac catheterization. Arterial blood is sampled from a systemic artery. Pulmonary blood flow, i.e. right ventricular output, is then calculated from the Fick equation above.

- **Indicator dilution** and **thermal dilution** methods have a better time resolution. A known mass of dye or cold saline is injected quickly into the right heart, and the concentration or temperature is recorded at a point downstream. Concentration or temperature is plotted versus time. Knowing the injected mass m, and the average downstream concentration C (or temperature), the volume of blood in which the indicator has distributed can be calculated; $V_D = m/C$. Volume V_D is divided by the time taken for the labelled blood to pass the sampling point. This equals the cardiac output.

- **Pulsed Doppler ultrasound** measures the average blood velocity across the aorta, millisecond by millisecond. The area under the velocity–time plot gives the distance advanced per ejection (stroke distance). Stroke volume is stroke distance × aortic diameter, which is measured by ultrasound.

- **Radionuclide ventriculography** measures the radioactive counts present in the ventricle during end-diastole and end-systole. The stroke volume and ejection fraction are calculated from the difference between counts.

- **Echocardiography (ultrasound cardiography)** records the changes in ventricular dimensions between diastole and systole, to estimate stroke volume and ejection fraction.

- With all methods that estimate stroke volume, the cardiac output is calculated as heart rate × stroke volume. The pulse rate can be monitored by **pulse oximetry** or **ECG**.

- **Peripheral pulse examination** is the simplest bedside method for assessing cardiac output. Heart rate is determined by counting the pulse. Sphygmomanometry measures the pulse pressure (systolic minus diastolic pressure). **Pulse pressure** is proportional to stroke volume, although the relation is complicated by runoff, non-linear aortic compliance, dependence on ejection rate and age-related arterial stiffening (arteriosclerosis). A computerized, continuous display of cardiac output based on finger pulse monitoring is used in intensive care units.

Further reading

Band DM, Linton RAF, O'Brien TK, Jonas MM, Linton NWF. The shape of indicator dilution curves used for cardiac output measurement in man. (Lithium dilution method.) *Journal of Physiology* 1997; **498**: 225–9.

Bogert LWJ, van Lieshout JJ. Non-invasive pulsatile arterial pressure and stroke volume changes from the human finger. *Experimental Physiology* 2005; **90**: 437–46.

Mehta N, Iyawe VI, Cummin ARC, Bayley S, Saunders KB, Bennett ED. Validation of a Doppler technique for beat-to-beat measurement of cardiac output. *Clinical Science* 1985; **69**: 377–82.

Nichols WW, O'Rourke MF. *McDonald's Blood Flow in Arteries*, 5th edn. London: Arnold, 2005. (Pulse pressure and arterial compliance.)

Schelbert HR, Verba IW, Johnson AD *et al.* Non-traumatic determination of left ventricular ejection fraction by radionuclide angiography. *Circulation* 1978; **51**: 902–9.

Sugawara J, Tanabe T, Miyachi M *et al.* Non-invasive assessment of cardiac output during exercise in healthy young humans; comparison between Modelflow method and Doppler echocardiography method. *Acta Physiologica Scandinavica* 2003; **179**: 361–6.

CHAPTER 8

Haemodynamics: flow, pressure and resistance

Learning objectives

After studying this chapter you should be able to:

- Use Darcy's law of flow to link mean arterial pressure, cardiac output and peripheral resistance (8.1).
- Sketch laminar and turbulent flow patterns and state where they occur (8.2).
- State the relation between arterial pulse pressure, arterial compliance and stroke volume (8.4, 7.4).
- Draw an arterial pressure pulse, label and scale it, and explain its main features (8.4).
- Explain how arterial stiffening raises cardiac work (8.4).
- Explain the cuff method for measuring human blood pressure (8.5).
- Use Poiseuille's law to explain how arteriolar radius regulates flow and arterial pressure (8.7).
- Show how Laplace's law contributes to aneurysm progression (8.7).
- State the factors governing blood viscosity and their clinical significance (8.8).
- Draw a graph showing blood flow as a function of arterial pressure in the absence and presence of autoregulation (8.9).
- Explain how gravity affects arterial and venous pressures on standing (8.11).
- List the key factors determining the volume of blood in peripheral veins (8.10).
- Explain how human central venous pressure can be estimated by inspecting neck veins (8.10).
- Describe the skeletal muscle pump and its three beneficial effects (8.12).

8.1 Hydraulic principles: the laws of Darcy and Bernoulli

The science of haemodynamics concerns the relation between blood flow, blood pressure and hydraulic resistance. The simplest guide to these issues is Darcy's law, which was introduced in Chapter 1.

Darcy's law relates flow to pressure difference

Darcy was a French civil engineer who studied the flow of water through the gravel beds of the fountains in Dijon. In 1856 Darcy reported that flow in the steady state, $\dot{Q}$, is linearly proportional to the pressure difference between two points, $P_1 - P_2$. That is to say:

$$\dot{Q} = K(P_1 - P_2) = \frac{(P_1 - P_2)}{R} \qquad (8.1a)$$

The proportionality coefficient K is called the hydraulic conductance, which is in effect the ease of flow. Its reciprocal is called the hydraulic resistance, R – the difficulty of flow. Darcy's law can be applied to channels of any geometry, including blood vessels.

For example, blood flow through the kidney is equal to the pressure in the renal artery minus the pressure in the renal vein, divided by renal vascular resistance.

The flow through the systemic circulation is the cardiac output, CO, and the pressure difference driving it equals mean aortic pressure $\bar{P}_a$ minus the central venous pressure CVP. The systemic resistance is called the total peripheral resistance or TPR. Putting these symbols into Darcy's law, we have:

$$CO = \frac{(\bar{P}_a - CVP)}{TPR} \qquad (8.1b)$$

All blood pressures are conventionally expressed as pressure above atmospheric pressure, and since CVP is close to atmospheric pressure, $CVP \cong 0$. Equation 8.1b therefore simplifies to $CO \cong \bar{P}_a / TPR$. This can be rearranged to answer the fundamental question, **What determines mean arterial blood pressure?** The answer is that mean arterial pressure is determined by the cardiac output and the total peripheral resistance;

$$\bar{P}_a \cong CO \times TPR$$

or in words,

> Mean arterial blood pressure =
> Cardiac output × Total peripheral resistance

Bernoulli's theory includes additional kinds of fluid energy

Darcy's law deals with pressure, but this is only one of three kinds of mechanical energy that affect flow. The other two are gravitational potential energy and kinetic energy, as recognized by Bernoulli, an eighteenth century Swiss physician who became a professor of mathematics at the age of 25. Bernoulli's theory states that the flow between points A and B, in the steady state, is proportional to the difference in the mechanical energy of the fluid; and the mechanical energy is the sum of the pressure energy, potential energy and kinetic energy.

- **Pressure energy** equals pressure × volume, $P \times V$
- **Potential (gravitational) energy** is the capacity of a mass to do work in a gravitational field by virtue of its height. The potential energy of blood relative to the heart is the blood mass (volume V × density ρ) × height above the heart h × gravitational force g.

- **Kinetic energy** is the energy of movement. It depends on mass and velocity, increasing in proportion to velocity squared (v^2). The kinetic energy of flowing blood is $\rho V v^2/2$, where V is blood volume.

Adding the three energies together we have:

$$\text{Mechanical energy of unit volume of blood} = \bar{P}_a + \rho gh + \rho v^2/2 \qquad (8.2)$$

Note that both the Darcy and Bernoulli laws apply to steady state flow, i.e. flow that is not varying with time. If the flow is pulsatile, as in arteries, the laws still apply to the mean flow; but they do not tell us how the flow varies instant by instant.

Application of Bernoulli's theory to the circulation

Pressure falls inside a stenosed artery. If blood passing along an artery encounters a stenosed (narrowed), atheromatous segment, the blood velocity increases in the narrow segment (Figure 8.1) – just as water velocity in a river increases when the banks narrow. Since v increases, some of the fluid energy is converted into kinetic energy, leaving less energy in the form of pressure (Bernoulli's theory). Consequently, pressure falls within the narrow segment, exacerbating its tendency to close. At the exit, blood flows into the wider segment despite a contrary pressure gradient – proving that flow occurs down a gradient of total energy rather than pressure alone.

A kinetic energy gradient aids cardiac filling. Kinetic energy accounts for ~12% of the total mechanical energy of venous blood in a resting

Figure 8.1 Basic Bernoulli hydraulics: flow is driven by the total mechanical energy gradient. For a given volume flow, velocity v increases where the cross-sectional area A narrows (e.g. arterial atheroma). Pressure energy is converted into kinetic energy KE at this point. Where the tube widens, KE is reconverted to pressure. Flow from the narrow section to wide section is against the pressure gradient but down the total energy gradient.

human. On entering the ventricle, blood velocity and hence kinetic energy fall virtually to zero. There is therefore a kinetic energy gradient between the central veins and ventricle, which aids ventricular filling. To put it another way, the momentum of the returning blood contributes to ventricular expansion.

Gravitational 'puzzles' in humans. Although Darcy's law is adequate for many purposes in vascular physiology, the more comprehensive Bernoulli theory can resolve a number of apparent puzzles. For example, during standing the mean arterial pressure is ~95 mmHg in the proximal aorta and 183 mmHg in the dorsalis pedis artery of the foot (Figure 8.2); yet blood flows from the aorta to the foot, seemingly in defiance of Darcy's law. The explanation, of course, is that proximal aortic blood has ~90 mmHg more gravitational potential energy than blood in the foot, so the energy of unit volume of aortic blood is 95 + 90 = 185 mmHg, compared with the foot's 183 mmHg. The small difference, 2 mmHg, suffices to drive flow from the aorta to the dorsalis pedis artery, because large arteries offer little resistance to flow.

8.2 Patterns of blood flow: laminar, turbulent, single-file

Three patterns of flow occur in the circulation: laminar flow, turbulent flow and single-file or bolus flow (Figures 8.3 and 8.4). Laminar flow occurs in normal arteries, arterioles, venules and veins. Turbulent flow occurs in the ventricles and stenosed arteries. Single-file flow occurs in capillaries.

Laminar flow has smooth, parallel streamlines

When a liquid flows through a smooth cylindrical tube at not too high a velocity, the liquid behaves like a set of infinitesimally thin concentric shells (laminae) that slide past each other (Figure 8.3a, right). The lamina in contact with the vessel wall has zero velocity due to molecular cohesive forces – the

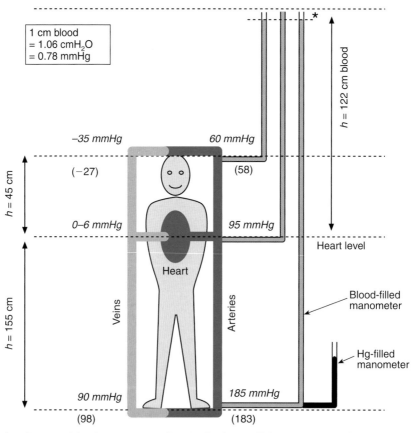

Figure 8.2 Effect of gravity on arterial and venous pressure in a standing human. Pink manometers are filled with blood, black (lower right) with mercury. Pressures in italics are central pressure plus pressure due to vertical fluid column. Pressures in brackets represents actual values for flowing blood, which are modified slightly by the arterial and venous resistances.

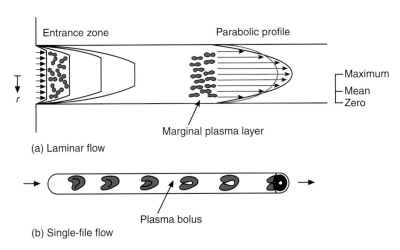

Entrance zone   Parabolic profile

Marginal plasma layer

(a) Laminar flow

Plasma bolus

(b) Single-file flow

Figure 8.3 Blood flow pattern in large vessel (a) or capillary (b). In (a), arrow length indicates the velocity of each lamina. For a Newtonian fluid in fully developed laminar flow, velocity ν is a parabolic function of radial position r, namely $\nu = \nu_{max} (1 - r^2/R^2)$, where R is tube radius. For non-Newtonian blood, the velocity profile is blunter (red line). The gradient of the velocity curve, called the 'shear rate', is greatest at the margins. (b) In capillaries the red cells deform into parachute/slipper configurations (left) and folded shapes (right). (After Chien S. *Microvascular Research* 1992; **44**: 243–54, with permission from Elsevier.)

Figure 8.4 Pressure–flow relation for a Newtonian fluid in a rigid tube. Darcy's law is the straight line through the origin. This breaks down when turbulence begins. Inset shows Sir Osborne Reynolds' apparatus for studying the onset of turbulence. The flow-pattern (top) was visualized by injecting dye into the fluid.

profile is more blunted (Figure 8.3a, red line). At the **entrance** to a tube, where there has been insufficient time for the parabolic profile to develop, the velocity profile is almost flat (Figure 8.3a, left). This is the situation in the **ascending aorta**, where the flat profile simplifies the estimation of aortic flow by Doppler ultrasound (Section 7.3).

Laminar shearing of blood creates a marginal plasma layer

The sliding motion of one lamina past another – like one hand rubbing over the other – is called **shear**. Shear causes the red cells to orientate preferentially in the direction of flow and drift a little towards the central axis (**axial flow of red cells**). This leaves a thin, cell-deficient layer of plasma next to the vessel wall called the **marginal plasma layer**, of thickness 2–4 µm. The marginal plasma layer is important, because it greatly facilitates the flow of blood through narrow resistance vessels (Fåhraeus–Lindqvist effect, Section 8.8). It also contributes to the low haematocrit in microvessels (Fåhraeus effect, Section 8.8).

Laminar shear stress tugs on the endothelium

The friction between the molecules in adjacent laminae causes each lamina to exert a dragging, tugging force on its neighbour, called **shear stress**. The shear stress increases with **shear rate** (rate of sliding) and fluid viscosity. At the vessel wall the **wall shear stress** tugs on the glycocalyx, a polymer coat rooted in the endothelium (Figure 9.2). This stresses the endothelium, with a mean shear stress of 0.5–1.5 Pa in human arteries, which stimulates endothelium to secrete regulatory, vasoactive agents such as nitric oxide (Chapter 9). In some

zero-slip condition. The adjacent lamina slides slowly past the zero-slip lamina. The third lamina slides past the second lamina, and since the second lamina is itself moving, the third lamina has a higher velocity relative to the tube wall – and so on until maximum velocity is reached in the centre of the tube. Blood in the centre of the vessel therefore has a higher velocity than blood near the wall. You can see the same effect during any riverside stroll – the current is faster in the centre than near the banks. For a simple fluid such as water, **the velocity profile across a cylindrical tube is a parabola**. For a particulate suspension, such as blood, the individuals with hypertension, atheroma or Marfan's syndrome, the high wall shear stresses in the proximal aorta (peak >4 Pa) can even tear the endothelium, creating a **dissecting aortic aneurysm**. Blood passes through the endothelial tear and tracks along the aortic wall in the subintimal plane, with potentially fatal results. An interim measure, prior to emergency surgery, is to reduce the cardiac output and hence shear stress, using cardio-inhibitory drugs.

Turbulence

If the pressure driving fluid through a tube is progressively increased, a point is reached where flow no longer increases linearly with pressure, but increases as the square-root of pressure (Figure 8.4). This marks the transition from laminar flow to a disorganized, turbulent flow. In turbulent flow, chaotic cross-currents dissipate more of the pressure energy as heat. The conditions that provoke turbulence were defined in 1883 by the engineer Sir Osborne Reynolds, who visualized turbulence using dyes. Turbulence is encouraged by a high fluid velocity ν, a large tube diameter D and a high fluid density (ρ, rho), because these factors increase fluid momentum and encourage the persistence of flow distortions. Turbulence is discouraged by a high viscosity (η, eta), which damps out flow deviations. The dimensionless ratio of the pro- to antiturbulence factors is called the **Reynolds number**, Re:

$$\mathrm{Re} = \frac{\nu D \rho}{\eta}$$

The critical Reynolds number for the onset of turbulence is ~2000 for steady flow down a rigid, straight, uniform tube, and less than 2000 in blood vessels, where the flow is pulsatile and the vessels are neither rigid nor straight. Even so, Re in most blood vessels is well below the critical value; for example, Re is ~0.5 in resistance vessels.

Turbulence occurs normally in the ventricles, where it mixes the blood to produce a uniform gas content. Turbulence can also occur in the human aorta and pulmonary artery during peak flow, creating an **innocent systolic ejection murmur** (Section 2.5). In the human aortic root, during peak ejection, Re reaches ~4600 (peak velocity ν = 70 cm/s, diameter D = 2.5 cm, blood density ρ = 1.06 g/cm³, blood viscosity η = 0.04 g cm^{-1}s^{-1}, or 4 mPa-seconds). An innocent ejection murmur may develop during exercise (because ejection velocity increases) and during pregnancy/anaemia (because blood viscosity falls).

Pathological turbulence can occur in leg arteries roughened by atheromatous plaques. The turbulence can cause a local murmur, audible through the stethoscope (a **bruit**), and sometimes a palpable **thrill**. By contrast, normal laminar blood flow is silent.

Single-file (bolus) flow occurs in capillaries

A capillary, diameter 5–6 μm, is narrower than a human red cell, 8 μm. Consequently, red cells have to bend into a folded, parachute-like configuration to pass through capillaries – a cartoon-like spectacle when seen *in vivo*. Since the deformed red cell spans the full width of the capillary, the cells are compelled to travel single file. The plasma trapped between each pair of red cells travels as a bolus at uniform velocity (**bolus flow**). This eliminates much of the internal friction associated with laminar flow, so bolus flow is a very low resistance type of flow. At the capillary wall, red cell friction is reduced by the 'shag-pile' of biopolymers coating the endothelium, i.e. the **glycocalyx** (Figure 9.2).

As explained above, capillary flow depends critically on the **deformability of red cells**. In **sickle cell anaemia**, red cells contain an abnormal haemoglobin that polymerizes in hypoxic situations. The polymerization causes the red cells to become sickle-shaped, rigid, and adhesive to endothelium and each other. These changes impair the passage of the red cells through microvessels, leading to tissue ischaemia, painful 'sickling crises' and strokes.

White cells (leukocytes) are rounder and much stiffer than red cells. A leukocyte therefore moves less freely along a microvessel, and often creates a little traffic jam of red cells behind it. During inflammation the leukocytes adhere to the endothelium, particularly in small venules, raising the resistance to flow and impairing tissue perfusion. This happens in inflammation, ischaemia, severe haemorrhagic hypotension and venous leg ulcers.

8.3 Measurement of blood flow

It is often necessary to measure blood flow for research or for clinical evaluation, e.g. of an ischaemic or ulcerated leg. The assessment of human coronary blood flow and other specialized circulation is covered in Chapter 15.

In anaesthetized animals, the velocity of blood in large vessels can be measured by a surgically implanted **electromagnetic velocity meter** (Section 7.5), or by **hot-wire anemometry**, in which the cooling of a heated wire in the bloodstream is proportional to the blood velocity. Blood flow in smaller regions can be assessed by giving a brief intra-arterial injection of **radiolabelled microspheres**, of diameter ~15 μm. The microspheres are washed into the tissue in proportion to local blood flow, and lodge in some of the terminal arterioles. The distribution of flow within the tissue is then assessed by excising the tissue, dicing it into small pieces and counting the radioactivity.

In humans, the method used to measure blood flow depends on the vessel or tissue of interest, as follows.

Doppler ultrasound measures large artery blood velocity

The use of pulsed Doppler ultrasound to measure human aortic blood flow was described in Section 7.3. This non-invasive approach is also widely used to assess placental perfusion in pregnancy, middle cerebral artery blood flow and arterial blood flow in the legs of patients with ischaemic or ulcerative limb disease. A variant of the method, the **laser-Doppler fluxmeter**, employs a laser light beam rather than ultrasound to record the flux of red cells through the superficial dermis.

Fick method measures organ blood flow

The Fick principle was introduced in Section 7.1 as a way of measuring pulmonary blood flow; but it can also be used to measure blood flow in several other organs. To measure **renal blood flow**, para-aminohippuric acid (PAH) is injected intravenously. PAH is almost completely cleared from the renal blood into urine, so the renal venous concentration is taken as zero and the arteriovenous concentration difference equated with the measured arterial concentration. Blood flow is calculated as PAH excretion rate in urine (mg/min) divided by PAH arterial concentration (mg/ml) (the Fick principle).

Venous occlusion plethysmography measures limb blood flow

Plethysmography is a non-invasive research technique that measures blood flow in a human limb, foot or digit (Figure 8.5). To measure forearm blood flow, an inflatable cuff is wrapped around the upper

Figure 8.5 Venous occlusion plethysmography. The 'congesting cuff' (upper arm) occludes venous return; the wrist cuff eliminates hand blood flow from the measurement. The extension of the strain gauge records the increase in forearm circumference due to the continuing arterial inflow; the pulsatile flow can be seen in the trace. The initial swelling rate (tangent to curve, dV/dt) measures forearm blood flow. Swelling rate tails off as venous back-pressure rises. After a few minutes, venous pressure exceeds cuff pressure, so venous outflow resumes and forearm blood volume stabilizes.

arm, overlying the brachial vein, and is inflated suddenly to 40 mmHg. This arrests the venous drainage out of the arm, but not the arterial inflow; so the forearm begins to swell with blood. The initial rate of swelling equals arterial inflow. The swelling is measured by recording the limb circumference, using an electronic strain gauge device wrapped around the forearm. In former years the limb swelling was measured by displacing air or water out of a rigid jacket around the limb, called a plethysmograph ('fullness record') – hence the method's gargantuan name.

Kety's tissue-clearance method measures microvascular blood flow

Microvascular blood flow in a small region of human tissue can be estimated from the rate of washout of a locally injected radioisotope. A rapidly diffusing, radioactive solute is injected as a local, interstitial depot (Figure 8.6). The solute is gradually cleared from the depot by diffusion into the

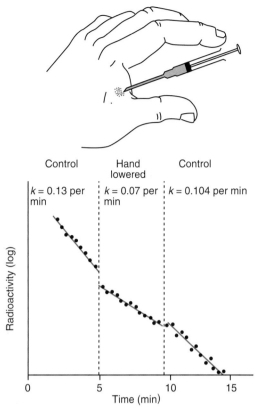

Figure 8.6 Kety's tissue clearance method. Xenon-133 was injected into the skin. With the hand at heart level, the washout slope k was 13% per min (half-life = $0.693/k$ = 5.3 min), from which blood flow was calculated to be 9 ml min^{-1} 100 ml^{-1}. Lowering the hand 40 cm below heart level reduced blood flow to 7 ml min^{-1} 100 ml^{-1}, due to arteriolar constriction (see Chapter 13). (After Lassen NA, Henriksen U, Sejrsen P. In: Shepherd JT, Abboud FM (eds). *Handbook of Physiology, Cardiovascular System*, Vol. 3, Part 1, Peripheral Circulation. Bethesda, MD: American Physiological Society, 1983: 21–64, with permission.)

neighbouring capillaries, which carry the solute away. Removal is recorded by a gamma-counter over the depot. If the solute diffusion rate is fast enough, clearance is limited solely by the capillary blood flow and is directly proportional to the blood flow ('Flow-limited exchange', Section 10.10). A small, lipid-soluble radioisotope, such as xenon-133 or krypton-85, is used to achieve the necessary high diffusion rate. Kety pointed out in 1949 that, given flow-limited exchange, the solute concentration declines exponentially with time, so a plot of the natural logarithm of concentration C against time t is linear (Figure 8.6). Its slope, k, is called the removal rate constant;

$$\log_e C = \log_e C_0 - kt$$

where C_0 is concentration at time zero. The removal rate constant k is proportional to the microvascular flow $\dot{Q}$:

$$k = \dot{Q}/V_D \lambda \qquad (8.3)$$

where V_D is the volume in which the solute is distributed and λ (lambda) is the solute equilibrium partition coefficient between blood and tissue. Microvascular blood flow per unit volume, $\dot{Q}/V_D$, is calculated from slope k.

8.4 The arterial pressure pulse

Basic shape of pulse in central systemic arteries

The ventricle ejects blood into the proximal elastic arteries, namely the aorta and subclavian vessels, faster than the blood can drain away. The resulting expansion of these elastin-rich vessels causes a steep increase in arterial pressure during systole (Figures 8.7 and 8.8). Around 67–80% of the stroke volume is temporarily stored in the elastic arteries during systole, while 20–33% runs off through the peripheral resistance. The mechanical energy stored in the stretched elastin serves to maintain the blood pressure during diastole.

As ventricular ejection wanes, runoff begins to outpace ejection, so blood volume and pressure in the proximal arteries begin to fall. When ejection ceases, a slight backflow closes the aortic valve. Valve closure produces a notch, the **incisura**, in the descending limb of the arterial pressure trace, followed by a brief, high frequency wavelet due to vibration of the tensed aortic valve cusps. In more peripheral arteries, such as the brachial artery, there is a pronounced notch, the dicrotic notch (Greek di[two], crotos[wave]) resulting from a diastolic reflected wave (Figure 8.7), as explained later. As the arterial blood continues to run off through the peripheral resistance vessels, central arterial pressure gradually decays towards its diastolic minimum. Since diastolic decay is slower than the systolic rise, the arterial pressure wave is asymmetrical.

Pulse pressure depends on stroke volume and arterial stiffness

The **pulse pressure** is the difference between diastolic and systolic pressure. The factors governing pulse pressure were explained in Section 7.4,

Figure 8.7 Pressure wave in human subclavian artery (similar to aorta) compared with brachial artery, recorded by electronic transducer over two cardiac cycles. Mean pressure is, formally, $\int(P.dt)/t$ – meaning the sum of (integral sign $\int$) the thousands of thin rectangular strips of individual area $P.dt$, divided by time t; dt is an infinitesimally small unit of time (bottom right). The pressure-time product above mean pressure (pink area above central dashed line) equals that below the mean. In central arteries, mean pressure is halfway between systolic and diastolic pressures. In the brachial artery, the mean is diastolic + one-third pulse pressure, due to the altered shape of the wave. Mean pressure falls by ~2 mmHg between the central artery and brachial artery, providing a mean pressure gradient for flow, even though systolic pressure is higher in the brachial artery. (*Insets*) Abnormal waveform in aortic valve stenosis (slow rise, prolonged plateau) and aortic incompetence (excessive pulse pressure, low diastolic pressure). (After Mills CJ, Gale IT, Gault JH *et al. Cardiovascular Research* 1970; **4**: 405, by permission of Oxford University Press; and Nichols WW, O'Rourke MF. *McDonald's Blood Flow in Arteries*, 5th edn. London: Arnold, 2005.)

but to recapitulate briefly, the primary determinants are:

- **stroke volume**, minus the runoff during the ejection phase; and
- **arterial stiffness (elastance)**, which is 1/compliance (Concept box 7.1).

Thus the greater the stroke volume, the bigger the pulse pressure (Figure 8.8, top); also, the greater the stiffness of the artery wall, the bigger the pulse pressure (Figure 8.8, bottom). Arterial stiffness increases with mean pressure, ejection velocity and age. As **mean pressure** rises, the arterial compliance curve gets steeper (stiffer), so a rise in mean pressure increases the pulse pressure, even if the stroke volume is unchanged (Figure 8.8, middle). Increased **ejection velocity** raises pulse pressure too, because the visco-elastic artery wall has less time to undergo viscous relaxation. This contributes to the increase in pulse pressure during exercise. Ageing is accompanied by **arteriosclerosis**, which increases artery wall stiffness and hence pulse pressure (Figure 8.8,

bottom). The pulse in **chronic hypertension** is described in Section 18.4.

The proximal pulse is transmitted rapidly to the peripheral arteries

If arteries had rigid walls, blood pressure would rise virtually instantaneously throughout the arterial system during systole. Arteries are not rigid, however, so the proximal pressure rise takes a finite time to spread to distal arteries, such as the radial artery. The pulse travels at around 4–5 m/s in young people and 10–15 m/s in the elderly – one of the few things the elderly do faster than the young!

The pulse transmission velocity, 4–15 m/s, is much faster than the blood velocity, which averages ~0.2 m/s in the ascending aorta. One is reminded at this point of the White Queen's suggestion that Alice should practise believing at least six impossible things before breakfast. The difference between pulse transmission velocity and blood velocity is, however, merely difficult to understand,

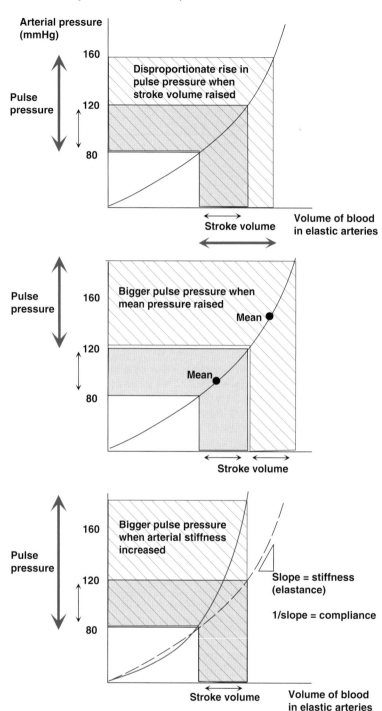

Figure 8.8 Non-linear pressure–volume relation of elastic arteries and effect on pulse pressure. (*Top*) A moderate increase in stroke volume increases pulse pressure disproportionately, because the artery gets stiffer with stretch, i.e. the curve gets steeper. (*Middle*) The same stroke volume ejected at a higher mean pressure (filled circles) causes a bigger pulse pressure, because distension increases the arterial stiffness (elastance). (*Bottom*) An increase in stiffness (e.g. arteriosclerosis of ageing) markedly increases the pulse pressure. Arterial compliance is the reciprocal of the slope.

not impossible (Figure 8.9). Since blood is incompressible, blood ejected into the proximal aorta has to create space for itself. It does this partly by distending the proximal aorta (which raises the blood pressure) and partly by pushing forwards the blood previously occupying the space. As the displaced blood moves forward, it too must make space for itself, which it does partly by distending the wall downstream (which raises the pressure there) and partly by displacing the blood ahead. This shunting sequence repeats itself in rapid succession along the arterial tree. The process can be likened to a railway

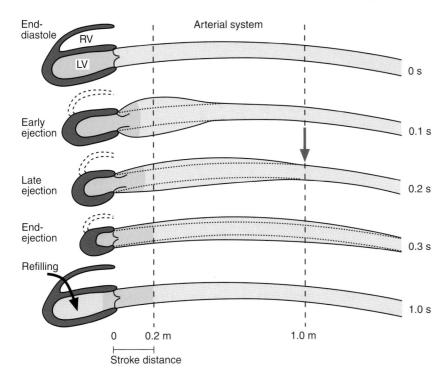

Figure 8.9 Transmission of pressure pulse along human arterial system at 5 m/s. In this example the left ventricle (LV) ejects 100 cm³ blood into an aorta of cross-sectional area 5 cm². The blood advances 20 cm in one beat (*stroke distance*). The wall distension, i.e. the arterial pulse, travels much faster (1 m in 0.2 s), as marked by the red arrow.

engine shunting trucks; the engine may only be moving at 3 mph, but the shunting shock wave travels down the line of wagons much faster. The pulse is thus transmitted by a wave of wall distension at 4–15 m/s, while the ejected blood itself advances just 20 cm (the **stroke distance**) in 1 second.

Since pulse propagation involves wall deformation, the stiffness of the wall affects the transmission velocity; **transmission velocity increases with wall stiffness**. As noted above, arterial stiffness increases with blood pressure and ageing. Consequently, pulse transmission is faster in hypertensive and elderly subjects. The pulse lag time between central and peripheral arteries can be used to estimate human arterial distensibility.

The shape of the pulse alters with ageing and pathophysiological state

Depending on age and pathophysiological status, the pressure wave in a human proximal artery may show two additional features, namely a **diastolic wave** or a **systolic inflection** (Figure 8.10). These features can affect cardiac performance, as explained later.

Reflection causes a diastolic wave in the young

In children, young adults and many mammals, the decay of pressure in diastole is interrupted by a small bump, i.e. a transient rise in pressure, called a diastolic or dicrotic wave. This is not present in older people, in whom pressure falls off exponentially after the incisura. The diastolic wave is caused by **wave reflection**. The initial systolic pressure wave travels rapidly down the arterial tree and reaches the major branches and resistance vessels in a fraction of a second. The branch points and resistance vessels partially reflect the wave, sending an attenuated pressure wave back up the arterial tree (inset, Figure 8.10). Since the wave velocity is ~4 m/s in young humans, and the distance to major reflection sites such as the aortic bifurcation is ~0.5 m, and the cardiac cycle lasts ~1 s, the reflected wave returns to the proximal arteries in time to interact with the initiating or **incident wave**. This creates the diastolic wave in young subjects (Figure 8.10b). An everyday analogy is the reflection of an incoming sea wave by a harbour wall; as the reflected wave travels back out to sea, it meets an incoming wave and the two waves summate briefly into a tall peak. The time interval between the foot (start) of the incident wave and the inflection marking arrival of the reflected wave can be used to estimate wave velocity, and hence arterial stiffness, in humans.

Reflection causes a systolic inflection in the elderly or hypertensive patients

The central arteries of ageing humans and hypertensive patients are stiffer than in young subjects,

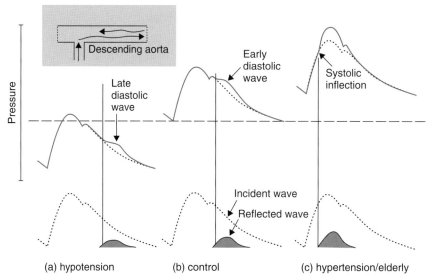

Figure 8.10 Changes in aortic pulse due to wave reflection. The observed pulse (red) is composed of two components, shown below: the basic or 'incident' wave and the reflected wave. Time from foot of incident wave to arrival of reflected wave depends on transmission velocity. (a) In hypotension, or after a vasodilator drug, the low pressure reduces arterial stiffness (Figure 8.8, middle). This slows pulse wave propagation, so the reflected wave occurs in late diastole. (b) At normal pressure and arterial stiffness in a young human or rabbit, faster pulse transmission causes an early diastolic reflected wave. (c) In hypertensive or elderly humans, or a normal subject after a vasoconstrictor drug, the raised arterial stiffness and transmission velocity cause a systolic reflected wave, which creates a systolic inflection. Pattern (b) can be generated from (c) by vasodilator drugs, e.g. glyceryl trinitrate. (*Inset*) Model of arterial system as an asymmetric T-tube. Short limb on left represents all arteries of upper body; long limb on right represents lower body; ends represent the average of all the reflection sites in the upper and lower body, respectively. (After Nichols WW, O'Rourke MF. *McDonald's Blood Flow in Arteries*, 5th edn. London: Arnold, 2005.)

so the incident and reflected waves travel faster. As a result, the reflected wave arrives back in the aorta in late systole rather than diastole (Figure 8.10c). Consequently, elderly humans lack a diastolic wave. Instead, the reflected wave adds to the late part of the incident systolic wave, raising the peak systolic pressure and creating a kink or **inflection** in the systolic wave.

The waveform alters in pathophysiological states

Whether the central pulse has a diastolic wave or a systolic inflection depends on (i) the degree of reflection by peripheral vessels, which is increased by vasoconstriction and reduced by vasodilatation; and (ii) pulse transmission velocity, which increases with ageing and mean blood pressure. Since clinical hypotension and vasodilator drugs lower blood pressure, and therefore artery wall stiffness (Figure 8.8), the reflected waves travel more slowly (Figure 8.10a). As a result, the systolic inflection of middle-aged/elderly humans is replaced by a diastolic wave during hypotension. This is also one of the effects of the anti-angina vasodilator, **glyceryl trinitrate** (see below). Conversely, raising blood pressure by a vasoconstrictor drug causes the reflected wave to return faster, which can transform a pulse with a low

systolic pressure and diastolic wave (Figure 8.10a or b) into one with a high systolic pressure, a systolic inflection and no diastolic wave (Figure 8.10c).

Why wave reflection matters

Reflected waves are important because they affect coronary blood flow and cardiac work. In young humans and many animals, the slow return of the reflected wave augments the diastolic pressure, which boosts coronary artery perfusion. By contrast, in elderly or hypertensive subjects the early return of the reflected wave increases systolic pressure (**systolic pressure augmentation**). The left ventricle therefore has to eject blood against an increased afterload, which increases cardiac work and O_2 demand. The properties of the artery wall thus affect cardiac O_2 demand.

Aortic stiffness increases cardiac O_2 demand

In young humans, the high distensibility of the aorta and proximal arteries keeps systolic pressure low, which in turn reduces cardiac work and O_2 demand. In older subjects, the stiff arterial system raises systolic pressure, both directly and through systolic pressure augmentation (Figure 8.10c), and this increases cardiac work and O_2 demand. It has been shown experimentally that the O_2 consumption of a dog heart ejecting through a rigid plastic tube is much higher than when ejecting through the aorta. The therapeutic benefit of **glyceryl trinitrate**, a vasodilator used to treat angina (cardiac pain due to oxygen demand exceeding supply), is partly due to the fact that it relaxes large arteries, as well as veins, and to a lesser degree resistance vessels. Large artery relaxation increases arterial compliance and reduces systolic augmentation by wave reflection. The resulting fall in systolic pressure reduces afterload and cardiac O_2 demand, and so contributes to the relief of angina (Section 15.1).

The shape of the pulse changes as it travels into peripheral arteries

As the pressure wave passes into the peripheral arteries, its shape changes in a surprising way; it grows taller in the named, peripheral arteries of young humans and dogs, rather than damping out as one might imagine (Figure 1.10, top; Figures 8.7 and 8.11). For example, systolic pressure is higher in the brachial artery than in the aorta, in young to middle-aged humans. Four features of the pressure wave change.

- The systolic pressure wave grows taller, rather like a sea wave approaching the beach. This **pressure amplification** can be as much as 60% in the femoral artery of young humans. Pressure amplification is less marked in middle-aged humans and is absent in the elderly (Figure 8.11).
- The incisura is damped out and disappears.
- The mean pressure falls only slightly, by ~2 mmHg between the ascending aorta and radial artery, showing that large arteries account for only ~2% of the total peripheral resistance.
- A new pressure wave appears in late diastole, the dicrotic wave, preceded by a pronounced dicrotic notch (Figures 8.7 and 8.11).

These complex changes are caused by a combination of factors: increased arterial stiffness with distance, faster transmission of the higher pressure components, aortic taper (the abdominal aorta is roughly half as wide as the ascending aorta) and wave reflection. The pulse pressure continues to increase as far as third- or fourth-generation arteries, such as the radial artery. Beyond this, the pulse becomes progressively damped out by the viscous properties of the vessel wall and blood (Figure 1.10, top). The pressure oscillations dwindle and the flow becomes more continuous as the blood enters the resistance vessels.

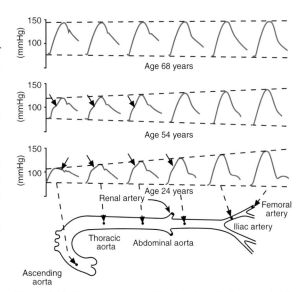

Figure 8.11 Pressure wave amplification along the human arterial tree, and its dependence on age. Distal pressure amplification is ~60% in the young but is negligible in the elderly. Arrows show systolic inflection, marking arrival of reflected wave. (After Nichols WW, O'RourkeMF. *McDonald's Blood Flow in Arteries*, 5th edn. London: Arnold, 2005.)

Clinical abnormalities of the pulse

Aortic valve stenosis. Narrowing of the aortic valve by fibrosis results in a slow, prolonged ejection phase. Arterial pressure rises sluggishly and has an abnormal plateau (Figures 2.8, top and 8.7, top).

Aortic valve incompetence. Diastolic reflux into the ventricle causes the arterial pressure to decay abnormally quickly. As a result the pulse pressure may be twice normal, causing relaxed limbs to jerk in time with the throbbing pulse (Figures 2.8, bottom and 8.7, top).

Pulsus paradoxus is a condition in which the pulse pressure falls by more than 10 mmHg during each inspiration. This is not really a 'paradox' at all; it is an exaggeration of the normal inspiratory fall (see 'Traube–Hering waves', next section). Pulsus paradoxus is generally caused by **cardiac tamponade** (pressure around the heart), due to constrictive pericarditis or an accumulation of a fluid in the pericardial cavity. Tamponade sets a fixed limit to the combined volume of the two ventricles inside the pericardial sac. During inspiration, the fall in intrathoracic pressure increases the flow of venous blood into the right ventricle, increasing the right ventricular volume. Since the total volume is limited by the tamponade, the rise in right ventricular volume reduces the left ventricular volume.

Thus left ventricular stroke volume and systolic pressure decline excessively during inspiration.

Pulsus alternans is a pulse that is alternately strong and weak; the pulse pressure is reduced every other beat. This is caused by oscillation of the size of the myocyte Ca^{2+} store, and is generally a sign of severe left ventricular failure.

8.5 Mean arterial pressure and pressure measurement

What does 'mean' pressure mean?

The time-averaged mean is the area under the pressure wave ($\int P.dt$) divided by time. In routine clinical practice, however, only systolic and diastolic pressures are measured, usually in the brachial artery rather than aorta. In the aorta, mean pressure $\overline{P}_a$ is approximately halfway between systolic and diastolic pressures, i.e. it is the arithmetic average (Figure 8.7, middle trace). In the brachial artery, however, the narrowing of the systolic peak, caused by distal transmission, shifts the time-averaged mean in the diastolic direction (Figure 8.7, bottom trace), and the mean pressure is approximately diastolic pressure plus one-third of the pulse pressure:

$$\text{Mean brachial artery pressure } \overline{P}_a = P_{diastolic} + \frac{P_{systolic} - P_{diastolic}}{3}$$

(8.4)

For example, if the brachial artery pressure is $110/80\,\text{mmHg}$, the pulse pressure is $30\,\text{mmHg}$ and the mean pressure is $90\,\text{mmHg}$. In the aorta, where the wave is less 'peaky', the mean is simply $(P_{diastolic} + P_{systolic})/2$.

What determines mean arterial blood pressure?

As explained in Section 8.1, Darcy's law tells us that two factors determine the mean arterial pressure, namely the cardiac output and the total peripheral resistance:

$$\text{Mean blood pressure } \overline{P}_a = \text{Cardiac output} \times \text{Total peripheral resistance TPR}$$

(8.5)

This is called the **mean blood pressure equation**. The mean blood pressure equation can be combined with the pulse pressure eqn 7.4 and brachial pressure eqn 8.4 to tell us how high the systolic pressure rises and how low the diastolic pressure falls for a given cardiac output and peripheral resistance. For example, the brachial systolic pressure is given by:

$$P_{systolic} = (SV.HR.TPR) + 2(SV - R_{off})/3C.$$

where SV is stroke volume, HR heart rate, R_{off} volume runoff during ejection and C arterial compliance.

Direct measurement of arterial pressure
Principle of manometry

Arterial pressure was first measured by Stephen Hales, the vicar of Teddington, near London, in 1773. Hales connected a 3-metre, vertical glass tube to the carotid artery of a horse via a goose trachea, and noted the height to which the blood rose in the tube (manometry). A century later, the French medical physicist JLM Poiseuille developed the smaller **mercury manometer**, which remained in routine use until very recently. The principle of manometry is that the column of fluid in a vertical tube exerts a downward pressure at the base, which is connected to the pressure source that is being measured (Figures 8.1 and 8.2). When the column height h is stable, the pressure at the bottom of the fluid column must be equal to the pressure to which it is connected. The pressure at the bottom of a column of fluid is ρgh (fluid density $\rho \times$ force of gravity $g \times h$). Since mercury is very dense, $13.6\,\text{g/ml}$, a column ~$100\,\text{mm}$ high is sufficient to balance the mean arterial blood pressure at heart level. Using his new mercury manometer, Poiseuille was the first to show that there is little change in mean pressure along the arterial system, and therefore little resistance to flow along named, macroscopic arteries.

Electronic pressure transducers

A mercury column has too much inertia to follow the rapidly changing waveform of a single pulse; it just records average pressure. To record the waveform, a fast-responding, electronic pressure transducer is connected, via a stiff, fluid-filled tube, to an intra-arterial cannula. The electronic pressure transducer was developed by the American scientists Lambert and Wood during aviation research in World War II. The transducer contains a thin metal diaphragm, which deforms slightly under pressure, changing the electrical resistance. The thin diaphragm is able to follow fast changes in pressure. The electrical signal, however, has to be calibrated against a column of liquid, so blood pressure is still reported in mmHg or cmH$_2$O rather than pascal. Conversion factors are given in Appendix 2 'Pressure'.

Indirect measurement of human blood pressure using the sphygmomanometer

Human blood pressure is usually measured in the brachial artery, using a non-invasive method called **sphygmomanometry**. This is based on the principle that a soft, healthy artery is readily compressed by external pressure (Figure 8.12). An inflatable rubber sac inside a cotton sleeve, called a **Riva–Rocci sphygmomanometer cuff**, is wound around the upper arm. The inflatable sac must be located medially over the brachial artery and the artery must be at heart level, with the subject seated. The cuff is inflated progressively, squeezing the soft tissues of the upper arm, until the brachial artery is occluded, as judged by the disappearance of a palpable radial pulse. This might require a pressure of >180 mmHg in an elderly subject. Until recently the cuff pressure was measured by a mercury manometer, but this has been replaced in modern instruments by a dial gauge, calibrated in mmHg by the manufacturer. A stethoscope is then placed over the brachial artery in the antecubital fossa (hollow of the elbow). No sound is heard at this stage, because no blood is flowing. Cuff pressure is then gradually lowered, using a screw-valve, until the following sequence of sounds is heard.

1 When cuff pressure falls just below systolic pressure, the artery opens briefly during each systole. The transient spurts of blood vibrate the artery wall, creating a dull tapping noise called a **Korotkoff sound**. The pressure at which the Korotkoff sound first appears is conventionally accepted as systolic pressure, though it is actually ~10 mmHg below the true value.

2 As the cuff pressure is lowered further, the Korotkoff sounds grow louder, because the intermittent spurts of blood grow stronger.

3 When cuff pressure is close to diastolic pressure, the artery remains patent for most of the cardiac cycle and the vessel vibration diminishes. This causes a rapid diminution of the Korotkoff sounds. The cuff pressure at which this happens used to be the accepted measure of the diastolic pressure, although it is ~8 mmHg higher than true diastolic pressure. A faint Korotkoff sound may persist below this and complete silence may not be attained until 8–10 mmHg below the true diastolic pressure. The British Hypertension Society currently recommends the point of silence as the reported diastolic pressure.

In some hypertensive patients there is a silent period within the systolic–diastolic pressure range, which could cause systolic hypertension to be missed. It is important, therefore, when first inflating the cuff, to palpate the radial artery and note the pressure at which the pulse disappears. This is a good measure of systolic pressure and guards against failure to diagnose a case of systolic hypertension.

The measured brachial artery pressure may differ from aortic pressure. As noted earlier, the pulse pressure is amplified as it travels along the arterial tree, except in the elderly (Figure 8.11). Consequently, brachial artery systolic pressure overestimates aortic systolic pressure, by up to 20 mmHg in resting, young to middle-aged subjects (Figure 8.7). When the blood pressure is altered by drugs, brachial artery measurements may underestimate the aortic pressure response, owing to changes in wave reflection.

Ankle-brachial pressure index (ABPI) assesses ischaemic leg disease. Human leg arteries are a common site for atheroma, leading to peripheral ischaemia. To assess the state of the leg arteries, blood pressure is measured in the foot. A Riva–Rocci cuff above the ankle is inflated to occlude the tibial artery, and blood flow in a distal artery such as the dorsalis pedis (foot) is recorded by

Figure 8.12 Measurement of human blood pressure. (a) Dashed line shows compression of brachial artery by sphygmomanometer cuff SC. Cuff pressure is controlled by the rubber bulb (RB). Cuff pressure was measured for generations by a mercury column, but recent instruments use a dial gauge. (b) Korotkoff sounds begin when cuff pressure is reduced to just below systolic pressure. They cease when cuff pressure is below diastolic pressure.

Doppler ultrasound as cuff pressure is lowered. The pressure at which distal flow restarts in the tibial artery is called the ankle systolic pressure. Ankle systolic pressure divided by brachial artery systolic pressure, the ABPI, is normally ≥1. An ABPI of <0.8 indicates substantial upstream arterial stenosis by atheroma. This leads to poor peripheral perfusion, pallor, **intermittent claudication** (pain on walking, relieved by rest) and **arterial ulcers**. An ABPI of ≤0.4 is associated with pain at rest and eventually **gangrene**. The ABPI is important for distinguishing between arterial ulcers and venous ulcers (ABPI ~1), since venous ulcers are treated by compression bandaging, which would be harmful in the presence of an impaired arterial supply. If the tibial artery is hardened, as in **diabetes**, a higher-than-normal cuff pressure has to be applied to compress the stiff artery, resulting in false high estimates of tibial artery pressure and an ABPI of >1.2.

Indirect, automated measurement of human blood pressure

Automated oscillometric cuff systems, such as the Dinamap, report brachial artery diastolic, systolic and mean pressure. An electronic system records not the Korotkoff sounds but the pulsing air pressure in the Riva–Rocci cuff, caused by the pulsation of the underlying brachial artery. An electrical pump first inflates the cuff to above systolic pressure. Since the artery is completely occluded, there is little oscillation in cuff pressure. The cuff is then automatically deflated. As the cuff pressure falls just below systolic pressure, the artery under the cuff begins to pulse, causing cuff pressure to oscillate. As cuff pressure is reduced further, the oscillation increases, reaching a maximum at mean arterial pressure. The pulsation drops to a minimum at diastolic pressure. These **oscillation criteria** are used to record the pressures electronically.

A different principle, called **volume clamp**, is used in intensive care units to record digital artery

What determines arterial pressure?

- Mean arterial pressure is determined by the cardiac output (CO) and the total peripheral resistance (TPR). From Darcy's law (Concept box 1.1), mean pressure = $CO \times TPR$. Clinical hypertension is caused by a rise in TPR, whereas hypotension is often due to a fall in CO.
- Systolic and diastolic pressures are determined by the size of the oscillation about the mean pressure.
- The size of the oscillation, or pulse pressure, is determined by the stroke volume SV and arterial compliance C. See Concept box 7.1.
- In the long term, the kidneys are crucial regulators of mean blood pressure, because they regulate the plasma volume and hence the cardiac filling pressure.

CONCEPT BOX 8.1

pressure continuously and non-invasively (the Finapress). The finger is enclosed in an inflatable cuff and changes in finger volume are monitored by infrared light transmission. Finger volume normally oscillates slightly with each arterial pulse. The volume signal is fed back to a pump, which increases its output to the finger cuff each time the artery pulses, just enough to 'clamp' the volume at a constant level. The cuff pressure is thus enslaved to the arterial pressure. The enslaved pressure is measured electronically and displayed continuously on a monitor, along with an estimate of cardiac output by the pulse pressure method (Section 7.4).

What is the 'normal' blood pressure?

That mythological polymath, 'every schoolboy', knows that 'normal' human blood pressure is 120/80 mmHg. For the brachial artery of a young adult under certain conditions, he would be right; but it is wrong to adopt 120/80 mmHg as the normal standard for a resting child, a pregnant woman in midterm or an elderly man. Blood pressure is actually quite labile over 24 hours (Figure 8.13), and the factors affecting it include the following.

Figure 8.13 Continuous record of human arterial blood pressure over 24 h. Sleep (red period) reduced blood pressure. A painful stimulus at 16.00 h and sexual intercourse at 24.00 h markedly raised pressure. (From Bevan AT, Honour AJ, Scott FH. *Clinical Science* 1969; **36**: 329, by permission.) © The Biochemical Society.

Age

Human blood pressure increases with age, averaging 105/65 mmHg at 10 years, 120/70 mmHg at 30 years and 140/75 mmHg at 70 years (Figure 17.10). The large increase in pulse pressure with age is caused by arteriosclerosis (not to be confused with atheroma, Table 17.4). As a very rough rule-of-thumb, systolic pressure is 90 mmHg plus age in years.

Activity; sleep and exercise

Blood pressure can fall as low as 80/50 mmHg during sleep (Figure 8.13). Conversely, in heavy, dynamic exercise, mean pressure increases by 10–40 mmHg. In heavy, resistive exercise, such as weightlifting, the pressure can increase by over 100 mmHg.

Gravity and standing: the giraffe's nightmare

Pressure increases equally in arteries and veins below heart level, due to the weight of the column of blood between the heart and blood vessel (Figure 8.2). For a fluid column of height h, the increase in pressure is $\rho g h$; see 'Principle of manometry' earlier. In the human foot ~115 cm below heart level, arterial blood pressure will increase by 122 cmH$_2$O (blood being 1.06 times denser than water). This is 90 mmHg (mercury is 13.6 times denser than water). Therefore, if mean aortic pressure at heart level is 95 mmHg, arterial pressure in the foot will be almost $90 + 95 = 185$ mmHg; it will actually be ~2 mmHg less than this, due to the slight arterial resistance to flow. Conversely, pressure falls in arteries above heart level, and is only 60 mmHg in the human brain during standing. Our gravitational problems are small, however, compared with the giraffe. Because the giraffe head is so far above heart level, the heart has to generate an aortic pressure of ~200 mmHg to ensure adequate cerebral perfusion.

Gravity and standing: indirect effects

On moving from lying to standing, changes in cardiac output and peripheral resistance lead to changes in arterial pressure. An initial, transient fall in arterial pressure can produce a passing dizziness (postural hypotension). This is followed by a small but sustained reflex rise in pressure (Section 17.1).

Emotion and stress

Anger, apprehension, fear, stress and sexual excitement are all potent 'pressor' stimuli, i.e. they elevate blood pressure (Figure 8.13). A formal meeting, such as visit to the doctor, can raise blood pressure by 20 mmHg ('white coat hypertension'), so a solitary high value is not diagnostic of clinical hypertension; the measurement must be repeated later, with the patient relaxed. The pressor effect of stress is particularly harmful to patients with ischaemic heart disease, as the cautionary tale of John Hunter in Section 6.14 illustrates.

Regular oscillations in mean arterial blood pressure

Mean blood pressure oscillates in time with breathing (**Traube–Hering waves**). Pressure falls by a few mmHg during each inspiration, because left ventricular stroke volume declines as the lung vascular bed expands. Although inspiration also raises the heart rate (sinus arrhythmia, Section 5.8), this compensates only partially for the fall in stroke volume, so human cardiac output and blood pressure fall during inspiration. In dogs, by contrast, the pressure rises during inspiration, because the inspiratory tachycardia outweighs the fall in stroke volume.

In addition to respiration-related oscillations, arterial pressure may show regular oscillations at a lower frequency of ~6/min (0.1 Hz), called **Mayer waves**. These are due to synchronous oscillations in sympathetic vasoconstrictor activity. The sympathetic oscillation is thought to result from a slow feedback by the baroreflex (Chapter 16).

Other factors

The **Valsalva manoeuvre**, which is a forced expiration against a closed or narrowed glottis, triggers a complex sequence of raised blood pressures (Section 17.2). In **pregnancy**, the blood pressure falls to a minimum at ~6 months, due to the expansion of the uterine and other vascular beds. Consequently, in obstetrical practice a pressure of 130/90 mmHg at 6 months gestation would cause grave concern. Many **pathological processes** also alter arterial pressure, such as dehydration, haemorrhage, shock, syncope (fainting), chronic hypertension, acute heart failure and valvular lesions, such as aortic incompetence.

It is clear from the above survey that **the criteria for assessing whether blood pressure is normal must be adjusted for the individual's age, physiological and psychological condition**.

8.6 Pulsatile flow

Blood flow is almost stop–go in the aorta and major arteries, e.g. femoral artery (Figure 8.14). Darcy's law cannot predict the flow at a given instant in the cardiac cycle, because Darcy's law is a steady-state expression; it can only describe mean flow over many cardiac cycles. When flow is pulsatile, the flow at a given instant is governed by Newton's second law of motion, namely acceleration = force/mass.

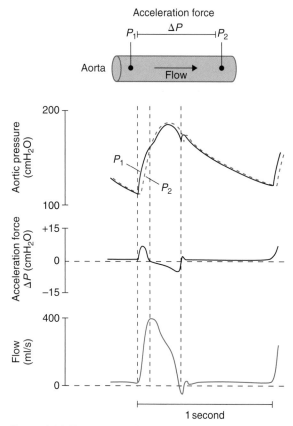

Figure 8.14 Flow, acceleration and pressure gradients in the human ascending aorta. The pressure difference ΔP at first accelerates flow along the aorta, then reverses and decelerates flow until a brief backflow closes the aortic valve. Proximal aortic flow is almost zero during diastole. (After Snell RE, Clements JM, Patel DJ, Fry DL, Luchsinger PC. *Journal of Applied Physiology* 1965; **20**: 691, with permission from the American Physiological Society.)

During systole, the pressure (force per unit area) rises first in the proximal aorta, creating a pressure gradient from the proximal aorta to the peripheral arteries (Figure 8.14, top trace). This accelerates the blood (Figure 8.14, middle trace). The pressure pulse then spreads distally, reaching the radial artery in ~0.1 s. At this moment in time, the distal pressure is transiently higher than the proximal pressure, which is tailing off. As a result, the pressure gradient is now reversed, and decelerates the flow. Thus, flow in the major arteries first accelerates and then decelerates over the initial third of the cardiac cycle. Proximal aortic flow actually reverses briefly as the aortic valve closes, and is very low throughout diastole (Figure 8.14, bottom trace).

The period of near zero flow gradually shortens as blood enters smaller arteries, and in the smallest arteries the flow becomes continuous, albeit still pulsatile (Figure 1.10, middle trace).

8.7 Peripheral resistance, Poiseuille's law and Laplace wall mechanics

The resistance of the systemic circulation to flow is located chiefly in the tiny terminal arteries and arterioles (Section 1.7; Concept box 1.1). Total peripheral resistance is the pressure drop required to drive unit flow through the systemic circulation (eqn 8.1b), namely ~1 mmHg per ml per second in a resting adult, or 1 peripheral resistance unit. But what factors determine the resistance to flow?

Poiseuille's law describes the hydraulic resistance of a tube

Resistance to flow arises exclusively from the internal friction within the fluid. It is not caused by friction at the tube wall, because there is no flow at the wall surface, owing to the zero-slip condition (Figure 8.3, laminar flow). Resistance is nevertheless greatly affected by tube radius, because the rate at which one lamina slides past the adjacent one (the shear rate) is greater in narrow tubes than wide tubes, for a given flow. High shear rates require more force and thus a bigger pressure gradient; and resistance is by definition the pressure gradient required to produce unit flow.

The factors governing tube resistance were first elucidated by the Parisian physician Jean Leonard Marie Poiseuille, around 1840, in a meticulous study of water flowing through glass capillary tubes. By studying the steady, laminar flow of a Newtonian fluid (water, plasma) along a straight cylindrical tube, Poiseuille established that the **resistance R is inversely proportional to tube radius raised to the fourth power, r^4.** Also, resistance is directly proportional to fluid viscosity η and tube length L:

$$R = \frac{8\eta L}{\pi r^4} \qquad (8.6)$$

Combining this expression with Darcy's law of flow (eqn 8.1a), and recalling that conductance K is $1/R$, we get an expression for flow through a tube called **'Poiseuille's law'**:

$$\dot{Q} = (P_1 - P_2)K = (P_1 - P_2)\frac{\pi r^4}{8\eta L} \qquad (8.7)$$

Poiseuille's law tells us that tissue blood flow is extremely sensitive to the radius of the resistance vessels, namely the terminal arteries and arterioles.

Figure 8.15 Basic rules of hydraulics. When vessels are linked in series (e.g. feed artery–terminal artery–arteriole), each adds to the resistance to the flow; net resistance is high. When vessels are linked in parallel, as in a capillary bed, their flow-transmitting capabilities (conductances) add up, so the net resistance is low.

Since these smooth muscle-rich vessels can change their radius actively, they can utilize the powerful Poiseuille relation to regulate local tissue perfusion.

Resistances in series versus in parallel

Poiseuille's law describes flow along a single tube. When several tubes are joined together in **series** (end-to-end), for example, a terminal artery and an arteriole, their total resistance R_{total} is the sum of the individual resistances (Figure 8.15, top). The sum of resistance is written as ΣR (Greek capital sigma, Σ, means 'sum of all individual values'). Thus in a series array, R_{total} equals ΣR.

If several tubes are arranged in **parallel**, as in a capillary bed, a given driving pressure will produce more flow than it would through a single tube, because the conducting capacities of the tubes summate (Figure 8.15, bottom). The net conductance is the sum of the individual conductances, ΣK. Since resistance is the reciprocal of conductance, the net resistance is $1/\Sigma K$. In parallel arrays, therefore, $R_{total} = 1/\Sigma K$. To summarize the rule, 'For series arrays, add the resistances; for parallel arrays, add the conductances'. The summation of huge numbers of conductances in parallel contributes to the surprisingly low hydraulic resistance of the capillary bed.

Armed with Poiseuille's law, plus the basic rules for vessels in series and in parallel, we can now consider the systemic resistance, which resides chiefly in the arterioles and tiniest arteries.

Arteriolar radius regulates both local blood flow and central arterial pressure

Vascular resistance is exquisitely sensitive to radius, due to the r^4 relation in Poiseuille's law. The difference in radius between the human aorta (1 cm) and a single arteriole (0.01 cm) represents a one hundred million-fold increase in resistance. This is why the arterioles and terminal arteries are the main sites of resistance. A mere 19% increase in the radius of the resistance vessels will double the low blood flow, due to the r^4 effect.

The radius of a resistance vessel is actively regulated by the tunica media smooth muscle. Contraction narrows the lumen (vasoconstriction) and relaxation widens it (vasodilatation). When constriction occurs throughout the body, the total peripheral resistance increases, raising **arterial blood pressure** at a given cardiac output (Figure 8.16). Conversely, widespread vasodilatation, as in endotoxin shock, lowers blood pressure. Widespread changes in resistance vessel tone are thus a powerful way of regulating arterial blood pressure (eqn 8.5). By contrast, if the changes in vessel tone are confined to a single organ or tissue, the **local blood flow** to that organ is altered (eqn 8.1a), without greatly affecting *TPR* or blood pressure. For example, during eating, a 1.8-fold dilatation of the salivary gland resistance vessels increases their perfusion ten-fold (the r^4 effect); but, since the salivary glands account for only a tiny fraction of the *TPR*, there is

Figure 8.16 Changes in pressure distribution across the circulation caused by widespread vasoconstriction/vasodilatation of resistance vessels (terminal arteries and arterioles, resistance R_a). Vasoconstriction raises arterial pressure (P_A), at a given cardiac output, because blood escapes less easily from the upstream arteries through the raised downstream resistance. Vasoconstriction also reduces capillary pressure P_C, because more pressure is lost as blood traverses the raised precapillary resistance R_a; less pressure 'gets through'. Conversely, a widespread vasodilatation tends to lower arterial pressure and raise capillary pressure.

no significant change in *TPR* or arterial blood pressure.

Capillaries are even narrower than arterioles, so the resistance of a single capillary is bigger than that of an arteriole. Yet the pressure drop across the whole capillary network, 20–30 mmHg, is less than that across the arteriolar network, 40–50 mmHg (Figure 8.16), i.e. the capillary network has the smaller resistance. How can this be? The low net capillary resistance is due to: (i) the vast number of capillaries arranged in parallel ($R_{total} = 1/\Sigma K$, Figure 8.15); (ii) the shortness of capillaries, ~500 µm (length L in eqn 8.7); and (iii) bolus flow in capillaries, which reduces the effective blood viscosity (η in eqn 8.7).

Laplace's law links radius, wall tension and pressure

The radius of a distensible tube depends on three mechanical factors (Figure 8.17):

- the **internal pressure** distending it (P_i)
- the **outside pressure** compressing it (P_o)
- the **circumferential wall tension**, i.e. force per unit length of vessel (T).

Flow through a tube; Poiseuille's law

- The conductance of a tube is the flow per unit pressure drop.
- Poiseuille's law states that the conductance of a tube of radius r is proportional to r^4, and inversely proportional to fluid viscosity η and vessel length L. The conductance is $\pi r^4/8\eta L$.
- For tubes connected in parallel, the conductances add up. Thus the conductance of the capillary bed is high.
- The inverse of conductance is resistance. Resistance is $8\eta L/\pi r^4$. For tubes connected in series, the resistances add up, e.g. small arteries and arterioles.
- Due to the r^4 relation, active changes in arteriolar calibre have a very powerful effect on local blood flow, and on total peripheral resistance and mean arterial pressure.
- Blood viscosity η depends chiefly on the haematocrit. The effective viscosity falls in microvessels (the Fåhraeus–Lindqvist effect), which reduces microvascular resistance and conserves cardiac energy.

CONCEPT BOX 8.2

When the radius is stable (a state called mechanical equilibrium), the circumferential wall tension exactly counteracts the transmural pressure difference,

Vasoconstriction

Vasodilatation

Figure 8.17 Wall mechanics in a tube of unit length. (*Upper panel*) Pressure equals force per unit area. Internal pressure P_i pushes outwards on area $2r$, driving the two halves of the cylinder apart with force $P_i 2r$. External pressure P_o exerts force $P_o 2r$ in the opposite direction. The net distending force, $P_i 2r - P_o 2r$, is countered by the wall tension T on each side of the cylinder. Thus $2T = P_i 2r - P_o 2r$, or $T = (P_i - P_o)r$ (Laplace's law). (*Lower panels*) Tension T is the sum of active tension in smooth muscle, T_a, and passive tension in elastin/collagen fibres, T_p, shown as a spring. The spring on the left is in its relaxed state and that on the right is stretched and tense. T_a and T_p change in opposite directions during vasoconstriction to achieve mechanical stability.

$P_i - P_o$ (Figure 8.17) . The equilibrium wall tension is given by **Laplace's law**, which we met earlier in relation to ventricular wall tension (Section 6.8). For a thin-walled tube, the Laplace equation is:

$$T = (P_i - P_o)r \qquad (8.8)$$

Laplace's law thus states that **the bigger the vessel radius, the bigger the wall tension** needed to counter a given transmural pressure difference. For example, wall tension is higher in the aorta than in named arteries with a similar pressure, and capillary wall tension is very low (Figure 8.18). Laplace's law helps us understand why an **aortic aneurysm** (bulging of a weak aortic wall) progresses inexorably, once started. The increase in r raises the tension T in the aneurysm wall; the high tension thins and weakens the wall. This increases r, and so on. The positive feedback eventually leads to wall rupture, with catastrophic consequences.

A slightly more elaborate version of Laplace's law, called Love's equation, takes into account wall thickness, w (Appendix 2). Wall thickness is important because it affects the **wall stress**, S, which is the force per unit wall area; $S = T/w$ for unit length of vessel. The aorta has a thick wall, so although the wall tension is high, it is shared between many cells, collagen and elastin fibres, reducing the stress on them. By contrast, the capillary wall is only $\sim 0.3\,\mu m$ thick, so capillary wall stress approaches that in many arteries, despite the low capillary blood pressure and wall tension (Figure 8.18, bottom). Indeed, capillary wall stress in the human foot during standing actually exceeds that in the aorta – highlighting the extraordinary strength of the capillary wall.

Changes in wall tension bring about constriction and dilatation

The total tension T in the artery wall has two components: the passive tension of the elastin and collagen fibrils, and the active tension exerted by smooth muscle cells. When the smooth muscle contracts, its immediate effect is to raise the wall tension T. This produces a temporary mechanical disequilibrium, so the radius begins to decrease. Laplace's law tells us that, if the transmural pressure $P_i - P_o$ is constant and radius r falls, a new mechanical equilibrium can only be attained by reducing the **net** (total) wall tension T. A fall in net wall tension is achieved by unloading the passive fibrils; the tension in the collagen and elastin fibres falls as the vessel radius is reduced (Figure 8.17). There is in effect a transfer of tension from the passive fibres to the active muscle cells. Without this, vasoconstriction would be an extremely unstable process.

Conversely, vasodilatation is brought about by smooth muscle relaxation. This reduces the active tension, creating a temporary mechanical disequilibrium. The internal distending pressure then pushes the wall out to a bigger radius, until a point is

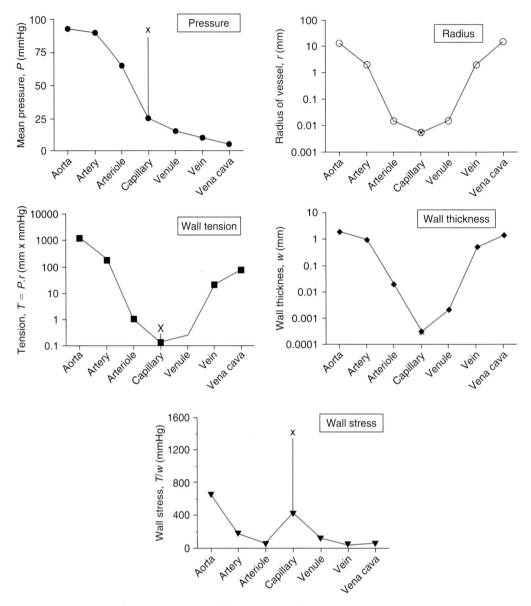

Figure 8.18 Pressure, radius, wall tension and stress in different categories of blood vessel at heart level (Laplace's law). Vessel wall thickness affects stress, which is tension/thickness. Crosses represent capillaries in foot during quiet standing, when gravity raises capillary pressure to ~90 mmHg.

reached where the increased tension of the stretched collagen and elastin re-establishes mechanical equilibrium (Figure 8.17).

8.8 Viscous properties of blood

Poiseuille's law tells us that vascular resistance depends not just on vessel geometry but also on the viscosity of the perfusing liquid, blood. Blood viscosity is altered in many haematological diseases, leading to changes in blood flow and pressure.

Viscosity represents the internal friction in a fluid

The word viscosity stems from 'viscum', Latin for mistletoe, because mistletoe berries contain a thick, glutinous fluid. Viscosity was defined by Isaac Newton as 'defectus lubricitatis', lack of slipperiness, because viscosity is really the internal friction within a moving fluid, analogous to the friction between two moving solid surfaces. Viscosity is defined formally as the shear stress required to generate one unit of shear rate (Appendix 2, Viscosity).

Shear stress is the sliding force applied to a unit area of contact between two laminae of fluid, and is proportional to the pressure gradient along the vessel. **Shear rate** is the change in fluid velocity per unit distance across the tube, i.e. the slope of the velocity profile in Figure 8.3. (To visualize these terms, imagine pushing one sheet of paper across the surface of another. The shear stress is the sliding force you apply, per unit area, and the shear rate is the speed with which the top paper slides over the lower one.) The absolute unit of viscosity is the Newton-s/m^2 or milliPascal-second. It is often more convenient, however, to cite **relative viscosity**, which is dimensionless. The relative viscosity of blood or plasma is the viscosity divided by that of water.

Plasma viscosity is dominated by plasma proteins

The voluminous albumin and globulin molecules of plasma raise plasma viscosity to 1.7 times that of water. In **myeloma**, a cancer of globulin-secreting cells, an increase in globulin concentration raises the plasma viscosity, and can cause the red cells to agglutinate (attach to each other) under cool conditions. The latter can raise blood viscosity to such a degree that tissue perfusion is badly impaired, leading to necrosis of the fingertips (tissue death).

Blood viscosity is dominated by haematocrit

Haematocrit is red cell volume as a percentage of blood volume. Red cells greatly increase the internal friction of blood, so blood viscosity is proportional to haematocrit (Figure 8.19). The relative viscosity of human blood is ~4 at a haematocrit of 47%. The haematocrit of a species represents a compromise between high O_2-carrying capacity and high viscosity, which impairs flow and raises blood pressure. In humans, the normal haematocrit is 40% (female) to 45% (male). In camels, the red cells are less flexible, so their viscous effect is greater and the camel's compromise haematocrit is lower, 27%.

Abnormalities of haematocrit have serious consequences, as follows.

Polycythaemia

Poly-(many)-cythaemia (blood cells) is a condition in which the haematocrit is higher than normal. In people living at **high altitude**, polycythaemia is a physiological adaptation to the chronic hypoxia; but in the disease **polycythaemia rubra vera** red cell overproduction by the bone marrow can raise the

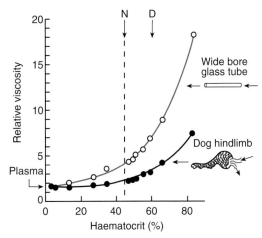

Figure 8.19 Effect of haematocrit on the viscosity of blood relative to water. Open circles: viscosity in a high-velocity, wide-bore glass viscometer. Closed circles: lower effective viscosity in an isolated, perfused dog hindlimb, due to the Fåhraeus–Lindqvist effect. N, normal haematocrit; D, haematocrit at which cells are packed so tightly that they deform even at rest. (After the classic experiment of Whittaker SRF, Winton FR. *Journal of Physiology* 1933; **78**: 339–69.)

haematocrit excessively, to 70%. At a haematocrit of 63%, the red cells are packed so closely that viscosity and resistance are doubled. As a result, polycythaemia rubra vera causes hypertension and a sluggish blood flow that predisposes to cerebral or coronary thrombosis (strokes and heart attacks).

Anaemia

Anaemia reduces the blood viscosity, and therefore *TPR*. To maintain the arterial blood pressure, cardiac output increases (eqn 8.5). If the anaemia is prolonged, a form of cardiac failure called high-output failure can ensue. Thus **homeostasis of blood viscosity is important for normal cardiovascular function**.

Blood viscosity is non-Newtonian: I. Flow through narrow tubes

The viscosity of a simple fluid, such as water or plasma, is unaffected by the radius of the conducting tube or shear rate. Such a fluid is called a **Newtonian fluid**. By contrast, whole blood shows bizarre, but physiologically helpful, non-Newtonian behaviour, as follows.

Viscosity decreases in microvessels (the Fåhraeus–Lindqvist radius effect)

In 1931 Fåhraeus and Lindqvist measured blood viscosity in a viscometer, consisting of a fine glass tube in which flow can be timed accurately. They discovered a strange phenomenon; blood viscosity is

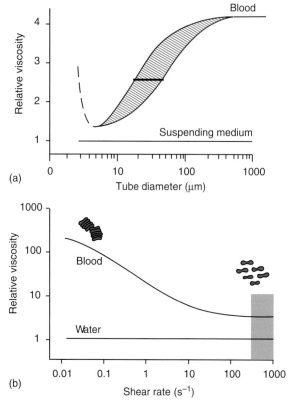

Figure 8.20 Anomalous viscosity of blood, demonstrated in glass tubing. (a) Blood viscosity falls as tube diameter is reduced (Fåhraeus–Lindqvist effect) but water viscosity is unchanged. The effective viscosity of blood in the circulation is ~2.5 (black bar), implying that the functional diameter of the resistance vessels is ~30 μm (arterioles). At diameters smaller than a blood capillary, viscosity rises again (dashed line). (b) Viscosity falls with increasing shear rate. Pink region shows typical shear rates *in vivo*. Sketches show red cell aggregation into rouleaux at low shear rates and disaggregation at high rates. ((a) After Gaetghens P. In: Gross DR, Wang NHC (eds). *The Rheology of Blood, Blood Vessels and Associated Tissues.* Amsterdam: Sijthoff and Noordhoff, with permission from Elsevier; (b) from Chien S, *Microvascular Research* 1992; **44**: 243–54, with permission.)

lower in a narrow-bore tube than a wide-bore tube (Figure 8.20a). The dependence of blood viscosity on tube radius evidently occurs in the circulation too, because the effective viscosity of blood perfused through a dog hindlimb is half that of blood in a wide-bore viscometer (Figure 8.19). Blood viscosity begins to fall in tubes less than 1 mm wide (small arteries), and falls to ~2.5 in tubes of arteriolar width, 30–40 μm. In tubes of capillary width, ~6 μm, blood viscosity reaches a minimum, almost as low as plasma viscosity. This 'Fåhraeus–Lindqvist effect' accounts for the surprisingly low effective viscosity of blood in the circulation (Figure 8.19). The Fåhraeus–Lindqvist effect is important because it greatly reduces microvascular resistance, and

therefore the arterial pressure needed to perfuse the microcirculation. Without this effect, arterial pressure and cardiac work would be much higher.

Several mechanisms underlie the Fåhraeus–Lindqvist effect. In capillaries, **bolus flow** reduces the effective viscosity (Section 8.2). In arterioles, the viscosity is reduced by the **peripheral plasma stream** generated by axial flow (Figure 8.3). Since shear rates are highest close to the vessel wall, a reduction in friction close to the wall has a marked, beneficial effect on net viscosity. The Fåhraeus–Lindqvist effect is not noticeable in tubes wider than 1 mm, because the thickness of the marginal plasma layer, 2–4 μm, becomes negligible relative to the tube width.

Haematocrit decreases in microvessels (Fåhraeus effect)

Robin Fåhraeus described an additional curious effect in narrow tubes. The concentration of red cells in flowing blood inside a narrow tube, the **dynamic** or **tube haematocrit**, is lower than the 'central' haematocrit in the feeding and draining vessels. If a tube of radius 15 μm is fed from a reservoir with a central haematocrit of 40%, the dynamic haematocrit of flowing blood in the tube is only ~24%. This is a little hard to digest at first acquaintance! The phenomenon is the result of the difference between axial and marginal stream velocity (Figure 8.3). Suppose, for example, that blood of central haematocrit 50% feeds an arteriole, in which the red cells have twice the velocity of the plasma, owing to their more axial location. This blood drains into a vein. If the haematocrit in the parent artery and vein are to remain the same, 50% (which must be the case, since the circulation is in a steady state), equal volumes of plasma and red cells must pass through the arteriole in a given time. Since the cell velocity is twice the plasma velocity in our example, equal volume flows are only possible if the concentration of red cells in the arteriole is half that in the parent blood. This is achieved by the red cells speeding away from the plasma at the tube entrance, thinning out like traffic entering a fast road from a congested slip road.

The dynamic haematocrit is particularly low in capillaries, because the glycocalyx makes the effective radius of the tube even narrower than its apparent radius.

Blood viscosity is non-Newtonian: II. Shear thinning

The viscosity of blood changes not only with vessel radius but also with flow velocity, or more accurately shear rate (Figure 8.20b). Shear rate, it will be recalled, is the change in fluid velocity per unit distance normal to the direction of flow, and it has the curious units of s^{-1} (cm/s per cm). Blood viscosity falls as flow and shear rate increase. This is called shear thinning – the same phenomenon as in non-drip paint.

The shear thinning of blood is attributed to the deformation and lining-up of red cells along the laminar flow lines, and to a tank-tread motion of the red cell membrane around its interior. At low flows in horizontal tubes, partial sedimentation of the cells within the tube also contributes to the rise in viscosity.

Shear rates are normally high in the circulation ($\sim 1000\,s^{-1}$), so blood is normally in a shear-thinned state. However, abnormally low flow allows the red cells to adhere to each other to form **rouleaux**, resembling stacks of coins. It is thought that such changes probably occur in veins *in vivo* if blood flow is sluggish. The tendency of red cells to aggregate in this way is related to the concentration of **fibrinogen** in the plasma.

8.9 Pressure–flow relations and autoregulation

Poiseuille's law applies to a steady flow (cf. pulsatile) of Newtonian fluid (cf. non-Newtonian blood) through a long, straight vessel (cf. branching, curved blood vessels) with rigid walls (cf. distensible blood vessels). Not surprisingly, therefore, blood flow through tissues can deviate from Poiseuille's law (Figure 8.21). For example, in perfused lungs, or a perfused dog hindlimb with little vascular tone, the pressure–flow relation is curved at low pressures, though nearly linear in the physiological range (Figure 8.21, 'blood' curve). The curvature at low pressures shows that resistance falls as pressure is raised. This is caused by the shear thinning of blood and, to a lesser degree, vessel distension. Shear thinning seems to be the chief factor, since the pressure–flow relation is almost linear when a dog hindlimb is perfused with saline, rather than blood (Figure 8.21).

Many vascular beds with a high, physiological level of arteriolar tone show a very different, physiologically important shape of pressure–flow relation, called an **autoregulation curve**, which deviates wildly from Poiseuille behaviour. Blood flow increases with perfusion pressure up to a certain point, beyond which the flow changes surprisingly little with pressure (the plateau), until pressure

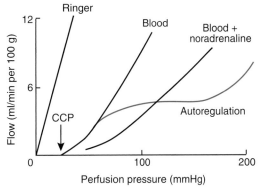

Figure 8.21 Pressure–flow curves in perfused skeletal muscle (canine). '*Autoregulation*' curve applies under physiological conditions, because arterioles respond myogenically to pressure changes (see text). '*Blood*' curve is observed if autoregulation is abolished. Near-zero flow occurs at a positive *critical closing pressure* (CCP) – probably due to increased blood viscosity at low shear rates. '*Blood + noradrenaline*' curve is less steep, because noradrenaline-induced vasoconstriction raises vascular resistance. '*Ringer*' line; perfusion with Ringer's solution, a physiological salt solution of low, Newtonian viscosity, produces a steep line that is almost straight, because the anomalous viscous effect of blood is absent. (From Pappenheimer JR, Maes JP. *American Journal of Physiology* 1942; **137**: 187–99; and Stainsby WN, Renkin EM. *American Journal of Physiology* 1961; **201**: 117–22, with permission from the American Physiological Society.)

exceeds $\sim 180\,mmHg$. An almost constant flow in the face of a changing pressure (autoregulation) is due to the vascular resistance changing in the opposite direction to pressure. For example, a rise in pressure triggers resistance vessels constriction, which prevents flow from rising (Section 13.6). Autoregulation is important, because it helps to stabilize the blood flow to an organ, such as the brain, in the face of fluctuating arterial pressures. Autoregulation occurs to a greater or lesser degree in most organs, except the lungs.

8.10 Venous pressure and volume

Peripheral veins and venules are thin-walled, contractile, voluminous vessels that contain about two-thirds of the blood pool. Due to their large, variable volume, the peripheral vessels act as an adjustable reservoir of blood. That is to say, they can contract and expel some of their blood to top up the central veins, and hence boost the CVP, stroke volume and arterial pressure. The volume of blood in the peripheral veins depends on the **venous blood pressure** and **smooth muscle tone** in the tunica media, as follows (Figure 8.22).

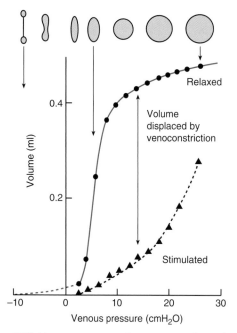

Figure 8.22 Venous pressure–volume curves, when veins are relaxed (circles) or maximally venoconstricted (triangles). Change in venous cross section with pressure in relaxed state shown above. Volume V at a given pressure P, called venous *capacitance*, is reduced by venoconstriction. *Compliance* (distensibility) is the slope dV/dP. (Canine saphenous vein, from Vanhoutte PM, Leusen I. *Pfluger's Archiv* 1969; **306**: 341–53, by kind permission from Springer Science and Business Media.)

The venous pressure–volume curve is sigmoidal due to changes in vessel profile

Blood pressure is ~12–20 mmHg in venules at heart level, falling to ~8–10 mmHg in named veins, such as the antecubital or femoral vein. Since venous resistance is small, 8–10 mmHg is enough to drive the cardiac output back to the right ventricle, where diastolic pressure is 0–6 mmHg.

Venous pressure depends very much on the position of the vein relative to heart level, due to the effect of gravity (Figure 8.2). Moreover, since the vein wall is thin and collapsible, the cross-sectional profile and volume change markedly with pressure (Figure 8.22). This results in large changes in peripheral venous blood volume with changes in body posture. When venous pressure is below zero (atmospheric pressure), as in a hand above heart level, the vein collapses into a dumb-bell shaped profile, and flow is confined to the narrow marginal channels. At a transmural pressure of +1 mmHg the vein assumes a narrow elliptical cross section. As pressure rises towards 10 mmHg, the elliptical profile becomes progressively rounder. These changes

in profile enable peripheral veins to accommodate a large volume of blood in response to a relatively small changes in pressure. The maximum distensibility (compliance) occurs at ~4 mmHg and is ~100 ml/mmHg for the human systemic venous system. This is some 50 times greater than arterial compliance.

Above 10–15 mmHg, the vein profile is fully circular, and since the collagen in the wall is relatively inextensible, venous volume becomes less sensitive to pressure. Due to the collapse of veins at low pressure and their relative stiffness at high pressure, the venous pressure–volume curve is sigmoidal (S-shaped).

Venous smooth muscle tone regulates venous volume

In the gastrointestinal tract, liver, kidneys and skin the venous tunica media is richly innervated by sympathetic vasomotor nerves. Sympathetic venoconstriction greatly reduces venous capacitance in these tissues, and the displaced blood moves into the thoracic compartment (Figure 8.22). In this way, the central nervous system is able to exert a degree of control over the filling pressure of the heart.

Human central venous pressure can be estimated by inspecting the neck veins

Central venous pressure (CVP) can be monitored directly in intensive care units by a catheter inserted into the subclavian vein or superior vena cava. During routine clinical examination, however, CVP is assessed indirectly by inspection of the neck veins (Figure 8.23). The external jugular vein runs over the sternomastoid muscle and the internal jugular vein runs deep to the muscle. When a human is semi-supine, the lower part of the jugular vein is normally distended but the upper part is collapsed, because blood in the upper part is at subatmospheric pressure, due to the effect of gravity (Figure 8.2). From the sigmoidal pressure–volume curve of veins, we know that **at the point of venous collapse, the transmural pressure is approximately zero**. The CVP must therefore equal the pressure exerted by the vertical column of blood between the point of jugular vein collapse and the right atrium.

A numerical example should make this clearer. Suppose that the point of jugular vein collapse, where venous blood pressure equals atmospheric pressure, is 7 cm vertical distance above the right

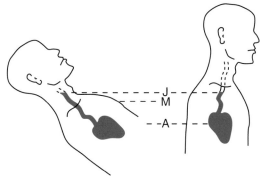

Figure 8.23 How to estimate central venous pressure (CVP) in a semirecumbent human. CVP is vena cava blood pressure at junction with the right atrium. It equals the vertical distance J–A, between the point of collapse of the jugular vein (J, blood at atmospheric pressure) and right atrium (A). Since A is not visible, the vertical height of J above the manubriosternal angle (M) is measured in cm, and an average vertical distance M–A (~5 cm) is added on. Thus CVP = (J–M) cm + 5 cm, in cm blood (almost same as cmH$_2$O). In the upright position, the entire jugular vein is normally collapsed, so is not visible.

atrium. The CVP must therefore be 7 cm of blood, which is 7.4 cmH$_2$O. The atrium is not visible, of course, but it is known to be ~5 cm lower than the manubriosternal angle, which can be palpated. Thus by measuring the vertical distance between the point of jugular vein collapse and the manubriosternal angle (2 cm in our example), and adding 5 cm, human CVP can be roughly estimated.

Although the accuracy of the inspection method is only about ±2 cm, it is good enough to detect the grossly elevated CVP that characterizes right ventricular failure (Chapter 18). In right ventricular failure, the CVP may be so high that the jugular venous pulse is visible even when the patient is upright. A normal subject has to be semi-supine for the jugular pulse to be visible, because in the upright position the transition point between collapse and distension is below the level of the clavicle.

CVP waves are visible in jugular veins in recumbent humans

The superior vena cava and jugular veins form a relatively direct tube into the right atrium, with no venous valves. Consequently, jugular venous pressure mirrors the pulsatile pressure wave in the right atrium (Section 2.3 and Figure 8.27). Although the jugular pulse pressure is only a few mmHg, it is sufficient to move the overlying skin. The 'x' and 'y' descents of the wave are normally visible as inward flickers of the skin in a semi-recumbent human.

Palpation readily distinguishes the jugular venous pulse (too weak to feel) from the carotid arterial pulse (easily felt).

8.11 Effects of gravity on the venous system

A change in posture from supine to standing triggers extensive changes in the human cardiovascular system (Section 17.1). The primary event that initiates these changes is the effect of gravity on venous blood distribution.

Orthostasis distends veins below heart level

In the standing position (**orthostasis**) pressure increases in all the blood vessels below heart level, and falls in all the vessels above heart level, due to the pull of gravity on the vertical column of fluid between heart and vessel (Figures 8.2 and 8.24). This particularly affects the distribution of blood in the venous system, owing to its steep, sigmoidal pressure–volume curve (Figure 8.22).

Upon tilting a human from the supine to upright position, a transitory closure of the venous valves in the limbs prevents any substantial venous backflow. Pressure in the dependent (below heart) veins then rises steadily over 30–60 s, as blood flows into them from the arterial system. As venous pressure rises, flow recommences up the limb veins and pushes open the venous valves. This re-establishes an uninterrupted column of blood. The weight of the continuous fluid column between heart and feet raises venous pressure in the feet nine-fold, from ~10 mmHg supine to ~90 mmHg in orthostasis (Figures 8.2, 8.24 and 8.26).

There is no counterbalancing rise in extramural pressure during orthostasis (unless the subject is immersed in water), so the dependent veins become greatly distended. Check for yourself – the effect is plainly visible in the back of the hand as the hand is moved above and below heart level. In a human adult about 500 ml of blood accumulate in the distended veins below heart level during orthostasis, over ~45 s (Figure 8.24). This is widely referred to as venous 'pooling', though the imagery here is misleading; a pool is static whereas **venous blood flows continuously** in the steady state. Most of the redistributed blood comes ultimately from the intrathoracic compartment, via arterial flow (not via venous backflow, since valves prevent this). The loss of blood from the intrathoracic veins reduces the

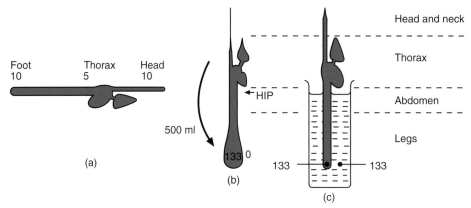

Figure 8.24 Venous blood displacement (red) on moving from supine (a) to standing (b). The thoracic compartment includes the central veins, heart and pulmonary blood. Numbers indicate cmH$_2$O pressure above atmospheric. Pressure surrounding extrathoracic veins is approximately atmospheric (zero baseline). The hydrostatic indifferent point (HIP) is the point where pressure does not change on tilting. (c) shows how upright immersion in water raises pressure outside the veins, displacing 'pooled' blood centrally and raising CVP. (After Gauer OH, Thron HL. In: Hamilton WF, Dow P (eds). *Handbook of Physiology, Circulation*, Vol. 3. Bethesda, MD: American Physiological Society, 1963: 2409–40.)

CVP, which impairs the stroke volume through the Frank–Starling mechanism. This causes a transitory arterial hypotension and sometimes dizziness, called **postural hypotension** (Section 17.1). A hand-count among medical students indicates that nearly all healthy individuals occasionally experience orthostatic dizziness, especially when warm and venodilated.

Gravity does not affect flow directly: the siphon principle

This short section deals with a common student misconception, namely that venous blood flow must decrease in the leg during standing 'because the blood has to go uphill against gravity'. This concept is wrong, because it ignores the fact that gravity exerts an equal and opposite 'downhill' pull on the arterial column. Gravity acts equally on the venous and arterial fluid columns, so the **pressure difference** between artery and vein at any level is not affected by orthostasis (Figures 8.2 and 11.5). Since flow is proportional to pressure difference, blood flow in the steady state is not directly affected by standing. The circulation through the leg or brain in fact resembles flow through a U-tube siphon (Figure 8.25). Flow through a rigid siphon is totally unaffected by the orientation of the siphon; flow is the same whether the siphon is horizontal, vertical, or upside down, for the reason given above. Similarly, if blood vessels were completely rigid, gravity would have no effect whatsoever on venous or arterial flow in the steady state.

Figure 8.25 The siphon principle. The pressure head in the feed-tank, 100 cmH$_2$O, drives flow through the open-ended tube. Pressure is 50 cmH$_2$O halfway along the tube when horizontal. If the tube is bent into a U shape, the pressure difference driving flow from tank to outlet is the same, so the flow is identical – irrespective of which way up the U tube is. Only the intermediate pressures are changed (numbers, cmH$_2$O); see Bernoulli principle. The middle sketch is equivalent to the situation in the leg vasculature during standing.

In reality, limb blood flow does decline in the steady state during dependency (Figure 8.6); but this is not because 'blood has to go uphill in the veins'. The reduction is caused by an active arteriolar contraction, which is partly a local response to the rise in pressure and partly a baroreceptor reflex.

Extracranial veins collapse above heart level

Gravity reduces the pressure of blood in vessels above heart level. When the transmural pressure falls to zero or less, unsupported superficial veins collapse (Figures 8.22, 8.23 and 8.24), as is easily observed in the back of one's hand. Deeper veins are better supported and do not collapse completely. Veins inside the cranial cavity are a special case. They do not collapse during orthostasis, despite their subatmospheric blood pressure, because gravity also reduces the pressure of the cerebrospinal fluid surrounding them. Thus the **transmural pressure** across the vein wall hardly changes. In the **venous sinuses of the dura mater**, however, the subatmospheric pressure does create one potential hazard. The walls of these sinuses are attached to the rigid interior of the skull and are therefore not collapsible. Consequently, if they are breached by an accident or surgery in the upright position, air can be sucked into the veins by the subatmospheric venous pressure, causing **air embolism**.

Immersion and other gravitational effects

When a human is partially immersed vertically in water, gravity acts on the water as well as the blood, so the extramural pressure at any point below heart level rises by almost the same amount as the intramural blood pressure. Consequently, transmural venous pressure barely changes in the lower limbs, unlike the situation in air. Upright immersion thus prevents venous pooling and maintains the intrathoracic blood volume and cardiac filling pressure. Due to the operation of Starling's law of the heart, the stroke volume increases by ~50% upon upright immersion to the neck.

Aeroplane pilots experience altered g forces during aerobatics. A pilot pulling out of a steep dive can experience $13-14g$ along the body axis. Venous pooling in the lower body is then so severe that CVP and stroke volume fall rapidly, leading to cerebral hypoperfusion and a blackout. To prevent this, an anti-gravity suit is worn; bags inflate automatically around the legs to raise extramural pressure and minimize venous distension during turns – mimicking immersion in water (Figure 8.24). Conversely, in an inverted loop-the-loop, a high negative g force is experienced, i.e. gravity is directed towards the head. This distends the retinal vessels and causes vision 'red-out'.

In space travel the circulation is subjected to zero gravity for long periods. As this is not dissimilar to a supine posture or water immersion (Figure 8.24, right panel), it presents no special problem for the cardiovascular system, until the return to positive gravity.

8.12 Venous blood flow and the accessory pumps

Venous blood flow is influenced by two accessory pumps, the exercise skeletal muscle pump and the respiratory pump.

The skeletal muscle pump has multiple roles

When a skeletal muscle contracts, it compresses the local veins and displaces their blood proximally, towards the central veins (Figure 8.26, top). The venous valves prevent retrograde flow and ensure that the emptied segments refill from the periphery when the muscle relaxes. Rhythmic exercise thus has a pumping effect on venous flow. Although this is not essential for venous return, it has the following beneficial effects:

- By redistributing venous blood from the periphery into the central veins, the muscle pump prevents CVP from falling during exercise, counteracting the cardiac pump effect of Figure 6.12. The muscle pump can even increase CVP slightly, shifting the ventricle up the Starling curve.

- Like any other pump, the muscle pump reduces pressure in its feed line (Figure 6.12). Each time the leg muscles relax, blood drains rapidly from the distal veins into the empty muscle veins, lowering venous pressure in the foot and ankle. At the same time, closure of the proximal valves interrupts the vertical column of blood between limb and heart. In this way, the leg muscle pump can reduce venous pressure in the lower leg from 70–90 mmHg during immobile standing to 20–40 mmHg during walking, running and cycling (Figure 8.26, bottom). This increases the arteriovenous pressure gradient driving blood through the calf muscle by 50–60% (Figure 15.8).

Figure 8.26 The skeletal muscle pump. Trace shows pressure in the dorsal vein of the author's foot (solid line), initially standing still, then rhythmically contracting the calf muscles (black bar). Insets show how the muscle pump operates. The author evidently had competent venous valves in his youth. Red line shows effect of failure of venous valves, as in varicose veins. (Unpublished results of Levick JR and Michel CC.)

• Since capillary pressure is close to venous pressure, the muscle pump lowers capillary pressure too, reducing fluid filtration into the feet and ankles. This helps prevent the feet and ankles from becoming swollen and oedematous (fluid filled) in the upright position.

Valvular incompetence leads to varicose veins and venous leg ulcers

The venous valves of the leg often become incompetent with ageing. As a result, the vertical column of venous blood cannot be broken up by the now ineffective muscle pump, and the distal leg veins are subjected to a chronically elevated pressure load during orthostasis (Figure 8.26, red recording). This leads to a permanent dilatation of the veins, the familiar **varicose veins**. The chronic venous hypertension also causes leukocytes to adhere in the dependent microcirculation, through mechanisms that are still being explored. The microvascular changes lead to trophic skin changes, namely discoloration and induration (hardening), followed by skin ulceration. **Venous leg ulcers** usually develop just above the medial malleolus of the ankle. They are common in the elderly, difficult to heal and a

great expense for national health services. Since venous ulcers are treated by compression bandaging while arterial ulcers are not, the ABPI is used to distinguish between arterial and venous disease prior to treatment (Section 8.5).

The respiratory pump and coughing

Inspiration increases the blood flow into the thoracic venae cavae by two mechanisms (Figure 8.27, inset). The fall in intrathoracic pressure expands the intrathoracic veins; and the descent of the diaphragm compresses the abdominal contents, raising the abdominal venous pressure and hence flow into the thorax. Conversely, expiration reduces flow into the thoracic venae cavae. The latter effect is greatly exaggerated during forced expiration, such as the **Valsalva manoeuvre** (Chapter 17) or coughing. **Coughing** can elevate intrathoracic pressure transiently to 400 mmHg, greatly impeding venous return. Indeed, **paroxysmal coughing** can impede venous return to such an extent that fainting ensues.

The respiratory pump has a dwindling effect on flow in more peripheral veins, though a small effect is still detectable in the femoral vein.

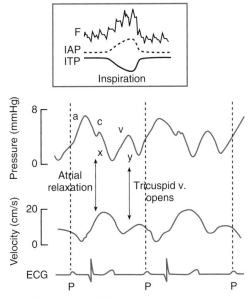

Figure 8.27 Pressure and flow in human superior vena cava over two cardiac cycles. (*Inset*) Effect of breathing on venous return. F, flow in thoracic inferior vena cava; IAP, intraabdominal pressure; ITP, intrathoracic pressure. a, c, v, x, y as in Figure 2.4 (Data from Brecher GA. *Venous Return*. New York: Grune and Stratton, 1956; and Wexler L, Bergel DL, Gabe T *et al. Circulation Research* 1968; **23**: 349–59.)

Flow is pulsatile in the great veins

Flow in the great veins is pulsatile, because there are no valves separating them from the right atrium. There are two venous spurts per cycle (Figure 8.27). **Peak flow** occurs during the *x* descent of the atrial pressure wave, as the atria begin to relax. Peak flow is aided by ventricular systole, which has a suction effect on the atria and central veins. As right ventricular systole shoots a mass of blood up into the pulmonary trunk, the ventricle itself is propelled downwards, like the ballistic recoil of a gun (Newton's law of action and reaction). This causes the annulus fibrosus (base of ventricle) to descend (Figure 2.2), stretching the atria and sucking blood into them. A **second flow-spurt** occurs during the *y* descent of the atrial pressure wave, due to the opening of the tricuspid valve in diastole. The second spurt is boosted by a second suction effect, mediated by the elastic recoil of the ventricular walls – especially when end-systolic volume is low during exercise. Thus flow through the great veins is driven primarily by the upstream (distal) pressure of ~8 mmHg (pressure from behind or *vis a tergo*) and is boosted by two transient reductions in downstream pressure due to the motion of the heart (suction from in front, *vis a fronte*).

SUMMARY

- The **pattern of blood flow** is **laminar** in healthy arteries and veins, **turbulent** in the ventricles and atheromatous arteries, and **bolus** (single file) in capillaries.

- **Darcy's law** states that laminar flow $\dot{Q}$ is proportional to the pressure drop along a tube, $P_1 - P_2$ and inversely proportional to resistance R. Thus $\dot{Q} = (P_i - P_o)/R$. **Bernoulli's theory** takes account of kinetic energy and gravitational potential energy as well as pressure energy. **Poiseuille's law** (below) defines the factors governing R in a tube.

- **Human blood flow** is measured in major arteries by Doppler ultrasound; in certain organs by the Fick principle (e.g. renal blood flow using PAH); in limbs by venous occlusion plethysmography; and in the microcirculation by Kety's radioisotope clearance method.

- **Human arterial pressure** is usually measured by brachial artery sphygmomanometry. It varies with age, exercise, emotional stress, sleep, pregnancy, orthostasis, gravity, hypovolaemia, hypertension and many other pathological conditions. The ankle-brachial pressure ratio tests for leg arterial disease.

- **Mean arterial pressure** equals cardiac output × total peripheral resistance. Mean pressure in the brachial artery is calculated as diastolic pressure + one-third of the pulse pressure.

- **Pulse pressure** is systolic minus diastolic pressure. Pulse pressure and systolic pressure depend on stroke volume, arterial stiffness (1/compliance) and wave reflection. Wave reflection adds a diastolic wave after the incisura in young subjects, but a systolic inflection before the incisura in older subjects, raising systolic pressure and cardiac work.

- The pressure wave **propagates** rapidly along the arterial tree. The propagation rate increases as ageing stiffens the artery wall (**arteriosclerosis**). Arterial stiffening also raises systolic pressure, hence cardiac work and O_2 demand.

- **Vascular resistance** is located chiefly in terminal arteries and arterioles, across which the pressure falls from ~80 mmHg to 35 mmHg. **Poiseuille's law** states that resistance depends on blood viscosity η, vessel length L and (inversely) radius r^4; $R = 8\eta L/\pi r^4$. Vascular radius is regulated by smooth muscle. Due to the r^4 effect, a small reduction in vascular tone increases local blood flow greatly. A widespread rise in vascular tone raises the total peripheral resistance and therefore arterial pressure.

- In many organs *in vivo*, flow is almost independent of arterial pressure in the physiological range, contrary to the classic laws of physics, because the arterioles actively regulate their resistance (**autoregulation**).

- **Laplace's law** shows that wall tension T in a thin tube at mechanical equilibrium increases with radius and transmural pressure; $T = \Delta Pr$. Wall tension and stress are therefore high in the aorta, which can lead to aneurysm formation.

- **Blood viscosity** η depends on haematocrit. This is raised in polycythaemia, leading to hypertension, strokes and heart attacks. Viscosity is reduced in anaemia. Blood viscosity falls in microvessels, facilitating microvascular perfusion (Fåhraeus–Lindqvist effect). Viscosity increases at low shear rates.

- **Venous pressure** is 8–10 mmHg in peripheral veins at heart level. CVP is 0–7 mmHg and can be estimated by inspection of the jugular veins.

- **Peripheral venous blood volume** is variable, and affects CVP and stroke volume. It depends on (a) venous smooth muscle tone, which is regulated by sympathetic fibres in the renal, splanchnic and cutaneous circulations; and (b) venous pressure, which depends on position of the vein relative to heart level (gravity). The venous pressure–volume curve is sigmoidal, due to vein profile changes.

- During **orthostasis**, gravity raises the venous and arterial pressures in the legs (principle of manometry, ρgh). Venous 'pooling' in distended leg veins reduces CVP and stroke volume, leading to transient postural hypotension. The muscle pump counteracts venous pooling during walking. Venous valve incompetence leads to chronic venous hypertension, varicose veins and venous leg ulcers.

Further reading

Reviews and chapters

Dormandy JA. Microcirculation in venous disorders: the role of the white blood cells. *International Journal of Microcirculation* 1995; **15** (Suppl 1): 3–8.

Fung YC. *Biomechanics*. New York: Springer, 2005.

Goldsmith HL, Cokelet GR, Gaehtgens P. Robin Fåhraeus: evolution of his concepts in cardiovascular physiology. *American Journal of Physiology* 1989; **257**: H1005–15.

Julien C. The enigma of Mayer waves: facts and models. *Cardiovascular Research* 2006; **70**: 12–21.

Lipowsky HH. Microvascular rheology and hemodynamics. *Microcirculation* 2005; **12**: 5–15.

Nichols WW, O'Rourke MF. *McDonald's Blood Flow in Arteries*, 5th edn. London: Arnold, 2005.

Pappenheimer JR. Contributions to microvascular research of Jean Leonard Marie Poiseuille. In: Renkin EM, Michel CC (eds). *Handbook of Physiology, Cardiovascular System*, Vol. 4, The Microcirculation. Bethesda, MD: American Physiological Society, 1984: 1–10.

Pickering TG. Physiological aspects of non-invasive ambulatory blood-pressure monitoring. *News in Physiological Sciences* 1990; **5**: 176–9.

Secomb T. Mechanics of blood flow in the microcirculation. In: Ellington CP, Pedley TJ (eds). *Biological Fluid Dynamics*. Cambridge: The Company of Biologists, 1995: 305–21.

Vowden KR, Goulding V, Vowden P. Hand-held Doppler assessment for peripheral arterial disease. *Journal of Wound Care* 1996; **5**: 125–8. (ABPI)

Research papers

See www.hodderplus.com/cardiovascularphysiology for a full list of Research papers for this chapter.

CHAPTER 9

The endothelial cell

Learning objectives

After reading this chapter you should be able to:

- Outline the structure of the glycocalyx, intercellular junction, vesicle system and actin cytoskeleton (9.2).
- Name the endothelial Ca^{2+}-conducting ion channels, and role of endothelial Ca^{2+} (9.3).
- List four vasoactive endothelial secretions (9.4, 9.5).
- Give the actions of endothelial NO and the factors regulating its production (9.4).
- State the effect of endothelium on blood (9.6).
- Outline how endothelium captures leukocytes during inflammation (9.8).
- Describe the other roles of endothelium in inflammation (9.8).
- Outline the factors that regulate capillary permeability (9.7).
- State the role of endothelium in angiogenesis (9.9).
- Describe the contribution of endothelial dysfunction to atheroma (9.10).

Endothelium is the monolayer of endothelial cells that lines the blood interface throughout the cardiovascular system, including the cardiac chambers. Its aggregate mass is several hundred grams in a human adult. The active nature of endothelium is much less obvious than that of cardiac myocytes, yet endothelium makes numerous, remarkably varied contributions to cardiovascular function. The enormous surface area of endothelium ($\sim$280 m^2 in human skeletal muscles, $\sim$90 m^2 in the lungs) facilitates the transfer of respiratory gases, nutrients and white cells between blood and tissue; the transfer of regulatory signals to vascular smooth muscle; and the modification of plasma composition (Figure 9.1).

9.1 Outline of endothelial functions

- **Endothelium regulates blood–tissue exchange**. The primary role of endothelium is to form a semipermeable membrane, in order to retain plasma and blood cells inside the circulation yet permit nutrient transfer into the tissues. Specialized, regulated intercellular junctions confer permeability to water and nutrients such as glucose, while an internal coating of biopolymers, the glycocalyx, restricts plasma protein escape.

- **Paracrine secretions regulate vascular tone**. Arterial endothelium expresses receptors to many vasoactive agents, such as acetylcholine, and it can also sense the shear stress generated by flowing blood. It responds to these signals by secreting vasoactive agents, namely nitric oxide, endothelium-derived hyperpolarizing factor, prostacyclin and endothelin. These agents act in a paracrine fashion (i.e. locally) on adjacent vascular smooth muscle cells to adjust local blood flow – for example, flow-induced arterial dilatation in exercising muscle (Section 13.7). More controversially, it has been suggested that local cardiac endothelial nitric oxide and endothelin may influence cardiac contractility.

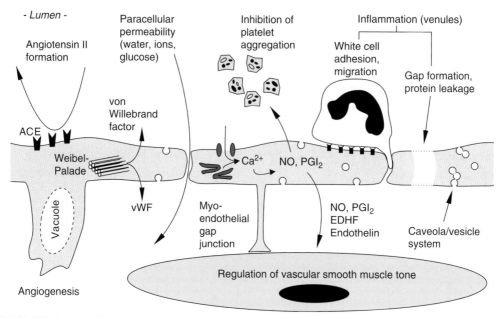

Figure 9.1 Multiple functions of endothelial cell; lumen is at top. NO, nitric oxide; PGI_2, prostacyclin; EDHF, endothelium-derived hyperpolarizing factor; ACE, angiotensin I-converting enzyme; vWF, von Willebrand haemostatic factor.

- **Endothelial surface enzymes modify vasoactive peptides in the bloodstream.** The luminal surface of endothelium possesses an enzyme, angiotensin-converting enzyme, which chemically modifies circulating, vasoactive peptides. The large surface area of the endothelium ensures the efficient conversion of substrate.
- **Endothelium secretes both antithrombotic and pro-clotting factor.** Nitric oxide and prostacyclin are not only vasodilators but also inhibitors of platelet aggregation. This prevents circulating blood from clotting (thrombosis). Endothelium also secretes von Willebrand factor, a component of the clotting cascade.
- **Endothelium participates in the inflammatory defence against pathogens.** In an inflamed tissue, venular endothelium inserts adhesion molecules into its surface membrane, in order to capture circulating leukocytes and promote their migration to the source of the inflammation. Also the endothelial cells change shape, forming large gaps that allow circulating immunoglobulins to access the inflamed tissue.
- **Endothelium initiates new blood vessel formation.** The sprouting of endothelial cells is the starting point for the development of all new blood vessels (angiogenesis). Angiogenesis is essential for tissue growth, pregnancy, wound repair and the growth of cancers. Anti-angiogenic drugs are now used to inhibit cancer growth.
- **Endothelial dysfunction contributes to atheroma.** The impairment of endothelial function appears to contribute to the development of arterial atheroma, the single biggest cause of morbidity and mortality in Westernized societies. Plasma-derived cholesterol and fibrin become trapped between the endothelium and tunica media, leading to the formation of the atheromatous plaque.

The roles of endothelium are thus many, diverse and vitally important. This chapter describes the cell biology underlying these roles. Solute exchange and fluid movement across endothelium are covered in Chapters 10 and 11, respectively. The regulation of vascular tone by endothelial secretions is integrated with the numerous other vascular control mechanisms in Chapter 13.

9.2 Structure of endothelium

Endothelium is a thin monolayer of polygonal, flattened endothelial cells. The cells are 0.2–0.3 µm thick, and are joined edge-to-edge in a 'crazy paving' pattern (Figures 1.11 and 9.2). Each cell contains a small store of Ca^{2+} in the endoplasmic reticulum, which can be as little as 8 nm or so from the surface. Endothelial cells also have a unique storage organelle, the Weibel–Palade body (Section 9.6).

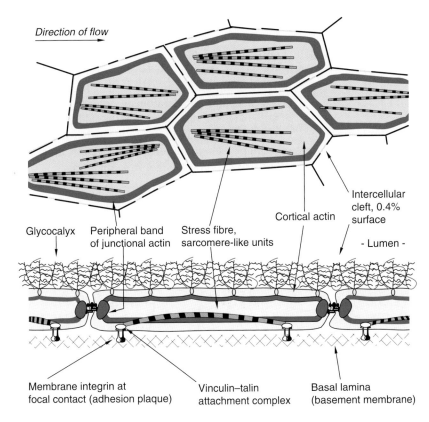

Figure 9.2 Organization of endothelial cytoskeleton and intercellular junctions, viewed *en face* (*top*) and in cross section (*bottom*). Black intercellular lines *en face* represent sealed region of cleft (~90%); the grey lines are the open, permeable parts of the cleft, at breaks in the junctional strands. Glycocalyx molecules form hairy tufts attached to the cell membrane and linked to cortical actin cytoskeleton at ~100 nm intervals (Adapted from Drenckhahn D, Ness W. In Born GVR, Schwartz CJ (eds). *Vascular Endothelium.* Stuttgart: Schattauer, 1997; and Weinbaum S, Tarbell JM, Damiano ER. *Annual Review Biomedical Engineering* 2007; **9**: 121–67.)

Labels on figure: Direction of flow; Intercellular cleft, 0.4% surface; Cortical actin; - Lumen -; Glycocalyx; Peripheral band of junctional actin; Stress fibre, sarcomere-like units; Membrane integrin at focal contact (adhesion plaque); Vinculin–talin attachment complex; Basal lamina (basement membrane)

Actin–myosin cytoskeleton provides shape and anchorage

Endothelial cell shape is maintained by an actin cytoskeleton, which is organized into three distinct systems: the cortical web, the junctional band and the basal stress fibres (Figure 9.2). The **cortical web** is a thin layer of actin filaments under the cell membrane, linked to membrane glycoproteins by filamin and other proteins. The cortical web helps anchor surface molecules, such as the glycocalyx and leukocyte-capturing selectins. The **junctional band** is a prominent ring of actin running around the cell perimeter (Figure 9.2). It is attached to the intercellular junction proteins via α-actinin and anchors them in place (Figure 9.3); if the junctional actin band is disassembled, using cytochalasin, gaps appear between the cells. **Basal stress fibres** are prominent in arterial endothelium and resist the shearing effect of the bloodstream. They comprise interdigitating myosin and actin filaments organized into 2–4 μm long, sarcomere-like units. The ends of the stress fibre are attached via a protein complex (α-actinin, vinculin, talin) to transmembrane dimers, called **integrins**. The integrins bind to extracellular laminin, collagen and fibronectin at **focal contacts** (adhesion plaques), thus gluing the cell down (Figures 9.2 and 9.3).

Intercellular clefts provide a pathway for water and nutrient transfer

Water and small, lipid-insoluble solutes, such as glucose, amino acids and drugs, can cross the endothelial barrier via the intercellular clefts, chiefly in capillaries. The clefts are 20 nm wide and occupy only 0.2–0.4% of the capillary surface (Figure 9.2, upper panel). Rows of protein particles in the cell membrane facing the cleft form **junctional strands**. Two or three junctional strands run around the cell perimeter. The strands on neighbouring cells meet across the intercellular cleft to form **tight junctions** (Figure 9.3). The tight junctions do not continue unbroken around the entire cell perimeter, however; there are occasional, 150–200 nm long **breaks in the junctional strands**, which provide a continuous, albeit tortuous, permeable pathway across the capillary wall (Figures 9.4 and 10.3). The number and width of the breaks greatly influence capillary permeability; postcapillary venules, for example, have fewer junctional strands and wider breaks than capillaries, so they have a higher permeability to water; whereas brain capillaries have numerous, complex junctional strands with no breaks, so their permeability is very low.

An additional, specialized transendothelial pathway, the **fenestrae** (windows), occurs in the capillaries of certain tissues, as described in Section 10.2.

Junctional proteins form a dynamic, regulated complex

In an epithelium, a tight or 'occludens' junction forms close to a distinct, separate anchoring or 'adherens' junction. The endothelial junction contains proteins associated both with occludens-type junctions (claudin-5, occludin, junctional adhesion molecule JAM, linker molecule ZO-1) and adherens-type junctions (VE cadherin, catenins) (Figure 9.3). Vascular endothelial (VE) cadherin is a membrane-spanning glycoprotein whose extracellular domain binds to the VE cadherin of the adjacent cell. Its intracellular domain binds to a complex of α, β and γ catenin, which is tethered by α-actinin to the junctional band of actin. A further junctional protein, platelet endothelial cell adhesion molecule (PECAM), promotes leukocyte emigration.

The junctional complex is a dynamic structure that can be regulated rapidly via intracellular

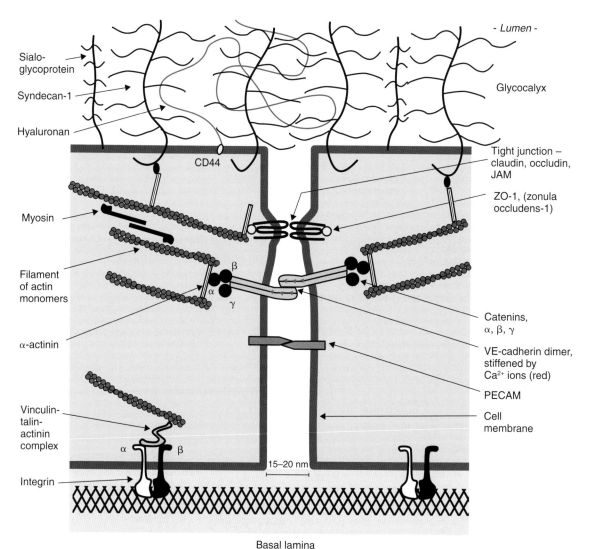

Figure 9.3 Organization of endothelial intercellular junction and glycocalyx. JAM, junctional adhesion molecule; PECAM, platelet–endothelial cell adhesion molecule; VE-cadherin, vascular endothelial cadherin. The cadherin extracellular domain requires Ca^{2+} ions (red triangles) for stiffness. Homocellular gap junctions in arterial endothelium not shown. The glycocalyx comprises linear core proteins to which are attached long heparan sulphate (and some chondroitin sulphate) side-chains (e.g. syndecan-1) or short sialic acid residues (sialoglycoproteins). Hyaluronan is an acetylglucosamine-glucuronic acid polymer with no core protein. (Based on Waschke J, Drenckhahn D, Adamson RH, Curry FE. *American Journal of Physiology* 2004; **287**: H704–11 with permission from the American Physiological Society; and Weinbaum *et al.* 2007, see Further reading.)

messengers. For example, agents that increase endothelial cAMP, such as isoprenaline, increase the number of junctional strands and thus reduce permeability. Conversely, during inflammation the phosphorylation of β catenin and breakdown of junctional actin rapidly weaken the junction, leading to gap formation.

Gap junctions in arterial endothelium transmit signals

Arterial endothelium has numerous gap junctions, as well as tight junctions. The gap junctions comprise connexins 37 and 40 assembled as aligned, conducting hemitubes, as in Figure 3.1 (bottom). **Homocellular gap junctions** are junctions between neighbouring endothelial cells; they transmit ions,

membrane potentials and small chemical messengers (≤1000 Da) along the endothelial sheet. **Heterocellular** or **myoendothelial gap junctions** convey signals between the endothelium and underlying vascular smooth muscle cells. Together the homo- and heterocellular gap junctions can conduct signals along small arteries, causing ascending vasodilatation (Section 13.7).

Glycocalyx is a negatively charged barrier to macromolecules

The luminal surface of endothelium is coated with a 60–570 nm thick, hydrated gel, the glycocalyx (Figures 9.2 and 9.5). The glycocalyx comprises negatively charged carbohydrate polymers, usually attached to a core protein, e.g. sialoglycoprotein, syndecan-1 (a heparan sulphate and chondroitin sulphate proteoglycan with a transmembrane 'root'; Figure 9.3) and glypican (a membrane-attached heparan sulphate proteoglycan). The long glycosaminoglycan, hyaluronan, is bound to the membrane receptor CD44. These various polymers protrude into the lumen in hairy, bush-like tufts and are connected intracellularly to the actin cytoskeleton at ~100 nm intervals. The functions of the glycocalyx are as follows:

- The luminal polymers, aided by bound albumin and orosomucoid, form a size-selective, charge-selective molecular sieve, that is permeable to water and small solutes, but not to plasma proteins or atherogenic low-density lipoproteins. The glycocalyx thus creates the all-important **semipermeability of endothelium**.
- The glycocalyx is a **mechano-sensor**, sensing changes in blood flow. For example, the flow-stimulated secretion of nitric oxide by endothelium is impaired if the glycocalyx is degraded by protease, heparinase or hyaluronidase.

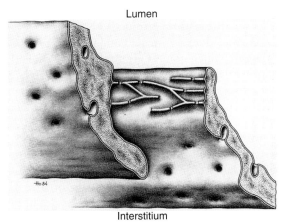

Figure 9.4 Three-dimensional reconstruction of capillary intercellular cleft, based on serial electron micrographs. The cleft is 500–1000 nm long (top to bottom) and 15–20 nm wide, except at the tight junctions. Water and small lipophobic solutes follow the tortuous pathway through the breaks in the junctional strands. (From Bundgaard M. *Journal of Ultrastructural Research* 1984; **88**: 1–17, with permission from Elsevier.)

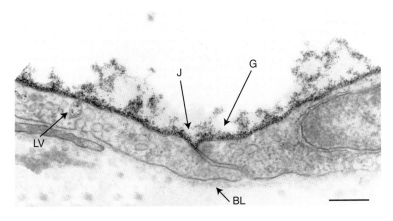

Figure 9.5 Electron micrograph of capillary after perfusion with cationized ferritin (ferritin with added positive charges). Each black dot is a ferritin molecule bound to the negatively charged glycocalyx (G). Binding causes a fall in permeability (Chapter 10, 'The protein effect'). Ferritin is excluded from the intercellular junction (J), but some enters the caveola–vesicle system (LV, labelled vesicle). Neutral ferritin does not bind to glycocalyx and does not reduce permeability. BL, basal lamina; Bar = 0.2 μm. (From Turner MR, Clough G, Michel CC. *Microvascular Research* 1983; **25**: 205–22, with permission from Elsevier.)

- The glycocalyx **lubricates** the deformed red cells as they squeeze in single file along a capillary.
- The glycocalyx can be **degraded and shed** into the bloodstream in response to ischaemia-reperfusion injury (reactive O_2 species), atrial natriuretic peptide, atherogenic oxidized low-density lipoprotein (LDL) and atheroma. This results in hyperpermeability, protein leakage, oedema, increased capillary dynamic haematocrit and leukocyte adhesion.

Caveolae and vesicles: specialized microdomains and transcytosis

Up to a quarter of the endothelial cell is occupied by membrane-bound **vesicles** of diameter ~70 nm. Although they look like detached spheres in a single section, serial sections show that 99% are connected to each other, and ultimately to the luminal/abluminal endothelial surface (Figure 9.6a). The surface vesicle resembles a little flask, or **caveola**, because the interior is connected to the plasma or interstitial fluid via a 20–30 nm wide neck (Figures 9.1 and 9.5). The vesicle system is thus a set of racemose invaginations of the cell membrane, resembling bunches of grapes dangling from each surface.

The caveola membrane is a highly specialized 'microdomain', of different composition to the rest of the cell membrane. The cytoplasmic face is covered by a striated coat of protein, caveolin, and the lipid membrane is enriched in nitric oxide synthase, cholesterol, sphingomyelin, and receptors for albumin (albondin), insulin, transferrin and caeruloplasmin. The concentration of so many proteins in a small lipid raft may facilitate local biochemical signalling.

The caveola–vesicle system can take up plasma macromolecules and transport them into the cell (**endocytosis** – the transfer of receptor-bound materials to endosomes). The vesicles can also transport small amounts of albumin, immunoglobulins and lipoproteins across the cell, from plasma to interstitium (**transcytosis**); but the quantitative significance of this is controversial. Vesicular transcytosis appears to involve the transient fusion of vesicles and transfer of contents (Figure 9.6). Also, very occasionally a row of fused vesicles and caveolae creates a continuous channel through the cell (Figure 9.6b, left). These rare 'multivesicular transendothelial channels' may likewise contribute to macromolecular permeation.

Capillary fragility: the basal lamina normally prevents rupture

The 50–100 nm thick basal lamina comprises a layer of lightly staining extracellular matrix next to the cell, the **lamina rara**, surrounded by a denser layer, the **lamina densa**. A major component is **type IV collagen**, which confers great mechanical strength. **Laminin**, an adhesive glycoprotein, and **perlecan**, a negatively charged heparan sulphate proteoglycan, are the other major constituents. The endothelial cell is attached to the collagen and laminin by β_1-**integrins** at the focal contact points (Figures 9.2 and 9.3). In most tissues the basal lamina is not a barrier to solutes, even those as large as plasma proteins.

Since capillaries lack a tunica media or adventitia, most of their mechanical strength resides in the basal lamina. The basal lamina prevents capillary rupture by blood pressure. **Tension** itself is low in the capillary wall, due to the small radius (Laplace's

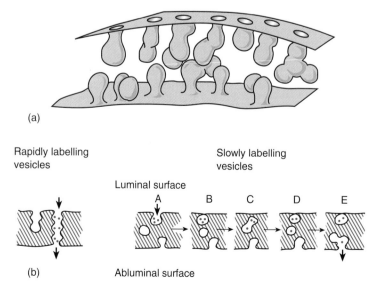

(a)

Rapidly labelling vesicles

Slowly labelling vesicles

Luminal surface

A   B   C   D   E

(b)   Abluminal surface

Figure 9.6 The caveola–vesicle system. (a) Reconstruction of serial sections show that most vesicles connect, directly or indirectly, with a surface via the caveolae (flask-shaped surface invaginations). Detached vesicles are rare. (b) Frames A–E show how transcytosis of macromolecules (red dots, ferritin) may occur by transient vesicular fusion and mixing of contents. Occasional abluminal vesicles that label unusually rapidly may be part of a multivesicular, transendothelial channel (left frame). ((a) From Frokjaer-Jensen J. *Progress in Applied Microcirculation* 1983; **1**: 17–34, by permission; and (b) from Clough G, Michel CC. *Journal of Physiology* 1981; **315**: 127–42, with permission from Wiley-Blackwell.)

law), but the tension per unit wall thickness, **wall stress**, is high, due to the extreme thinness of the wall. Indeed, capillary wall stress is comparable to artery wall stress (Figure 8.18). In **Goodpasture's syndrome**, autoantibodies against type IV collagen weaken the basal lamina, and the fragile capillaries bleed into the lung alveoli and renal glomeruli.

Endothelium differs between vessels

Not all endothelium is the same; it differs between types of blood vessel and between tissues. In **arteries**, where haemodynamic stresses are high, the endothelial cells are elongated in the direction of flow and have prominent stress fibres. **Postcapillary venules** have extensive breaks in the junctional strand, raising their permeability. Venular endothelium also abundantly expresses receptors to inflammatory mediators, and has a large reserve of leukocyte 'glue' (P-selectin); so venular endothelium is the primary site of the inflammatory response. In **lymph nodes**, postcapillary venules have unusually tall endothelial cells, called 'high endothelium', which

entice lymphocytes to recycle from blood to lymph node. In **glandular tissues, intestinal mucosa and the kidney**, the capillary endothelium is perforated by circular windows called fenestrations, which boost permeability (Figure 10.2). At the other extreme, **brain microvessels** have no fenestrations, no breaks in the junctional strands and few vesicles, creating a blood–brain barrier to many solutes (Section 15.4).

9.3 Ion channels, Ca^{2+} and endothelial function

Endothelial cells express a variety of ion channels, many of which influence intracellular Ca^{2+} ion concentration. Calcium ions regulate several endothelial functions, including nitric oxide production and the hyperpermeability of inflammation. Basal cytosolic Ca^{2+} concentration, 30–100 nM, is much lower than extracellular Ca^{2+} concentration, 1 mM, and can be increased five- to ten-fold (e.g. by histamine), partly by the influx of extracellular Ca^{2+} through ion channels, and partly by the release of Ca^{2+} stored in the endoplasmic reticulum (Figure 9.1). In the following account it is assumed that the reader is familiar with the electrophysiological concepts introduced in Chapter 3.

Membrane potential affects endothelial responses

Endothelial cells are not excitable, i.e. they cannot generate action potentials, because they do not express sufficient voltage-gated Na$^+$ or Ca^{2+} channels. They do, however, have a regulated, negative intracellular potential of -30 to -68 mV, which is generated mainly by the outward diffusion of K$^+$ ions through **inward rectifier K$^+$ channels (K$_{ir}$)** and **K$_{Ca}$ channels** (Figure 9.7). Also, the electrogenic 3Na$^+$–2K$^+$ pump contributes about -8 mV. Membrane potential magnitude is important, because it affects the electrochemical force driving extracellular Ca^{2+} into the endothelial cell; abolition of the potential greatly attenuates Ca^{2+}-mediated responses (Figure 11.29). Also, changes in endothelial membrane potential can be conducted through gap junctions to serve as a signal, as in ascending vasodilatation (Section 13.7).

Endothelium expresses TRPC Ca^{2+}-conducting channels

Although endothelium lacks voltage-gated Ca^{2+} channels, the surface membrane has two other types of Ca^{2+}-conducting channel: receptor-operated

Endothelium is a selectively permeable membrane

- The lipid membrane of endothelial cells permits the rapid permeation of lipid-soluble molecules, such as O$_2$, CO$_2$ and anaesthetics between blood and tissue.
- The endothelial intercellular cleft is an aqueous, paracellular pathway that transmits water and small lipophobic solutes, such as glucose – except in the brain, where there are no breaks in the intercellular junctional strands.
- The permeability of the intercellular cleft is reduced by the β adrenoceptor–cAMP pathway, which enhances junctional strand formation. Intercellular permeability is increased by flow and by atrial natriuretic peptide, acting through cGMP.
- The glycocalyx, a coating of biopolymers on the luminal surface, forms a semipermeable layer; it reflects plasma proteins, but permits the passage of smaller solutes and water.
- Cytoplasmic vesicles transfer plasma proteins slowly across endothelium by a poorly understood process.
- In inflammation, wide gaps form between and through venular endothelial cells. The rapid transfer of plasma proteins and water through the gaps causes inflammatory swelling.

Figure 9.7 Endothelial electrophysiology and Ca^{2+} regulation. The coupling between receptor and membrane phospholipase C (PLC) differs between receptors. Classic G-protein-coupled receptors are heptahelical proteins (seven transmembrane loops) that on activation cause the dissociation of the trimeric G protein $G_{q/11}$. The released $G\alpha$ component diffuses in the membrane to activate the PLC-β isoform. Other receptors (e.g. to growth factors) are dimeric transmembrane proteins called receptor protein tyrosine kinases, which activate the PLC-γ isoform. Either PLC isoform generates intramembrane diacyl glycerol (DAG) and cytosolic inositol trisphosphate (IP$_3$). eNOS, endothelial nitric oxide synthase; IK_{Ca}, SK_{Ca} intermediate and small conductance calcium-activated potassium channels; K_{ir}, inward rectifying K^+ channel; PIP_2, phosphatidyl inositol bisphosphate (an inner membrane phospholipid); PLC, phospholipase in membrane, linked by G protein (grey) to agonist receptor; ROC, receptor-operated Ca^{2+} channel; SOC, store-operated Ca^{2+} channels.

channels and store-operated channels. When the cell is stimulated by an agonist, such as histamine, these Ca^{2+} channels are activated and raise the intracellular free Ca^{2+} concentration five- to ten-fold.

Receptor-operated channels (ROCs) are cation-conducting channels that are activated via a biochemical cascade when an extracellular agent, the 'agonist', binds to its specific membrane receptor. Endothelial agonists include histamine, bradykinin, thrombin, serotonin, ATP and acetylcholine. The agonist receptor activates a G-protein, which activates the membrane-bound enzyme **phospholipase C** (Figure 9.7). Phospholipase C splits a phospholipid, phosphatidyl inositol bisphosphate (PIP$_2$), into **diacyl glycerol (DAG)** and **inositol trisphosphate (IP$_3$)**. The DAG activates the ROC ion channel, and the IP$_3$ releases a small store of Ca^{2+} from the endoplasmic reticulum. ROCs are poorly selective cation channels that conduct Ca^{2+} and also some Na^+ and K^+. Since there is a large electrochemical gradient for Ca^{2+} influx, ROC activation causes a rapid rise in cytosolic [Ca^{2+}]. The ROC constituent proteins were recently identified as members of the TRPC family (transient receptor potential, canonical subtype).

Store-operated channels (SOCs) are again Ca^{2+}-conducting channels in the surface membrane, but their activation is associated with Ca^{2+} store release. There are two main types of SOC. Human endothelium expresses SOCs composed of TRPC1

protein. These are low-selectivity, cation-conducting channels that are activated by IP$_3$ as it releases the endoplasmic reticulum store (Figure 9.7). A second type of SOC is composed of Orail proteins. This channel is exquisitely Ca^{2+}-selective, and is activated by an endoplasmic reticulum protein, STIM1, following Ca^{2+} store release; so it is also called the CRAC channel (calcium-release activated channel). SOC activation leads to an influx of extracellular Ca^{2+}, called capacitative or store-operated Ca^{2+} entry. This raises the free Ca^{2+} level, as well as restocking the SR store. SOCs are thought to be more abundant than ROCs in many types of endothelium.

As a result of these multiple pathways, an agonist usually evokes a biphasic change in endothelial Ca^{2+} concentration. There is an initial high spike in free Ca^{2+} concentration, brought about by IP$_3$-mediated store release and DAG-mediated ROC activation. This is followed by a lesser but more sustained Ca^{2+} elevation due to SOC activation. Endothelial cells may also possess **stretch-activated channels**, which allow Ca^{2+} entry in response to shear stress.

Calcium-activated K$^+$ channels (K$_{Ca}$) can hyperpolarize endothelium

A rise in endothelial free Ca^{2+} activates a special type of K^+ channels, the calcium-activated potassium channels K$_{Ca}$ (Figure 9.7). This increases the

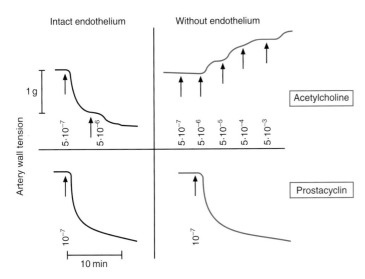

Figure 9.8 Recording of force exerted by a strip of canine artery *in vitro*. Addition of acetylcholine or prostacyclin caused relaxation (*left panels*). When endothelium was rubbed away, the response to acetylcholine changed to contraction (*top right*). Thus, the relaxation was endothelium dependent. In the unrubbed vessel, the response depends on the balance between endothelium-mediated relaxation (dominant) and the direct constrictor action of acetylcholine on smooth muscle. The response to added prostacyclin was not endothelium dependent (*bottom right*). (Redrawn and modified using data from Altura B. *Microcirculation, Endothelium and Lymphatics* 1988; **4**: 97–110, by permission.)

membrane permeability to K^+, leading to hyperpolarization, i.e. a more negative potential (eqn 3.4). Hyperpolarization serves two functions. It increase the electrochemical force drawing extracellular Ca^{2+} into the cell; and it can be transmitted through myoendothelial gap junctions to induce arteriolar relaxation (Sections 9.5 and 13.7).

There are three subtypes of K_{Ca} channel: small conductance (**SK$_{Ca}$**), intermediate conductance (**IK$_{Ca}$**) and big conductance (**BK$_{Ca}$**). SK$_{Ca}$ and IK$_{Ca}$ occur exclusively in endothelium (Figure 9.7), while BK$_{Ca}$ occurs in vascular smooth muscle. The channels are pharmacologically distinguishable: SK$_{Ca}$ is blocked by apamin, a constituent of bee stings; IK$_{Ca}$ and BK$_{Ca}$ are blocked by charybdotoxin, a constituent of scorpion stings; and BK$_{Ca}$ is blocked by iberiotoxin.

9.4 Nitric oxide production by endothelium

Nitric oxide (NO) is a freely diffusible, dissolved gas with vasodilator properties. It is generated continuously by arterial endothelium at a low basal rate. The discovery that endothelium secretes vasoactive agents was a relatively late one, and arose as follows.

The discovery that endothelium modulates vascular tone

- **Prostacyclin**. The role of the endothelium as a regulator of vascular tone began to emerge when Vane and colleagues discovered in 1976 that blood vessels secrete a vasodilator substance, prostacyclin (PGI$_2$). Prostacyclin-induced dilatation is illustrated in Figure 9.8, lower panels.

- **Nitric oxide (NO)**. A second endothelium-derived vasodilator agent was discovered in 1980 by Furchgott and Zawadski, who noted that the vasodilatation of large arteries by an acetylcholine analogue, carbachol, changed into vasoconstriction when the endothelial lining was rubbed away (Figure 9.8, upper panels). It emerged that agonists, such as acetylcholine, stimulate endothelium to secrete a vasodilator substance, initially dubbed 'endothelium–derived relaxing factor' (EDRF) and now identified as nitric oxide. The vasodilator action of the endothelium-derived nitric oxide overrides the direct vasoconstrictor action of acetylcholine on arterial muscle.

- **Endothelium-derived hyperpolarizing factor (EDHF)**. A third vasodilator, EDHF, was discovered when it was realized that endothelium-dependent vasodilatation persists in some small vessels after blocking nitric oxide and prostacyclin production. The response involves smooth muscle hyperpolarization (Figure 9.9).

- **Endothelin**. A fourth endothelial secretion, a vasoconstrictor peptide called endothelin, was discovered in 1989 by a Japanese group using molecular biology techniques.

All four substances are released as they are produced, rather than being stored for later secretion.

Endothelial nitric oxide has multiple functions

NO is soluble in both lipid and water, so it diffuses freely from the endothelium into the neighbouring vascular smooth muscle and bloodstream, with multiple local effects.

Figure 9.9 (a) Endothelium-dependent relaxation of guinea-pig coronary artery (black line) in response to acetylcholine (bar). The relaxation is mediated partly by hyperpolarization of the vascular smooth muscle (red line). (b) Blockage of NO production, using nitroarginine methyl ester (NAME), and prostacyclin, using indomethacin, abolishes the late part of the response. The early phase of hyperpolarization and relaxation, which is mediated by EDHF, persists. (From Parkington HC, Tona MA, Coleman HA, Tare M. *Journal of Physiology* 1995; **484**: 469–80 with permission from Wiley-Blackwell.)

- NO **lowers vascular tone in veins, and in large muscular arteries**, such as the coronary artery (Figure 9.9a). NO also dilates small resistance vessels, though EDHF is relatively more important in these vessels. Arterial NO production is stimulated by shear stress, leading to **flow-induced dilatation in large arteries**, which helps increase the blood flow to exercising muscles (Sections 13.3 and 13.7). NO production is also stimulated by inflammatory mediators, such as bradykinin, leading to the characteristic **vasodilatation of inflammation**. The NO-releasing drug **glyceryl trinitrate** relieves angina partly through venous dilatation, which reduces central venous pressure and therefore cardiac work; and partly through large artery relaxation, which reduces wave reflection and therefore systolic pressure and cardiac work (Figure 8.10). Since basal NO production is continuous, inhibitors of NO production cause vasoconstriction.

- NO contributes to **gap formation in venules during inflammation**.
- NO **inhibits vascular myocyte proliferation**, a component of atheroma.
- NO **inhibits platelet aggregation** and thus protects blood vessels from thrombosis.
- NO **inhibits the transcription of leukocyte-binding adhesion molecules**, such as endothelial VCAM.

The inhibition of smooth muscle proliferation, platelet activation and leukocyte adhesion by NO are all anti-atheroma actions, and reduced NO availability is thought to contribute to atheroma formation (Section 9.10).

NO is generated from L-arginine by nitric oxide synthase (eNOS)

Nitric oxide is generated continuously and survives only seconds before degradation. It is produced by a constitutively expressed enzyme, endothelial nitric oxide synthase, eNOS (NOS-III). eNOS is a haem-containing enzyme located on the inner surface of the caveolar membrane, in a complex with caveolin, high-density lipoprotein (HDL) and oestrogen receptors. eNOS cleaves the nitrogen group from the amino acid L-arginine and combines it with oxygen to form NO (Figure 9.10). Inactive analogues of arginine, such as nitroarginine methyl ester (NAME), compete with normal arginine for the eNOS binding site, and therefore act as eNOS blockers. There are also non-endothelial isoforms of nitric oxide synthase (inducible iNOS, neural nNOS), as described in Section 13.3.

NO production is stimulated by shear stress and agonists

As noted above, eNOS activity is stimulated tonically by the shear stress exerted by flowing blood, and can be enhanced by agonists such as acetylcholine and inflammatory mediators.

Shear stress stimulates eNOS via PI3 kinase

Basal shear stress (Figure 8.3) provides an important, tonic drive for NO production. Moreover, during exercise, increased blood flow in the arteries feeding the active skeletal muscles raises the shear stress and NO production. This results in **flow-induced vasodilatation** in large, conduit arteries supplying active muscle groups (Section 13.4). The shear stress

Figure 9.10 Regulation of NO production and its effect on neighbouring vascular smooth muscle. Key as for Figure 9.7; eNOS endothelial nitric oxide synthase; ER endoplasmic reticulum; PDE-5 phosphodiesterase 5 (inhibited by sildenafil, Viagra); PI-3 kinase, phosphatidyl inositol-3 kinase; PKB protein kinase B (akt).

is probably transduced into a biochemical signal by the glycocalyx, since glycocalyx-degrading enzymes reduce NO production. Transduction activates the enzyme **phosphatidyl inositol-3 kinase** (PI3 kinase), leading to the activation of protein kinase B (akt), which phosphorylates eNOS (Figure 9.10). Phosphorylation renders eNOS more sensitive to background Ca^{2+}-calmodulin, the intracellular activator of eNOS.

Agonists stimulate eNOS via Ca^{2+}–calmodulin

Agonist such as acetylcholine raise endothelial free Ca^{2+} concentration via the PLC–ROC/SOC pathway (Figure 9.7). Some of the Ca^{2+} binds to an intracellular Ca^{2+}-binding protein, calmodulin. The Ca^{2+}–calmodulin complex enhances eNOS activity and hence NO production (Figure 9.10). Agonists that act in this way include bradykinin, thrombin, substance P, ATP, ADP, acetylcholine (via muscarinic M_3 receptors), vasoactive intestinal polypeptide, insulin and in some tissues/species histamine. Several of these agents are released during inflammation, so NO contributes to the characteristic redness (vasodilatation) of inflamed tissue.

NO causes vasodilatation by two mechanisms

(i) Endothelial NO diffuses rapidly into neighbouring vascular smooth muscle cells, where it binds to the haem group of a soluble enzyme, guanylyl cyclase (Figure 9.10). N-O is chemical cousin to O-O, oxygen, hence its high affinity for haem. The activated guanylyl cyclase catalyses the production of **cyclic guanosine monophosphate (cGMP)** from guanosine triphosphate. The cGMP activates kinases (enzymes that phosphorylate other proteins to alter their activity) that promote vascular relaxation, as detailed in Section 12.7. (ii) High concentrations of NO directly activate big conductance **BK_{Ca} channels** in the smooth muscle membrane (Figure 9.10). This hyperpolarizes the smooth muscle, leading to vascular relaxation (Figure 9.9a).

NO is inactivated rapidly

NO is inactivated within seconds by two mechanisms: (i) NO reacts with a by-product of oxidative metabolism, the superoxide anion O_2^-, to form peroxynitrite, $ONOO^-$. Peroxynitrite is then converted into ordinary nitrite (NO_2^-) and nitrate (NO_3^-) for excretion in the urine. (ii) Some NO diffuses into the bloodstream, where its similarity to oxygen (O-O) causes it to bind to red cell haemoglobin.

9.5 Other vasoactive endothelial products: EDHF, prostacyclin, endothelin

Endothelium-derived hyperpolarizing factors (EDHF)

NO exerts its main physiological effects in large vessels, where eNOS is abundant. If NO and prostacyclin production are blocked in **small arteries and arterioles**, agonists such as acetylcholine and bradykinin still evoke endothelium-dependent dilatation, which is mediated by smooth muscle hyperpolarization (Figure 9.9b). Also, in some tissues saline washed through agonist-stimulated vessels picks up a chemical that can hyperpolarize isolated vascular muscle – an 'endothelium-derived hyperpolarizing factor', EDHF.

The **stimuli for EDHF** production include the classical parasympathetic transmitter acetylcholine, inflammatory agents such as bradykinin, and possibly shear stress. The **roles of EDHF** are thought to be:

- to help increase blood flow to exercising muscle, by dilating small, feed arteries (ascending, conducted vasodilatation; Section 13.7);
- to contribute to the cholinergic vasodilatation of small resistance vessels in certain tissues with a cholinergic autonomic innervation (Sections 14.2 and 14.3);
- to contribute to the vasodilatation of inflammation.

The **identity of EDHF** is controversial. Although endothelium-derived hyperpolarization can indeed be brought about by released, chemical factor(s) in some tissues, it can also be brought about by direct, electrical coupling between the endothelium and vascular muscle. Electrical transmission may be the primary hyperpolarizing mechanism, with released, soluble EDHFs serving to boost the myocyte hyperpolarization.

(i) **Direct electrical transmission of endothelial hyperpolarization to vascular myocyte** has been demonstrated in arterioles and small arteries (diameter $\sim 100\,\mu m$), where myoendothelial gap junctions are abundant (Figure 1.11). When an agonist raises the endothelial free Ca^{2+} concentration, the activated SK_{Ca} and IK_{Ca} channels hyperpolarize the endothelial cell (Figure 9.7). The endothelial

hyperpolarization then spreads through the myoendothelial (heterocellular) gap junctions to hyperpolarize and relax the vascular myocytes. This form of 'EDHF' is inhibited by gap junctions blockers, and by apamin and charybotoxin, the blockers of endothelial SK_{Ca} and IK_{Ca} channels.

(ii) **Released chemical factors**. Activated endothelial SK_{Ca} and IK_{Ca} channels release **K^+ ions** into the interstitial spaces around neighbouring vascular myocytes. The rise in extracellular K^+ reinforces myocyte hyperpolarization, by stimulating the myocyte $3Na^+-2K^+$ pump and by activating myocyte K_{ir} channels (Section 13.4). Also, in small coronary, renal and skeletal muscle arteries, **epoxyeicosatrienoic acid (EET)** may be an additional EDHF. In these vessels, the agonist bradykinin activates endothelial phospholipase A_2, which generates arachidonic acid. Arachidonic acid is converted by endothelial cytochrome P450 epoxygenase to diffusible EET. Myocyte EET receptors trigger a pathway that activates myocyte BK_{Ca} channels, leading to hyperpolarization and vasodilatation (Section 12.7). Additional candidate EDHF factors are hydrogen peroxide and c-natriuretic peptide.

Prostacyclin (PGI$_2$)

Like NO, prostacyclin causes vasodilatation and inhibits platelet aggregation. It is produced by endothelium constitutively (i.e. without needing stimulation), and also in response to agonists, such as thrombin. **Phospholipase A_2** converts membrane phospholipids into the unsaturated fatty acid, **arachidonic acid**. The arachidonic acid is then converted by **cyclo-oxygenases** into prostacyclin. Prostacyclin production is greatly increased in inflammation and contributes to the associated vasodilatation. It also contributes to the cutaneous vasodilatation associated with sweating.

Endothelins

The endothelins are a family of peptides related to the snake venom sarafotoxin. Endothelin-1, the main isoform secreted by the endothelium, causes a powerful, unusually sustained vasoconstriction, lasting 2–3 hours. Endothelin-1 activates myocyte ET_A receptors, which are coupled via a G protein to the myocyte phospholipase C–IP$_3$ system. The resulting rise in myocyte Ca^{2+} triggers vasoconstriction. Over a longer time scale, endothelin also stimulates vascular and cardiac myocyte proliferation.

Endothelin is produced continuously and makes a small contribution to basal vascular tone in humans. Its production can be increased by vibration, hypoxia, angiotensin II, vasopressin and thrombin. Plasma endothelin levels are raised in pre-eclamptic toxaemia (the hypertension of pregnancy) and heart failure. Endothelin also contributes to cerebral artery vasospasm in patients with haemorrhagic strokes.

9.6 Actions of endothelium on blood

Endothelium catalyses angiotensin II production

Angiotensin I is a relatively inactive, circulating decapeptide formed in renal plasma (Section 14.8). It is converted into angiotensin II, an octapeptide with strong vasoconstrictor properties, by **angiotensin-converting enzyme (ACE)**, a zinc carboxypeptidase expressed on the luminal surface of endothelium (Figure 9.1). Conversion occurs mainly in the lungs, the first large area of endothelium encountered by angiotensin I after its production in renal venous plasma. ACE inhibitors, such as captopril, reduce angiotensin II levels and are widely used to treat hypertension and heart failure (Chapter 18).

Lung ACE also rapidly degrades the circulating vasoactive agents bradykinin and serotonin. These are pro-inflammatory substances, so occasional side effects of ACE inhibitors are oedema formation and cough.

Endothelium secretes a haemostatic agent, von Willebrand factor

Endothelial cells contain a unique, rod-shaped, storage organelle, the Weibel–Palade body, which consists of numerous, stacked tubules composed of a glycoprotein, **von Willebrand factor** (vWF) (Figure 9.1). The vWF is secreted constitutively into the bloodstream, and has two roles in blood clotting. (i) vWF is a carrier for clotting factor VIII. (ii) During blood clotting, plasma prothrombin is converted into thrombin. Thrombin not only converts fibrinogen into insoluble fibrin (a crucial step in blood clotting), but also activates endothelial thrombin receptors, which triggers a rapid, local exocytosis of vWF (Figure 9.1). Some of the vWF binds to subendothelial collagen and promotes platelet adhesion, another crucial step in blood clotting. **von Willebrand disease**, which is a common, inherited failure to synthesize vWF, is characterized by prolonged bleeding after injury.

The Weibel–Palade body also contains a store of the leukocyte-adhesive protein **P-selectin**. When endothelium is activated by an inflammatory agonist, the P-selectin is translocated to the surface and initiates the capture of passing leukocytes (Figure 9.11).

Platelet aggregation is inhibited by NO and prostacyclin

Platelet aggregation, an important step in thrombosis and blood clotting, is inhibited by NO and prostacyclin. When blood clots, activated endothelial thrombin receptors not only cause vWF exocytosis but also stimulate NO and prostacyclin production. This limits the spread of platelet aggregation. The endothelial secretions thus contribute to a limited, well-regulated haemostatic process, rather than a runaway vascular thrombosis.

9.7 Endothelial permeability and its regulation

The endothelial intercellular cleft of capillaries is the main pathway for the transfer of water and nutrients from blood to tissue (Figures 9.3 and 9.4). The permeability of this pathway is not fixed; it can be modulated by blood velocity and by chemical messengers, as outlined below. For a fuller account, see Chapters 10 and 11.

Increased permeability

An increase in **plasma velocity** raises capillary intercellular permeability, which facilitates the transfer of glucose from blood into exercising muscle (Section 10.11). The increased permeability is mediated by flow-stimulated NO production, since it is blocked by eNOS inhibitors. Permeability can also be increased by **atrial natriuretic peptide**, a hormone involved in the regulation of plasma volume (Section 14.9). Both NO and atrial natriuretic peptide raise endothelial cGMP, which activates pathways that raise intercellular permeability. **Endothelial cGMP** also has a key role in raising permeability during inflammation (Sections 9.8 and 11.11). **Vascular endothelial growth factor** (VEGF, originally called 'vascular permeability factor') is a protein secreted by growing or healing tissues, that increases endothelial permeability and stimulates microvessel growth (Section 9.9).

Reduced permeability

Beta$_2$-adrenoceptor agonists, such as isoprenaline and terbutaline, reduce basal capillary

CONCEPT BOX 9.2

Endothelium mediates many aspects of inflammation

- Inflammation is characterized by redness, heat, swelling, pain, loss of function and leukocyte migration. Endothelium has key roles in these changes.
- The *redness* and *heat* are caused by vasodilatation. Many mediators of inflammation (bradykinin, substance P, thrombin and cytokines) increase endothelial production of the vasodilator, nitric oxide (NO).
- The *swelling* is due to the formation of large gaps in venular endothelium. The gaps allow a rapid efflux of water and plasma proteins, including immunoglobulins.
- *Leukocyte capture* occurs when specific 'glue' molecules (P-selectin, E-selectin, ICAM, VCAM) are inserted into the luminal membrane of venular endothelium under the influence of cytokines (IL-1β, TNFα). The arrested leukocytes migrate through the intercellular junctions to attack the cause of the inflammation.

permeability. These agents raise **endothelial cAMP** (cyclic adenosine monophosphate), which activates pathways that enhance junctional strand formation. Thus cAMP is a barrier-enhancing messenger and cGMP is a barrier-reducing messenger. cGMP may act in part by activating a phosphodiesterase that degrades cAMP (Section 11.11).

9.8 Endothelium and the inflammatory response

Endothelium contributes to the classic signs of inflammation

Inflammation is a group of defensive responses to infection, burns, trauma and autoimmune diseases, such as rheumatoid arthritis. Celsus (30BC to 38AD) defined inflammation as a combination of redness (rubor), heat (calor), swelling (tumor) and pain (dolor), to which Galen (130–200AD) added a fifth criterion, loss of function. This definition remains lucid and valid today, and endothelium has a central role in the redness, heat and swelling.

The **redness** and **heat** are the results of vasodilatation, which is induced by a host of inflammatory mediators (histamine, bradykinin, prostacyclin, substance P, platelet activating factor, superoxide radicals and cytokines). Most of these agonists produce

vasodilatation by raising endothelial $[Ca^{2+}]$, which stimulates NO and EDHF production.

The characteristic **swelling** of inflammation is caused by the rapid escape of plasma from the circulation through the newly formed gaps in venular endothelium. These inflammatory gaps are triggered by the agonist-induced rise in endothelial $[Ca^{2+}]$ and NO (Figures 9.7 and 11.30).

A sixth fundamental feature of inflammation, discovered by Addison and Waller between 1843 and 1846, is the **emigration of leukocytes**, which in its most gross form leads to pus formation. Endothelium has a crucial role in leukocyte emigration, as follows.

Venular endothelium induces circulating leukocytes to emigrate (diapedesis)

During acute inflammation, polymorphonuclear neutrophils migrate from the bloodstream into the inflamed tissue, followed by monocytes and eventually lymphocytes. Leukocyte migration involves three, sequential steps: rolling capture, arrest and emigration.

Rolling capture. The capture of circulating leukocytes begins in venular endothelium, where inflammatory agonists, such as histamine and thrombin, trigger the transfer of **P-selectin** from the Weibel–Palade body to the surface membrane. P-selectin is a carbohydrate-binding protein ('lectin') that renders the surface sticky to leukocytes. The leukocyte itself has microvilli that penetrate the glycocalyx, and oligosaccharides on the microvilli bind loosely to the P-selectin. Since the adhesion is weak, the 'marginated' leukocyte continues to roll slowly over the endothelium, driven by the bloodstream. Rolling, marginated leukocytes appear within minutes of applying an inflammatory stimulus.

The inflamed tissue produces not only acute inflammatory agonists such as histamine, but also the cytokines interleukin-1 (IL-1), tumour necrosis factor (TNFα) and interferon γ, which act more slowly. These cytokines stimulate endothelium to produce a second type of leukocyte glue, **E-selectin**, which can maintain rolling margination for several hours.

Arrest. Tight-binding proteins are then activated on both the endothelium and leukocyte. The endothelial binding proteins are **ICAM** (intercellular adhesion molecule) and **VCAM** (vascular cell adhesion molecule). The ICAM and VCAM bind firmly to β_2-**integrins**, which

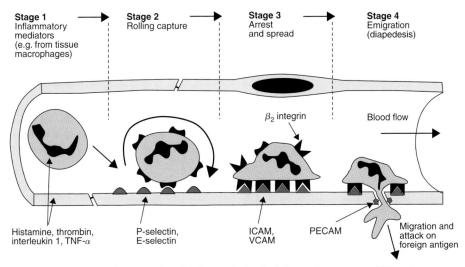

Figure 9.11 Rolling capture, arrest and extravasation of leukocyte during the inflammatory response. TNF-α, tumour necrosis factor α; ICAM, VCAM, PECAM: see text.

appear on the surface of slowly rolling leukocytes. This brings the leukocytes to a halt, 'like so many pebbles or marbles over which a stream runs without disturbing them', as Waller vividly reported in 1846. In the rare genetic condition of '**leukocyte adhesion deficiency**', a lack of β₂-integrins results in a failure of leukocyte arrest, leading to a life-threatening susceptibility to bacterial infection.

Emigration. Once arrested, the leukocyte inserts a thin foot into the endothelial intercellular junction and squeezes through into the tissue (diapedesis). This process depends on a high local concentration of ICAM-1 and platelet–endothelial cell adhesion molecule (PECAM). In genetically engineered, knock-out mice lacking PECAM, leukocytes become trapped at the basal lamina, reducing emigration. This indicates that PECAM is needed to activate the leukocyte to break through the basal lamina.

The intercellular junction reseals rapidly, in seconds, after leukocyte migration. Not infrequently, leukocytes also migrate through holes in the endothelial cell itself, rather than the intercellular junctions. These transcellular holes likewise reseal quickly.

9.9 Endothelium and angiogenesis

The endothelial cell has a lifespan of months to years, so cell division is normally infrequent. However, when there is a need for new vessels (angiogenesis), endothelial cells can multiply rapidly, forming a simple endothelial tube in a few days. The tube then matures into an artery, vein or capillary. In adults, angiogenesis is essential for tissue growth, adaptation (e.g. increased number of capillaries in trained muscle) and wound healing. Endothelium also grows over the artificial grafts used in vascular surgery. On the downside, angiogenesis contributes to cancer growth, rheumatoid arthritis and diabetic eye disease.

New vessels arise from capillary sprouts and splits

New vessel formation begins with the degradation of the endothelial basement membrane by proteases in an existing capillary or venule. This is followed by an outward **sprouting** of the endothelial cells (Figure 9.1). Vacuolation of the cell interior creates a lumen, and further cell division extends the tube, until it connects up with another new vessel. The new vessels are hyperpermeable at first, and allow fibrinogen to extravasate into the tissues. This creates an oedematous, fibrin-rich, vascular matrix called **granulation tissue**, which is a favourable environment for cell growth and wound healing. With maturity the microvessel permeability declines to normal, probably due to an increase in the cAMP:cGMP ratio. In addition to sprouting, new vessels can be formed by **splitting**. In this process, an endothelial septum grows inwards along a length of a capillary, partitioning the lumen into two.

The maturation of new endothelial tubes into arterioles and venules is brought about by the recruitment of smooth muscle cells and connective tissue cells, driven by **platelet-derived growth factor** (PDGF-BB) and **angiopoietins**. The final fate of the vessel, i.e. whether it becomes an artery or vein, is determined by the expression of the protein **ephrin B** and its receptor.

Angiogenesis is initiated by VEGF and other growth factors

Angiogenesis is initiated by tissue growth factors that induce endothelial gene expression. The principal endothelial growth factors are the **vascular endothelial growth factors** (VEGF for capillary sprouting, VEGF-C for lymphatic sprouting) and acidic and basic fibroblast growth factors. VEGF is abundant wherever tissues are forming new vessels, e.g. fetus, placenta, healing wounds, tumours, psoriatic plaques, rheumatoid pannus, myocardium adjacent to infarcts and the diabetic retina (a leading cause of blindness in the West). The endothelial VEGF receptor is linked to a tyrosine kinase that activates a cascade of MAP kinases. This activates nuclear transcription factors, which switch on the angiogenesis genes.

What regulates VEGF secretion in such a way as to produce a capillary within 20–50 μm of most cells, and the highest capillary density in the most active tissues? The answer is that a shortage of O_2 stimulates cells to produce **hypoxia-inducible factor** (**HIF**), a gene-regulating protein. HIF stimulates the transcription of the VEGF gene, which in turn leads to angiogenesis. When sufficient new vessels have formed, the O_2 supply becomes adequate, so HIF levels fall and VEGF production is switched off. If VEGF production fails to switch off, the result is a haemangioblastoma – a tumour composed largely of a dense mass of blood vessels.

Angiogenesis is restrained by thrombospondin and angiostatin

Endothelial growth is normally held in check by the anti-angiogenic proteins thrombospondin and angiostatin. For angiogenesis to occur, the levels of thrombospondin and angiostatin have to fall, as well as VEGF rising. The discovery of anti-angiogenic factors has led to anti-angiogenic drugs to restrict cancer growth. Once a tumour grows above ~1 mm in size, it depends on angiogenesis for an adequate nutrient supply. Anti-angiogenic drugs are therefore now used to complement cytotoxic drugs in the treatment of some cancers.

9.10 Endothelium and atheroma

Atheroma, the commonest cause of serious morbidity and death in Westernized societies, is a patchy, cholesterol-rich deposit in the subendothelial intima of large arteries. Atheroma is known alternatively as atherosclerosis – a rather self-contradictory term meaning 'gruel-like hardening'. The atheroma forms a plaque that narrows the artery lumen, leading to tissue ischaemia and thrombosis. In the heart, this results in **angina** and **heart attacks**; in the brain, **transient ischaemic attacks** and **thrombo-embolic strokes**; and in the legs, **intermittent claudication** (ischaemic pain on walking), **arterial ulcers** and **gangrenous necrosis** (tissue death, requiring amputation). The chief predisposing factors are high plasma levels of low-density lipoprotein (LDL – cholesterol bound to a carrier protein, $\sim 3 \times 10^6$ Da), high plasma fibrinogen, smoking, diabetes and hypertension. Shear stress disturbances too are atherogenic, since atheroma commonly develops at branches and bends. A moderate, regular intake of any alcoholic drink reduces the incidence of ischaemic heart disease by 20–30%, and red wine may be particularly beneficial.

Atheroma is rich in plasma-derived cholesterol

The atheromatous plaque begins as an intimal, subendothelial accumulation of LDL (mainly cholesterol) and fibrin, both derived from the plasma. The early lesion is also characterized by foam cells, which are lipid-laden macrophages derived from circulating monocytes. Later, proliferating vascular smooth muscle cells migrate into the lesion and a fibrous cap is laid down over the lipid deposit. Rupture of the cap can lead to platelet aggregation and thrombosis. Since the lesion involves the transendothelial passage of LDL and fibrinogen, and often platelet aggregation, endothelial dysfunction is thought to contribute to the pathogenesis. More specifically, impaired NO levels appear to be a contributory factor, as follows.

Reduced NO levels facilitate atheroma formation

Endothelial nitric oxide is anti-atherogenic, because it inhibits vascular smooth muscle migration, platelet aggregation and endothelial expression of the monocyte glue, VCAM (source of atheroma foam cells) (Section 9.4). There is now considerable

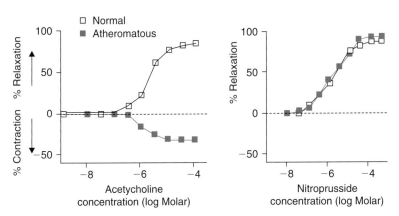

Figure 9.12 Reduced NO availability in atheromatous arteries of monkey. Response of normal (open squares) and atheromatous iliac artery (red filled squares) to acetylcholine (left panel) and to the NO donor nitroprusside (right panel). The NO-dependent vasodilator response to acetylcholine becomes a constrictor response in atheromatous arteries. Sketch shows proposed explanation – high levels of endothelial superoxide radicals in atheromatous vessels react with NO, reducing the amount of transferable NO. (Redrawn from Freiman PC, Mitchell GC, Heistad DD *et al. Circulation Research* 1986. **58**: 783–9.)

evidence that reduced NO levels contribute to atheroma formation. For example, atheroma formation in hypercholesterolaemic rabbits is reduced by L-arginine, which boosts NO production. Conversely, eNOS inhibitors increase the uptake of LDL and fibrinogen into the artery wall. Smokers and diabetics, who are especially prone to atheroma, have low NO levels and show impaired NO-dependent arterial vasodilatation. Diabetics have low insulin levels, or are insulin-resistant, and insulin is normally a significant tonic stimulus to NO production.

NO is depleted by increased superoxide production

Healthy arteries respond to acetylcholine by endothelium-dependent vasodilatation, but atheromatous arteries show impaired dilatation or even constriction (Figure 9.12). This indicates that endothelial NO levels are low in atheromatous arteries. In early lesions, this is due to reduced endothelial NO generation, while in more advanced lesions, there is also increased inactivation of NO. Increased inactivation is caused by an overproduction of the superoxide radical O_2^- by oxidases involved in oxidative metabolism. Superoxide inactivates NO by reacting with it, to form peroxynitrite, $ONOO^-$ (Appendix 2, Free radicals). Superoxide generation is increased three-fold in the aorta of cholesterol-fed rabbits, and is increased by smoking and diabetes. Moreover, superoxide dismutase, an enzyme that scavenges (removes) superoxide radicals, improves the endothelium-dependent vasodilatation of atheromatous vessels. It appears, therefore, that excessive superoxide production reduces NO concentration and hence the NO-based protection against atherogenesis.

Peroxynitrite is itself harmful, because it undergoes further reactions that produce hydroxyl radicals, which damage cell membranes and oxidize LDL. Oxidized LDL reduces NO production further, by displacing eNOS from its caveolar, cholesterol-rich binding site. By contrast, the 'good' high-density lipoprotein (HDL) promotes eNOS localization in caveolae and boosts NO production.

SUMMARY

- Endothelium is a monolayer of flattened cells tethered to the basal lamina by integrins. The collagen IV-rich basal lamina prevents capillary rupture. Adjacent cells are joined by circumferential strands of junctional proteins, tethered internally to the actin cytoskeleton. Breaks in the junctional strands allow the intercellular passage of water and small solutes. Plasma proteins are prevented from entering the intercellular cleft by a semipermeable luminal coat, the glycocalyx. Some plasma protein is transported slowly across endothelium by a caveola–vesicle system.

- Endothelium has an intracellular potential of -30 to $-60\,\text{mV}$, due chiefly to inward rectifier K^+ channels. Receptors to inflammatory agonists (e.g. histamine, bradykinin) activate phospholipase C, which leads to the activation of receptor-operated and store-operated Ca^{2+} channels. The influx of extracellular Ca^{2+} triggers NO secretion and raises microvascular permeability. The Ca^{2+} also activates SK_{Ca} and IK_{Ca} channels, which increases the negative potential to boost Ca^{2+} entry.

- Endothelium regulates local vascular tone by secreting the vasoconstrictor peptide endothelin and three vasodilator agents: nitric oxide, endothelium-derived hyperpolarizing factor and prostacyclin.

- Endothelin causes a long-lasting vasoconstriction. Circulating endothelin is elevated in hypoxia, pre-eclamptic toxaemia, heart failure and haemorrhagic strokes.

- NO is generated continuously from L-arginine by Ca^{2+}–calmodulin-dependent endothelial nitric oxide synthase (eNOS). eNOS activity can be increased by (i) shear stress, leading to flow-induced vasodilatation in large arteries; and (ii) agonists such as acetylcholine, bradykinin and other inflammatory agents. The angina-relieving action of glyceryl trinitrate is due to its NO-like vasodilatation of large veins and arteries.

- EDHF dilates smaller arterial vessels. It mediates ascending (conducted) vasodilatation of feed arteries in exercising muscle. Prostacyclin, like nitric oxide, causes vasodilatation and inhibits platelet aggregation.

- Endothelium also influences blood. Angiotensin-converting enzyme (ACE) on the endothelial surface catalyses angiotensin II formation. Von Willebrand factor, released from the endothelial Weibel–Palade body, carries clotting factor VIII. NO and prostacyclin inhibit platelet aggregation to prevent/limit clotting.

- Venular endothelium contributes to the inflammatory response. Adhesive proteins (selectins, ICAM, VCAM) are inserted into the luminal membrane to capture circulating leukocytes. Also the formation of wide intercellular gaps in venular endothelium speeds up the transfer of immunoglobulins and water, and leads to inflammatory swelling.

- Capillary permeability is regulated via changes in the organization of junctional proteins. Permeability is raised by flow and atrial natriuretic peptide, acting through cGMP. Conversely, agents that increase endothelial cAMP enhance the intercellular barrier.

- Vascular endothelial growth factor stimulates capillary sprouting (angiogenesis). Angiogenesis is necessary for tissue and tumour growth. Angiogenesis is inhibited by thrombospondin, angiostatin and anti-cancer angiostatic drugs.

- The trapping of plasma-derived low-density lipoprotein and fibrin under arterial endothelium gives rise to atheroma, the biggest killer in Westernized societies. Endothelial NO normally protects against atheroma by reducing LDL and fibrinogen uptake, VCAM expression, smooth muscle proliferation and platelet aggregation. NO levels are low in atheromatous arteries, due in part to a reaction with superoxide.

Further reading

Reviews

Bazzoni G, Dejana E. Endothelial cell-to-cell junctions: molecular organization and role in vascular homeostasis. *Physiological Reviews* 2004; **84**: 869–901.

Carmeliet P. Angiogenesis in life, disease and medicine. *Nature* 2005; **438**: 932–36.

Cohen AW, Hnasko R, Schubert W, Lisanti MP. Role of caveolae and caveolins in health and disease. *Physiological Reviews* 2004; **84**: 1341–79.

Curry FE. Regulation of capillary permeability in single perfused microvessels. In: Reed RK, Rubin K (eds). *Connective Tissue Biology, Integration and Reductionism.* London: Portland Press, 1998: 195–206.

Davies PF. Flow-mediated endothelial mechanotransduction. *Physiological Reviews* 1995; **75**: 519–60.

De Wit C, Wolfle SE. EDHF and gap junctions: important regulators of vascular tone within the microcirculation. *Current Pharmaceutical Biotechnology* 2007; **8**: 11–25.

Fisslthaler B, Dimmeler S, Hermann C, Busse R, Fleming I. Phosphorylation and activation of the endothelial nitric oxide synthase by fluid shear stress. *Acta Physiologica Scandinavica* 2000; **168**: 81–8.

Kvietys, PR, Sandig M. Neutrophil diapedesis: paracellular or transcellular? *News in Physiological Sciences* 2001; **16**: 15–19.

Nilius B, Droogmans G. Ion channels and their functional role in vascular endothelium. *Physiological Reviews* 2001; **81**: 1415–59.

Parekh AB, Putney JWJ. Store-operated calcium channels. *Physiological Reviews* 2005; **85**: 757–810.

Reitsma S, Slaaf DW, Vink H, van Zandvoort MAMJ, oude Egbrink MG. The endothelial glycocalyx: composition, functions and visualization. *Pfluger's Achiv* 2007: **254**: 345–59.

Shaul PW. Endothelial nitric oxide synthase, caveolae and the development of atherosclerosis. *Journal of Physiology* 2003; **547**: 21–23.

Thurston G, Baluk P, McDonald DM. Determinants of endothelial cell phenotype in venules. *Microcirculation* 2000; **7**: 67–80.

Tiruppathi C, Ahmed GU, Vogel SM, Malik AB. Ca^{2+} signaling, TRP channels and endothelial permeability. *Microcirculation* 2006; **13**: 693–708.

Walzog B, Gaehtgens P. Adhesion molecules: the path to a new understanding of acute inflammation. *News in Physiological Sciences* 2000; **15**: 107–13.

Research papers

See www.hodderplus.com/cardiovascularphysiology for a full list of Research papers for this chapter.

CHAPTER 10

The microcirculation and solute exchange

Learning objectives

After reading this chapter you should be able to:

● Explain how terminal arterioles regulate capillary perfusion (10.1).
● Sketch the key structural differences between three main types of capillary (10.2).
● Distinguish between the laws governing solute exchange (diffusion) and water exchange (hydraulic flow) (10.3).
● List the factors governing the rate of diffusive transport (Fick's law) (10.3).
● Define 'solute permeability' and explain how a porous membrane affects it (10.4).
● Name three main categories of solute, based on capillary permeability (10.5–10.7).
● Outline the special features of the blood–brain barrier (10.8).
● Sketch the concentration profile of a metabolized solute (e.g. glucose) along a capillary. Use the sketch to define 'the Fick principle' (cf. law), 'extraction' and 'plasma clearance' (10.9).
● Explain the difference between flow-limited and diffusion-limited exchange (10.10).
● Describe 'capillary recruitment', and list other factors that enhance solute exchange in exercising muscle (10.11).

A single, inescapable necessity has driven the evolution of the cardiovascular system – the need to deliver metabolic substrates, such as oxygen and glucose, rapidly to the cells of a large organism (Section 1.1). The delivery hatch, so to speak, is the capillary wall. The exchange of materials across the capillary wall is the payload for the entire, hugely complex system of pumps, valves, tubes and electrical potentials that we call the cardiovascular system – the sole reason for its existence.

10.1 Organization and perfusion of exchange vessels

The term 'exchange vessel' embraces not only the capillaries but also, strictly speaking, the microvessels immediately upstream and downstream, since some oxygen transfer occurs through the walls of terminal arterioles, and some fluid transfer across the walls of pericytic (postcapillary) venules. Nevertheless, capillaries account for the great majority of solute and fluid exchange.

Supply and drainage of a capillary bed

The smallest, terminal arteries branch into first-order arterioles, and further divisions give rise to **terminal arterioles**, the last arterial vessels with smooth muscle in the wall. Each terminal arteriole divides into a cluster or **module of capillaries** (Figure 10.1). **Capillary** means 'hair-like', a typical capillary being 500–1000 μm long and 4–8 μm wide – hence invisible to the naked eye. The existence

Figure 10.1 Capillary bed of relaxed cremaster muscle (rat), with a terminal arteriole feeding a module of ~14 capillaries. Numbers are means of observations. (From Smaje LH, Zweifach BW, Intaglietta M. *Microvascular Research* 1970; **2**: 96–110, with permission from Elsevier.)

of capillaries was inferred by William Harvey, from his demonstration that blood flows from arteries into veins; but it was not until the invention of the microscope that Malpighi, in 1661, first observed capillaries, in the frog lung.

The venous ends of capillaries reunite to form **pericytic venules** (postcapillary venules). These are thin-walled vessels, ~15 μm wide, with pericytes but not smooth muscle surrounding the endothelium. Pericytic venules are highly permeable to water and play a major role in inflammation. Smooth muscle reappears in the walls of venules of width 30–50 μm.

Arteriovenous anastomoses are muscular microvessels, 20–130 μm wide, that link arterioles directly to venules, bypassing the capillary network. They are found chiefly in the skin of the extremities (fingers, nose, lips, earlobes), where they are important for temperature regulation (Section 15.3).

Capillary density is adapted to tissue function

The number of capillaries packed into unit volume of tissue is called the capillary density, and is regulated by the HIF–VEGF mechanism (Section 9.9). Skeletal muscle contains 300–1000 capillaries per mm² cross section, or 1–3 capillaries per muscle fibre. Endurance training stimulates angiogenesis and can raise the capillary:fibre ratio to 6–8. In the myocardium and brain, where the metabolic rate is both high and sustained, the capillary density is correspondingly high, ~3000 per mm². This has two advantages:

- A high capillary density increases the endothelial surface area available for gas and nutrient exchange. Capillary surface area increases from ~100 cm² per gram in skeletal muscle to ~500 cm² per gram in myocardium or brain.
- A high capillary density reduces the distance between the bloodstream and tissue cells. This is important, because distance profoundly affects the time needed for diffusive transport (see Section 1.1).

The lungs provide the most extreme example of capillary packing; here, the capillary surface area is a staggering 3500 cm² per gram, for obvious functional reasons.

Terminal arterioles regulate the number of perfused capillaries

The contractile state of the terminal arterioles controls the number of capillaries that are well perfused with blood at any one moment. The relaxation of an individual arteriole allows a brisk perfusion of the associated capillary module, and such capillaries are referred to as 'open'. The contraction of a terminal arteriole slows or halts the blood flow through its associated capillary module, and such capillaries are referred to as 'closed'. In skeletal muscle at rest, some arterioles are relaxed and others are contracted at any one moment. As a result, a substantial fraction of the capillaries are 'closed' at any one instant, and the distribution of flow is uneven. This **heterogeneity of tissue perfusion** is characteristic of many resting tissues. When arteriolar tone decreases, capillary perfusion becomes more uniform; in other words, vasodilatation improves the homogeneity of tissue perfusion.

The regulation of the number of perfused capillaries used to be ascribed to a largely mythical beast, the 'precapillary sphincter'. In reality, **there is no discrete sphincteric ring of muscle at the capillary entrance** in most tissues. It is the terminal arteriole that regulates the numbers of open and closed capillaries in general.

Capillary blood flow varies with time, due to vasomotion

An individual arteriole does not usually remain relaxed or contracted for long – its muscle tone changes constantly. This is called **vasomotion**. In some tissues, such as resting skeletal muscle, vasomotion has a regular rhythm, with a cycle time of $\sim 15\,s$; in other tissues, such as skin, vasomotion is less regular. As a result of arteriolar vasomotion, blood flow in an individual capillary tends to fluctuate; it may wax and wane every $15\,s$ or so, and can stop for a while in 'closed' capillaries.

Capillary transit time governs the time available for exchange

The time that it takes a red cell to pass through the capillary bed, from entrance to exit, is called the **transit time**. Transit time represents the time available for each unit of blood to unload O_2, glucose, etc. and load up with CO_2, urea, etc. Vasomotion causes transit times to vary, but a typical transit time in a well-perfused capillary is 0.5–2 s (blood velocity 300–1000 μm/s). The transit time can fall to around 0.25 s during exercise, because the arterioles dilate and blood velocity increases. During extreme human exercise, when cardiac output is very high, the transit time through the lung capillaries can become so short that the blood emerges without having had time to achieve full O_2 saturation.

10.2 Three types of capillary

Electron microscopy has revealed three basic types of capillary. They are, in order of increasing permeability to water, the continuous capillary, the fenestrated capillary and the discontinuous capillary.

The continuous capillary

Continuous capillaries occur in skeletal muscle, myocardium, skin, lung, connective tissue and fat. Also a specialized form, the tight capillary, occurs in the central nervous system and testis. The circumference comprises a ring of one to three endothelial cells surrounded by a continuous basement membrane (Figure 10.2a). Due to the thinness of the

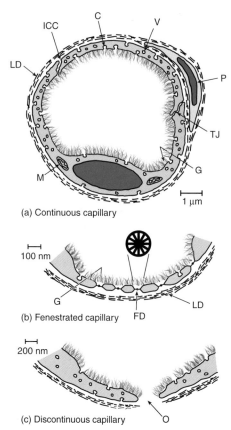

Figure 10.2 Sketches of capillary wall in transverse section, based on electron micrographs. C, caveola (open surface vesicle); FD, fenestral diaphragm; inset shows diaphragm viewed *en face*; G, glycocalyx; ICC, intercellular cleft; LD, lamina densa of basal lamina; M, mitochondrion; O, open gap; P, pericyte; TJ, tight part of intercellular junction; V, vesicle.

cells, the transcapillary diffusion distance is only $\sim 0.3\,\mu m$. **Pericytes**, formerly called Rouget cells, partly envelop the outside of the capillary. Recent genetic knock-out studies in mice indicate that the pericytes regulate capillary diameter and structure. Pericytes are unusually well developed around retinal capillaries, and seem to be contractile in this tissue.

The structural features of continuous capillaries that influence solute exchange are primarily the following. (i) The **intercellular cleft** transmits water and small lipid-insoluble solutes, e.g. glucose. These small molecules weave their way through the breaks in the junctional strands (Figures 9.2, 9.4 and 10.3); (ii) The luminal **glycocalyx** excludes plasma proteins from access to the cleft, but is permeable to water and small solute (Figure 9.3). (iii) The **caveola–vesicle** system transfers large molecules slowly across the wall (Figures 9.5 and 9.6).

View of intercellular cleft *en face*

Junctional strand   Lanthanum ions

Interstitium Face of endothelial Capillary
cleft lumen

0.2 µm

Figure 10.3 Three sections of same intercellular cleft (left). The capillary was perfused with a solution of lanthanum ions (black) for 10 s before fixation. The cleft is depicted *en face* on the right. The tight junction (red lines on right, arrows on left) blocks the cleft in Section 1, but a break in the junctional strands creates an open pathway in Section 3. The intermediate Section 2 gives the false impression that the tight junction is permeable. L, lumen; E1 and E2, endothelial cells. (Redrawn from Adamson and Michel. *Journal of Physiology* 1993; **466**: 303–27, with permission from Wiley-Blackwell.)

Fenestrated capillaries are specialized for rapid fluid filtration

Fenestrated capillaries are at least an order of magnitude more permeable to water and small lipid-insoluble solutes than are continuous capillaries. They are found in tissues that specialize in fluid exchange (kidneys, exocrine glands, intestinal mucosa, synovial lining of joints, choroid plexus, ciliary body of the eye) and in endocrine glands. The endothelium is perforated by clusters of small, circular windows, or fenestrae, of diameter 50–60 nm (Figure 10.2b). Each fenestra is bridged by an extremely thin membrane, the diaphragm, of thickness 4–5 nm, except in renal glomerular capillaries, where the diaphragm is absent. The diaphragm resembles a cartwheel, with wedge-shaped apertures between the spokes, through which water, nutrients and hormones can pass very rapidly to reach the surrounding tissue. The only currently known diaphragmatic constituent is a glycoprotein, PV-1.

Fenestrae appear to form when VEGF from neighbouring cells causes a local removal of the endothelial F-actin cytoskeleton. This closely approximates the luminal and abluminal membranes. Renal glomerular capillaries have an exceptionally high density of fenestrae and the surrounding cells (podocytes) express very high levels of VEGF. Conversely, in heterozygous knock-out mice with low VEGF levels, fenestrae fail to develop.

Discontinuous capillaries allow blood cell turnover

Discontinuous or sinusoidal capillaries have endothelial gaps over 100 nm wide, with a corresponding discontinuity in the basal lamina, so these capillaries are highly permeable, even to plasma proteins. Discontinuous capillaries occur in organs where red cells and/or white cells need to migrate between the blood and tissue, namely in the bone marrow, spleen and liver.

10.3 Diffusion, convection and reflection across a porous membrane

Before dealing with solute permeation through the capillary wall, a brief overview of passive transport through porous membranes may be helpful.

Solutes diffuse, whereas water flows

Water and solutes (e.g. glucose) cross the capillary wall by **passive** transport, i.e. without any energy expenditure by endothelium. Solutes, however, cross the wall by an entirely different physical process from water. Water **flows** across the wall down a **pressure gradient**, whereas a metabolized solute, such as glucose or O_2, **diffuses** across the wall down its **concentration gradient** (Figure 10.4). The Danish physiologist August Krogh established as long ago as 1919 that passive diffusion accounts for O_2 transfer from blood to muscle.

Figure 10.4 Timed sequence showing diffusion of Evans blue (small, lipid-insoluble solute, radius ~1 nm) out of a perfused frog mesenteric capillary. Dye-filled micropipette (arrow) is visible at arterial end of capillary in first frame; other arrows show direction of flow. The arteriovenous gradient of permeability is obvious; venous capillaries are normally more permeable than arterial capillaries. (From Levick JR, Doctoral thesis, Oxford.)

It is true that solutes such as glucose are also swept along in the water that is continuously flowing out through the capillary wall – a process called **convective transport**. The flow of water is so slow, however, that it generally contributes little to the transport of a metabolite or drug; diffusion is much faster over capillary-to-cell distances. (For proof, see footnote to Table 10.2.). A further source of confusion is the common textbook statement that water molecules can cross the wall very quickly by diffusion. While this is true, it is a red-herring, because water diffusion is bidirectional and achieves no net transport.

Thus, to understand the transcapillary movement of glucose, amino acids, drugs and other lipid-insoluble metabolites in most tissues (except brain, Section 10.8), we need to focus on passive, non-carrier-mediated diffusion through a porous membrane.

Fick's law describes free diffusive transport in a fluid

The basic physics of diffusive transport was worked out by Adolf Fick, Professor of Physiology at Wurzburg in Germany. **Fick's first law of diffusion** (1855) states that the mass of solute transferred by diffusion per unit time, J_s, across a body of liquid depends on four factors (Figure 10.5a):

- J_s is directly proportional to **concentration difference**, $C_1 - C_2$ or ΔC (delta means 'a difference in').
- J_s is inversely proportional to **diffusion distance**, Δx. The ratio $\Delta C/\Delta x$ is called the concentration gradient.

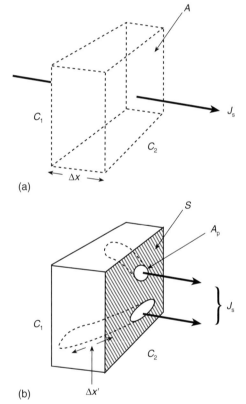

Figure 10.5 (a) Free diffusion in bulk solution. The solute diffuses through an unimpeded layer of fluid of thickness Δx and surface area A, driven by concentration difference ($C_1 - C_2$). J_s is the diffusion rate (mole/s). (b) A porous membrane reduces J_s by confining the solute to pores of total area A_p. The pore pathlength $\Delta x'$ is usually greater than the membrane thickness Δx.

- J_s is directly proportional to **surface area**, A.
- J_s is directly proportional to the solute **diffusion coefficient** or diffusivity, D.

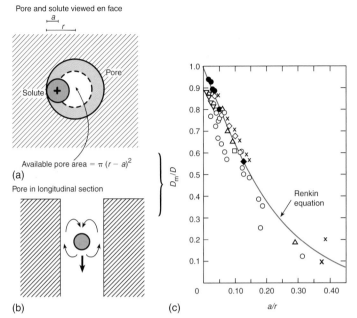

Pore and solute viewed en face

Available pore area = $\pi (r - a)^2$

(a)

Pore in longitudinal section

(b)

(c)

Figure 10.6 Difficulties encountered by a spherical molecule of radius 'a' (grey) diffusing through a water-filled cylindrical pore of radius r. (a) End-on, bird's-eye view of pore, showing steric exclusion of solute centre from an annulus of fluid (pink). The solute can only move around in the central clear area, reducing the available pore area to $\pi(r - a)^2$. (b) Longitudinal section through the pore. As solute molecule diffuses down the pore (thick arrow), water molecules must squeeze past it, through the narrow gap between wall and solute. This increases the hydrodynamic drag on the solute (restricted diffusion). (c) Plot of reduced diffusion across a membrane, D_m, as fraction of free diffusion coefficient D, against ratio of solute to pore size, a/r. The Renkin equation (see Appendix 2, 'Diffusion') predicts D_m/D from the steric exclusion and restricted diffusion phenomena. (From Beck RB, Schultz JS. *Biochimica Biophysica Acta* 1972; **255**: 273–303, with permission from Elsevier.)

Fick's law can thus be written:

$$J_s = -DA\Delta C/\Delta x \qquad (10.1)$$

The negative sign, which often puzzles students, is a mathematical convention to show that transport is 'downhill', i.e. down the concentration gradient. The **diffusion coefficient** is a measure of the ease with which a given molecular species slips through the solvent. Since big molecules encounter more friction than little ones, D is inversely related to solute size; small molecules, such as glucose, have a large D and diffuse faster than big molecules, such as albumin. See 'Diffusion' and 'Stokes–Einstein radius' in Appendix 2 for details.

Pores impede diffusive transport

When a solute diffuses through a large body of solvent, the distant walls of the container do not affect the solute and the process is called free diffusion. By contrast, when a solute diffuses through very narrow pores in a membrane, as in the capillary wall, diffusion is slowed down by three distinct factors.

(i) Reduction of area available for diffusion

When a solute is confined to water-filled pores, the maximum area available for diffusion is the total pore area A_p, which is usually a very small percentage of the total surface area of the membrane S (Figure 10.5b). This reduces the transport rate by the factor A_p/S. A further effect, **steric exclusion**, can reduce the available area to less than A_p/S (Figure 10.6a). For a solute molecule of radius 'a', the closest the centre of the molecule can get to the pore wall is a. Consequently, in a cylindrical pore of radius r the diffusive movements are confined to the central column of fluid, of radius $r - a$. The area available for diffusion is now only a fraction of the total pore area A_p.

(ii) Restricted diffusion inside a pore

When the solute radius is $\geqslant 1/10$th of pore radius, the close proximity of the pore wall impedes diffusion by a hydrodynamic mechanism. For the solute molecule to advance along the pore, water molecules ahead of it have to slip back through the narrow gap between the pore wall and solute, to make space for the advancing solute particle (Figure 10.6b). The narrower the gap between the solute and the pore wall, the less easily the water slips past; in biophysical terms, the hydrodynamic drag of water on the solute increases as the solute size approaches the pore diameter. As a result, the solute diffusion coefficient inside a narrow pore, D_{res}, is smaller than the free diffusion coefficient in bulk solution, D. This is called **restricted diffusion**, and can be a substantial reduction. For example, D_{res} is half D_{free} when solute radius a is 15% of pore radius r.

(iii) Increased pathlength

Most endothelial junctions pass obliquely through the capillary wall (Figures 9.4 and 10.3). Consequently the true diffusion distance, $\Delta x'$, is greater than the membrane thickness Δx (Figure 10.5b).

As a result of the above three effects, the transcapillary diffusion of lipid-insoluble solutes, such as glucose, lactate, amino acids, peptides, hormones and drugs, is slowed down by more than two orders of magnitude. **Membrane permeability** is an index of this depression of diffusion (Section 10.4).

Narrow pores cause molecular reflection; the reflection coefficient

In the above account, there was no solvent flow across the membrane, so solute transport was purely diffusive. If there is also pressure-driven fluid filtration across the membrane, solute transport is partly by filtration and partly by diffusion, and we need a new membrane parameter to deal with this – the reflection coefficient, σ (sigma). The reflection coefficient is the fraction of solute molecules reflected by the membrane during filtration at a high rate, and is an index of the difficulty a solute experiences in passing through a pore, relative to water. When a small solute (radius a) is washed into a large pore (radius r), steric exclusion is negligible, so the solute passes through the pore as freely as water. Its reflection is zero ($\sigma = 0$, Figure 10.7c) and the solute exerts no osmotic pressure across the membrane. At the other extreme, if the solute is wider than the pore ($a > r$), steric exclusion is total, so all the solute molecules are reflected ($\sigma = 1$) and the ultrafiltrate contains no solute (Figure 10.7a). The solute exerts its full osmotic potential in these circumstances. In the intermediate state, where a/r is >0.1 but <1, the solute is partially excluded from the pore (Figure 10.6a), so a fraction is reflected (σ is >0 but <1) and the ultrafiltrate has a reduced solute concentration, $1 - \sigma$ (Figure 10.7b). The solution exerts a fraction of its osmotic pressure in these circumstances (Section 11.1).

Since the reflection coefficient depends simply on a/r, it has been measured in capillaries, using solutes of known radius a, in order to estimate the equivalent radius r of the transendothelial channels at their narrowest point. The result was 4–5 nm (Appendix 2, Reflection coefficient). That is to say, the capillary wall is perforated by water-filled channels with similar properties to cylindrical channels of radius 4–5 nm. The channels are not cylindrical in reality, being the inter-fibre spaces of the glycocalyx (Figure 9.3).

The reflection coefficient and permeability, though related, are distinct; permeability depends on the number and length of pores, as well as their width, whereas reflection depends solely on pore width.

$\sigma = 1.0$ (a) $\sigma = 0.5$ (b) $\sigma = 0$ (c)

Figure 10.7 The osmotic reflection coefficient σ is a measure of the molecular selectivity of a pore. It depends on the ratio of solute width to pore width.

10.4 The concept of 'permeability'

Definition of permeability

Because a membrane impedes diffusion by multiple, hard-to-measure effects (steric exclusion, restricted diffusion, porous area and pathlength), it is convenient to encapsulate them in one, catch-all parameter, namely permeability. The permeability of a membrane P is the rate of diffusion of solute (J_s) across unit area of membrane per unit concentration difference across the membrane ΔC, in the absence of fluid filtration. If we write the definition out in symbols, using S for capillary surface area, we have the permeability equation:

$$P = J_s/S\Delta C \qquad (10.2)$$

Rearranging the permeability equation, we see that it is actually a simplified version of Fick's first law of diffusion (eqn 10.1);

$$J_s = PS\Delta C \qquad (10.3)$$

Permeability has the units of velocity, cm/s. The product PS is called the capillary diffusion capacity of a tissue and has units of cm^3/s.

Permeability and local concentration gradient determine solute flux

The rearranged permeability eqn 10.3 tells us that the amount of solute transported across a segment of capillary in a given time depends on three factors (Figure 10.8):

- endothelial permeability
- surface area
- the transcapillary concentration difference for that particular segment.

It is necessary to consider each segment separately, rather than the whole capillary, because solute concentration changes non-linearly as blood passes

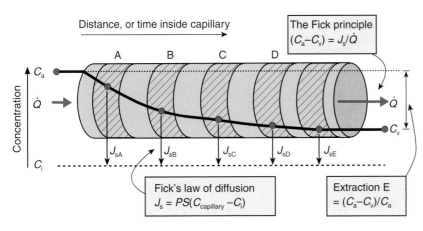

Figure 10.8 Concentration of a rapidly diffusing solute falls non-linearly along a capillary, from arterial concentration C_a to venous concentration C_v. Black arrows indicate size of diffusional fluxes J_s. PS, permeability–surface area product; $\dot{Q}$, blood flow. The concentration profile is exponential, if the interstitial concentration C_i is zero or uniform. For mean intracapillary concentration, see Appendix 2, Capillary concentration profile.

Table 10.1 Capillary permeability to different types of solute

Solute	M (Dalton)	Diffusivity $D\,(\times 10^{-5}\,\mathrm{cm}^2/\mathrm{s})$	Radius a (nm)	Membrane	Permeability $(\times 10^{-6}\,\mathrm{cm/s})$
Oxygen	32	2.11	0.16	Continuous capillary	~100 000
Urea	60	1.90	0.26	Continuous capillary	26–28
Glucose	180	0.91	0.36	Continuous capillary	9–13
Sucrose	342	0.72	0.47	Continuous capillary	6–9
				Cerebral capillary	0.1
				Fenestrated capillary	>270
Albumin	69 000	0.085	3.55	Continuous capillary	0.03–0.01
				Fenestrated capillary	0.04

M, molecular mass; D, free diffusion coefficient in water at 37°C; a, Stokes–Einstein diffusion radius. (After Renkin EM. *Circulation Research* 1977; **41**: 735–43; Clough GE, Smaje LH. *Journal of Physiology* 1984; **354**: 445–55; Landis EM, Pappenheimer JR. Exchange of substances through the capillary walls. In: Hamilton WF, Dow P (eds). *Handbook of Physiology, Cardiovascular System, Circulation*, Vol. II. Bethesda, MD: American Physiological Society, 1963: 961–1034.)

along the capillary, due to diffusion (Figure 10.8). Consequently, ΔC is different in each successive segment along the capillary.

Permeability depends on the properties of both membrane and solute

If we compare Fick's free diffusion eqn 10.1 with the transcapillary diffusion eqn 10.3 (as in Appendix 2, Diffusion), we see that endothelial permeability P to a lipid-insoluble solute depends on both **pore geometry** and **solute properties**, namely:

- the restriction to diffusivity D caused by the solute/pore width ratio, a/r;
- the pore area A_p per unit endothelial area S, which is determined by the extent of the breaks in the junctional strands;
- the non-excluded fraction of the pore area, which is again determined by a/r;
- the path length Δx, which is governed by the length of the intercellular cleft.

For example, when the number of junctional strands is increased by cAMP (Section 9.7), fractional pore area A_p/S falls, so permeability falls.

The key solute properties are **size**, which influences exclusion and restricted diffusion, and **lipid solubility**. Lipid-soluble solutes, such as O_2, diffuse through the entire lipid cell membrane, and therefore have a vastly greater area for diffusion than lipid-insoluble solutes, such as glucose, which are confined to the aqueous pores. Solutes therefore fall into three main permeability categories, namely **lipid-soluble molecules** (e.g. O_2), **small lipid-insoluble molecules** ($a \ll r$, little restriction or exclusion, e.g. glucose, electrolytes) and **large lipid-insoluble molecules** ($a \gtrsim r$, major restriction and exclusion, e.g. plasma proteins). Capillaries are many thousand times more permeable to lipid-soluble O_2 than to lipid-insoluble glucose; and nearly 1000 times more permeable to glucose (180 Da) than to albumin (69 000 Da; Table 10.1). We therefore need to consider each class of solute separately.

10.5 Lipid-soluble molecules diffuse extremely rapidly across endothelium

The permeability of endothelium to lipophilic ('fat-loving') molecules increases in proportion to their oil-to-water partition coefficient. Since virtually the entire capillary surface is available for diffusion, the permeability is extremely high. Respiratory gases, general anaesthetics and the blood flow tracer xenon are examples of lipophilic solutes. The oil:water partition coefficient is ~5 for **oxygen** and 1.6 for **carbon dioxide**. The permeability to O_2 is so high that there is a significant diffusion of O_2 out of arterioles, reducing the haemoglobin saturation to ~80% by the time blood enters the capillary. However, only part of the deoxygenation is due to O_2 transfer into the tissue. The rest is caused by **diffusive, countercurrent shunting** of O_2 from the supplying arterioles into the draining venules, which commonly run alongside the arterioles.

10.6 Small lipid-insoluble molecules permeate the small pore system

Lipophobic (fat-hating), hydrophilic (water-loving) solutes include the plasma electrolytes, glucose, lactate, amino acids, vitamins such as B_{12}, hormones such as adrenaline and insulin, and many drugs. These solutes cannot diffuse through the lipid endothelial membrane; they are confined to the water-filled pathways through the intercellular junctions and fenestrae. The intercellular clefts occupy only 0.2–0.4% of the capillary surface, so the permeability of a continuous capillary to small lipophobic solutes is a fraction of its permeability to lipophilic solutes, though still high.

Restricted diffusion provided the first clue to capillary pore size

In 1951 Pappenheimer, Renkin and Borrero proposed the seminal 'small pore theory' of capillary permeability. Their measurements of lipophobic solute permeation indicated that the capillary wall is perforated by narrow, aqueous channels that occupy only 0.01–0.04% of the capillary surface (about one-tenth of the cleft area), of width equivalent to 3–5 nm radius pores. The estimate of pore size was based on their discovery that, as lipophobic solute radius increases, capillary permeability falls faster than the free diffusion coefficient (Figure 10.9). Pappenheimer and colleagues realized that this must be due to steric exclusion and restricted

Figure 10.9 Effect of Stokes–Einstein radius of solute molecule on capillary permeability. Except for oxygen the points denote lipophobic solutes. Dashed line of slope −1 shows effect of fall in free diffusion coefficient with increasing molecular size. Red line shows decline in permeability for cylindrical pores of radius 5 nm, as discovered by Pappenheimer, Renkin and Borrero in 1951. A small but persistent permeability to solutes larger than albumin reveals the existence of a small number of larger pores. Data from mammalian skeletal muscle and skin, except for oxygen (lung). (After Renkin EM, Curry FE. In: Giebisch G, Tosteson DC, Ussing HH (eds) *Membrane Transport in Biology*, Vol. IV. Berlin: Springer-Verlag, 1978: 1–45. With kind permission of Springer Science and Business Media.)

diffusion in narrow pores (Figure 10.6), and from the degree of restriction they calculated the equivalent pore size to be 3–5 nm (Appendix 2, Diffusion). As noted in Section 10.3, pore size has also been calculated from capillary reflection coefficients. Taking a broad average, the transcapillary channels in myocardium, skeletal muscle and intestine have similar restrictive and reflective properties to cylindrical, water-filled pores of radius 4–5 nm. It must be emphasized, however, that nobody believes that the small pores are actually cylindrical tubes – only that some of their properties resemble those of narrow tubes.

Differences in permeability between capillaries often result from differences in pore numbers, not size

The permeability of capillaries in the different tissues of the body to a given lipophobic solute or water spans a very wide, ~100-fold range. Fenestrated capillaries are 10–100 times more permeable than continuous capillaries, because each fenestra contains a collection of small pores of very short pathlength, namely the gaps between the cartwheel spokes (Figure 10.2). However, there are up to ten-fold differences in permeability even amongst continuous capillaries (e.g. muscle versus mesenteric capillaries) with no immediately obvious anatomical cause. An important clue to the cause is that the solute permeability and the hydraulic conductance of the capillary wall correlate linearly, i.e. if one is ten-times higher, so is the other. This indicates that permeability differences are not caused by differences in pore radius − since hydraulic flow is proportional to r^4 (Poiseuille's law, eqn 8.7), whereas diffusion is proportional to pore area and hence πr^2 (Fick's law). Physiological differences in permeability must therefore be caused by differences in **pore numbers**. It appears that the proportion of the intercellular cleft that is 'open for business', due to breaks in the junctional strands, varies from tissue to tissue (Figures 9.2, 9.4 and 10.3). The open fraction is typically ∼10%. A vessel with more extensive breaks in the junctional strands (equivalent to more pores) has a higher permeability, as in the postcapillary venule. Conversely, less extensive breaks produce a vessel of lower permeability, such as the arterial capillary. Ultrastructural investigations using markers such as ferrocyanide ions, lanthanum ions and microperoxidase confirm that small lipophobic solutes do indeed permeate the intercellular cleft through breaks in the junctional strands (Figure 10.3).

The glycocalyx is the site of the size-selective small pores

Although the intercellular cleft is undoubtedly the pathway through which water and small solutes cross the capillary wall, the cleft itself is unlikely to be the size-limiting structure, i.e. the small pore of radius 4–5 nm, because it is ∼20 nm wide. Moreover, discrepancies between the estimates of small pore size from hydraulic data versus diffusion data indicate that the small pore is unlikely to have a continuous, solid wall. This led Curry and Michel to suggest, in 1980, that the size-limiting pores are located in the glycocalyx, the luminal coat of biopolymers that spans the entrance to the intercellular cleft (Figures 9.3 and 9.5). This is the **fibre-matrix theory of capillary permeability**.

The fibre matrix theory (Figure 10.10) proposes that the glycocalyx biopolymers form a fine network that acts as a size-selective sieve, i.e. the small pore system. There is now considerable evidence supporting this view. For example, the glycocalyx excludes fluorescent macromolecules perfused through a capillary. Also, enzymatic digestion of the glycocalyx increases endothelial permeability. Conversely, the binding of albumin to the glycocalyx greatly reduces endothelial permeability (the **protein effect**), as does cationized ferritin (Figure 9.5); whereas macromolecules that do not bind to the glycocalyx do not reduce capillary permeability. It is thought that bound albumin regulates the pore size within the network (Figure 10.10a). The highly anionic plasma protein orosomucoid likewise binds to the glycocalyx, increasing the negative charge density and the exclusion of negatively charged plasma proteins.

The modern view, then, is that **two different structures, the glycocalyx and the breaks in junctional strands, together determine the permeability** of continuous endothelium to solutes and water. The **area** available for the passage of water and small solutes, and hence the permeability, depends on the extent of the breaks in the junctional strands. The **size- and charge-selectivity** of the pathway, however, is determined by the spacing and charges within the glycocalyx polymer network covering the entrance to the clefts. The uniform coating of the intercellular junctions and fenestrae by glycocalyx (Figure 10.10b) also explains the remarkable constancy of the reflection coefficient to plasma proteins (0.8–0.95) across different capillary beds with a 400-fold range in hydraulic permeability.

The concepts of John Pappenheimer and Gene Renkin, the originators of pore theory, and Charles Michel and Roy Curry, the originators of the fibre matrix theory, might be summarized as follows:

The Pappenheimer pore's so small
You cannot make it out at all,
Though many sanguine doctors hope
To see one through the microscope −
Rectangular or round in shape
With many nanometres gape.
Some say the pore is made of fluff,
A glycocalyxacious stuff,
Whose fibres subdivide the space
Constructing there a random lace
'Til albumin, a protein, lands
And tidies up those tangled strands,
Through which there flows dilute saline.
All this has never yet been seen,
But Scientists, who ought to know,
Assure us that it must be so.
Oh let us never, never doubt
What nobody is sure about.

(With apologies to Hilaire Belloc's *The Microbe*)

(a)

(b)   Basal lamina

Figure 10.10 Fibre matrix model of capillary permeability. Glycocalyx covers the endothelium (E) and fenestrae (F) and intercellular junction (J) and sieves out plasma proteins. Number of open junctions and fenestrae determines net permeability to smaller lipophobic solutes and water. The multivesicular transcellular channel (MVC) or vesicles (V) may represent the large pore system. Large pores are few in number. (Adapted from Michel CC. *Journal of Physiology* 1980; **309**: 341–55; by permission.) Inset outlines key features of glycocalyx. Negatively charged proteoglycan fibres (PG) and sialoglycoproteins (SGP) bind to the positively charged arginine groups of albumin (red ellipsoids). This creates a 3-dimensional sieve that reflects plasma proteins. Reflection is governed primarily by the glycocalyx mesh size, secondarily by its net negative charge. PM, plasmalemma membrane; ICC, intercellular cleft. (After Curry FE. *Circulation Research* 1986; **59**: 367–80.)

In addition to its role as a semipermeable, size-selective ultrafilter, the glycocalyx has **haemodynamic effects** in microvessels, and contributes to **endothelial mechanosensitivity** in larger vessels (Section 9.2).

Specific transporters generally contribute little to transcapillary exchange

In most tissues carrier-mediated solute transport by integral membrane proteins and water transport through membrane aquaporins (water channels) contribute negligibly to transcapillary transport, because their transport capacities are orders of magnitude lower than that of the intercellular cleft. There are important exceptions, however. Brain endothelium has a very low intercellular permeability, and therefore relies on integral membrane proteins to transport solutes such as glucose (Section 10.8). Also, carrier-mediated urea transport is important in the descending vasa recta of the kidney (medullary capillaries).

10.7 Large lipid-insoluble molecules pass through a large pore system

The permeability of continuous and fenestrated endothelium to plasma proteins is around one millionth of their permeability to oxygen. Nevertheless, there is a small but important flux of plasma proteins into the tissues, as demonstrated by their presence in lymph at 20–70% of the plasma concentration. This flux is needed for immunoglobulins to exercise their defence role, and for the transfer of protein-bound substances, such as iron, copper, vitamin A, thyroxine, testosterone, oestradiol, lipids and short-chain fatty acids.

The permeability versus molecular size plot reveals a large-diameter transport system

As solute radius approaches 3.6 nm (albumin), which is approximately the size of the small pores (glycocalyx mesh size), solute permeation falls off steeply (Figure 10.9). Indeed, one might expect zero permeability to solutes bigger than the small pores, namely the plasma proteins. In reality, however, there is still a finite, albeit low permeability to plasma protein of radius >4 nm. This led Grotte to propose, in 1956, the existence of a second transport pathway, with properties equivalent to a small number of large pores, of radius 20–30 nm. Reflection coefficient measurements support this view; macromolecule reflection coefficients are less than 1, even for fibrinogen (radius 10 nm). Nevertheless, the permeability to macromolecules is very low, showing that the large pores are few in number – around one large pore per 4000 small pores in continuous capillaries, and essentially none in cerebral and renal glomerular capillaries.

Macromolecular permeation depends on charge as well as size

Large plasma proteins such as fibrinogen cross the endothelial layer less readily than smaller proteins such as albumin. Moreover, negatively charged macromolecules, such as albumin, permeate the endothelial barrier less readily than neutral or positively charged ones of similar size. This is due to electrical repulsion by the fixed negative charges of the glycocalyx.

The identity of large pores: continuous channels and/or vesicular transport?

The large pore system is a functional concept, inferred from permeability data (Figure 10.9). There is controversy as to whether the system consists of true pores, i.e. hydraulically continuous channels, in the form of multivesicular channels (Figures 9.6b and 10.10) or glycocalyx gaps, or whether it is really the caveola–vesicle transport system.

'True pore' protagonists point out that the rate of transport of macromolecules across the capillary wall is proportional to the pressure driving fluid across the wall, as expected for a hydraulically continuous large pore. Moreover tissue cooling, which should inhibit active vesicular transport, has only a small effect on macromolecular permeation. Also, caveolin knock-out mice lack endothelial caveolae, yet show no impairment of transendothelial protein permeation.

Nevertheless, vesicular transport may contribute significantly to macromolecular transfer at low filtration rates. Macromolecules such as gold-labelled albumin and ferritin (radius 5.5 nm) undoubtedly enter the luminal caveolae and appear soon afterwards in the abluminal caveolae (Figures 9.5 and

9.6). It remains unclear, however, how much this contributes to total protein transport. It is possible that, at normal, low capillary filtration rates, conductive channels and vesicular transport both contribute to protein permeation.

Our current understanding of the various parallel pathways for solute movement across the capillary wall is summarized in Figure 10.11.

10.8 Blood–brain barrier and carrier-mediated transport

Cerebral capillaries form a tight blood–brain barrier

Brain capillaries, like all capillaries, are highly permeable to lipophilic solutes (O_2, CO_2, general anaesthetics); but they are exceptionally impermeable to lipophobic solutes, such as L-glucose, catecholamines and plasma proteins. This is called the blood–brain barrier. The function of the barrier is to protect the neurons from circulating stimulants, such as catecholamines, and to prevent the washout of neurotransmitters from the brain parenchyma by the bloodstream. The blood–brain barrier is formed by complex, multiple junctional strands between the endothelial cells, with no breaks; the strands form a continuous, unbroken seal around the cell perimeter. The caveola–vesicle system is also very scanty. Breakdown of the barrier is common in pathological conditions such as local cerebral ischaemia (strokes), cerebral haemorrhage and cerebral inflammation, and leads to cerebral oedema.

Specific endothelial carriers transport solutes into the brain parenchyma

In stark contrast to most capillaries, cerebral capillaries rely on specific carrier proteins in the endothelial cell membrane to transport essential, lipid-insoluble solutes between the blood and brain parenchyma. There are specific carrier proteins for D-glucose (the natural, dextrose form of glucose; carrier GLUT-1), lactate, pyruvate, amino acids and adenosine. This form of transport is **transcellular**, as opposed to paracellular. The transport is not active, but is brought about by the diffusion of the carrier-bound solute down its concentration gradient (facilitated diffusion). In addition, cerebral endothelium can regulate the K^+ concentration of cerebral interstitial fluid by active transport, via Na^+–K^+-ATPase in the abluminal membrane (Section 15.4).

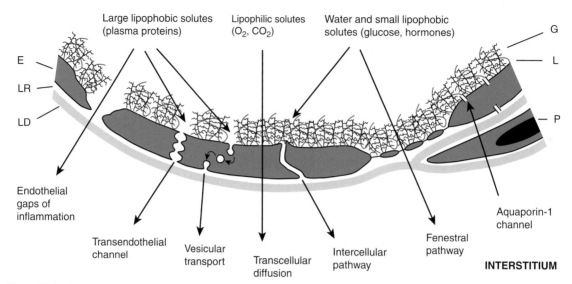

Figure 10.11 Main transport pathways across the capillary wall. Water flows mainly through the small pore system, i.e. glycocalyx overlying intercellular clefts and fenestrae. Only a little passes through membrane aquaporin-1 channels or the scanty large pore system. Note large gap and break in glycocalyx in inflammation. E, endothelium; G, glycocalyx; L, lipid plasma membrane; LR and LD, lamina rara and lamina densa of basement membrane, respectively; P, pericyte.

10.9 Extraction and clearance in capillaries

The concentration of a consumed solute, such as oxygen, glucose or a drug, falls along the capillary (Figure 10.8), and this decay is crucial to understanding the effect of blood flow on solute transfer. This section describes the concentration profile along a capillary and the related concepts of extraction and clearance; Sections 10.10 and 10.11 build on this to explain the effects of blood flow and exercise on solute exchange. To illustrate the capillary concentration profile, let us consider glucose transfer into active muscle. The interstitial glucose concentration is lower than the arterial concentration, because the muscle is consuming glucose; and for simplicity we will assume that the interstitial glucose concentration is uniform.

Concentration decays non-linearly along a capillary

At the start of the capillary, plasma glucose concentration is close to arterial level and the difference in concentration across the capillary wall is high (point A, Figure 10.8). Consequently, glucose diffuses rapidly out of the first part of the capillary, as dictated by Fick's law of diffusion (arrow J_{sA}, Figure 10.8). Due to this solute efflux, the plasma concentration falls off steeply at first, e.g. from A to B in Figure 10.8. Further along the capillary the

concentration difference across the wall is smaller (point C), so the solute efflux is slower (flux J_{sC}). As a result, the plasma concentration falls off less steeply, as from C to D. In the case of lactate or CO_2, where the concentration is higher in the tissue than the capillary, the concentration increases rather than decays along the capillary axis, but again in a curvilinear fashion. The capillary concentration profile is thus a curve, and mean capillary concentration is less than the average of the arterial and venous concentrations (Appendix 2, Capillary concentration profile). If the curvature is pronounced, with a steep initial decay, almost all the solute exchange happens near the start of the capillary, with little downstream. The degree of curvature depends on the permeability and the blood flow (Section 10.10).

The Fick *principle* (cf. Fick's law) describes exchange across the whole capillary bed

The net solute exchange across an entire capillary bed is easily worked out using the Fick *principle* (Section 7.1) – which should not be confused with Fick's law of diffusion! The Fick principle states that the solute exchange rate equals the arteriovenous concentration difference $C_a - C_v$ multiplied by the blood flow $\dot{Q}$:

$$J_s = \dot{Q}(C_a - C_v) \tag{10.4}$$

For example, the glucose flux into a muscle can be evaluated by measuring the blood flow, the arterial glucose concentration and the local venous concentrations. Conversely, the Fick principle can be used to work out the concentration drop $C_a - C_v$ that will be produced by any particular combination of solute consumption and blood flow (Figure 10.8).

Extraction (E) is the fraction of solute removed from plasma during one capillary transit

Let us suppose that glucose enters a capillary bed at an arterial concentration of 5 mM and leaves at a venous concentration of 4.5 mM. Clearly, 0.5 mM has been removed by diffusion into the tissues. This is 10% of the amount delivered in the arterial blood (0.5/5.0), so the 'extraction' is 10%. Extraction is defined as the arteriovenous concentration difference, $C_a - C_v$, as a fraction of the arterial concentration C_a : $E = (C_a - C_v)/C_a$ (Figure 10.8 and Appendix 2, Extraction). Oxygen extraction in many tissues is ~25% at rest, rising to 80–90% in heavily exercising muscle.

Solute extraction following an intra-arterial injection is illustrated in Figure 10.12. The solute was vitamin B_{12} in this case, and the injected solution also contained a non-exchanging or 'reference' solute, namely radiolabelled albumin. Samples of the venous effluent showed that the diffusible solute concentration fell below the reference solute concentration, due to diffusion out of the capillaries. The reference solute concentration shows what the test solute concentration would have been if no exchange had taken place. The extraction of vitamin B_{12}, calculated from the difference between the test and reference solute concentrations, was initially ~40% (Figure 10.12b). Extraction then declined, because the interstitial concentration increased, reducing the concentration gradient across the capillary wall. This pattern of extraction shows that solute exchange is a diffusive process that obeys Fick's law of diffusion.

Clearance (Cl) is the volume of plasma cleared of solute per unit time

The plasma clearance is the volume of plasma that has been emptied of a specified solute per minute, due to the extraction of that solute. The clearance equals the plasma flow multiplied by extraction E:

$$Cl = \text{plasma flow} \times E \qquad (10.5a)$$

(a)

(b)

Figure 10.12 Diffusion of vitamin B_{12} (cyanocobalamin, radius 0.8 nm) out of the fenestrated microcirculation of the cat salivary gland, following a bolus arterial injection. Albumin (radius 3.6 nm) served as a non-extracted reference solute (see text). (a) Amount of vitamin B_{12} and albumin in successive venous samples as a percentage of the initial arterial dose. The lines cross after 3 seconds because the interstitial concentration of B_{12} is now higher than the falling level in the blood, causing a net back-diffusion into the blood. (b) Extraction of B_{12} is high at first, then falls as interstitial concentration rises. Permeability can be calculated from the extraction and blood flow, using the Renkin–Crone relation, eqn 10.6. (From Mann GE, Smaje LH, Yudilevich DL. *Journal of Physiology* 1979; **297**: 335–54, with permission from Wiley-Blackwell.)

For example, if the plasma flow through an exercising muscle is 100 ml/min and the glucose extraction is 10%, then 10 ml of plasma are cleared of glucose per minute.

Note that the units of clearance are plasma volume/time, not solute mass/time; the mass of solute removed per unit time is called the solute flux (J_s, eqn 10.1). Solute flux equals plasma clearance $\times$ arterial concentration; $J_s = Cl \cdot C_a$. Therefore, clearance can also be defined as solute flux per unit arterial concentration ($Cl = J_s/C_a$), which again has the units of volume/time. The relationships between clearance, extraction and solute flux may thus be summarized as:

$$Cl = \text{Plasma flow} \times E = \text{Plasma flow} \times (C - C_v)/C_a = J_s/C_a \quad (10.5b)$$

The concept of plasma clearance is used a great deal in renal physiology. For example, the renal clearance of the waste product creatinine from plasma is $\sim$140 ml/min in young humans and declines in renal failure. The concept of 'clearance' can also be applied to any other organ or solute. For example, the pulmonary clearance of CO_2 is $\sim$370 ml/min in a resting human.

10.10 How blood flow affects solute transfer

Raising the blood flow through a tissue can boost solute exchange – or have virtually no effect at all! This is because there are two basic exchange states, called flow-limited exchange and diffusion-limited exchange. Each state has a different, distinctive capillary concentration profile. In **flow-limited exchange** the solute concentration decays very steeply in the first part of the capillary (Figure 10.13, red curves), and the transcapillary solute flux is limited by the rate at which blood delivers solute to the capillary (see below). In **diffusion-limited exchange** the solute concentration profile is relatively flat (Figure 10.13, black curves) and the transcapillary solute flux is limited by the rate at which the solute can permeate the capillary wall.

In flow-limited exchange, solute transfer rate is proportional to blood flow

If capillary permeability to the solute is very high (e.g. CO_2 in lung capillaries), the solute crosses the wall so quickly that its plasma concentration equilibrates with the concentration outside the capillary (pericapillary interstitial fluid or alveolar gas) long before the blood reaches the end of the capillary (Figure 10.13a, curve 1). This is usually the case for lipophilic solutes such as O_2 and CO_2, and for small lipophobic solutes in fenestrated capillaries. It can also be true for small lipophobic solutes such as urea and glucose in continuous capillaries if blood flow is slow. Since the plasma

Figure 10.13 Effect of blood flow on diffusive transport across capillary wall. (a) Decay of plasma concentration along capillary at low to high blood flows (curves 1–7), for a constant or zero pericapillary concentration C_i. C_a, C_v, arterial and venous concentrations. Slow transits allow time for equilibration ($C_v = C_i$) before the end of the capillary (curves 1–3). This is flow-limited exchange. With fast transits, there is not enough time for equilibration across the diffusion barrier; C_v is $>C_i$ (curves 5–7). This is diffusion-limited exchange. (b) Resulting effect of blood flow on transcapillary exchange, expressed as plasma clearance (solute flux/C_a, eqn 10.5b). Plateau clearance value equals the capillary diffusion capacity PS. Data are for urea in muscle capillaries. (Data of Renkin EM. In: Marchetti G, Taccardi B (eds). *International Symposium on Coronary Circulation*. Basel: Karger, 1967: 18–30.)

concentration quickly falls to that of the surrounding interstitial fluid, only the initial part of the capillary contributes to exchange. When the blood flow is raised, the time available for exchange shortens but equilibration may still occur before the capillary exit, albeit further downstream (curves 2 and 3). Since the arteriovenous difference ($C_a - C_v$) is unchanged yet blood flow has increased, transcapillary solute flux J_s has increased (Fick's principle, eqn 10.4, $J_s =$ blood flow $\times (C_a - C_v)$). In fact the solute flux increases in direct proportion to the blood flow, as shown by points 1–3 in panel (b) of Figure 10.13.

Gas exchange in the lungs is a prime example of flow-limited exchange, of major physiological importance. The CO_2 and O_2 in the pulmonary capillary blood equilibrate with the alveolar gas long before the end of the capillary is reached. Consequently, an increase in pulmonary blood flow, i.e. cardiac output, causes a directly proportional increase in capillary O_2 uptake and CO_2 removal.

In flow-limited exchange the solute clearance rate is a measure of blood flow, not capillary permeability. This is the basis of the Kety xenon clearance method (Figure 8.6). It is not possible to measure capillary permeability P when exchange is flow-limited, because the fraction of the capillary wall that is contributing to exchange is unknown, i.e. S is unknown.

In diffusion-limited exchange, solute transfer rate is little affected by blood flow

Diffusion-limited exchange is at the opposite end of the spectrum to flow-limited exchange. In diffusion-limited exchange the solute transfer is limited by endothelial permeability rather than by solute delivery rate, i.e. blood flow. The plasma solute concentration has not equilibrated with the pericapillary space by the time the end of the capillary is reached, and the concentration profile is relatively flat, as in curve 5 of Figure 10.13a. Medium–to–large lipophobic solutes, such as inulin and cyanocobalamin (vitamin B_{12}), behave in this way. So too do small solutes, such as urea and glucose, when the transit time is shortened by high blood flows; diffusion-limited exchange occurs with big molecules at normal flow and with small molecules at high flows.

In diffusion-limited exchange, raising the blood flow causes relatively little increase in solute exchange, because the blood is already spending too little time in the capillary to unload its solute fully. If the transit time is shortened further by raising blood flow, the extraction fraction falls and the venous concentration rises (curves 6 and 7 of Figure 10.13a). The arteriovenous concentration difference $(C_a - C_v)$ therefore declines. Applying the Fick principle (eqn 10.4), we find that solute exchange J_s increases relatively little; the effect of the rise in $\dot{Q}$ is largely offset by the fall in $(C_a - C_v)$. Thus points 5–7 in Figure 10.13b show little increase in solute clearance with increasing blood flow.

Ratio of diffusion capacity to blood flow, $PS/\dot{Q}$, determines whether exchange is flow-limited or diffusion-limited

The nature of the exchange process – whether diffusion-limited or flow-limited – is determined by

---

Capillary permeability and blood flow influence solute exchange

- Permeability P (cm/s) is the diffusive solute transfer J_s (g/s) across unit area of membrane S (cm^2) per unit concentration difference ΔC (g/cm^3): $P = J_s/S\Delta C$.
- Solute transfer rate depends on the diffusion capacity of the capillary bed PS (cm^3/s) and the mean concentration difference between plasma and tissue: $J_s = PS\Delta C$. This is Fick's law of diffusion adapted for a membrane.
- Capillary permeability depends on solute properties (lipid solubility, molecular size, charge) and membrane porosity. Pore size is determined by the fibre-spacing within the glycocalyx, while porous area is determined by the extent of the breaks in the intercellular junctional strands (the paracellular pathway) and by fenestrae.
- If capillary diffusion capacity PS (cm^3/s) exceeds blood flow (cm^3/s) by $\geq$5-fold, solute equilibrates with the pericapillary fluid before the end of the capillary. Raising blood flow therefore increases the solute transfer rate, as in pulmonary gas exchange (flow-limited exchange).
- If PS is less than the blood flow ($PS/\dot{Q} < 1$), the solute does not equilibrate with the pericapillary space by the end of the capillary (diffusion-limited exchange). Extraction is low and solute exchange is not appreciably increased by raising flow.

CONCEPT BOX 10.1

---

the ratio of the permeability–surface area product of the capillary bed, PS (the diffusion capacity), to blood flow $\dot{Q}$. Both factors have the same units, cm^3/s, so $PS/\dot{Q}$ is dimensionless. If the diffusion capacity substantially exceeds the blood flow $(PS/\dot{Q} > 5)$, equilibration is reached before the end of the capillary and the exchange is flow-limited. If flow exceeds the diffusion capacity $(PS/\dot{Q} < 1)$ equilibration is not achieved and the exchange is diffusion-limited. This follows from the non-linear relation between extraction E and blood flow, the **Renkin–Crone relation** (see Appendix 2, Capillary concentration profile):

$$E = 1 - \exp(-PS/\dot{Q}) \qquad (10.6)$$

Renkin and Crone pointed out that at $PS/\dot{Q} = 5$ the solute extraction E is >99%, so there is almost complete equilibration and exchange is flow-limited. By contrast, when $PS/\dot{Q}$ is $\leq$1, the extraction is $\leq$63%, so equilibration is not achieved and exchange is diffusion-limited. Typical $PS/\dot{Q}$ values for glucose in skeletal muscle capillaries are ~5 at rest, because blood flow is low in resting muscle, and ≤1 during exercise, because blood flow is raised.

It is clear from the Renkin–Crone equation and Figure 10.13b that flow-limited exchange and diffusion-limited exchange are really just the extremes of a continuous spectrum. There are many **intermediate states** (Figure 10.13b, the region between points 3 and 5) where raising the blood flow does increase the solute flux, via an increase in mean capillary concentration (Fick's law of diffusion), but fails to increase it proportionally (as in purely flow-limited exchange), because C_v rises. This is illustrated by the increase in solute flux between point 4 and point 5 in Figure 10.13b (intermediate regime).

An increase in blood flow can also trigger an increase in permeability

The preceding section describes the purely passive, biophysical effect of blood flow on solute exchange. Recent work indicates, however, that blood flow can also induce active increases in endothelial permeability to lipophobic solutes. This is described in the next section, because it is one of several ways in which the body adjusts the rate of solute transfer to meet increased demand during exercise.

10.11 Physiological regulation of solute transfer

The transfer of O_2 and nutrients across the capillary wall should, ideally, match tissue demand; when demand increases, as in exercising muscle or myocardium, transfer needs to increase too. If the supply artery is narrowed by atheroma, however, solute delivery is restricted and transfer may lag behind the increased demand. In patients with coronary artery disease, this results in exercise-induced angina, while in patients with femoral artery disease it results in calf pain during exercise (intermittent claudication).

The O_2 consumption of skeletal muscle can increase up to 20–40-fold during exercise, and a matching increase in the transcapillary flux of O_2 is normally brought about by three mechanisms:

- more uniform perfusion of the capillary bed, due to capillary recruitment
- an increase in the concentration gradient from plasma to tissue
- an increase in local blood flow.

Additional factors include an increase in the O_2 diffusion velocity through muscle myoglobin as intracellular oxygen partial pressure falls; and, in the case of small lipophobic solutes such as glucose, probably an increase in capillary permeability with flow.

Capillary recruitment improves solute exchange in exercising muscle

In skeletal muscle each capillary supplies a cylindrical envelope of surrounding muscle fibres, called a Krogh cylinder (Figure 10.14). The number of muscle fibres supplied by one capillary, and hence the radius of the Krogh cylinder, depends on the anatomical capillary density and the fraction that is well perfused at any moment in time. The injection of visible particles or dyes has shown that, in resting skeletal muscle, half to three-quarters of the capillaries are not perfused, or are perfused only sluggishly, at any one moment, because the terminal arterioles supplying them are in the constricted phase of their vasomotion cycle (Section 10.1). Since a relatively small number of capillaries is well perfused at rest, each capillary has to supply a large zone of surrounding muscle fibres. In resting muscle, therefore, the Krogh cylinder radius is large.

During exercise the terminal arterioles are dilated by metabolites released by the contracting muscle fibres (Section 13.7, Metabolic hyperaemia). This increases the number of well-perfused capillaries, a process termed **capillary recruitment**. Capillary recruitment increases the **surface area** of endothelium available for exchange (S) and at the same time reduces the Krogh cylinder radius and hence the solute **diffusion distance**, Δx (Figure 10.14). These changes improve the uniformity of the oxygen supply, i.e. they reduce the heterogeneity present in resting muscle (Section 10.1); and the increase in $S/\Delta x$ greatly increases the rate of diffusive transport, as dictated by Fick's law (eqn.10.1).

Increased metabolic consumption steepens the concentration gradient

The increased metabolic rate of an active tissue lowers the tissue concentration of glucose and oxygen, and therefore increases the concentration difference between the capillary blood and the tissue. For example, the mean concentration difference for glucose across the capillary wall is estimated to increase from ~0.3 mM in resting muscle to ~3 mM during heavy exercise (Table 10.2). The increased concentration difference, coupled with the shortening of

REST

Terminal arteriole 1, dilated.
VSM relaxed.
Capillary module perfused.

Oxygen flux

r_K

Krogh
cylinder
of muscle

Terminal arteriole 2, constricted.
VSM contracted.
Capillary module not perfused.

EXERCISE - metabolic hyperaemia

$\updownarrow r_K$

Reduced
distance for
diffusion

Terminal arteriole 2, dilated.
VSM relaxed.
Capillary module now perfused.

Increased surface area for diffusion

Figure 10.14 The Krogh muscle cylinder and capillary recruitment. In resting skeletal muscle, contraction of terminal arteriole 2 arrests the perfusion of one capillary module (dashed lines). Each perfused capillary therefore has to supply a broad cylinder of muscle (Krogh cylinder). The radius of the Krogh cylinder r_K is the maximum diffusion distance. When exercise commences, metabolic vasodilatation dilates terminal arteriole 2, leading to perfusion of the previously closed-off capillaries. This improves the homogeneity of O_2 supply, increases the perfused capillary surface area, reduces the radius of each Krogh cylinder, and thus reduces the maximum diffusion distance r_K. VSM, Vascular smooth muscle.

Table 10.2 Transport of glucose from blood to 100 g skeletal muscle *in vivo*

	Notation	Units	Rest	Heavy exercise	Fractional change (exercise/rest)
Glucose consumption rate[a]	J_s	μmol/min	1.4	60	43×
Arterial concentration	C_a	mM	5.0	5.0	–
Venous concentration	C_v	mM	4.44	4.0	0.9×
Extraction	E	%	11.2%	20%	1.8×
Blood flow	$\dot{Q}$	ml/min	2.5	60	24×
Perfused capillary density		number/mm²	250	1000	4×
Diffusion capacity[b]	PS	cm³/min	5	20	4×
Mean concentration difference across capillary wall	ΔC[c]	mM	0.3	3	10×
Mean pericapillary concentration	C_i	mM	4.7	2	0.4×
Krogh cylinder radius	r_K	μm	36	18	0.5×

[a]Diffusion accounts for most of the transcapillary transport of glucose and other small metabolites, not fluid filtration. *Proof*: resting skeletal muscle consumes 1.4 μmol glucose/min (100 g)$^{-1}$. Net transcapillary filtration rate is 0.005 ml/min (100 g)$^{-1}$ and glucose concentration is 5 μmol/ml, so convective glucose transport is 0.025 μmol/min. This is only 2% of the total glucose flux. (After Crone C, Levitt DG. In: Renkin EM, Michel CC (eds). *Handbook of Physiology, Cardiovascular System*, Vol. IV, Microcirculation. Bethesda, MD: American Physiological Society, 1984: 431.)
[b]Recent evidence shows that some of the increase in PS may be due to increased capillary permeability as flow increases (see text), as well as recruitment.
[c]ΔC is calculated as J_s/PS (see eqn 10.3).

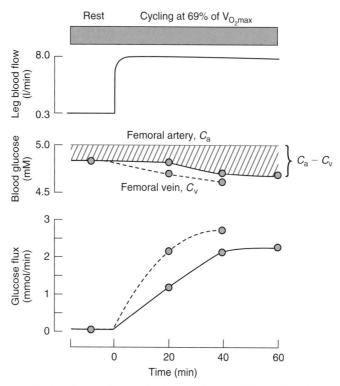

Figure 10.15 Increase in glucose flux from blood to leg muscles during cycling, calculated by Fick principle (solute flux = blood flow × arteriovenous concentration difference). At first the muscle utilizes both stored glycogen and extracted glucose. As the glycogen store is depleted, blood glucose extraction $(C_a - C_v)/C_a$ increases. When muscle glycogen was depleted prior to exercise, glucose extraction is increased (dashed lines with grey circles). $\dot{V}_{O_2max}$ is subject's maximum oxygen consumption rate. (From data of Blomstrand E, Saltin B. *Journal of Physiology* 1999; **514**: 293–302.)

diffusion distance by capillary recruitment, can increase the concentration gradient $\Delta C/\Delta x$ by more than an order of magnitude.

Blood flow increases with increased metabolic activity

Blood flow increases in direct proportion to metabolic rate in most organs, including skeletal muscle (Figure 10.15), myocardium (Figure 15.4) and brain (Figure 15.15). The metabolic hyperaemia increases the rate of delivery of O_2 and glucose and prevents the transcapillary exchange from becoming flow-limited. Metabolites such as glucose are diffusion-limited at the high flows that occur during exercise, so solute transfer is not limited by solute delivery rate.

Endothelial permeability increases in response to flow

Recent measurements of K^+, Na^+, urea and fluorescein exchange show that an increase in blood flow not only increases the delivery of solute to the capillaries but also triggers a rapid rise in capillary permeability to these solutes. The flow-mediated rise in permeability involves an active endothelial response mediated by nitric oxide. The raised permeability helps to explain the large increase in transcapillary glucose flux into exercising muscle.

To draw together the various concepts introduced in this chapter, let us finish with two specific examples of how solute flux is increased to meet an increase in demand.

How glucose transfer is increased in exercising muscle

Human muscle contains ~400 grams of glycogen (1–2% by weight), providing an internal source of glucose in the early stages of exercise. As exercise proceeds, muscle glycogen levels fall and glucose transport from blood to muscle increases (Figure 10.15). During 25 min of cycling, the glucose consumption of leg muscles is proportional to the exercise intensity. Arterial plasma glucose itself is kept constant through increased glucose production by the liver and other tissues. The factors that increase the transfer of blood glucose to the exercising muscle fibres are brought together in Table 10.2 and Figure 10.15. **Capillary recruitment** reduces the radius of the Krogh cylinder and hence **diffusion distance** Δx. Recruitment also enhances the **surface area** for diffusion, S, and the effect of flow on capillary permeability P may further raise the net capillary diffusion capacity, PS. A fall in tissue glucose concentration raises the **concentration gradient** across the capillary wall, and the resulting increase in diffusive flux raises the fractional extraction and arteriovenous concentration difference $(C_a - C_v)$ (Figure 10.15). Increased **blood flow** delivers glucose faster to the capillary and prevents a major fall in the mean intracapillary plasma concentration, thereby avoiding flow-limitation of exchange. The Fick principle (Figure 10.8) tells us that the new transcapillary glucose flux equals the increased blood flow multiplied by the increased $(C_a - C_v)$ (Figure 10.15).

How oxygen transfer is increased in exercising muscle

Oxygen diffuses through endothelial cells so rapidly that the capillary wall offers no significant resistance to its transport. The main factor impeding O_2 transport into a muscle fibre is the length of the extravascular pathway, $\sim 20\,\mu m$ – over 60 times longer than the transcapillary pathway, $0.3\,\mu m$. The main O_2 concentration gradient is therefore from pericapillary space to muscle mitochondria, rather than from plasma to pericapillary space (Figure 10.16a). Net transfer is intermediate between flow- and diffusion-limited exchange, as in curve 4 of Figure 10.13a; the end-capillary P_{O_2} of 40 mmHg (oxygen partial pressure, resting muscle) is lower than arterial P_{O_2}, 100 mmHg; but has not equilibrated to mitochondrial P_{O_2}, namely ~ 20 mmHg in resting muscle (Figure 10.16a).

During exercise, **capillary recruitment** occurs, as described above for glucose. This raises the **surface area** available for exchange and reduces the **diffusion distance**. Mitochondrial P_{O_2} is estimated to fall to <5 mmHg, due to increased oxygen consumption, and this **raises the concentration gradient** from arterial blood to muscle. Consequently, the oxygen extraction increases and the end-capillary P_{O_2} can fall as low as ~ 15 mmHg. **Increased blood flow**, and hence increased oxygen delivery, prevents the end-capillary P_{O_2} from falling lower (Figure 10.16, bottom). If flow did not increase, oxygen

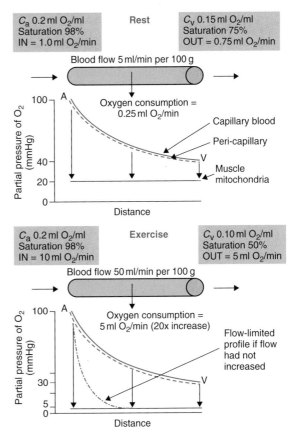

Figure 10.16 Oxygen exchange along a capillary in resting versus exercising skeletal muscle. Mitochondrial P_{O_2} is estimated from myoglobin saturation data. Note that the O_2 demand of the exercising muscle, 5 ml O_2/min, exceeds the total resting arterial supply, 1 ml O_2/min. If blood flow did not increase, the oxygen content of the blood would approach zero soon after it entered the capillary (dot–dash line). A, arterial end of exchange microvessels (strictly, the terminal arteriole); V, venous end of exchange system.

exchange would become severely flow-limited, since a moderately exercising muscle consumes more oxygen per minute than its total resting arterial supply.

An additional factor that speeds up O_2 transport in exercising muscle is the partial deoxygenation of the **myoglobin**, which is present at up to 7 g/kg in the sarcoplasm of red muscle. Although there is a large oxygen gradient from the blood to a point just inside the sarcoplasm, the P_{O_2} is surprisingly uniform across the muscle fibre itself, despite the considerable transport distance, and this is due to the transport-enhancing effect of myoglobin. Partially deoxygenated myoglobin greatly speeds up the rate of O_2 diffusion through the sarcoplasm, because the O_2 molecules can 'hop' from one unoccupied myoglobin binding site to the next. This is called **facilitated diffusion**.

SUMMARY

- A dense network of fine, thin-walled capillaries subserves nutrient and water exchange between blood and tissue.

- Solutes such as O_2 and glucose **diffuse rapidly** across the capillary wall down **concentration gradients**. Water, by contrast, **flows slowly** across the wall down a **pressure gradient** across the intercellular cleft and fenestrae.

- **Fick's law of diffusion** states that the amount of solute transferred per unit time by diffusion is proportional to concentration gradient (concentration difference/distance), area available for diffusion and solute diffusion coefficient.

- A **porous membrane**, such as the capillary wall, limits the area available for diffusion and restricts the intrapore diffusivity. These effects are lumped together in the parameter '**membrane permeability**'. Diffusive transport rate J_s equals permeability P × membrane area S × concentration drop across the membrane ΔC; $J_s = P S \Delta C$.

- Capillary permeability depends on both **ultrastructure** and **solute properties**. Three types of capillary – continuous, fenestrated and discontinuous – form a hierarchy of increasing permeability to lipid-insoluble solutes. Solutes fall into three classes:

  (i) **Lipid-soluble molecules**, such as O_2, CO_2 and general anaesthetics, diffuse across the entire endothelial cell membrane; so they permeate capillaries extremely rapidly.

  (ii) **Small, lipid-insoluble molecules**, such as salts, glucose, amino acids and many drugs, diffuse through an aqueous pathway, namely the **intercellular cleft** and fenestrations. The intercellular space is small, so permeation is much slower than for lipid-soluble molecules. The entrance to the intercellular pathway is guarded by **small pores** (equivalent radius 4–5 nm) that exclude and reflect the plasma proteins. The pores are the tiny spaces between the polymers of the endocapillary coat, the **glycocalyx. Blood–brain barrier** capillaries have exceptionally tight intercellular junctions, so glucose and amino acid transfer is mediated by specific carrier proteins, through facilitated diffusion.

  (iii) **Large, lipid-insoluble molecules**, such as plasma proteins (radius >4 nm), cross endothelium slowly through a limited large-pore system, the identity of which is controversial. Both vesicular transport and porous channels may contribute.

- **Solute extraction** E is the fraction of the arterial solute that is extracted by the tissue during capillary transit. $E = (C_a - C_v)/C_a$, where C_a and C_v are the arterial and venous plasma concentrations. For oxygen, E averages ~25% in a resting human. **Plasma clearance** (ml/min) = plasma flow × E. **Solute transfer rate** J_s can be determined by applying the **Fick principle**; J_s = plasma flow × $(C_a - C_v)$.

- **Solute transfer rate** can be increased hugely, e.g. in exercising muscle, through a combination of (i) **an increase in the blood-to-tissue concentration difference** ΔC, due to increased metabolic consumption by the tissue; (ii) **recruitment** of underperfused capillaries by arteriolar dilatation, which raises S, reduces diffusion distance Δx across the Krogh cylinder and improves perfusion homogeneity; and (iii) **increased capillary blood flow**.

- The **effect of increased blood flow** depends on whether solute exchange is **flow-limited**, **diffusion-limited** or **intermediate**. If capillary diffusion capacity PS is $\geqslant 5$ times blood flow $\dot{Q}$, blood equilibrates with pericapillary fluid before the capillary exit is reached. Such exchange is flow-limited; raising the blood flow increases the exchange rate proportionately – as with O_2 uptake by pulmonary capillaries. If $PS/\dot{Q}$ is <1, equilibration is not achieved before the end of the capillary and exchange is diffusion-limited (e.g. glucose in exercising muscle); transfer is not limited by solute delivery rate.

Further reading

Reviews and chapters

Abbott NJ. Inflammatory mediators and modulation of blood–brain barrier permeability. *Cellular and Molecular Neurobiology* 2000; **20**: 131–47.

Duelli R, Kuschinsky W. Brain glucose transporters: relationship to local energy demand. *News in Physiological Sciences* 2001; **16**: 71–6.

Ellsworth ML, Ellis CG, Popel AS, Pittman RN. Role of microvessels in oxygen supply to tissue. *News in Physiological Sciences* 1994; **9**: 119–23.

Firth JA. Endothelial barriers: from hypothetical pores to membrane proteins. *Journal of Anatomy* 2002; **200**: 541–8.

Hudlicka O, Egginton S, Brown MD. Capillary diffusion distances – their importance for cardiac and skeletal muscle performance. *News in Physiological Sciences* 1988; **3**: 134–8.

Intaglietta M, Johnson PC. Functional capillary density: active and passive determinants. *International Journal of Microcirculation* 1995; **15**: 213–76.

Jürgens KD, Papadopoulos S, Peters T, Gros G. Myoglobin: just an oxygen store or also an oxygen transporter? *News in Physiological Sciences* 2000; **15**: 269–74.

Michel CC. Microvascular permeability, ultrafiltration and restricted diffusion. *American Journal of Physiology* 2004; **287**: H1887–8.

Tuma PL, Hubbard AL. Transcytosis: crossing cellular barriers. *Physiological Reviews* 2003; **83**: 871–932.

Wittenberg JB, Wittenberg BA. Myoglobin function reassessed. *Journal of Experimental Biology* 2003; **206**: 2011–22.

Wolf MB. A three-pathway pore model describes extensive transport data from mammalian microvascular beds and frog microvessels. *Microcirculation* 2002; **9**: 497–511.

Research papers

See www.hodderplus.com/cardiovascularphysiology for a full list of Research papers for this chapter.

CHAPTER 11

Circulation of fluid between plasma, interstitium and lymph

Learning objectives

After reading this chapter you should be able to:

- Name the factors determining capillary fluid exchange and relate them using the Starling equation (11.1).
- Define 'osmotic reflection coefficient' and explain its importance (11.1, 11.3, 11.11).
- Outline the factors determining capillary pressure (11.2).
- Give typical values for human capillary pressure and plasma colloid osmotic pressure (11.2, 11.3).
- Sketch how extravascular protein concentration alters with filtration rate, and explain its importance (11.4).
- Outline how Starling pressures and fluid flux change along the capillary axis (11.6).
- State the circumstances under which capillaries absorb interstitial fluid (11.6).
- Explain why normal tissue does not 'pit' but oedematous tissue does (11.7).
- Draw an interstitial pressure–volume relation, marking the normal and oedematous zones (11.7).
- List the functions of the lymphatic system and outline how lymph is moved (11.8).
- Categorize the causes of oedema and explain the 'safety margin' (11.10).
- List the changes that bring about inflammatory swelling (11.11).

Capillary blood pressure causes fluid to filter slowly across the capillary wall into the interstitial space. From here, the fluid drains into the lymphatic system, which returns it to the bloodstream. Although this fluid turnover is usually very slow, the cumulative turnover over many hours is substantial; in fact **the entire plasma volume completes an extravascular circulation in under one day**, except for the plasma proteins. Consequently, the distribution of fluid between the plasma and interstitial compartment can be distorted relatively quickly by changes in capillary or lymphatic function. For example, increased capillary filtration during prolonged standing or exercise reduces the plasma volume by up to 20%; and increased capillary filtration during cardiac failure drives an excess of water in the tissues (oedema). To understand such fluid shifts, we must first identify the forces that determine fluid exchange.

11.1 The Starling principle of fluid exchange

Transcapillary fluid movement is a process of **plasma ultrafiltration across a semipermeable membrane**. That is to say, water and electrolytes pass through the wall more easily than plasma proteins, producing an ultrafiltrate with a substantially reduced protein content – the interstitial fluid. The ultrafilter is the endocapillary coating of biopolymers, the glycocalyx (Figures 9.3, 9.5 and 10.10). The glycocalyx interpolymer spaces function as a system of small pores (radius 4–5 nm), that are permeable to water and small solutes but are too narrow to transmit plasma proteins readily. The glycocalyx is thus a semipermeable membrane, and it covers the entrance to the intercellular cleft, through which the plasma ultrafiltrate flows to reach the pericapillary, interstitial space (Figure 11.1b). In fenestrated capillaries, the fenestrae provide an additional, subglycocalyx pathway permeable to water (Figures 10.10 and 10.11). In discontinuous capillaries the gaps further enhance permeability (Figure 10.2).

Blood pressure drives filtration; plasma colloid osmotic pressure opposes it

The primary force driving plasma ultrafiltration is the **capillary blood pressure**, as Carl Ludwig

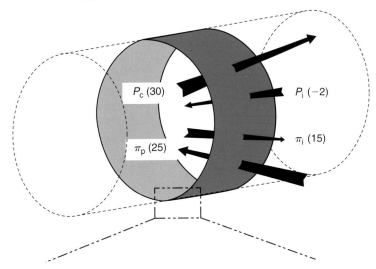

(a) *Traditional Starling principle: filtration force = $(P_c - P_i) - \sigma(\pi_p - \pi_i)$*

P_c (30) P_i (−2)

π_p (25) π_i (15)

(b) *Revised Starling principle: filtration force = $(P_c - P_i) - \sigma(\pi_p - \pi_g)$*

P_c π_p

Plasma

Small pore system, glycocalyx network

Subglycocalyx space π_g Large pore system, transporting plasma proteins (grey)

Endothelium

Intercellular cleft

Interstitial fluid   Plasma ultrafiltrate

P_i π_i

Figure 11.1 (a) Four classic Starling pressures influencing fluid exchange across capillary wall. P_c, capillary blood pressure (mmHg, human skin, heart level). P_i, interstitial fluid pressure. π_p, plasma colloid osmotic pressure (COP). π_i, interstitial fluid COP. Pressures are relative to atmospheric pressure (760 mmHg), so $P_i = -2$ mmHg means an absolute pressure of 758 mmHg – hence arrow direction. (Data from Levick JR, Michel CC. *Journal of Physiology* 1978; **274**: 97–109; Bates DO *et al. Journal of Physiology* 1994; **477**: 355–63.) (b) Cross section of intercellular cleft to show gradient of extravascular plasma protein extending into subglycocalyx space (COP $= \pi_g$); concentration indicated by shade of grey. Gradient is result of battle between upstream diffusion of extravascular plasma protein (solid curves) and its washout by plasma ultrafiltrate emerging from the glycocalyx small pore system (dashed line). (Adapted from Levick JR. *Journal of Physiology* 2004; **557**: 704.) At a fenestration, the difference between π_g and π_i is less extreme, because the small pore outlets are less confined (Levick JR. *Microvascular Research* 1994; **47**: 90–125.)

recognized in 1850. The primary force opposing ultrafiltration is the **osmotic pressure of the plasma proteins**, which tends to suck fluid into the capillary, as shown by Ernest Starling in 1896. Starling injected isotonic saline or serum into the tissues of a dog hindlimb and found that the saline was absorbed into the bloodstream, as revealed by haemodilution – whereas serum was not. He concluded that the capillary wall is a semipermeable membrane, across which the plasma proteins ('colloids') exert an absorptive force, the colloid osmotic pressure. This is the **Starling principle of fluid exchange**.

Colloid osmotic pressure (COP) and oncotic pressure are synonyms for the osmotic pressure of the plasma proteins. Students unfamiliar with osmosis should note that osmotic pressure is a **suction** force, not a pushing force (Section 11.3). Plasma COP is of major importance because **plasma COP is the sole force retaining water within the plasma compartment**. Starling's discovery led to the use of solutions of artificial colloids to replace lost plasma in wounded soldiers during World War I, and more recently to the development of plasma substitutes such as urea-linked gelatin solution – a nice example of practical benefit arising from 'pure' research.

Rate and direction of fluid exchange are governed by four pressures

The Starling principle of fluid exchange (not to be confused with Starling's law, Section 6.4) states that the transcapillary filtration rate is proportional to the hydraulic pressure difference across the wall minus the opposing colloid osmotic pressure difference (Figure 11.1a). In other words:

Capillary filtration rate ∝ [Hydraulic push −
Osmotic suction].

When hydraulic push exceeds osmotic suction, fluid filters from the bloodstream into the interstitium. This is the normal state of affairs. If, however, osmotic suction exceeds hydraulic push, the filtration rate becomes negative, i.e. fluid is absorbed from the interstitial compartment into the plasma, as happens after a haemorrhage.

We can easily convert the above statement into an equation that predicts the volume filtered per unit time, J_v. The net hydraulic push equals capillary blood pressure P_c minus interstitial fluid pressure P_i. The net osmotic suction equals plasma COP, π_p, minus the COP of fluid on the downstream side of

the semipermeable membrane, the glycocalyx, π_g. So, replacing words with symbols:

$$J_v \propto [(P_c - P_i) - (\pi_p - \pi_g)] \qquad (11.1a)$$

P_c, P_i and π_p have all been measured. Unfortunately, π_g cannot be measured at present, only computed. However, interstitial fluid COP (π_i) can be measured, and the interstitial fluid is connected to the subglycocalyx fluid via the intercellular cleft (and fenestrae, when present) (Figure 11.1b). Therefore π_i has traditionally been substituted for π_g (for caveats, see Section 11.6). This gives us the traditional formula:

$$J_v \propto [(P_c - P_i) - (\pi_p - \pi_i)] \qquad (11.1b)$$

The proportionality factor depends on capillary surface area S and the hydraulic conductance of the wall, L_p, so we can write:

$$J_v \cong L_p S[(P_c - P_i) - (\pi_p - \pi_i)] \qquad (11.1c)$$

This equation still lacks one crucial term, however; it neglects the fact that endothelium is as an **imperfect** semipermeable membrane – that is to say, it is slightly leaky to plasma proteins. This is dealt with by introducing the reflection coefficient, as follows.

The reflection coefficient quantifies imperfect semipermeability

When a membrane is leaky to a solute, the solute's potential osmotic pressure is not exerted fully (Figure 10.7). The ratio of the effective osmotic pressure across a leaky membrane ($\Delta\pi_{effective}$) to the full osmotic pressure across a perfect semipermeable membrane ($\Delta\pi_{ideal}$) is called the osmotic reflection coefficient σ:

$$\sigma = \frac{\Delta\pi_{effective}}{\Delta\pi_{ideal}} \qquad (11.2)$$

Endothelial σ for plasma proteins is 0.80–0.95, so 80–95% of the plasma COP is exerted at the capillary wall. (NB The reduction is not caused by protein outside the membrane. The effective osmotic pressure of extravascular protein is likewise reduced by factor σ.) Thus the osmotic pressures in eqn 11.1 must be reduced by fraction σ, giving us the **classic Starling equation for fluid filtration**.

$$J_v = L_p S[(P_c - P_i) - \sigma(\pi_p - \pi_i)] \qquad (11.3)$$

As we shall see, the Starling equation is central to understanding disorders such as oedema, inflammatory swelling and posthaemorrhagic fluid absorption. It must be remembered, however, that π_i is a rough substitute for the true factor π_g, and in some circumstances the distinction is important (Section 11.6).

Key features of the Starling principle have been proved in single capillaries

Transcapillary fluid movement was first measured in an individual capillary by an American medical student, Eugene Landis, in 1926. The capillary is cannulated with a micropipette and blocked downstream by a glass rod (Figure 11.2a). If ultrafiltration occurs out of the blocked segment, the lost fluid is replaced from the pipette, sweeping the trapped red cells towards the blocker. Conversely, if interstitial fluid is absorbed into the capillary, the red cells are pushed back towards the pipette. The flow is calculated from the red cell velocity, and the capillary pressure is measured through the micropipette.

The Landis red cell method established that the capillary filtration rate increases linearly with pressure P_c, as the Starling equation predicts (Figure 11.2b). The slope equals endothelial hydraulic conductance, L_p. The results also prove that the capillary wall is a semipermeable membrane, because filtration rate is zero when capillary pressure is close to the plasma colloid osmotic pressure π_p, and reverses direction to absorption when capillary pressure is lowered below π_p. The transient nature of fluid absorption is considered later (Section 11.6).

Filtration rate increases with venous pressure in humans limbs

Capillary filtration rate can be measured in human limbs and isolated perfused organs using the slow rise in volume or weight that occurs when capillary pressure is raised. Capillary pressure can be raised in a human limb by inflating a proximal sphygmomanometer cuff to ~40 mmHg, thereby raising distal venous pressure. After the vascular volume has stabilized, the limb swells slowly due to increased capillary filtration (Figure 11.3a). A **deep venous thrombosis** of the leg causes leg oedema in this way. The swelling rate increases linearly with venous pressure (Figure 11.3b), and the slope of the relation, the **capillary filtration capacity**, equals the sum of the capillary area × wall conductance values, $\Sigma(L_p S)$, in a given volume of tissue.

(a)

(b)

Figure 11.2 (a) Landis–Michel red cell method to measure fluid exchange in a single capillary. Filtration rate in the blocked vessel (J_v) equals axial shift in red cell per unit time × vessel cross-sectional area. Measurements are made at several capillary pressures. (b) Initial filtration rate per unit wall area (J_v/A) increases with capillary pressure. The 'plasma' here was an infused albumin solution of COP (π_p) 22 cmH$_2$O. The pressure intercept at zero filtration, 15 cmH$_2$O, is the effective osmotic pressure of the albumin *in vivo*, $\sigma\pi_p$. P_i and π_i were probably close to zero, because the tissue was continuously washed with saline. The slope is the endothelial hydraulic conductance, L_p. (From Michel CC. *Journal of Physiology* 1980; **309**: 341–55, with permission from Wiley-Blackwell.)

The effect of venous pressure on capillary filtration raises the question 'What determines capillary pressure?' The next section addresses this issue.

11.2 Capillary blood pressure (P_c) and its regulation

Capillary blood pressure is the most variable of the four Starling pressures and is the only factor under nervous control. It is affected by arterial and venous pressures, vascular resistance, gravity and distance along the capillary axis.

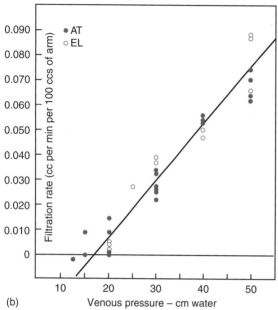

Figure 11.3 Capillary filtration in the human forearm. (a) Forearm volume was measured by plethysmography (Figure 8.5). Arrows mark inflation of venous congesting cuff around upper arm to 40 cmH$_2$0 and deflation after 15 min. After the initial phase of venous distension (~2 min), the slow swelling is caused by capillary filtration. (b) Capillary filtration rate at a series of venous pressures. The slope, 0.003 ml min^{-1}mmHg^{-1} per 100 ml forearm, is called the capillary filtration capacity. (From the classic study of Krogh A, Landis EM, Turner AH. *Journal of Clinical Investigations* 1932; **11**: 63–95.)

Pre- to postcapillary resistance ratio (R_A/R_V) regulates capillary pressure

Capillary pressure lies between arterial pressure and venous pressure, and is usually closer to venous than arterial pressure. How close the capillary pressure is to arterial or venous pressure depends on the ratio of precapillary, arteriolar resistance R_A to postcapillary, venular resistance R_V (Figure 11.4). If R_A/R_V is high, the pressure drop across the arterioles is large, so the pressure reaching the capillary is much attenuated, as in the 'vasoconstriction' curve of Figure 8.16. As a result, capillary pressure is close

to venular pressure. Conversely, if R_A/R_V is low, as it is during inflammation, capillary pressure is high (Figure 8.16, vasodilatation curve). R_A/R_V is normally quite large, ~4, so capillary pressure is normally low and four times more sensitive to venous pressure than to arterial pressure. This is why venous hypertension causes oedema but arterial hypertension does not.

Since capillary pressure is regulated by R_A/R_V, **the sympathetic vasomotor nerves can influence fluid exchange**. After a haemorrhage, sympathetic-mediated arteriolar vasoconstriction raises R_A/R_V, which reduces capillary pressure. Plasma colloid osmotic pressure now predominates over capillary pressure, so interstitial fluid is absorbed into the capillary bloodstream, topping up the depleted circulation (Section 18.2). The active regulation of capillary pressure by R_A/R_V is a daily occurrence in the human leg during standing, as described next.

The rise in capillary pressure below heart level is attenuated by precapillary vasoconstriction

Due to gravity, arterial and venous pressures increase with vertical distance below heart level, to ~180 mmHg and ~90 mmHg, respectively, in the feet of a standing human (Figure 8.2). Capillary pressure increases too, to ~95 mmHg in the foot. This is why oedema is common in the feet and ankles, or over the sacrum if bed-ridden. Capillary pressure does not increase as steeply, however, as the arterial and venous pressures (Figure 11.5). This is because a local, arteriolar vasoconstriction, the **veni–arteriolar response**, raises R_A/R_V to 20–30 (Figure 11.5, top right). The large rise in precapillary resistance shifts the capillary pressure towards the lower, venous limit of its range. In this way, the veni–arteriolar response attenuates the fluid filtration rate and helps prevent postural oedema.

Blood pressure decays along a capillary

Due to the capillary's hydraulic resistance, blood pressure falls along a capillary, from ~32–36 mmHg at the arterial end to 12–25 mmHg at the venous end of human skin capillaries at heart level. Capillary pressure is considerably lower in the lungs (~10 mmHg) and portal circulations (renal tubular capillaries ~14 mmHg, hepatic sinusoids ~6–7 mmHg).

$$P_c = \frac{P_V[R_A/R_V] + P_A}{1 + [R_A/R_V]}$$

Metabolic and inflammatory vasodilatation ⟷ Sympathetic vasoconstriction

Normal arteriolar tone

Figure 11.4 Control of capillary pressure by resistance vessels in cat skeletal muscle. Pressure was measured towards the venous end of capillary bed; venous pressure P_V was 7 mmHg, arterial pressure P_A 100 mmHg. Peripheral resistance (unit PRU) is generated mainly by precapillary, arteriolar resistance. *Inset* shows how ratio of precapillary resistance R_A to postcapillary resistance R_V regulates capillary pressure P_c. Blood flow from artery to mid-capillary equals $(P_A - P_c)/R_A$. Flow from mid-capillary to vein equals $(P_c - P_V)/R_V$. Since the two flows are virtually equal, $(P_A - P_c)/R_A = (P_c - P_V)/R_V$. Rearranging, we get the Pappenheimer–Soto Rivera equation for capillary pressure in the box. (Data from Maspers M, Björnberg J, Mellander S. *Acta Physiologica Scandinavica* 1990; **140**: 73–83, by permission.)

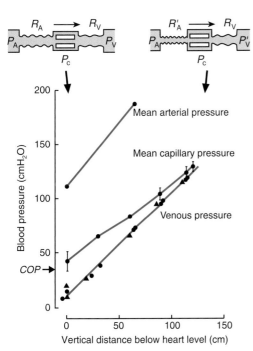

Figure 11.5 Capillary blood pressure in nail-fold skin of human foot, measured by micropuncture, with foot at various distances below heart level. Popliteal artery pressure and dorsal foot vein pressure increase with distance below heart level in the simple way predicted by physics (effect of gravity), but capillary pressure increases less than expected. *Top insets* show how the rise in capillary pressure is attenuated by a vasoconstrictor response. This 'veni-arteriolar response' may be mediated by the Bayliss myogenic response, but also requires an intact sympathetic innervation. (From Levick JR, Michel CC. *Journal of Physiology* 1978; **274**: 97–109, by permission.)

Next we must consider the main force opposing capillary filtration, the plasma colloid osmotic pressure.

11.3 Osmosis across capillaries: plasma COP (π_p)

Capillaries can absorb interstitial fluid by osmosis under certain circumstances (Figure 11.2), so let us consider next the process of osmosis.

Osmosis is the flow of water molecules across a semipermeable membrane from a dilute to a stronger solution

The total pressure acting on the entrance to a pore in a semipermeable membrane is the result of the bombardment of the pore entrance by both solvent molecules and solute molecules, which are in a state of continuous, thermodynamic motion (Figure 11.6). If the solution is at, say, atmospheric pressure, the sum of the solvent and solute bombardments equals one atmosphere. The solvent itself, therefore, must exert less than one atmosphere of pressure – just as, in a mixture of gases at 1 atmosphere, each gas has a partial pressure of less than 1 atmosphere. The solute thus reduces the solvent free energy (Figure 11.6, red line). If the opposite side of the membrane is exposed to pure solvent or a less

Figure 11.6 Osmotic flow from solvent (right) to solution (left), both at atmospheric pressure, P_0. The solute lowers the 'partial pressure' P' of the solvent in the solution (i.e. its free energy), so P' is less than P_0. The resulting pressure gradient across the pore drives the osmotic flow of solvent into the solution. Osmosis is a process of hydraulic flow, not water diffusion. (After Mauro A. In: Ussing HH, Bindslev N, Lassen LA, Sten-Knudsen D (eds). *Water Transport Across Epithelia*. Copenhagen: Munksgaard, 1981: 107–10, with permission from Wiley-Blackwell.)

Figure 11.7 Osmotic pressure of human plasma proteins in isotonic saline (pH 7.4, 37°C). Pink region shows normal human range. Dashed line is van't Hoff law prediction for albumin. COP is bigger than predicted and is described (in mmHg) by polynomial equations:

albumin $\pi = 0.28C + 1.8 \times 10^{-3}C^2 + 1.2 \times 10^{-5}C^3$,
plasma $\pi = 0.21C + 1.6 \times 10^{-3}C^2 + 0.9 \times 10^{-5}C^3$,
globulins $\pi = 0.16C + 1.5 \times 10^{-3}C^2 + 0.6 \times 10^{-5}C^3$,

where C is g/l. (From Scatchard G *et al.*, summarized by Landis EM, Pappenheimer JR. In: Hamilton WF, Dow P (eds). *Handbook of Physiology 2*, Circulation III. Washington: American Physiological Society, 1963: 961–1034, by permission)

concentrated solution at atmospheric pressure, there is now a difference in solvent energy level across the pore. This drives a hydraulic flow of solvent through the pore into the more concentrated solution – osmotic flow. The osmotic flow can be halted by applying pressure to the concentrated solution, to raise its solvent free energy to the same level as on the opposite side. **The hydrostatic pressure that halts the osmotic flow from pure solvent into a solution is called the 'osmotic pressure' of the solution.** This way of measuring osmotic pressure accounts for the fact that a suction effect is referred to as a 'pressure'.

Note that, during osmosis, the solvent flows hydraulically through the pore. Contrary to a popular belief, perpetuated in some textbooks, the net water movement is **not by diffusion**. Experiments half a century ago proved that osmotic flow through pores of known radius r obeys Poiseuille's law of hydraulic flow (flow $\propto r^4$, Section 8.7), not Fick's law of diffusion (flux $\propto$ area $\propto r^2$, Section 10.3).

Albumin contributes disproportionately to colloid osmotic pressure π_p

As a rough rule, the plasma colloid osmotic pressure (COP) in different types of vertebrate equals mid-capillary blood pressure – both are high in humans and low in amphibia. Human plasma contains 65–80 g protein per litre, and its COP is 21–29 mmHg (Figure 11.7). Albumin, which accounts for half the plasma protein mass, generates about two-thirds of the COP. Albumin's osmotic pressure greatly exceeds the 'ideal' osmotic pressure predicted by van't Hoff's law (see Appendix 2, van't Hoff's law), partly because the albumin molecule has 17 negative charges at physiological pH. These attract extra Na^+ ions into the solution (**Gibbs–Donnan effect**), which contribute about one-third of albumin's osmotic pressure.

Colloid osmotic pressure differs massively from crystalloid osmotic pressure

The total osmotic pressure of plasma is extremely high, ~5800 mmHg, but 99.6% is due to the 300 millimoles of 'crystalloids' per litre, chiefly sodium chloride. The crystalloid osmotic pressure, though massive, does not affect capillary fluid exchange under most circumstances, because the salt concentration in interstitial fluid and plasma is almost identical and the endothelial reflection coefficient for crystalloids is only ~0.1. Plasma protein concentration is only ~1 mM, but plasma proteins exert a sustained osmotic pressure of ~25 mmHg, due to their high reflection coefficient. The plasma proteins are thus responsible for retaining fluid in the circulation. There are a few circumstances, however, in which crystalloid osmotic pressure influences transcapillary fluid exchange, as follows.

Aquaporins provide a water-only, transcellular pathway of low conductance

The endothelial glycocalyx–intercellular cleft pathway provides a high-conductance pathway for both water and crystalloids. Continuous capillaries also have low-conductance channels in the cell membrane, formed by the transmembrane glycoprotein aquaporin-1. Aquaporin channels conduct water but not crystalloids. Their main role is cell volume regulation. Aquaporins normally contribute little to transcapillary flow, due to their low hydraulic conductance and the absence of a significant transcapillary crystalloid gradient. If interstitial crystalloid concentration increases, however, flow through the aquaporin pathway can become significant, since crystalloids exert their full osmotic pressure on the water-only aquaporin channels ($\sigma = 1$). Interstitial crystalloid concentration increases in the following situations.

- **Exercising muscle fibres** release lactate and K^+ ions into the interstitial fluid, raising the local crystalloid osmotic pressure. This draws water from the plasma compartment through the aquaporin-1 channels. Consequently, muscles swell during exercise, and plasma volume falls (Section 11.9).
- The **renal outer medulla** has long capillaries (descending vasa recta) with abundant aquaporin-1 channels. A gradient of sodium chloride created by the renal tubules draws water through these channels.
- In **peritoneal dialysis** a concentrated glucose solution is infused into the peritoneal cavity of renal failure patients. The glucose, a crystalloid, sucks fluid osmotically from the plasma into the peritoneal cavity, enabling the physician to control the plasma volume. Mercuric chloride, which blocks aquaporin-1 channels, blocks this fluid transfer.

11.4 Magnitude and dynamics of extravascular COP (π_i, π_g)

Having considered plasma COP, we must next consider the smaller but by no means insignificant extravascular COP. As noted earlier, the underside of the semipermeable glycocalyx is exposed to the subglycocalyx fluid of the intercellular cleft and fenestrations, which connects with the interstitial fluid compartment (Figures 10.10 and 11.1b). If the filtration rate is slow, interstitial albumin and other escaped plasma proteins can diffuse upstream in the intercellular cleft to influence the colloid osmotic pressure π_g at the outer face of the semipermeable membrane (Section 11.6). We must therefore consider the interstitial fluid plasma protein concentration and the factors that change it.

Interstitial plasma protein concentration and COP are *not* insignificant

There is widespread, time-hallowed misconception that the plasma protein content and COP of interstitial fluid are insignificant. This is simply not true for most tissues. Mean interstitial plasma protein concentration is ~20–30 g/l, and since interstitial fluid is 16% of the body weight, over half of the entire plasma protein mass is actually extravascular. Interstitial fluid composition has been determined by collecting fluid from prenodal lymphatics and implanted wicks. Human leg lymph contains 15–35 g/l plasma protein, intestinal lymph 30–40 g/l and lung lymph 40–50 g/l, representing 23% (leg) to 70% (lung) of the plasma concentration (Table 11.1). Since the interstitial plasma proteins

Table 11.1 Starling pressures in human subcutaneous tissue (mmHg)

	Normal	Congestive cardiac failure
Chest		
Plasma COP	26.8	23.3
Interstitial fluid COP	15.6	10.5
Interstitial fluid pressure	−1.5	−1.4
Ankle		
Plasma COP (arterial)	26.8	23.3
Interstitial fluid COP	10.7	3.4 (mild oedema)
Interstitial fluid pressure	0.1	0.4 (mild oedema)

COP, colloid osmotic pressure. Interstitial fluid COP measured in soaked wick fluid. Interstitial fluid pressure measured by wick-in-needle.
(From Noddeland H, Omvik P, Lund-Johansen P *et al. Clinical Physiology* 1984; **4**: 283–97.)

can diffuse into the subglycocalyx space, they can affect the COP gradient across the semipermeable glycocalyx, and hence fluid exchange (Section 11.6). So what determines the interstitial plasma protein concentration?

Interstitial protein concentration and COP are a dynamic function of filtration rate

Plasma protein concentration in the bulk interstitial fluid is not a fixed quantity; it varies with fluid exchange rate, due to the following simple relation. Plasma proteins pass slowly from plasma to interstitium through the large pore system, which is spatially separate from the main filtration pathway (intercellular clefts, fenestrae – Figures 10.11 and 11.1b). If the large pores transmit a plasma protein mass m into the interstitium in time t (flux J_s), and the small pores transmit a water volume V over the same period (flow J_v), the interstitial protein concentration C_i is given by the **interstitial dilution relation**:

$$C_i = \frac{m/t}{V/t} = \frac{J_s}{J_v} \qquad (11.4)$$

In other words, interstitial protein concentration equals the rate of arrival of protein divided by the rate of arrival of water, in the steady state (Figure 11.8, top panel). Interstitial protein concentration is thus a **dynamic variable**, governed by two continuous influxes, one of which (J_v) varies with capillary pressure. When capillary pressure is raised, the water transfer rate increases more than the protein transfer rate, since small pores sieve out the plasma proteins. Consequently, **interstitial protein concentration varies inversely with capillary filtration rate** (Figure 11.8, lower panel). This is sometimes called the 'protein wash-down' effect. Conversely, if the water filtration rate were reduced to zero, the interstitial protein concentration would eventually equilibrate with the plasma level, due to protein permeation through the large pores.

In Section 11.1 we saw that the pericapillary COP (COP just outside the membrane) can be a **determinant** of filtration rate (eqn 11.3), while here we have seen that pericapillary COP is also **dependent** on filtration rate (eqn 11.4). The interdependence of filtration rate and pericapillary COP has important consequences (Section 11.6), but before tackling these we must review the fourth Starling pressure, the interstitial fluid pressure.

(a)

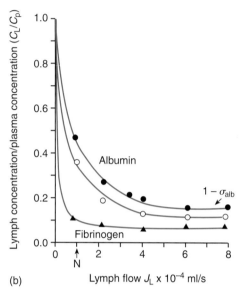

(b)

Figure 11.8 Effect of capillary filtration rate on interstitial protein concentration. (a) Mass of protein entering the interstitium in a given time (m'/t or J_s) is diluted by the volume of filtrate produced over the same time interval (V'/t or J_v); so interstitial protein concentration $C_i = J_s/J_v$. This drains away as lymph ($C_i = C_L$). (b) Effect of filtration rate on lymph/plasma concentration ratio, C_L/C_p, in dog paw. Filtration rate was measured as lymph flow J_L and was varied by venous congestion. N is normal value. Curves are for albumin (●, radius 3.55 nm), γ-globulin (○, radius 5.6 nm) and fibrinogen (▲, radius 10 nm). At high flows C_L/C_p falls to a limit, the transmitted fraction $1 - \sigma$. (From Renkin EM *et al.* 1977, plotted by Curry FE. In: Renkin EM, Michel CC (eds). *Handbook of Physiology, Cardiovascular System*, Vol. IV, Part II, Microcirculation. Bethesda, MD: American Physiological Society, 1984: 309–74, by permission.)

11.5 Interstitial matrix and interstitial fluid pressure (P_i)

Interstitium is a biphasic, porous material composed of fluid and biopolymers

Interstitium, or extracellular matrix, is the complex substance between the parenchymal cells of a tissue; it is not just a pool of liquid bathing the cells (Figure 11.9). **Collagen fibrils** provide tensile strength, and in skin and large arteries **elastin**

Hyaluronan chain

GAG   CP
Proteoglycan   Collagen fibril

Figure 11.9 Interstitial matrix is a network of fibrous biopolymers with interstitial fluid in the tiny spaces between the chains. The hyaluronan chain acts as the 'string' to which proteoglycan 'pearls' are anchored (string-of-pearls model). Cutting the string with hyaluronidase raises interstitial hydraulic permeability about five-fold. GAG, sulphated glycosaminoglycan chain (long, chondroitin sulphate; short, keratan sulphate); CP, core protein of proteoglycan. Microfibrils and glycoproteins, such as fibronectin, not shown.

confers elasticity (Figure 1.11). The interfibrillar spaces contain **glycosaminoglycan chains** (GAGs), which are long-chain polymers of amino-sugars, up to 40 nm long, mostly rich in negative sulphate groups (chondroitin, keratan, dermatan and heparan sulphates). Multiple sulphated GAG chains are anchored to a linear core protein, forming a large, brush-shaped molecule, the **proteoglycan**. Multiple proteoglycans are anchored to an enormously long chain of non-sulphated GAG, **hyaluronan** (length ~5000 nm, size 2–3 million dalton). All GAGs have fixed negative charges in the form of carboxyl groups ($-COO^-$) and most also have sulphate groups, $-SO_4^-$. **Glycoproteins**, such as the cell-attachment 'glue' fibronectin, add further to the structural complexity. The interstitium thus comprises a three-dimensional network of negatively charged biopolymer fibres, the solid phase, and a space-filling solution of electrolytes and escaped plasma proteins, the fluid phase.

GAGs reduce interstitial permeability; interstitial fluid is not easily displaced

The GAGs have two major roles: they are **water-attracting, expansion elements**, and they determine **interstitial permeability**. Regarding the latter role, interstitial water and solutes occupy the minute spaces within the GAG matrix. The effective radius of these spaces, or mean hydraulic radius, ranges from a mere 3 nm in cartilage, which has a very high GAG concentration, to 300 nm in the vitreous body of the eye, which has a very low GAG concentration. Because the spaces are tiny, their resistance to flow is high. As a result, interstitium has a gel-like consistency, as exemplified by umbilical cord Wharton's jelly (mean hydraulic radius 30 nm). The low mobility of interstitial water stabilizes tissue shape, prevents interstitial fluid displacement by gravity, and impedes bacterial spread.

GAGs expand the interstitial compartment

GAGs are responsible for the large volume of the interstitial compartment, because they attract water and swell. If a slice of connective tissue, or Wharton's jelly from the umbilical cord (almost pure interstitium), is placed in saline, the interstitial matrix imbibes the saline and swells. The swelling can be halted by lowering the saline pressure to a sufficiently subatmospheric value. The subatmospheric pressure that exactly counteracts the suction effect of the GAGs is called the **gel swelling pressure**. As with osmosis, this kind of 'pressure' is really a suction force, not a pushing force. The gel swelling pressure is caused by the osmotic activity of the GAGs, which is due chiefly to Na^+ ions attracted by their fixed negative charges (the **Gibbs–Donnan** effect). *In vivo*, the interstitial matrix is under-saturated – that is to say, it still has a swelling tendency, despite the continuous input plasma ultrafiltration by capillaries. The unsaturated state is due to the operation of the lymphatic system, which pumps water away from the interstitium, leaving the interstitial fluid at a subatmospheric pressure.

In some tissues, such as skin, the swelling tendency of the interstitial matrix is partly counteracted by fibroblasts. The fibroblasts exert tension on the collagen fibrils through $\alpha_2\beta_1$-integrins at their membrane focal contact points, and the tensed collagen fibrils help to limit the matrix swelling.

Interstitial fluid pressure P_i is often subatmospheric

Interstitial fluid pressure is difficult to measure, due to the low mobility of fluid in interstitium. This problem was first overcome in 1960 by the American physiologist Arthur Guyton, who implanted a hollow perforated capsule under the skin of dogs (Figure 11.10). Over several weeks

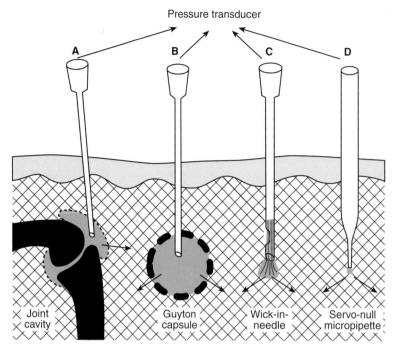

Pressure transducer

A   B   C   D

Joint cavity
Guyton capsule
Wick-in-needle
Servo-null micropipette

Figure 11.10 Measurement of interstitial fluid pressure. (A) Cannulation of a free fluid space in contact with interstitium, e.g. joint cavity, epidural space. (B) Guyton's chronic capsule method. (C) Acute wick method of Fadnes, Reed and Aukland; fine cotton filaments conduct interstitial pressure into a hypodermic needle. (D) Acute micropipette method; micropipette filled with 1 M NaCl, a good electrical conductor, is connected to a motorized pump that varies the intra-pipette pressure until fluid neither enters nor leaves the tip (null flow) as indicated by its electrical resistance. All four methods rely on equilibrating a small volume of free fluid (pink) to interstitial fluid pressure. Arrows show how the linking fluid is absorbed by the interstitial matrix until its subatmospheric pressure equals that in the matrix.

the **Guyton capsule** filled with interstitial fluid, and the fluid pressure was subatmospheric, around $-5\,\mathrm{mmHg}$. This evoked considerable controversy, since interstitial fluid pressure was previously thought to be positive. Subsequently, acute techniques, such as the **wick-in-needle** and **servo-null micropipette** methods (Figure 11.10), confirmed that interstitial fluid pressure is slightly subatmospheric in the skin, subcutis, relaxed muscle, joint spaces and the epidural space (-1 to $-3\,\mathrm{mmHg}$). Interstitial pressure is above atmospheric in the kidney ($+1$ to $+10\,\mathrm{mmHg}$), myocardium, resting salivary gland, bone marrow, tooth pulp and flexed joints.

Like interstitial COP, **interstitial fluid pressure is not a fixed quantity**, but varies with fluid exchange. In the small intestine, for example, water absorption from the gut lumen raises mucosal P_i from $1\,\mathrm{mmHg}$ to $5\,\mathrm{mmHg}$, which promotes water transfer into the fenestrated mucosal capillaries. Conversely, in salivary glands, secretion reduces P_i from $3\,\mathrm{mmHg}$ to $-0.8\,\mathrm{mmHg}$, which boosts capillary filtration and thus supplies the extra water needed for saliva formation. Interstitial fluid pressure is also influenced by fibroblasts, which exert a mild compressive effect on the interstitial matrix via integrin bonding to collagen fibres – a point we will return to when considering inflammation (Section 11.11).

11.6 Tissue fluid balance: filtration versus absorption

Having covered the forces affecting fluid exchange, we are in a position to address the problem of volume homeostasis – that is to say, how does the interstitium avoid accumulating plasma ultrafiltrate? The most important factor is the drainage of interstitial fluid by the lymphatic system. A second possibility, long believed and still taught tenaciously in most textbooks, yet clearly disproved by a large body of evidence over the past 20 years (see below), is that venous capillaries continuously reabsorb the filtrate generated by arterial capillaries.

Lymphatics drain away the capillary filtrate

Almost all tissues form lymph; indeed, the lungs generate lymph even though pulmonary capillary pressure is less than plasma COP (see later). Lymph formation shows that there is normally a net filtration of fluid from the microcirculation into the interstitium, from where the fluid drains into lymphatics. The ratio of lymph flow to plasma flow tells us the fraction of the plasma water that escapes during one transit through the capillary – the **filtration fraction**. The filtration fraction is tiny, ~0.1–0.3% in most tissues. Over a day,

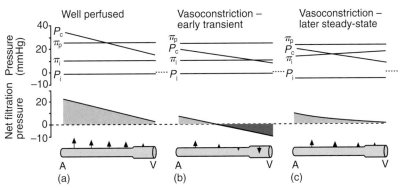

Figure 11.11 Pressure gradients from arterial end of capillary (A) to venule (V). Shaded line shows sum of four classic Starling pressures, $(P_c - P_i) - \sigma(\pi_p - \pi_i)$, as measured in skin, muscle and mesentery at heart level. Arrows show fluid flux inferred from Starling forces. A broadly similar pattern is predicted when differences between π_i and π_g are taken into account. (a) Net filtration along entire length of a well-perfused capillary. Note that neglect of measured π_i and P_i would lead to the spurious prediction of absorption in downstream half of capillary. (Data from Levick JR. *Experimental Physiology* 1991; **76**: 825–57.) (b) Transient absorptive force immediately after a haemorrhage and/or arteriolar constriction, which lower P_c. (c) Loss of absorptive force with time, due to progressive rise in π_i and π_g and fall in P_i. See text for symbols.

however, some 4000 litres of plasma pass through the human microcirculation, so the tiny filtration fraction generates a substantial volume of lymph, ~4–8 litres/day. In some microcirculations, such as the fenestrated vessels of the renal glomerulus and salivary glands, or the capillaries of the foot during standing, the filtration fraction can be a hundred times higher, e.g. 20% in glomerular capillaries.

Filtration rate decays along the capillary axis

Blood pressure falls as the blood passes along a capillary, so the filtration rate dwindles along the capillary (Figure 11.11). Arterial capillary pressure (~35 mmHg in human skin at heart level) exceeds plasma COP (25 mmHg), whereas venous capillary pressure (~15 mmHg) is below plasma COP (Figure 11.11, top left). This led to the traditional view that arterial capillaries are in a filtration state, while venous capillaries continuously reabsorb most of the filtrate, thus preventing tissue swelling. This line of reasoning, however, ignores the by no means negligible interstitial force. The Starling equation (11.3) tells us that, at the balance point for zero filtration, filtration pressure P_c equals the sum of the opposing pressures $\sigma(\pi_p - \pi_i) + P_i$. (We can temporarily ignore differences between interstitial and subglycocalyx protein concentrations, because at zero filtration rate they will equilibrate by diffusion.) Measurements in human skin, muscle and mesentery show that the factor $\sigma(\pi_p - \pi_i) + P_i$ is

~12.5 mmHg. This is lower than venous capillary pressure, ~15 mmHg. There is thus a small net filtration pressure in venous capillaries, and even in venules (Figure 11.11, bottom left). Figure 11.12 summarizes similar data for 12 tissues. In all cases the venular blood pressure exceeds the opposing force $\sigma(\pi_p - \pi_i) + P_i$. The Starling forces thus indicate that a **well-perfused capillary is normally in a state of filtration along its entire length**, in most tissues.

Venous capillaries absorb fluid transiently when pressure falls

Although venous capillaries do not normally have a net absorptive force, they can absorb interstitial fluid for a while if the Starling pressures are changed. This was demonstrated in Starling's seminal experiment (Section 11.1) and in the studies of Figures 11.2 and 11.13. In a clinical setting, a fall in blood pressure coupled with precapillary vasoconstriction, as during haemorrhage and other form of **hypovolaemic shock**, can reduce the capillary pressure sufficiently for osmotic absorption to occur transiently (Figure 11.11b). Absorption gradually tails off, however, because (i) ultrafiltration of the absorbed interstitial fluid at the underside of the glycocalyx raises subglycocalyx plasma protein concentration, π_g and π_i; and (ii) interstitial pressure P_i falls as fluid is removed from the interstitium. The changes in π_g and P_i gradually abolish the net absorptive force, so the absorption rate decays, until finally a steady state of slight filtration is restored (Figure 11.11c).

Figure 11.12 Comparison of venular blood pressure and the net pro-absorption Starling pressures in 12 tissues, showing a moderate net filtration force in venules. When differences between π_i and π_g are taken into account, the net filtration force is smaller. Tissues include muscle, skin, joints, lung (lowest left point) and mesentery (highest right point) (filled circles). Filled square shows fasting rat intestinal mucosa. Unfilled square shows the switch to absorption into mucosal capillaries after the rat drank water, mediated by a fall in π_i and rise in P_i. These changes illustrate the importance of interstitial forces in determining the direction of fluid movement (Data from many laboratories, reviewed in Levick JR, Mortimer PS. Fluid balance between microcirculation and interstitium in skin and other tissues; revision of classical filtration-reabsorption scheme. In: Messmer K (ed.). *Progress in Applied Microcirculation*. Basle: Karger, 1999: 42–62.)

Figure 11.13 Demonstration that lowering capillary pressure below plasma COP (32 cmH$_2$O here) causes a transient but not sustained fluid absorption. Method as for Figure 11.2. Upon lowering capillary pressure to venular levels, there was transient fluid absorption (open circles); but after several minutes of perfusion at low pressure, the absorption ceased (closed circles). *Lower inset* shows extravascular plasma protein (red dots) reflected by capillary wall during water absorption (long arrows). This raises extravascular protein concentration (*upper sketch*). (Adapted from Michel CC, Phillips ME. *Journal of Physiology* 1987; **388**: 421–35, with permission from Wiley-Blackwell.)

Proof that **absorption is not sustained at capillary pressures below the plasma COP** was provided by the seminal study of Figure 11.13. Capillary pressure was lowered to venular levels and held there. At first there was a transient absorption of fluid, in agreement with the Starling principle. Within a few minutes, however, absorption ceased, as predicted by modern exchange theory (see Glycocalyx–cleft model below).

Fluid exchange in the lung. As pointed out earlier, the lung generates lymph (i.e. capillary filtrate) even though pulmonary capillary pressure, ~10 mmHg, is much lower than plasma COP, 25 mmHg. Pulmonary capillaries are in a filtration state because pulmonary interstitial protein concentration is high, ~70% of plasma level, creating an interstitial COP of 16–20 mmHg. As a result, the difference in COP across the capillary wall is smaller than the hydraulic pressure difference. Fluid exchange

in the lung thus falls on the flat part of the steady-state line of Figure 11.13.

Venous capillaries are NOT normally in a state of sustained absorption

The antiquated view that venous capillaries are normally in a state of sustained absorption is still widely taught as an established fact – based usually on inaccurate interstitial force values derived from differing tissues. This view has now been disproved by:

- measurement of all four Starling forces in the same tissue (Figure 11.12)
- direct measurement of fluid exchange at venous capillary pressures (Figure 11.13)
- experimental and theoretical proof that extravascular COP is inversely related to filtration rate (Figure 11.8).

The traditional dogma must therefore be abandoned for most tissues. Its dogged persistence, despite extensive contrary evidence, is characteristic of the antisocial behaviour of factoids! As William Harvey aptly put it in his seminal work *De Motu Cordis*: 'I tremble lest I have mankind for my enemies, so much has wont and custom become second nature. Doctrine once sown strikes deep its root, and respect for antiquity influences all men.'

Michel–Weinbaum glycocalyx–cleft theory of fluid exchange

The modern form of the Starling principle recognizes that the capillary wall is a two-layer membrane, comprising a thin semipermeable membrane, the glycocalyx, over a more coarsely porous sheet, the endothelial intercellular cleft +/− fenestrae. Many commercial semipermeable membranes are constructed similarly. The Michel–Weinbaum theory (Figure 11.1b and 11.14) states that (a) since the endocapillary glycocalyx is the semipermeable

membrane, the Starling equation must incorporate the subglycocalyx COP, π_g:

$$J_v = L_p S[(P_c - P_i) - \pi(\pi_p - \pi_g)] \quad (11.5)$$

(b) the low subglycocalyx protein concentration, and hence the osmotic absorption gradient $(\pi_p - \pi_g)$, depends on the continuous, outward ultrafiltration of plasma. If filtration declines or ceases, plasma proteins entering the interstitium via the large pore system accumulate there, raising the interstitial protein concentration (Figure 11.8). When the filtration stream in the intercellular cleft is slow, zero or reversed, the interstitial protein can diffuse more easily up the cleft into the subglycocalyx space, raising π_g and reducing absorption force $(\pi_p - \pi_g)$ (Figure 11.14, dashed line). The glycocalyx–cleft model thus predicts that absorption at low capillary pressure should dwindle and cease with time − as demonstrated experimentally in Figure 11.13.

Figure 11.14 Michel–Weinbaum glycocalyx–junctional break model of fluid exchange in a continuous capillary. The colloid osmotic pressure acting on the underside of the semipermeable glycocalyx, π_g, can differ from that in the interstitium, π_i, because the diffusion of interstitial plasma proteins up the cleft is opposed by the outward stream of ultrafiltrate, particularly where it converges in the narrow break between junctional strands ($\pi_g < \pi_i$). Conversely, during interstitial fluid absorption, the reversed intercellular flow causes reflected protein to accumulate in the subglycocalyx space ($\pi_g > \pi_i$). (Based on Adamson *et al. Journal of Physiology* 2004; **557**: 889–907, with permission from Wiley-Blackwell.)

How is net filtration rate kept so low?

Continuous capillaries generate lymph very slowly, indicating a low net filtration rate. For example, the foot of a supine human produces only 0.22 ml lymph per 100 g per hour overnight. To explain the low filtration rates, the Starling pressure imbalance has to be very small, ~1 mmHg or less. This has been attributed to two factors, pore exit gradients and vasomotion.

Pore exit gradients; differences between π_g and π_i. The glycocalyx small pore system transmits essentially protein-free plasma ultrafiltrate into the subglycocalyx space, upstream of the intercellular junctional strands. From the subglycocalyx space, the ultrafiltrate has to converge and pass through narrow breaks in the strands, creating a rapid local current – like a lake draining through a narrow gorge. Interstitial plasma proteins diffuse up the filtration stream, against the current, to act osmotically on the glycocalyx underside (Figure 11.14). This 'race' between upstream diffusion and downstream washout results in a subglycocalyx protein concentration that is lower than the interstitial concentration. Consequently, the true transmembrane osmotic difference, $\pi_p - \pi_g$, is greater than the classical one, $\pi_p - \pi_i$. This helps explain the low rate of filtration and lymph production.

In support of the cleft gradient model, recent studies showed that raising π_i around rapidly filtering capillaries has much less effect on filtration rate than predicted by the classic Starling equation – because π_g is ~10% of π_i in such capillaries. At normal capillary pressure and filtration rate, π_g may be 70–90% of π_i, because diffusion makes better progress against a slow current of filtrate. Under these conditions π_g mirrors π_i more closely.

Vasomotion is the cycling of arterioles between dilatation and constriction. In some tissues, such as skeletal muscle, vasomotion occurs rhythmically, several times per minute. Since capillary pressure depends partly on precapillary resistance (Figure 11.4), each contraction phase reduces capillary pressure, allowing a transient absorption of interstitial fluid. Under these conditions the microcirculation alternates between states (a) and (b) in Figure 11.11, reducing the rate of lymph formation.

Tissues with an independent fluid input can sustain fluid absorption

Fluid absorption is sustained (cf. transient) in **intestinal mucosa fenestrated capillaries** after drinking water (Figure 11.12, unfilled square). It is also sustained in **renal peritubular fenestrated**

The Starling principle of fluid exchange

- Capillary filtration rate depends on four classic Starling pressures, namely *capillary blood pressure* minus *interstitial fluid pressure*, and the opposing *plasma colloid osmotic pressure* (COP) minus *extravascular COP* (or more accurately, subglycocalyx COP).
- Filtration rate also depends on the *hydraulic conductance* and *osmotic reflection coefficient* of the endothelial layer.
- In most tissues the Starling pressures add up to a *net filtration force*, even in venous capillaries and lungs. This generates interstitial fluid, which drains away as lymph.
- *Osmotic absorption* occurs transiently when capillary pressure is reduced by hypovolaemia and/or precapillary vasoconstriction. Absorption is transient, because it raises extravascular COP and lowers interstitial pressure.
- *Oedema* is caused by increased capillary pressure (e.g. heart failure), or reduced plasma COP (e.g. malnutrition), or increased endothelial conductance and reduced reflection coefficient (inflammation), or reduced lymphatic drainage (e.g. postmastectomy arm oedema).

---

capillaries and in **lymph node continuous capillaries**. Sustained absorption becomes possible when the interstitial compartment receives an independent fluid input, i.e. fluid from a source other than capillary filtration – such as water absorbed by the gut lumen or renal tubules or supplied by afferent lymphatics. Much of the fluid is absorbed, while the remainder flushes the interstitial space, washing away the interstitial plasma proteins so that they do not accumulate and abolish the absorption gradient. In the intestinal mucosa, 80% of the water absorbed from the gut lumen is absorbed by the microcirculation. The remaining 20% acts as the flushing solution, lowering π_i and raising P_i to maintain a net transendothelial absorption force. This abolishes the inverse link between interstitial protein concentration and capillary filtration rate, which halts absorption in other tissues (Figure 11.8).

11.7 Interstitial compliance and conductivity: effect of oedema

The human interstitial compartment contains 10–12 litres of fluid and serves as a reservoir for the plasma compartment (3 litres). If the plasma volume is reduced by a haemorrhage, a transient absorption of fluid from the interstitial compartment helps top up the depleted plasma compartment. Conversely, if the plasma compartment is over-expanded, due to renal fluid retention or over-transfusion, some of the excess fluid spills over into the interstitium, raising the interstitial volume. The relationship between interstitial fluid volume and pressure – the interstitial compliance curve – is as follows.

Interstitial compliance is normally low, but is raised in oedema

Normal hydration. In subcutaneous interstitium, where clinical oedema commonly accumulates, the interstitial volume–pressure relation is sigmoidal (Figure 11.15). At normal interstitial hydration, the interstitial fluid pressure P_i is subatmospheric and is very sensitive to fluid addition or removal. The normal compliance (volume change required for unit pressure change) is small, because a change in interstitial water content alters the glycosaminoglycan concentration, and hence the gel swelling pressure (Section 11.5).

Oedematous tissue. When excess fluid is added, acutely, to the interstitium, dilution of the glycosaminoglycans reduces the swelling pressure to essentially zero, eliminating this influence on the compliance curve. Interstitial pressure P_i is close to atmospheric pressure at this point (Table 11.1). In an acutely oedematous limb, ~98% of the excess fluid is in the subcutis, stretching the overlying skin. Since skin is very stretchy, P_i increases relatively little with

further volume expansion; the oedema pressure–volume relation is relatively flat, and interstitial compliance is ~20-fold normal. By contrast, in tissues bounded by an inelastic fibrous capsule, such as the muscle compartments of the limbs, the pressure–volume curve is steeper and P_i can reach high levels.

The pitting test for increased interstitial conductivity in oedema

Depending on the tissue, water makes up 65–99% of normally hydrated interstitial matrix by weight. The interstitial water is not easily displaced, because the glycosaminoglycans massively reduce interstitial hydraulic conductivity (Section 11.5 and Figure 11.9). Interstitial hydraulic conductivity depends on the fraction of the interstitial matrix that is water (the 'porosity' ε) relative to the surface area of the fixed biopolymers (S), which create hydraulic resistance. The ratio ε/S is called the **mean hydraulic radius** and ranges from 3 nm in articular cartilage to 300 nm in the vitreous body of the eye. When the mean hydraulic radius is raised by increased tissue hydration, as in clinical oedema, interstitial conductivity increases dramatically. This is the basis of the clinical **pitting test** for subcutaneous oedema. When finger pressure is applied to normal skin for 1 min, then removed, little to no indentation remains, because interstitial fluid mobility is normally low and little fluid is displaced. In oedema, by contrast, the interstitial conductivity is high and fluid is rapidly displaced by the applied pressure, leaving a distinct pit in the tissue (Figure 11.16).

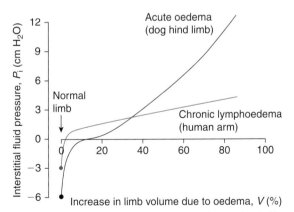

Figure 11.15 The interstitial compliance curve of limb subcutis. The steeper relation was observed in dog hind limbs made acutely oedematous by intravenous saline infusion; pressure was recorded in subcutaneous capsules. Pressure gradually declines with time, for a given degree of swelling ('creep'). Consequently, in the chronically swollen human arm (lymphoedema caused by breast cancer surgery) the interstitial compliance curve is flatter. Human subcutis interstitial pressure was measured by the wick-in-needle technique. (Drawn from data in Bates, Levick and Mortimer. *International Journal of Microcirculation Clinical & Experimental* 1992; **11**: 359–373, and Guyton, Taylor and Granger. *Circulation Physiology II; Dynamics and control of the Body Fluids*. WB Saunders: Philadelphia. 1975.)

Figure 11.16 Human calf showing pitting oedema (arrow) in a patient with cardiac failure. The oedema was exacerbated by dependency. Note the skin damage (arrowhead, top left) caused by an oedema blister. The ankle is off lower edge of picture. (Courtesy of Professor P Mortimer, Department of Dermatology, St. George's Hospital, London.)

Solute transport and exclusion in interstitium

Small solutes, such as O_2 and glucose, diffuse freely through the spaces between the negatively charged interstitial proteoglycans. Macromolecules, such as albumin, experience restricted diffusion and partial exclusion in the interstitial matrix. See Section 10.3 for an explanation of these terms. Albumin is excluded from 20–50% of the water in subcutaneous and muscle interstitium, due to its size (steric exclusion) and net negative charge (electrical exclusion). Consequently the effective interstitial protein concentration, i.e. protein mass divided by available water volume, is higher than the apparent concentration (protein mass/total water volume). Protein is transported through the interstitium to the lymphatic system by convection, i.e. it is washed along by the stream of capillary filtrate.

11.8 Lymph and the lymphatic system

Parts of the lymphatic system were recognized in the early seventeenth century by Aselli, Pecquet, Rudbeckius and Bartholin, but it was not until the eighteenth century that William Hunter concluded 'lymphatic vessels are the absorbing vessels all over the body … they constitute one great and general system dispersed throughout the whole body for absorption.' The three main functions are as follows.

- **Preservation of fluid balance.** Lymph vessels return the capillary ultrafiltrate and escaped plasma proteins to the bloodstream, by draining into the neck veins (Figure 1.8). This completes the extravascular circulation of fluid and protein and maintains tissue volume homeostasis (Figure 11.17). If lymphatic function is impaired, the tissue develops a severe, intractable form of oedema called **lymphoedema**.
- **Nutritional function.** Intestinal lymph vessels, or 'lacteals', take up and transport tiny globules of digested fat (chylomicra) that have been absorbed by the mucosa, as Aselli noted in 1627 (Figure 11.18).
- **Defence function.** As interstitial fluid drains into the lymphatic system, it carries foreign materials, such as antigens, viruses, bacteria and inhaled carbon particles, to the lymph nodes – an effective, economical method of immuno-surveillance (Figure 11.18). The lymph nodes phagocytose particulate matter, which accounts for the blackened nodes in the lungs of smokers and coal miners. Bacterial and viral antigens activate nodal lymphocytes, which are released into the efferent (postnodal) lymph for transport to the bloodstream. Efferent lymph thus has a higher white cell count than afferent (prenodal) lymph.

Genetic disorders can impair lymphatic development

During embryogenesis the lymphatics sprout from the venous system and join up with a superficial lymphatic plexus (network) formed by mesenchymal lymphangioblasts. This is why lymph drains, ultimately, into the large veins of the neck (Figure 11.18). Lymphatic growth is driven by an isoform of vascular endothelial growth factor, VEGF-C, and by the transcription factors FOXC2 and PROX1. Inherited defects in the VEGF-C receptor or FOXC2 cause different forms of hereditary lymphoedema.

- **VEGF-C** is crucial for lymphatic growth, and acts on the lymphatic endothelial receptor VEGFR-3, a receptor tyrosine kinase. **Milroy disease** is an autosomal dominant form of human hereditary lymphoedema, caused by heterozygous mutation of VEGFR-3. This results in a severely hypoplastic (underdeveloped) peripheral lymphatic plexus and leg lymphoedema.

Figure 11.17 Estimate of extravascular circulation of fluid and plasma protein in a 65 kg human. (After Renkin EM. *American Journal of Physiology* 1986; **250**: H706–10, with permission from the American Physiological Society.)

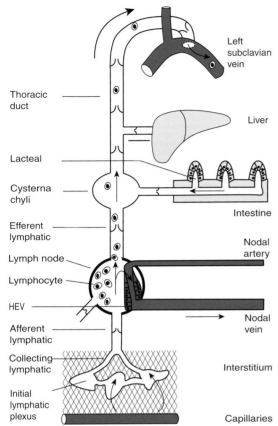

Figure 11.18 The lymphatic system. Curved arrow within node indicates absorption of some of the fluid by nodal capillaries. HEV, high endothelial venule, where circulating lymphocytes re-enter the node.

Labels on figure:
Thoracic duct
Lacteal
Cysterna chyli
Efferent lymphatic
Lymph node
Lymphocyte
HEV
Afferent lymphatic
Collecting lymphatic
Initial lymphatic plexus
Left subclavian vein
Liver
Intestine
Nodal artery
Nodal vein
Interstitium
Capillaries

- **FOXC2** is a transcription factor promoting the maturation of primary lymphatics into lymphatics with valves. FOXC2 $-/-$ knock-out mice still develop a lymphatic system, but the main lymphatics lack valves; also, the finest lymphatics, normally simple endothelial tubes, acquire smooth muscle. **Lymphoedema distichiasis** is an autosomal dominant form of human hereditary lymphoedema caused by heterozygous, loss-of-function point mutations of the FOXC2 gene. This results in leaky lymphatic valves, leg lymphoedema and a double row of eyelashes (distichiasis). Leg venous valves are leaky too, emphasizing the common ancestry of lymphatics and veins.

- **PROX1** is a transcription factor whose deletion in mice results in a total aplasia (absence) of the lymphatic system and perinatal death.

Structure of lymphatic vessels

Lymphatic capillaries
The initial lymphatic vessels are microscopic lymphatic capillaries (diameter 10–50 μm), which form a network of anastomosing tubes in most tissues,

and blind-ended sacs in the intestinal villi (Figure 11.18). The wall is a single layer of endothelial cells with an incomplete basement membrane. Some of the endothelial intercellular clefts are 14 nm or more wide, so interstitial proteins and fine particles readily enter lymphatic capillaries. Due to its oblique orientation, the intercellular cleft is thought to act as a flap valve, allowing fluid into the lumen when lymph pressure is low, but closing when lymph pressure is raised above interstitial pressure by local tissue movements (Figure 11.19). The outer surface of the wall is tethered to the surrounding tissues by radiating microfibrils, the **anchoring filaments**, composed of the protein fibrillin. In swollen, oedematous tissue, tension in the anchoring filaments helps to dilate the initial lymphatics.

Collecting and afferent lymphatics
The initial lymphatic network drains into collecting vessels, which feed into afferent lymph trunks running beside major blood vessels. **Semilunar valves** direct the lymph centrally. From the collecting vessel onwards the lymphatic wall acquires a coat of smooth muscle and is actively contractile. Lymphatic smooth muscle is abundant in man and ruminants, but scanty in dogs and rabbits. The contractile segment between successive pairs of valves is called a **lymphangion**.

Lymph nodes
The lower vertebrates have a lymphatic system but no lymph nodes; nodes evolved in mammals, marsupials and some aquatic birds. Lymph enters the node at its hilum through multiple afferent vessels. The node is a mass of lymphocytes and phagocytic cells, permeated by a network of sinuses carrying the lymph flow. The sinuses are endothelial tubes, with gaps to allow lymphocytes to join the lymph. Nodal blood vessels supply O_2 and nutrients, and the blood capillaries drain into **high-endothelial venules** involved in lymphocyte trafficking. High-endothelial venules express a receptor for L-selectin on circulating lymphocytes. The captured lymphocytes penetrate the venule intercellular junctions to re-enter the node, thus completing their own unique circulation, i.e. efferent lymph → blood → node.

Efferent lymphatics and the thoracic duct
Lymphocyte-rich efferent lymph from the legs and viscera is actively pumped into a large lymphatic vessel on the posterior abdominal wall. A saccular dilatation of the vessel, the **cisterna chyli**, receives chyle, the fatty lymph formed in intestinal lacteals after a fatty meal. The ultimate lymphatic trunk, the thoracic duct, carries about three-quarters of the total efferent lymph and drains into the left subclavian

Figure 11.19 Lymphatic transport mechanisms. (a) Interstitial fluid enters the initial lymphatic through the intercellular cleft flap valves down a pressure gradient. Each muscular segment then pumps lymph into the next segment and ultimately into the venous system. (b) Proposed operation of initial lymphatic endothelial junctions as flap valves (see text). P_i, interstitial pressure; P_L, lymph pressure.

vein, near its junction with the jugular vein. Smaller cervical and right lymphatic trunks carry lymph from the head, neck and upper right quadrant, and drain into the neck veins. There may also be minor, small lymphovenous communications at more peripheral sites. The brain, uniquely, has no lymphatic system, but has a specialized fluid drainage system (Section 15.4).

Initial lymphatics may fill by a squeeze-and-recoil mechanism

The composition of prenodal lymph (water, salts, diluted plasma proteins) shows that it is simply interstitial fluid that has drained into the lymphatic capillaries. The filling mechanism is not certain, but probably resembles that of a Pasteur (rubber teat) pipette. To fill the pipette, one first squeezes the rubber bulb empty (phase 1), then one allows its elastic recoil to suck up fluid (phase 2). Similarly, it is thought that tissue movements compress the initial lymphatic plexus, driving fluid proximally; the intercellular flap valves prevent backflow into the interstitium (phase 1). Then, when the tissue compression ceases, the elastic recoil of the tissue and tethering filaments reduce the intralymphatic pressure below interstitial fluid pressure. This opens the intercellular flap valves and draws interstitial fluid into the initial lymphatics, re-expanding them (phase 2) (Figure 11.20).

Figure 11.20 Suction of interstitial fluid into initial lymphatics of bat wing. (*Top*) Micropipettes were inserted into the interstitium and into a contractile lymphatic to record the interstitium-to-lymph pressure gradient. (*Bottom*) Interstitial pressure (I) exceeded lymph pressure (II) for 43% of the time, because lymph pressure fell to subatmospheric levels during lymphatic relaxation. (From Hogan RD. In: Hargens AR (ed.). *Interstitial Fluid Pressure and Composition*. Baltimore, MD: Williams and Wilkins, 1981: 155–63.)

Figure 11.21 Effect of raising tissue fluid pressure on lymphatic drainage rate from pleural and peritoneal spaces in rabbit. The coupling of lymph drainage to interstitial pressure is essential to prevent fluid accumulation in the extravascular compartment. (Based on data from Miserocchi G, Negrini D, Mukenge P, Turconi P, Del Fabbro M. *Journal of Applied Physiology* 1989; **66**: 1579–85; and Miserocchi G, Negrini D. In: Crystal RG *et al.* (eds). *The Lung*. Philadelphia, PA: Lippincott-Raven, 1997, with permission of the American Physiological Society.)

Lymph flow is coupled to capillary filtration rate

The rate of lymph formation depends on interstitial fluid pressure and volume; the higher they are, the greater the lymph flow, up to a limit (Figure 11.21). Since interstitial fluid pressure and volume depend on capillary filtration rate, these interstitial parameters couple lymph flow to capillary filtration rate. This coupling is essential, because lymph drainage rate must match capillary filtration rate if oedema is to be avoided.

Extrinsic and intrinsic mechanisms contribute to lymph flow

Lymph cannot drain passively along the lymphatic system, because the pressure at the venous outlet is higher (~3 mmHg) than in the initial lymphatics (~0). Lymph is therefore pumped. Collecting lymphatics and the more proximal vessels have smooth muscle to pump the lymph along – the intrinsic pump. Initial lymphatics, however, lack smooth muscle in most tissues, so extrinsic pumping is needed here. Since the initial lymphatics are in series with the muscular lymphatics, both intrinsic and extrinsic propulsion are necessary overall.

Extrinsic propulsion

Flow in the non-contractile lymph vessels is induced by tissue movements, which intermittently compress the lymphatics, e.g. skeletal muscle contractions, intestinal peristalsis, pulsation of adjacent arteries. Extrinsic propulsion accounts for the large increase in lymph flow from the leg of an anaesthetized animal when the leg is cycled passively.

Intrinsic propulsion

Lymphatic contraction was first described by Heller in 1869. Lymphatic vessels with abundant encircling smooth muscle, such as those in the human leg, exhibit spontaneous, rhythmic contractions at ~8–15 cycles per minute (Figure 11.22a). Successive regions, comprising one or more lymphangia, behave like mini-hearts linked in series, and the pumping cycle of each region bears a striking resemblance to the cardiac cycle. Each region has longitudinally running **pacemaker cells**, that trigger local action potentials in the circumferentially orientated smooth muscle, leading to rhythmic contractions. As in the heart, the pacemaker cells express the 'funny' pacemaking current i_f and T-type Ca^{2+} channels. The smooth muscle action potentials are generated by L-type Ca^{2+} channels and fast Na^+ channels. As in the cardiac ventricle, a diastolic filling phase, with the distal valve open and the proximal valve closed, is followed by an isovolumetric contraction phase (all valves closed), then an ejection phase (proximal valve open; ejection fraction ~25%) and an isovolumetric relaxation phase (all valves closed). Thus each contractile segment traces out a pressure–volume loop analogous to that of the ventricle (Figure 11.22b). Human limb lymphatics can pump to 40–50 mmHg against a resistance – an important point when dealing with **envenomation** by a snake or spider bite. To prevent venom transmission by active lymphatic pumping, the tourniquet pressure needs to be >40–50 mmHg.

Lymphatic contraction is regulated by filling pressure, sympathetic nerves and vasoactive agents

Lymphatic contractile frequency, and to a lesser degree stroke volume, are increased by **distension**. In this way, a lymphatic segment can increase its output in response to an increased input from a more distal segment. Maximal output occurs at a diastolic filling pressure of ~4–8 cmH$_2$O in isolated lymphatics; at higher pressures the stroke volume and output begin to fall.

Large lymphatics are innervated by an outer plexus of **sympathetic noradrenergic fibres** and an inner plexus of peptidergic fibres. Sympathetic activity and circulating adrenaline both increase contractile frequency. Following a haemorrhage, lymphatic contractile frequency rises and ejection fraction increases to ~40%, boosting the transfer of interstitial fluid into

(a)

2 sec

(b)

Figure 11.22 Electrical and contractile properties of lymphatic smooth muscle. (a) Periodic bursts of action potentials and contraction in isolated bovine lymphatic trunk. (From McHale N and colleagues. *Journal of Physiology* 1977; **272**: 33P–4P; and *Journal of Physiology* 1991; **438**: 168P, with permission from Wiley-Blackwell.) (b) Pressure–volume cycle of contracting sheep mesenteric lymphatic vessels at various diastolic distensions (TP, transmural pressure). Dashed loop shows increased contractility and ejection fraction after a haemorrhage. Note analogy with cardiac pressure–volume loops of Figure 6.11b. (From Li B, Silver I, Szalai JP, Johnston MG. *Microvascular Research* 1998; **56**: 127–38, with permission from Elsevier.)

the depleted circulation (Figure 11.22b, dashed loop). Substance P, a chemical mediator of inflammation, stimulates lymphatic contraction, whereas nitric oxide inhibits lymphatic contraction.

Lymph nodes absorb some lymph: postnodal versus prenodal lymph

The concentration of plasma proteins in postnodal lymph from the legs of dogs and sheep is up to twice that in the prenodal lymph, due mainly to the absorption of water by nodal blood capillaries. Postnodal lymph composition is unrepresentative, therefore, of interstitial fluid composition, and postnodal lymph flow underestimates capillary filtration rate. In light of this, our estimate of fluid turnover in humans, based on thoracic duct lymph flow, has been revised upwards (Figure 11.17). However, the exact proportion of afferent lymph that is absorbed in human lymph nodes is unknown, and probably depends on posture, since capillary pressure in the nodes must increase with dependency.

Table 11.2 Postnodal lymph flow and composition in man

	Flow (%)[a]	L/P[b]
Thoracic duct	1–3 litre/day	0.66–0.69
Liver	30–49%	0.66–0.89
Gastrointestinal	~37%	0.50–0.62
Kidneys	6–11%	0.47
Lungs	3–15%	0.66–0.69
Limbs and cervical trunks	<10%	0.23–0.58

[a]Expressed as percentage of total thoracic duct flow.
[b]Protein concentration in postnodal lymph (L) relative to plasma (P). (From Joffey JM, Courtice FC. *Lymphatics, Lymph and the Lymphomyeloid Complex*. London: Academic Press, 1970.)

Lymph flow and composition differs from tissue to tissue

Postnodal lymph flow in the human thoracic duct averages 1–3 litres per day, of which the **liver** contributes 30–50% (Table 11.2). Hepatic lymph is particularly rich in plasma protein, due to the

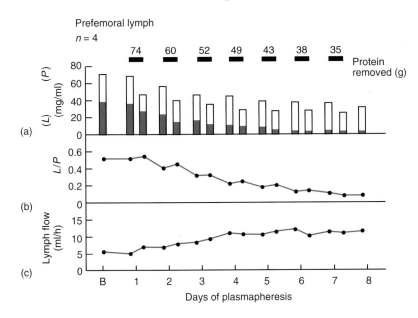

Figure 11.23 Effect of hypoproteinaemia on fluid exchange. (a) Protein was removed from sheep by daily plasmapheresis (removal of blood, re-injection of cells, water and electrolytes). This progressively lowered the plasma protein concentration P (top of white bars). (b) The protein concentration fell relatively more in postnodal leg lymph (L, red bars) than plasma, so the ratio L/P declined. (c) Lymph flow, a measure of capillary filtration rate in the steady state, more than doubled. Two of the safety factors against oedema are seen operating here, the dilution of interstitial protein (reducing extravascular COP, π_i) and increased lymphatic drainage rate. (From Kramer G *et al.* In: Renkin EM. *American Journal of Physiology* 1986; **250**: H706–10, with permission from the American Physiological Society.)

discontinuities in hepatic capillary endothelium. The **intestine** makes the second greatest contribution to total lymph flow, especially after a meal. **Lung** and **renal** lymph flows are substantial too. The **limbs** contribute a variable quantity of lymph, depending on exercise intensity. The concentration of plasma protein in lymph varies from tissue to tissue; it depends on protein size and charge, capillary permeability, reflection coefficient and capillary filtration rate (Figures 11.8 and 11.23).

The **brain**, unusually, lacks a lymphatic system. Cerebral interstitial fluid is in contact with the cerebrospinal fluid, which drains into the cerebral venous sinuses through specialized structures called arachnoid granulations. Some cerebrospinal fluid also drains along perineural sheaths around the olfactory nerve, passing through the bony cribriform plate to reach lymphatics in the nasal submucosa.

11.9 Challenges to tissue fluid balance: orthostasis and exercise

Two physiological events can increase the capillary filtration rate so much that plasma volume falls. They are orthostasis (upright posture) and physical exercise.

Orthostasis causes dependent swelling and a fall in plasma volume

During standing/sitting, blood pressure is raised in all the capillaries below heart level (Figure 11.5).

This increases their filtration rate, especially in the most dependent (lowermost) tissues. The foot, for example, swells at a rate of ~30 ml/h, driving people to unlace their shoes during long-haul flights or long films. During a 15–40 min period of standing, the increased plasma ultrafiltration into dependent tissues reduces plasma volume by 6–20%, with a concomitant haemoconcentration and rise in plasma COP. The latter increased from 25 mmHg to 29 mmHg in university students over an 8-h period of sitting in lectures, reading, etc. These changes would be considerably worse, were it not for the following attenuating mechanisms.

- **Postural vasoconstriction**. Strong precapillary vasoconstriction in dependent tissues raises R_A/R_V, which attenuates the increase in capillary pressure (Figure 11.5). Dependent vasoconstriction is a local reaction, mediated by the myogenic response (Section 13.2) and veniarteriolar response (Section 15.3).

- **Local haemoconcentration**. Postural vasoconstriction reduces blood flow through the dependent tissues (Figure 8.6), while the increased capillary pressure raises the filtration rate. Together, these changes can greatly increase the filtration fraction, from ~0.1–0.3% at heart level to 20–27% in the foot during standing. The resulting local haemoconcentration raises the plasma COP in the venous capillaries to 35–44 mmHg. This attenuates filtration in these vessels, which have a higher L_p than arterial capillaries.

- **Reduced capillary filtration capacity.** The contraction of some terminal arterioles may stop flow completely through capillary modules for short periods, thereby reducing the capillary filtration capacity. The evidence for this in human limbs is conflicting, however.
- **The skeletal muscle pump.** Dynamic exercise in the upright position reduces venous pressure in the active limbs (Figure 8.26), which in turn reduces capillary pressure and hence filtration rate. Movement also enhances **lymph transport**.

Exercise causes muscle swelling and a fall in plasma volume

People working out at the gym notice that intensively exercised skeletal muscles becomes swollen and tense. Likewise rock-climbers, for reasons not unconnected with their well-being, become keenly aware of swollen, pumped forearm muscles during steep, fingery climbs. A temporary 20% increase in muscle volume is not uncommon. The causes are as follows.

- **Increased interstitial osmolarity** is the main cause of the acute swelling. The contracting muscle fibres release small solutes, such as lactate and K^+ ions, which raise the local interstitial fluid osmolarity by 7–10% (20–30 mmol/litre) – a rise in crystalloid osmotic pressure of 380–580 mmHg (van't Hoff's law, Appendix 2). The increased crystalloid osmotic pressure is exerted across endothelial **aquaporin channels**, which are strongly expressed in the continuous capillaries of muscle. Although aquaporin conductance is low, the increase in interstitial osmotic suction is large, so capillary filtration rate increases substantially. Since aquaporins are water-only channels, the NaCl concentration rises in the venous blood of active muscle. Muscle sarcoplasm osmolarity increases too during exercise, due to the creatine phosphate breakdown and lactate formation. Consequently, **intracellular swelling** contributes to the muscle swelling.
- **Vasodilatation** of the resistance vessels in exercising skeletal muscle not only increases blood flow but also reduces R_A/R_V. This raises capillary pressure, which contributes to the increased filtration rate (Figure 11.4).
- **Capillary recruitment** in the exercising muscle not only boosts O_2 transport but also

raises the capillary filtration capacity. This too contributes to the increased filtration rate (Figure 10.14).

During prolonged heavy exercise involving multiple, large muscle groups, such as strenuous cycling, net muscle volume can increase by up to 1100 ml and plasma volume falls by ~600 ml (20%). The relative preservation of plasma volume is brought about by a compensatory absorption of interstitial fluid from the non-exercising tissues into the plasma compartment.

11.10 Oedema

Oedema is an excess of interstitial fluid. Clinical oedema can develop in the subcutis (peripheral oedema), lungs (pulmonary oedema), abdominal cavity (ascites) or other body cavities (synovial, pleural and pericardial effusions). Inflammation can cause oedema in almost any tissue.

In **subcutaneous oedema**, the tissue has reached the flat part of the interstitial compliance curve (Figure 11.15); so there is little further rise in interstitial fluid pressure to oppose ongoing capillary filtration and volume expansion. The oedema is not usually detected until interstitial volume has doubled, which corresponds to ~10% limb swelling. Peripheral oedema causes discomfort, impaired limb mobility, impaired cell nutrition (due to increased diffusion distance), and may lead to cellulitis, ulceration or blistering (Figure 11.16).

Pulmonary oedema is often secondary to left ventricular failure, which raises left ventricular filling pressure and hence pulmonary venous pressure (Section 18.5). The congested, oedematous lung is difficult to inflate, causing **dyspnoea** (difficulty in breathing). In the most severe cases, the interstitial oedema spills over into the alveolar spaces, impairing O_2 exchange, with potentially fatal consequences.

Causes of oedema

Oedema develops when capillary filtration rate exceeds lymphatic drainage rate for a sufficient period. The key relation is:

Tissue swelling rate = Capillary filtration rate
$$- \text{Lymphatic drainage rate.}$$

From this relation we see that oedema can result from a raised capillary filtration rate and/or a low lymph drainage rate. Since capillary filtration is governed by the Starling principle (eqn 11.3), the Starling factors allow a logical classification of oedema, as follows.

Raised capillary pressure, P_c

Capillary pressure is elevated when venous pressure is chronically raised, as in the oedema of:

- cardiac failure
- over-transfusion
- deep venous thrombosis
- dependent tissues, such as the ankles, or the sacral area during recumbency.

Pressures of 20–40 mmHg have been recorded in the venous limbs of skin capillaries at heart level during right ventricular failure; cf. normal 12–15 mmHg. The resulting oedema fluid has a low protein concentration, 1–10 g/l, due to the interstitial dilution relation (Figure 11.8).

Reduced plasma COP, π_p

Clinical oedema develops when the plasma protein concentration falls below ~30 g/l, because the fall in plasma COP raises the capillary filtration rate. The oedema fluid again has a low protein concentration, 1–6 g/l, lowering the interstitial COP. This, along with an increased lymph flow (Figure 11.23), helps to limit the severity of the oedema. The hypoproteinaemia can be caused by:

- malnutrition (inadequate protein intake);
- intestinal disease (malabsorption and protein loss);
- nephrotic syndrome (albumin leakage into urine, >20 g/day, due to a breakdown of the glomerular ultrafilter);
- hepatic failure (failure to synthesize albumin, fibrinogen, α- and β-globulins). Hepatic failure is often caused by alcoholic cirrhosis. The attendant fibrosis raises portal vein pressure, and hence intra-abdominal capillary pressures. As a result, the oedema is predominantly peritoneal (**ascites**).

Increased capillary permeability ($\uparrow L_p$, $\downarrow \sigma$, $\uparrow P_{protein}$)

In **inflammation** there is a major breakdown of the capillary barrier, due to the formation of wide gaps and glyocalyx disruption (Figure 10.11). The hydraulic conductance L_p and protein permeability $P_{protein}$ increase and the protein reflection coefficient σ falls. These changes cause severe oedema with a raised protein content, >30 g/l. Section 11.11 describes the signal pathways involved.

Lymphatic insufficiency

Lymph is the only way of returning escaped plasma proteins to the circulation, so an impairment of lymphatic drainage causes both water and plasma proteins to accumulate in the interstitium. Lymphoedema is thus characterized by a protein content of >30 g/l. Chronic lymphoedema provokes the gradual deposition of a fibrous, adipose tissue in the interstitium, as a result of which long-standing lymphoedema may not pit easily ('brawny' non-pitting oedema). In Western countries the commonest cause of lymphatic insufficiency is damage to the lymph nodes during **cancer** surgery and radiotherapy (Figure 11.24). The rarer **hereditory lymphoedemas** are due to inadequate limb lymphatic development, as in **Milroy disease** and

Figure 11.24 Lymphoedema caused by surgery to treat testicular cancer. (Courtesy of Professor P Mortimer, Department of Dermatology, St. George's Hospital, London.)

lymphoedema distichiasis (see earlier). The commonest cause of lymphoedema worldwide, however, is **filariasis**, a nematode worm infestation transmitted by mosquitoes. The nematodes impair lymphatic function in the limbs and scrotum, causing a gross lymphoedema associated with hyperkeratotic, elephant-like skin (**elephantiasis**).

Oedema only develops when a 'safety margin' is exceeded

Clinicians have long recognized that oedema does not appear until the plasma COP or venous pressure has changed by ~15 mmHg. There is thus a 15 mmHg margin of safety against oedema. The safety margin is attributed to three factors that 'buffer' the capillary filtration rate – namely, a fall in extravascular COP, rise in interstitial fluid pressure and rise in lymph flow as filtration rate increases (Figure 11.25).

- **Fall in extravascular COP**. A rise in capillary filtration rate reduces the extravascular plasma protein concentration (Figure 11.8) and opposes the diffusion of extravascular plasma protein up the intercellular cleft into the subglycocalyx space (Figure 11.14). Consequently, the subglycocalyx COP π_g falls and the absorptive force $\pi_p - \pi_g$ rises (Figure 11.25a). This attenuates the capillary filtration rate. This buffering mechanism is most effective in tissues with a normally high extravascular protein concentrations, such as the lung ($\pi_i \cong 18$ mmHg).
- **Rise in interstitial fluid pressure**. In normally hydrated tissue, a small rise in interstitial volume causes a relatively large rise in interstitial pressure (Figures 11.15 and 11.25b). This reduces the pressure drop across the capillary wall, $P_c - P_i$. If P_i is normally -2 mmHg and clinical oedema becomes apparent at around $+1$ mmHg, the change in P_i provides a safety margin of 3 mmHg. In oedematous interstitium, by contrast, large volumes of capillary filtrate can accumulate with little further rise in the opposing pressure P_i.
- **Rise in lymph flow**. Lymphatic drainage rate increases as interstitial pressure and volume increase, helping prevent oedema formation (Figures 11.21 and 11.25c). For example, lymph flow increases 20-fold in response to a 30 mmHg elevation of venous pressure in the cat intestine. There comes a point, however, at which lymph flow cannot keep pace with capillary filtration, and oedema then develops.

Figure 11.25 Three safety factors against oedema. Stars indicate normal state. (a) When capillary filtration rate increases, the COP difference opposing filtration, ($\pi_p - \pi_g$), increases, because extravascular plasma protein concentration falls in the interstitial and subglycocalyx compartments. (b) Interstitial fluid pressure changes markedly with hydration in normal subcutis. Once oedema develops, however, interstitial compliance becomes very large, so there is little further rise in the supra-atmospheric pressure. (NB This is Figure 11.15 turned on its side.) (c) Lymphatic drainage rate increases with increasing interstitial hydration, thereby opposing oedema formation. Dashed lines indicate that lymph flow reaches a limit in stationary tissue, but perhaps not in moved limbs. (After Taylor AE, Townsley MI. *News in Physiological Science* 1987; **2**: 48–52, with permission from the American Physiological Society.)

11.11 The swelling of inflammation

The six definitive characteristics of inflammation are tissue swelling, redness, heat, pain, loss of function and leukocyte migration. The swelling is caused by a protein-rich oedema, which can form very rapidly.

(a)

(b) Intercept = $\sigma\Delta\pi$ Venular pressure (cmH₂O)

Figure 11.26 (a) Gap formation, oedema and leukocyte migration in acutely inflamed, postcapillary venule. (b) Effect of an inflammatory agonist, serotonin, on permeability of a single venule (rat). Hydraulic permeability increases (slope, Lp) and osmotic reflection coefficient decreases (intercept at zero filtration, $\sigma\Delta\pi$). Although serotonin was infused continuously, the hyperpermeability was transient and returned towards baseline by 9 min. (Adapted from Michel CC, Kendall S. *Journal of Physiology* 1997; **501**: 657–62, with permission from Wiley-Blackwell.)

Examples include blisters, rashes, swollen joints, pleural, pericardial and peritoneal effusions and cerebral oedema. The key change precipitating the swelling is the formation of gaps in the endothelial barrier, as follows.

Chemical mediators initiate gap formation in venules

When a tissue is damaged, whether by trauma, infection, ischaemia or allergy, numerous pro-inflammatory chemicals are released by the tissue cells. These agents include histamine, bradykinin, prostaglandins, serotonin, thrombin, substance P, platelet activating factor, superoxide radicals, leukotrienes and cytokines. The cytokines interleukin-1β and tumour necrosis factor α are pro-inflammatory agents secreted by monocytes/macrophages, fibroblasts and endothelial cells, and they induce leukocyte adhesion and migration (Figure 9.11).

Figure 11.27 Three-dimensional reconstruction of an inflammatory gap in frog endothelium, induced by mild heat injury. The gap is transcellular; it passes through the cell on the left, close to but separate from the intercellular junction. Part of an underlying, third cell is visible through the gap (stippled grey). (Based on 18 serial electron-micrograph sections by Neale CR, Michel CC, with permission from Wiley-Blackwell.)

Most chemical mediators of inflammation act primarily on receptors expressed by the **postcapillary venule** to cause **endothelial gap formation** (Figures 11.26 and 11.27). The endothelial gaps create holes in the normally continuous glycocalyx,

Figure 11.28 Hyperpermeability of venules in cremaster muscle induced by inflammatory agonist PAF (platelet activating factor), applied for 3 min in wild-type mice. Intravenous fluorescein-labelled dextran (77 000 Da) leaked out rapidly following inflammation, as shown by the integrated optical intensity (IOI) of the images. In eNOS $-/-$ knockout mice, the hyperpermeability response was greatly reduced, demonstrating the obligatory role of nitric oxide in the inflammation signalling pathway. (From Hatakeyama T, Pappas PJ, Hobson RW, Boric MP, Sessa WC, Duran WN. *Journal of Physiology* 2006; **574**: 275–81, with permission from Wiley-Blackwell.)

disrupting the semipermeable barrier. Consequently, water and plasma proteins leak out rapidly into the tissue (Figure 11.28). The greater the inflammatory stimulus, the greater the number of the leakage spots. In ischaemia-reperfusion injury (Section 6.12), glycocalyx damage may possibly raise permeability without gap formation. A common pharmacological test for inflammation, the **skin blueing test**, is based on the raised protein permeability. The dye Evans blue is injected into the plasma of a rat. Little escapes into normal skin, because the dye binds to circulating plasma albumin; but if an inflammatory agent is injected into the skin, the dye–albumin complex leaks out, producing a blue skin patch.

The inflammatory response to an agonist often shows two phases. Over the first 10–30 min there is a large but transient rise in permeability, which then decays (Figures 11.26 and 11.28). This is followed by a second, more sustained increase lasting hours. Histamine, serotonin and bradykinin cause only a transient rise in permeability, whereas thrombin and VEGF cause more prolonged rises.

The extravasated fluid has a high fibrinogen content

Due to the barrier breakdown, inflammatory oedema has a high plasma protein concentration ($\geqslant 30$ g/l). This is termed an **exudate**, to distinguish it from the low protein oedema, or **transudate**, of cardiac failure, venous thrombosis, etc. ($\leqslant 15$ g/l). One of the exuded proteins is **fibrinogen**. The formation of extravascular, insoluble fibrin clots can lead

to serious complications, such as intestinal adhesions following peritonitis or abdominal surgery.

Net filtration force and permeability both increase

Exudation is rapid and severe because the chemical agonists alter almost every factor in the Starling principle (eqns 11.3 and 11.5).

- **Capillary pressure**, P_c. Many inflammatory agonists cause arteriolar vasodilatation, leading to the characteristic **redness** and **heat** of inflamed tissue. The vasodilatation reduces R_A/R_V, which raises capillary filtration pressure (Figure 11.4).
- **Interstitial fluid pressure**, P_i. In established swelling P_i is increased to ~2 mmHg, and serves as a minor check on filtration. At the onset of the inflammation, however, in skin and submucosa, P_i falls transiently to a more subatmospheric level, before rising as oedema accumulates. This curious effect is mediated by fibroblasts. Normally, fibroblasts slightly tense the surrounding collagen fibrils, to which they adhere through transmembrane $\alpha_2\beta_1$-**integrins**. The collagen tension slightly compresses the interstitial matrix, reducing its swelling tendency (Section 11.5). Release of the fibroblast's gel-compressing bonds at the onset of inflammation lowers P_i by several mmHg, which in turn enhances the initial swelling rate. In **burns** P_i can fall more dramatically, to -30 mmHg transiently, so plasma extravasation is very rapid in burn injuries. The large

suction force is attributed to the denaturation of collagen by heat to gelatin, which is water-soluble and has a large swelling pressure.

- **Extravascular osmotic pressure, π_i, π_g.** Interstitial protein concentration increases as plasma proteins leak out through the endothelial gaps. This reduces the difference in COP across the capillary wall and thus increases the filtration rate.
- **Osmotic reflection coefficient, σ.** The residual difference in COP across the endothelium itself becomes less effective, because σ is reduced to $\sim$0.4 by the impairment of the glycocalyx barrier. The fall in σ is evident from the leftward shift of the intercept in the filtration rate-versus-pressure plot (Figure 11.26), and from the outpouring of plasma macromolecules (Figure 11.28).
- **Hydraulic conductance of the wall, L_p.** The changes in P_c, P_i, π_i and σ greatly increase the net filtration force across the venules (term inside the square brackets in eqns 11.3 and 11.5). The effect of the increased filtration force is amplified many times by the increase in wall hydraulic conductance caused by gap formation. L_p can increase around seven-fold. The increase in L_p is evident from the increase in slope of the filtration rate-versus-pressure plot (Figure 11.26).

The net effect of the above five changes is a 50–100-fold rise in fluid extravasation rate. This rapid leakage, along with flow obstruction by marginating leukocytes (Section 9.8), can lead to plugging of the microvessels by packed columns of red cells (**stasis**).

Endothelial gaps can be intercellular and/or transcellular

During inflammation gaps up to 1-μm wide form in the endothelial lining of the postcapillary venules, with accompanying breaks in the glycocalyx layer. The venular gaps can be **intercellular**, resulting from a separation of the junction between two endothelial cells, or **transcellular**, resulting from the formation of a hole directly through the endothelial cell, close to but not through the intercellular junction (Figure 11.27). Histamine, serotonin, substance P and platelet activating factor induce mainly intercellular gaps, whereas vascular endothelial growth factor, heat injury, pressure overload, psoriasis and encephalomyelitis induce relatively more transendothelial gaps.

A biochemical cascade leads to gap formation

Inflammatory mediators, such as histamine, bradykinin, serotonin and thrombin, trigger multiple signalling pathways that lead to cytoskeletal reorganization and gap formation. Different mediators may trigger different pathways. Many mediators, such as histamine, act via a NO pathway (see below); but bradykinin may act via reactive oxygen species. The signal pathway leads to loosening of the intercellular junctions and endothelial cell contraction, as described next.

Increased cytosolic Ca^{2+} is an early step in the signal cascade

Agonists, such as histamine, activate their cognate endothelial receptor, which is coupled by Gq-protein to phospholipase C. The latter generates two chemical messengers, inositol trisphosphate (IP_3) and diacylglycerol (DAG). IP_3 releases the endothelial Ca^{2+} store and triggers **store-operated Ca^{2+} entry** (SOC) (Figure 9.7). DAG activates **receptor-operated Ca^{2+} entry channels** (ROCs). Consequently, extracellular Ca^{2+} passes into the cell, raising its cytosolic Ca^{2+} concentration four- to tenfold within a minute (Figure 11.29). DAG also activates **protein kinase C (PKC)**, which activates a MAP kinase cascade implicated in some inflammatory responses (Figure 11.30). The **extracellular Ca^{2+} influx is obligatory for the inflammatory response**; if it is reduced, the change in hydraulic conductance is likewise reduced (Figure 11.29). But the rise in Ca^{2+} does not directly initiate gap formation, since Ca^{2+} still increases when nitric oxide production is blocked, yet permeability hardly changes (Figure 11.28). The Ca^{2+} must act, therefore, by stimulating nitric oxide formation.

Nitric oxide, cGMP and cAMP continue the signal cascade

The increased cytosolic Ca^{2+} raises the Ca^{2+}-calmodulin level, which stimulates endothelial nitric oxide synthase activity (eNOS, Section 9.4). Although small amounts of NO can lower permeability (by scavenging toxic oxygen radicals), **high levels of NO are pro-inflammatory** (Figure 11.28). Nitric oxide activates soluble guanylyl cyclase, which produces cGMP (cyclic guanosine monophosphate). **cGMP is a permeability-raising messenger** that activates phosphodiesterase 2 and protein kinase G (PKG) (Figure 11.30). Since phosphodiesterase 2 is more abundant in venular than arterial endothelium, this helps localize the

Figure 11.29 Parallel changes in free cytosolic Ca^{2+} (a) and hydraulic permeability (b) during the inflammatory response of frog venule to inflammatory agonist ATP. ATP was used because frogs do not respond to mammalian agonists such as histamine. Endothelial depolarization by a high K^+ solution (open symbols) reduced the Ca^{2+} transient and conductance changes in parallel (see text). (Redrawn from work of He P, Zhang X, Curry FE. *American Journal of Physiology* 1996; **271**: H2377–87 with permission from the American Physiological Society.)

Figure 11.30 Simplified summary of current understanding of signal transduction cascade leading to endothelial gap formation in inflammation. Major second messengers are in grey boxes, enzymes in red. PIP_2, phosphatidyl inositol bisphosphate; PKC, protein kinase C – this activates a MAP kinase cascade (not shown) implicated in some inflammatory responses; Epac, exchange protein activated by cAMP; Rap1, Rac1, small GTPases that promote cortical actin stability.

inflammatory response to venules. Phosphodiesterase 2 degrades **cAMP, an anti-inflammatory, barrier-enhancing messenger**, so a fall in cAMP raises permeability. Conversely, cAMP-raising agonists, such as the β-adrenoceptor agonists isoprenaline and terbutaline, attenuate gap formation and inflammation. cAMP's anti-inflammatory action is mediated by two pathways: (i) cAMP activates protein kinase A, which inhibits myosin contraction (Section 9.7);

(ii) cAMP activates Epac ('exchange protein activated by cAMP'), which activates pathways that stabilize the junctional strands and actin cytoskeleton. A fall in cAMP therefore favours gap formation by **loosening the intercellular junction** and by **endothelial contraction** (retraction). In intact venules, junction loosening seems the more important factor, since inhibitors of myosin light chain kinase, a key initiator of contraction (see below), do not block the inflammatory response. By contrast, active contraction is important in cultured endothelial cells, a much used but potentially misleading research 'model'.

Intercellular junctions are loosened by junctional protein redistribution

Intercellular gaps form when the key transmembrane protein, **VE-cadherin**, diffuses away from the junction (Figure 9.3). The duration of a VE-cadherin bond is only about half a second, so cadherins can dissipate quickly by lateral diffusion in the cell membrane. This is normally prevented by their attachment to catenins, which in turn are held in place by the actin cytoskeleton. During inflammation **fragmentation of the anchoring peripheral F-actin band**, along with **altered phosphorylation of the VE-cadherin and β-catenin**, weakens the junction, facilitating its separation. A fall in cAMP and Epac activity appears to mediate the changes in F-actin and junctional proteins.

Endothelial cell contraction may contribute to gap formation

Endothelial contraction was originally inferred from the nuclear wrinkling seen in inflamed venules, and it certainly occurs in inflamed, cultured endothelial cells. The contractile process is unlike that in the heart, and resembles that in smooth muscle (Chapter 12). The rise in endothelial Ca^{2+}–calmodulin activates **myosin light chain kinase**, which activates actin–myosin contraction. Since myosin light chain kinase is inhibited by cAMP-activated PKA, the fall in cAMP during inflammation may increase the tension on the weakened junction (Figure 11.30).

Transcellular gaps are thought to arise from a thinning of the cell, brought about by actin–myosin contraction. As the cell thins, vacuoles and vesicles fuse across the cell to form fenestrations, transcellular gaps and breaks in the glycocalyx.

Cytokines, VEGF and leukocytes mediate longer-lasting hyperpermeability

The above account describes acute inflammation. In chronically inflamed tissue, such as rheumatoid arthritis, psoriasis and cancer, the microvascular permeability is raised for months or years, sustained by continuous **cytokine** production. The chronic hyperpermeability is mediated partly by **vascular endothelial growth factor** (VEGF), which used to be called 'vascular permeability factor'. **Leukocytes** too contribute to chronic inflammation. Leukocyte migration through endothelium (Section 9.8) does not in itself raise permeability, because the endothelium reseals quickly behind the migrating leukocyte; but activated leukocytes raise permeability by releasing pro-inflammatory agents, such as the potent leukotrienes and platelet activating factor (Section 13.5). Other leukocyte products, such as superoxide anions, hydrogen peroxide and elastase (a potent protease), damage the endothelium directly and increase its permeability.

Steroids (glucocorticoids) are often used to suppress chronic inflammatory states, such as rheumatoid arthritis. Steroids suppress leukocyte migration, cytokine production, gap formation and vasodilatation.

SUMMARY

- The transcapillary filtration of ~4–8 litres/day (humans) affects plasma and interstitial fluid volumes, and washes escaped plasma proteins and antigens into the lymphatic system. The filtration fraction is low in continuous capillaries (0.1–0.3%) but high in fenestrated capillaries (renal glomerulus 20%).

- The capillary wall is coated internally by a **semipermeable membrane, the glycocalyx**, which overlies the intercellular clefts and fenestrae. The glycocalyx reflects the plasma proteins, which therefore exert a colloid osmotic pressure (COP). The **Starling principle** states that the filtration rate, per unit surface area, equals the hydraulic conductance of the wall, L_p, multiplied by the sum of the pressures acting on the wall, namely the hydraulic pressure drop across the wall, [capillary blood pressure P_c − interstitial fluid pressure P_i], minus the effective colloid osmotic pressure difference, $\sigma \times$ [plasma COP π_p − interstitial COP π_i (or more accurately subglycocalyx COP, π_g)]. The protein reflection coefficient σ is 0.8–0.95.

- **Human capillary pressure** P_c is ~35 mmHg at the inlet, falling to ~12 mmHg at the outlet (heart level). P_c depends on arterial pressure, venous pressure and precapillary, arteriolar resistance, which is under sympathetic nervous control. Gravity increases capillary pressure greatly in dependent tissues (ankles, sacral region), which are therefore prone to oedema.

- **Human plasma COP** π_p is 21–29 mmHg. Albumin contributes disproportionately, due to Na^+ ions attracted by its net negative charge (Gibbs–Donnan distribution).

- **Interstitial COP** π_i is typically about one-third of plasma COP, due to escaped plasma proteins. Interstitial protein concentration and π_i are not fixed quantities. They fall as filtration rate increases, thereby attenuating the filtration rate. Conversely, when interstitial fluid is absorbed by capillaries after a haemorrhage, π_i and subglycocalyx π_g rise and eventually halt the absorption process.

- **Interstitial fluid pressure** P_i is slightly subatmospheric in many tissues. P_i increases to ~2 mmHg in oedema. Interstitial fluid mobility is normally low, due to interstitial glycosaminoglycans. In oedema, glycosaminoglycan dilution results in a high mobility (clinical pitting test). The P_i-versus-hydration curve (compliance curve) is steep at physiological hydrations, but flat in the oedema range.

- The Starling pressures generally cause **filtration**, even in postcapillary venules, contrary to traditional teaching. If capillary pressure is reduced, by hypovolaemia and/or precapillary vasoconstriction, capillaries **absorb** interstitial fluid transiently; but absorption tails off as π_i and π_g rise and P_i falls. Absorption is only sustained in tissues where the interstitium is flushed by an independent stream of liquid (intestinal mucosa during water absorption; renal peritubular capillaries; lymph nodes).

- In **orthostasis**, capillary pressure is high in the dependent tissues, so filtration rate increases and plasma volume falls. **Exercise** too reduces plasma volume, because interstitial crystalloids released by the active muscle fibres (lactate, K^+) exert osmotic pressure across endothelial, water-only aquaporin channels, promoting filtration into the active muscle.

- **The lymphatic system** preserves tissue volume homeostasis by returning escaped plasma proteins and fluid to the circulation. Flow in the non-contractile initial lymphatics is driven by extrinsic compression, whereas the contractile main lymphatic vessels pump lymph actively. Pumping is enhanced by distension and sympathetic activity. Some lymph can be reabsorbed by blood capillaries in the lymph nodes. The rest drains via efferent lymph trunks (chiefly the thoracic duct) into neck veins. Impaired lymph transport, whether hereditary, post-surgical or infective (filariasis), results in high-protein **lymphoedema**.

- **Clinical oedema** develops when capillary filtration rate exceeds lymphatic drainage rate. Increased capillary filtration can cause a low-protein oedema (transudate, <15 g/l) following capillary pressure elevation (dependent oedema, cardiac failure, deep venous thrombosis) or plasma COP reductions (malnutrition, intestinal disease, hepatic failure, nephrotic syndrome); or a high protein oedema (exudates, >30 g/l) following inflammation.

- **Inflammatory swelling** is caused by increases in venular permeability to water and plasma proteins ($\uparrow L_p, \downarrow \sigma$). Also, net filtration force is increased by vasodilatation ($\uparrow P_c$), an initial dip in interstitial pressure ($\downarrow P_i$, especially in burns) and plasma protein leakage ($\uparrow \pi_i, \pi_g$).

- The inflammatory hyperpermeability is due to the formation of intercellular and transcellular **gaps** in the venular endothelium and glycocalyx. Inflammatory mediators, such as histamine, bradykinin and thrombin, raise endothelial **cytosolic Ca^{2+}**, which activates a pathway involving nitric oxide, cGMP and cAMP. This leads to gap formation by loosening intercellular junctions, possibly aided by endothelial cell contraction. Also, the cytokines IL-1β and TNFα initiate **leukocyte** margination and emigration. The activated leukocytes release endothelium- and glycocalyx-damaging agents such as free oxygen radicals and proteases.

Further reading

Reviews and chapters

Alitalo K, Tammela T, Petrova T. Lymphangiogenesis in development and human disease. *Nature* 2005; **438**: 946–53.

Aukland, K. Why don't our feet swell in the upright position? News in Physiological Sciences, 1994; **9**: 214–19.

Aukland K, Reed RK. Interstitial–lymphatic mechanisms in the control of extracellular volume. *Physiological Reviews* 1993; **73**: 1–78.

Aukland K. Arnold Heller and the lymph pump. *Acta Physiologica Scandinavica* 2005; **185**: 171–80.

Comper WD. *Extracellular Matrix*. Amsterdam: Harwood Academic Publishers, 1996.

Curry FE. Microvascular solute and water transport. *Microcirculation* 2005; **12**: 17–31.

Levick JR. Flow through interstitium and other fibrous matrices. *Quarterly Journal of Experimental Physiology* 1987; **72**: 409–38.

Levick JR. Revision of the Starling principle: New views of tissue fluid balance. *Journal of Physiology* 2004; **557**: 704.

Mehta D, Malik AB. Signaling mechanisms regulating endothelial permeability. *Physiological Reviews* 2006; **86**: 279–367.

Michel CC. Starling: The formulation of his hypothesis of microvascular fluid exchange and its significance after 100 years. *Experimental Physiology*, 1997; **82**: 1–30.

Sabolic I, Brown D. Water channels in renal and nonrenal tissues. *News in Physiological Sciences* 1995; **10**: 12–17.

Varani J, Ward PA. Mechanisms of neutrophil-dependent and neutrophil-independent endothelial cell injury. *Biological Signals* 1994; **3**: 1–14.

Weinbaum S, Tarbell JM, Damiano ER. The structure and function of the endothelial glycocalyx layer. *Annual Review Biomedical Engineering* 2007; **9**: 121–67.

Wiig H, Rubin K, Reed RK. New and active role of the interstitium in control of interstitial fluid pressure: Potential therapeutic consequences. *Acta Anaesthesiologica Scandinavica* 2003; **47**: 111–21.

Zawieja D. Lymphatic biology and the microcirculation: Past, present and future. *Microcirculation* 2005; **12**: 141–50.

Research papers

See www.hodderplus.com/cardiovascularphysiology for a full list of Research papers for this chapter.

CHAPTER 12

Vascular smooth muscle: excitation, contraction and relaxation

Learning objectives

After reading this chapter you should be able to:

- Outline the ultrastructural basis of vascular contraction (12.2).
- Contrast contraction in vascular and cardiac myocytes (12.1, 12.3).
- Outline the roles of Ca^{2+} channels, K$^+$ channels and Cl$^-$ channels in vascular tone regulation (12.4).
- State the roles of myosin light chain kinase, myosin phosphatase, phospholipase C, inositol trisphosphate and diacylglycerol in excitation–contraction coupling (12.5).
- Explain the difference between depolarization-dependent and depolarization-independent contraction (12.5, 12.7).
- State the role and mechanism of Ca^{2+}-sensitization during tonic contraction.
- Explain how sympathetic nerve activity evokes vasoconstriction (12.6).
- Outline four mechanisms mediating vasodilatation (12.7).

12.1 Overview

The tunica media (middle coat) of arteries, arterioles, venules and veins consists mainly of vascular smooth muscle cells (VSM, vascular myocytes). These are spindle-shaped cells, 20–60 μm long by ~4 μm wide at the centre, wrapped helically around the vessel (Figure 1.11). Changes in their contractile tension (tone) cause the vessel to constrict or dilate as required. There are substantial differences in the way contraction is regulated in different blood vessels – making this a tricky subject for teacher and student alike. Nevertheless, two principles apply to nearly all vessels; (i) **contractile tension is governed primarily by cytosolic Ca^{2+} concentration**; and (ii) **contractile tension is also regulated by changes in sensitivity to Ca^{2+}**.

Other key features, often contrasting sharply with cardiac contraction, are as follows.

- **Membrane depolarization may/may not initiate VSM contraction**. In many blood vessels, contraction is not driven by action potentials (cf. heart and skeletal muscle). Depending on the vessel, three types of activation can be discerned. (i) Vascular myocytes may show a graded, sustained depolarization upon activation, but no action potential generation. This causes a graded, sustained contraction (Figure 12.1). (ii) In some vessels, vascular myocytes fire action potentials on top of the underlying depolarized state. This evokes twitch increments of the underlying contractile tension (Figures 12.2a and 12.2b). (iii) In large vessels,

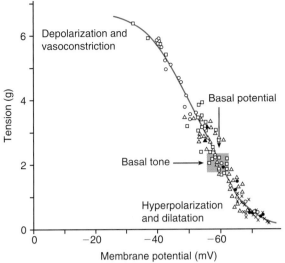

Figure 12.1 Dependence of contractile tone on membrane potential in isolated canine carotid artery. Membrane potential was altered by extracellular H^+ ($\triangle$), extracellular K^+ ($\square$), extracellular Ca^{2+} ($\bullet$), noradrenaline ($\bigcirc$) and hypoxia ($\times$). The highlighted box indicates membrane potential and tone in the 'resting', basal state. (Data from Siegel G *et al. Journal of Vascular Medicine and Biology* 1991; **3**: 140–9.)

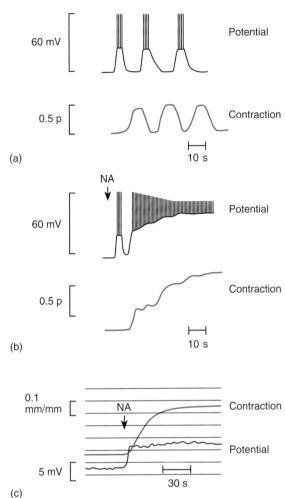

Figure 12.2 Diverse characteristics of vascular smooth muscle. (a) (*Upper trace*) Membrane potential in spontaneously active portal vein of guinea pig, showing automaticity. Regular, slow depolarizations trigger bursts of action potentials. (*Lower trace*) Contractions followed the membrane depolarization (p is tension). (b) Response of portal vein to noradrenaline (NA), showing further depolarization-dependent contraction. (c) Contrasting response of sheep carotid artery to noradrenaline. There are no action potentials and the sustained contraction is not dependent on the slight accompanying depolarization (depolarization-independent contraction). ((a) and (b) From Golenhofen K, Hermstein N, Lammel E. *Microvascular Research* 1973; **5**: 73–80, with permission from Elsevier. (c) From Keatinge WR, Harman CM. *Local Mechanisms Controlling Blood Vessels*. London: Academic Press, 1980, by permission.)

contraction is often induced by biochemical pathways, with little change in membrane potential; any associated change in membrane potential is secondary, and not the cause of contraction (Figure 12.2c). Patterns (i) and (ii) have been called **electromechanical coupling**, while pattern (iii) is **pharmacomechanical coupling**.

- **Myosin activation causes contraction.** Cardiac contraction occurs when Ca^{2+} binds to troponin on the actin filament. By contrast, VSM contraction is brought about primarily by the activation of the myosin filament. The VSM myosin isoform is activated by a phosphorylating enzyme, **myosin light chain kinase (MLCK)**, which is itself activated when cytosolic Ca^{2+} rises.

- **Active tension (tone) is regulated not only by Ca^{2+} concentration but also by Ca^{2+} sensitivity.** In the heart, an agonist such as adrenaline increases contractile force by increasing the cytosolic Ca^{2+} concentration. In VSM, agonists can increase contractile force by increasing $[Ca^{2+}]$ and by increasing the sensitivity of the contractile apparatus to Ca^{2+}.

- **Contraction duration can be very long.** A cardiac contraction lasts ~ 300 ms, whereas many blood vessels are in a partially contracted state, called **basal tone**, throughout life. Vascular dilatation results from a reduction in the tone, constriction from an increase in the tone.

To understand these features, we must consider the structure of VSM and its varied expression of ion channels and signal pathways. To avoid undue repetition, it is assumed that the reader is familiar with the electrophysiology basics introduced in Chapter 3.

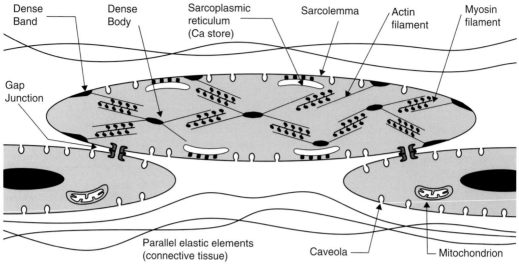

Figure 12.3 Structure of vascular myocyte. Fine, periodic, dark-staining elements extend from the subsarcolemmal sarcoplasmic reticulum towards the sarcolemma, thought to be Ca^{2+} release channels. The local, subsarcolemmal region may therefore experience higher Ca^{2+} concentrations than the cytosol. General organization of tunica media and myoendothelial gap junctions is shown in Figure 1.11. (Based partly on Gabella G. *Physiological Reviews* 1984; **64**: 455–77, with permission of the American Physiological Society.)

12.2 Structure of a vascular myocyte

Actin–myosin filaments form the contractile machinery

As in the heart, contraction depends on crossbridge formation between thick myosin filaments (2.2 μm × 0.315 μm) and overlapping, parallel thin actin filaments (1.5 μm × 0.037 μm) (Figure 12.3). The similarities end here, however. The smooth-muscle thin filament is longer than in cardiac muscle, allowing greater shortening; and it lacks troponin, the cardiac Ca^{2+}-sensitive regulatory protein. Troponin is replaced by the proteins caldesmon and calponin on VSM thin filaments. The myosin too differs from that in the heart, and only participates in contraction when **phosphorylated**, i.e. when phosphate groups are added to it, by the enzyme **myosin light chain kinase**. VSM contraction therefore depends primarily on thick-filament activation, rather than thin-filament activation.

VSM lacks the Z lines that align the filaments in a cardiac myocyte. Instead, the actin filaments are rooted in **dense bands** on the inner cell membrane and in **dense bodies** in the cytoplasm. These structures are composed of α-actinin, the protein forming the cardiac Z lines. The dense bodies are not aligned across the cell, so VSM lacks the striated appearance of cardiac and skeletal muscle. A third kind of filament, the intermediate filament (meaning intermediate in thickness) acts as a cytoskeletal element; it links the various dense bodies and dense bands, so that the cell contracts as a whole. Vascular intermediate filaments are composed mainly of the proteins desmin and vimentin.

VSM sarcoplasmic reticulum is a Ca^{2+} store with two kinds of Ca^{2+}-release channel

The smooth endoplasmic reticulum of VSM, or sarcoplasmic reticulum (SR), contains a releasable store of Ca^{2+} ions. Since the SR is relatively poorly developed (1–4% of the cell volume), the Ca^{2+} store is not very big, especially in small resistance vessels. Indeed, tonic vasoconstriction in resistance vessels requires not only store release but also extracellular Ca^{2+} influx – so Ca^{2+}-channel blockers, such as nifedipine, are good resistance vessel dilators. The close proximity of the SR to the cell membrane (sarcolemma), ~15 nm in places, facilitates store release by agonists, such as noradrenaline. The activation of the sarcolemmal agonist receptor triggers the formation of soluble factor, inositol trisphosphate (IP$_3$), which quickly diffuses to the nearby SR, where IP$_3$ receptors are linked to Ca^{2+} release channels (**IP$_3$–Ca^{2+} release channels**). IP$_3$ thus releases the SR Ca^{2+} store. This raises cytosolic Ca^{2+} 'globally' (i.e. throughout the cell) and thereby increases vascular tone.

The SR membrane also has a second type of Ca^{2+} release channel, the **ryanodine receptor** (RyR), as in cardiac myocytes. In the basal state, ryanodine receptors spontaneously release brief bursts of Ca^{2+}, called Ca^{2+} sparks. A Ca^{2+} spark only raises the Ca^{2+} concentrations locally (cf. globally), in the subsarcolemmal region. This activates nearby sarcolemmal Ca^{2+}-dependent K^+ channels, leading to hyperpolarization (Section 12.4); so the RyR Ca^{2+} spark does not cause contraction.

Gap junctions transmit ionic currents

Vascular myocytes are connected to each other by ion-permeable, electrically conductive gap junctions (**homocellular gap junctions**) (Figure 12.3). The gap junction, or nexus, is composed of the protein connexin, as in the heart. Six connexin molecules form a hemi-tube (connexon), and the hemi-tubes of adjacent cells join end-to-end, connecting the cytoplasm of the two cells. This allows ionic currents to transmit depolarization from cell to cell. The spread is decremental, however, and extends only ~1 mm along the vessel longitudinally.

The innermost myocytes of the tunica media also form gap junctions with the endothelial cells. These **heterocellular** or **myoendothelial gap junctions** transmit hyperpolarizing signals from the lining endothelium to the vascular myocytes, as described under 'Endothelium-derived hyperpolarizing factor' (Section 9.5).

Caveolae

The cell surface is heavily invaginated with tiny flask-shaped pits, called caveolae ('little flasks'). The caveolae are so numerous that they increase the total membrane area by up to 75%. The cytoplasmic surface of each caveola has a striated coat of protein, caveolin-1, and the caveolar membrane is enriched in cholesterol and sphingomyelin. The functions of caveolae are only just emerging. Since they contain high concentrations of β adrenergic receptors, G proteins, L-type Ca^{2+} channels, K_{ATP} channels and signal pathway proteins such as adenylyl cyclase and protein kinase $C\alpha$, caveolae are thought to be 'signalosomes' where biochemical pathways are integrated.

12.3 Contractile properties and role of Ca^{2+}

Resistance vessels and large arteries are normally in a state of partial contraction called **basal tone**. Regulatory mechanisms exist to increase the tone (**vasoconstriction** – this section) or reduce it (**vasodilatation** – Section 12.7). Vasoconstriction

Figure 12.4 Contraction and cytosolic free Ca^{2+} concentration in rabbit mesenteric artery. (a) Contraction in response to noradrenaline was well sustained (upper black line). The effect of a depolarizing concentration of extracellular KCl was less sustained (lower, dashed black line). 'Global' cytosolic Ca^{2+} concentration over the whole tunica media (upper red line) is average of hundreds of asynchronous Ca^{2+} waves in individual myocytes (lower red line). After the initial, transient phase of store release, Ca^{2+} wave frequency and magnitude decline, reducing the global average $[Ca^{2+}]$; yet the noradrenaline-induced contraction is maintained (tonic phase). This shows that the noradrenaline-triggered pathway raises the sensitivity to Ca^{2+}. (b) Dependence of contractile force on mean cytosolic free $[Ca^{2+}]$ in phase 2. Noradrenaline steepens the relation, demonstrating Ca^{2+} sensitization. (Based on Ito T, Kajikuri J, Kurigama H. *Journal of Physiology* 1992; **457**: 297–314, with permission from Wiley-Blackwell; and Wier WG, Morgan KG. *Reviews of Physiology, Biochemistry and Pharmacology* 2003; **150**: 91–139.)

can be induced by depolarizing the cell, e.g. by isotonic KCl in the laboratory (Figure 12.4), or more physiologically by:

- sympathetic vasomotor fibres releasing noradrenaline;
- circulating hormones, such as adrenaline (acting on α-adrenoreceptors), angiotensin II (AT_1 receptors) and vasopressin;
- paracrine agents, such as endothelin (ET_A and ET_B receptors), serotonin ($5HT_{2A}$ receptors), histamine (H_1 receptors) and thromboxane.

The receptor type is specified above, because agonists can have an opposite effect when bound to a different receptor type, due to the linkage of the receptor to a different signalling pathway within the cell. For example, adrenaline bound to α-adrenoreceptors causes vasoconstriction, but adrenaline bound to β_2-adrenoreceptors causes vasodilatation. Likewise histamine H_1 receptors elicit vasoconstriction, whereas H_2 receptors elicit vasodilatation. Vasoconstriction is illustrated in Figures 12.2, 12.4 and 12.9, and has the following characteristics.

Vascular contraction is slow but sustained

- **Speed of contraction.** The vascular myocyte has evolved for slow, sustained contraction (Figure 12.4a), unlike the brief twitch of a cardiac myocyte. The shortening velocity is about one-tenth that of striated muscle, because the myosin crossbridges form and break much more slowly in VSM than in striated muscle.
- **Degree of shortening.** The vascular myocyte can shorten by a half or more, whereas striated muscle fibres shorten by only about one-third. The enhanced shortening of VSM is due to the greater actin filament length and a difference in myosin filament structure. The myosin heads on one side of the filament all face the same direction, and those on the opposite side face the opposite direction (Figure 12.3) – unlike the arrangement in cardiac myosin filaments (Figures 3.13 and 6.3).
- **Contractile force.** This is regulated by agonists, as listed above.
- **Duration of contraction.** The sustained nature of vascular contraction is remarkable; many arterioles and arteries maintain tone throughout life. This is vitally important to support arterial blood pressure, and is a prerequisite for vasodilatation, which is simply a reduction in tone. In vessels with a high tone, each myocyte is tonically contracted, and excessive ATP consumption is avoided by means of a special 'latch state' (see below). In vessels with low tone, individual myocytes show asynchronous, recurring contraction–relaxation cycles, associated with Ca^{2+} waves (Figure 12.4a).

Contraction is mediated by Ca^{2+}–calmodulin, leading to myosin phosphorylation

As noted earlier, vascular contraction depends primarily on global cytosolic Ca^{2+} ion concentration (Figure 12.4), which triggers myosin filament activation as follows.

Myosin light chain kinase (MLCK) activates the myosin motor

A rise in cytosolic Ca^{2+} concentration causes the formation of Ca^{2+}–calmodulin complex; calmodulin is a cytoplasmic protein, related to troponin C, that binds 4 Ca^{2+} ions. The Ca^{2+}–calmodulin complex activates the enzyme, myosin light chain kinase (MLCK). The light chain is a component of the myosin head involved in crossbridge formation with actin, and vascular myosin only forms crossbridges when the light chain is phosphorylated (unlike striated muscle myosin). MLCK transfers a phosphate group from ATP to the myosin light chain, enabling the myosin head to form a crossbridge with actin. The myosin head then rotates to generate tension, as in striated muscle. Instead of quickly detaching, however, as it would in cardiac muscle, the crossbridge remains attached in the tense, flexed state for a prolonged period (see 'latch state', below).

Myosin light chain phosphatase inactivates the myosin motor, causing relaxation

The phosphate group can be removed by the enzyme, myosin light chain phosphatase (Figure 12.7). When intracellular Ca^{2+} concentration falls, MLCK activity declines and the competing myosin phosphatase dominates, dephosphorylating the myosin. Since dephosphorylated myosin cannot form new crossbridges, the phosphatase in effect turns off the myosin motor. As existing crossbridges detach, new ones cannot form, so the myocytes relax, leading to vasodilatation. Increased myosin phosphatase activation may explain cases of vascular relaxation with little fall in cytosolic Ca^{2+} concentration, e.g. hypoxic vasodilatation (Figure 13.5).

Slow crossbridge cycling (the latch state) maintains vascular tension economically

The energy cost of maintaining vascular tone throughout the body would be substantial, were it not for the ability of VSM to maintain tension with just 1/300th of the energy expenditure of striated muscle. This is due to a difference in crossbridge duration. In a skeletal muscle fibre, crossbridge duration is very short, so tension can only be maintained by the continuous, rapid making and breaking of crossbridges – consuming one ATP molecule per crossbridge cycle. In smooth muscle, a crossbridge lasts much longer, so tension maintenance consumes much less ATP. This is called the **latch state**. The muscle is in effect locked into the crossbridged state, in a similar way to the latch muscle of a bivalve shell. VSM can thus maintain tension for a

Figure 12.5 Ion channels, pumps, exchangers and co-transporters in sarcolemma of vascular myocyte. For channel abbreviations see text. Crosses denote transport blockers. The Na^+–HCO_3^- co-transporter and Na^+–H^+ exchanger combat intracellular acidosis during a sustained contraction. The $Na^+K^+2Cl^-$ co-transporter and HCO_3^-–Cl^- exchanger generate a high intracellular chloride concentration, which affects the Cl^- electrochemical gradient (see text).

long period with little ATP consumption and without fatiguing.

Cytosolic free [Ca^{2+}] depends on rate of influx versus removal

The cytosolic free Ca^{2+} concentration regulating VSM tone is typically in the range 100–350 nM (Figure 12.4), and is determined by three factors (Figure 12.5).

1 **Extracellular Ca^{2+}** enters the myocyte through Ca^{2+}-conducting channels in the sarcolemma. These fall into three functional classes: **voltage-sensitive Ca^{2+} channels, receptor-operated channels** (ROCs) and **store-operated channels** (cat-SOCs); see next section. The voltage-sensitive Ca^{2+} channels have a low but finite open-state probability under basal conditions, allowing a small extracellular Ca^{2+} influx that contributes to **basal tone**.
2 **Stored Ca^{2+}** is released from the SR store through the IP_3-dependent Ca^{2+} release channels, when the myocyte is stimulated by noradrenaline. The released Ca^{2+} can spread across the cell as a Ca^{2+} wave. At the same time, the activation of sarcolemmal store-operated channels increases extracellular Ca^{2+} entry.

3 **Ca^{2+}–ATPase pumps** in the sarcolemma and SR membrane continuously pump Ca^{2+} out of the cytoplasm. SR uptake is called **Ca^{2+} sequestration** and extracellular transfer is called **Ca^{2+} expulsion**. A sarcolemmal Na^+–Ca^{2+} exchanger also contributes to Ca^{2+} expulsion (Figure 12.5). Due to the small but continuous influx of Ca^{2+} through Ca^{2+} channels in the basal state, the sarcolemmal Ca^{2+} pumps have to expel Ca^{2+} continuously – otherwise, Ca^{2+} would accumulate in the cell.

Since Ca^{2+} channels and membrane potential are major factors influencing VSM contraction, we must next consider the mix of ion channels in the VSM membrane.

12.4 Vascular ion channels

This section introduces the players in the game. In a pressurized arterial vessel exhibiting basal tone, the myocyte membrane potential is -50 mV to -60 mV (Figure 12.1). This is a more depolarized state than the cardiac myocyte, owing to differences in the ion channel population. The VSM sarcolemma has, rather dauntingly, four types of K^+-conducting channel, four types of Ca^{2+}-conducting channel and a Cl^--conducting channel (Figures 12.5 and 12.6). These channels are expressed to different degrees in different vessels and tissues, so VSM shows very diverse electrical behaviour (Figure 12.2). Voltage-operated Na^+ channels, which are of major importance in cardiac electrophysiology, generally play no role in VSM. The key channels are as follows.

K^+ channels generate the negative membrane potential

Like all cells, the vascular myocyte has a high intracellular K^+ concentration, generated by the sarcolemmal Na^+–K^+ pump (Figure 12.5). The sarcolemma also has ~50 000 K^+ channels, a substantial fraction of which is open at any one moment, transmitting a small outward current of K^+ ions down their electrochemical gradient (Table 12.1). The negative charges left behind create the negative basal membrane potential. Also, the Na^+–K^+ pump, by expelling three Na^+ ions in exchange for two K^+ ions, contributes around -11 mV to the membrane potential.

Since the Nernst equilibrium potential for K^+, E_K, is -90 mV, whereas the membrane potential is only -50 mV, the sarcolemma clearly has a significant basal conductance to other ions too, notably Na^+ ions (due to TRP channel constitutive activity, see below) and chloride ions (due to Cl_{Ca} channels). The chemical gradient and equilibrium potential for these ions are listed in Table 12.1. The influx of Na^+ and slight efflux of Cl^- down their electrochemical gradients accounts for the low membrane potential.

K^+ channel status (open/closed) is important, because it determines the membrane potential, which in turn controls voltage-sensitive Ca^{2+} channels and hence vascular tone. For example, **hypoxia**

increases the fraction of open K^+ channels, leading to hyperpolarization (a more negative potential) and therefore closure of the voltage-sensitive Ca^{2+} channels. This reduces Ca^{2+} influx, which contributes to hypoxic vascular relaxation (Figure 12.1, crosses).

The four main types of K^+ channel expressed by VSM are the inward-rectifier channel (K_{ir}), its biochemical relative the ATP-dependent K^+ channel (K_{ATP}), the voltage-dependent K^+ channel (K_V) and its relative the calcium-dependent K^+ channel (K_{Ca}) (Table 12.2). Their properties differ markedly, and each makes a specific contribution to vascular behaviour, as follows.

Inward-rectifier channel K_{ir} senses extracellular K^+ and contributes to vasodilatation in exercising muscle, myocardium and brain

The structure of the inward rectifier channel is shown in Figure 3.12 (top left). The channel serves as a sensor of external K^+ concentration, being the only K^+ channel whose **open probability is increased by a rise in extracellular [K^+]**, in the range 5–25 mM. The increased K^+ conductance shifts the membrane potential towards E_K, causing hyperpolarization and hence vasodilatation. This is important in exercising muscle, myocardium and active areas of the brain (Figure 15.15), where increased metabolic activity raises the local interstitial [K^+]. The resulting vascular hyperpolarization and vasodilatation helps raise blood flow, to match demand ('metabolic hyperaemia', Section 13.4). By contrast, a very high, non-physiological extracellular K^+ concentration will depolarize the myocyte, because it abolishes the [K^+] gradient responsible for the membrane potential. The depolarization activates Ca^{2+} channels, leading to contraction (Figure 12.4).

ATP-dependent channel K_{ATP} senses ischaemia and contributes to hypoxic vasodilatation

The ATP-dependent K^+ channel comprises four α subunits of K_{ir} protein, each surrounded by a sulphonylurea receptor unit that confers sensitivity to ATP and sulphonylurea-related drugs (Figure 3.12, top right). The channel open probability is increased by a fall in intracellular ATP, as in severe ischaemia; and by a rise in ADP, GDP, adenosine and H^+ concentration, which occurs during moderate hypoxia. The K_{ATP} channel thus helps link vascular tone to tissue oxygen status; ischaemia and hypoxia increase

Table 12.1 Ionic composition of vascular smooth muscle

Ion	Intracellular fluid (mM)	Extracellular fluid (mM)	Nernst equilibrium potential (mV)[d]
K^+	165	5	-89
Na^+	9	137	$+69$
Ca^{2+}	0.0001[b]	1.2[c]	$+124$
Cl^- [a]	54	134	-23
HCO_3^-	7.3	15.5	-19
H^+	8.7×10^{-8} (pH 7.06)	4.0×10^{-8} (pH 7.40)	-20

[a]Chloride concentration is unusually high is VSM.
[b]Relaxed state.
[c]Total plasma calcium is ~2.5 mM, but only 1.2 mM is in unbound, ionic form.
[d]See Section 3.3.

Table 12.2 Ion channels in sarcolemma (plasma membrane) of vascular smooth muscle (VSM)

Channel	Properties	Roles
Potassium conducting channels		
Inward rectifying, K_{ir} (2T)[a]	Expressed in arterioles. Open at basal membrane potential. Open state increased by K_o^+ Blocked by Ba^{2+}	Supplies part of outward current for basal membrane potential. Mediates vasodilatation by interstitial K^+ in exercising muscle, myocardium, brain.
ATP-dependent, K_{ATP} (K_{NDP}) (2T, specialized form of K_{ir})[b]	Opened by low ATP, raised ADP, GDP, adenosine A_1 receptors and $[H^+]$. Inhibited by α_2 adrenoceptors. Blocked by glibenclamide $\rightarrow$ contraction. Activated by diazoxide, pinacidil, cromakalim, nicorandil, CGRP, VIP $\rightarrow$ dilatation.	Links vascular tone to metabolic state in exercise and hypoxia. Low, basal open state due to basal PKA activity. Open state raised in cAMP-PKA-mediated vasodilatation.
Voltage-dependent (delayed rectifying), K_v (6T)[c]	Opens slowly on depolarization beyond $-30\,mV$. Blocked by 4-aminopyridine (4-AP).	Part of outward current for basal potential in resistance vessels. Action potential repolarization.
Calcium-activated, K_{Ca} (BK) (6T, specialized form of K_v)	Open state promoted by Ca_i^{2+} and depolarization. Big conductance type (BK) strongly expressed in large artery VSM (cf. small and intermediate conductance isoforms, SK, IK, in endothelium). Blocked by tetraethyl ammonium(TEA), iberiotoxin, charybdotoxin, ethanol.	Contributes to basal membrane potential and repolarization. If abundantly expressed, BK suppresses action potentials. Provides a 'brake', e.g. on myogenic contraction. Implicated in action of NO.
Selective calcium-conducting channels		
Voltage-sensitive Ca^{2+} channel, VSCC	Mainly L-type, meaning large conductance, Long opening. Abundant in resistance vessels. Blocked by dihydropryidines, e.g. nifedipine.	Supplies inward current for action potentials, graded electromechanical coupling and Bayliss myogenic response.
Non-selective cation-conducting TRP channels (Ca^{2+} channels)		
Receptor-operated channel, ROC (TRPC proteins, e.g. TRPC3, TRPC6)	Poorly selective between Ca^{2+}, Na^+, K^+. Activated by diacylglycerol when α_1-. adrenoceptor and other G_q-protein-coupled receptors activated. Insensitive to nifedipine.	Mediates pharmacomechanical coupling by NAd, angiotensin, vasopressin, 5HT, histamine. Related channel contributes depolarizing current i_{cat} of slow excitatory junction potential (EJP).
Store operated cation channel, cat-SOC (TRPC1 protein)	Activated when IP_3 discharges the SR Ca^{2+} store.	Conducts extracellular Ca^{2+} into VSM when Ca^{2+} store released.
Stretch-activated cation channel, SAC (TRPV?)	Activated by stretch. Inward Na^+ and Ca^{2+} currents $\rightarrow$ depolarization $\rightarrow$ VSCC activation.	Contractile response of VSM to stretch (myogenic response). Autoregulation of blood flow.
Chloride conducting channels		
Calcium-activated chloride channel, Cl_{Ca}	Open state promoted by Ca_i^{2+} at $>200\,\mu M$.	Contributes 'inward' current $i_{Cl(Ca)}$ (efflux of negative ions) for slow EJP. Modulates membrane potential. Contributes to vasomotion.

[a] 2T, 2 transmembrane helices per α subunit. 4 α subunits make up one conducting channel.

[b] An octamer. Four $K_{ir}6.1$ α subunits form the pore, and four sulphonylurea receptor subunits (SUR2B) surround them, confering sensitivity to ATP and drugs.

[c] 6T, 6 transmembrane helices per α subunit; each α unit is a K_v protein produced by the *KCNA* gene. Four α subunits make up the conducting channel. The channel is a hetero-tetramer i.e. a mix of different K_v α isoforms, e.g. K_v 1.2/1.5 (rat cerebral artery) , K_v 1.3/1.6 (mouse cerebral artery), K_v 1.5/1.6 (rabbit pial artery).

the K_{ATP} open probability, leading to vascular hyperpolarization, vasodilatation and increased O_2 delivery (Figure 12.1, crosses). An alternative name for the channel, emphasizing its ADP sensitivity, is 'nucleotide diphosphate-dependent channel', K_{NDP}.

Even under normal, non-hypoxic conditions, some K_{ATP} channels are open, due to phosphorylation by background levels of active protein kinase A (Section 12.7). Consequently, the K_{ATP}-blocker **glibenclamide** causes partial depolarization and vasoconstriction. Conversely, the K_{ATP}-activating drug **nicorandil** causes vasodilatation; it is also a nitrodilator, and is used to treat angina.

Voltage-dependent K$^+$ channel K$_v$ and Ca-dependent K$^+$ channels K$_{Ca}$ (BK) contribute to resting potential and prevent vasospasm

The **voltage-dependent K$^+$ channel** K_v is a heterotetramer (Figure 3.12). K_v is activated by depolarization, and thus brings about repolarization after an action potential. It also contributes to the basal membrane potential.

The **calcium-dependent K$^+$ channel** K_{Ca} is a specialized form of K_v that is activated by intracellular Ca^{2+} as well as depolarization. VSM expresses a K_v isoform of big conductance, BK, unlike the endothelial isoforms of small and intermediate conductance (SK, IK). Under basal conditions the BK channels are activated intermittently by the spontaneous SR Ca^{2+} sparks (see earlier), generating 'spontaneous transient outward currents' (STOCs) that contribute to the membrane potential. BK channels reduce vascular excitability and prevent vasospasm, because, as Ca^{2+} enters the myocyte, BK activation makes the membrane potential more negative, which reduces the voltage-sensitive Ca^{2+} channel open probability. For the same reason, vessels with a high BK density do not generate action potentials, except after treatment with the BK blockers iberiotoxin and charybdotoxin (a component of scorpion venom). In mice, BK channel knock-out raises vascular tone and blood pressure. Conversely, gain-of-function mutations in human BK protect against diastolic hypertension. Thus BK functionality appears to influence our susceptibility to hypertension.

Voltage-sensitive Ca^{2+} channels (VSCCs) mediate depolarization-dependent contraction

The voltage-sensitive Ca^{2+} channel (also known as voltage-operated, voltage-gated or voltage-dependent Ca^{2+} channel) is highly selective for divalent cations (Ca^{2+} and Ba^{2+}), and its open probability is increased by depolarization. As a result, **vascular tension is a graded function of membrane depolarization in many vessels** (Figure 12.1). The predominant VSCC is the L-type Ca^{2+} channel (Figure 4.3). Since the open probability is a continuous, graded function of membrane potential, there is a very low, but finite, open state probability at the basal potential of $-50\,mV$ to $-60\,mV$. This, along with some constitutive TRP channel activity (see below), allows a small flux of extracellular Ca^{2+} into the myocyte under basal conditions. The resulting cytosolic Ca^{2+} concentration, though low, activates sufficient myosin heads to generate **basal vascular tone**.

L-type Ca^{2+} channels are expressed more abundantly in arterioles and terminal arteries (~1000 per myocyte) than in large arteries, so their contribution to vasoconstriction is most pronounced in small, resistance vessels. Many arterioles and small arteries express L-type Ca^{2+} channels so abundantly that they fire Ca^{2+}-based **action potentials** following sympathetic stimulation (Figure 12.6a). The inward calcium current, i_{Ca-L}, generates the upstroke of the action potential. The dihydropyridine **nifedipine** inhibits L-type Ca^{2+} channels, leading to the vasodilatation of resistance vessels; nifedipine is therefore used to treat clinical hypertension.

Ca^{2+}-conducting TRP channels mediate depolarization-independent contraction and contribute to agonist-induced electrical excitation

If the VSM membrane potential of an artery is abolished by extracellular isotonic KCl solution, noradrenaline can still evoke a contraction, provided that Ca^{2+} ions are added to the extracellular solution. This finding showed that VSM expresses channels that are permeable to extracellular Ca^{2+}, but are not classic, voltage-operated channels; rather, they are activated by agonist receptors. The channel was called a receptor-operated channel, and was recently shown to be composed of TRP protein (see below).

Receptor-operated channels (ROCs) are cation-conducting channels that are about three- to five-fold more permeable to Ca^{2+} than Na^+. A lag of $\sim0.1-1.0\,s$ between agonist application and channel activation indicates that a relatively slow, biochemical pathway leads to channel activation (Figure 12.6b). When the agonist binds to its G-protein coupled receptor – for example, noradrenaline to the α_1-adrenoceptor – the activated receptor splits trimeric

Depolarization-dependent contraction

(a)

Depolarization-independent contraction

(b)

Figure 12.6 Pathways by which noradrenaline α_1-receptors evoke depolarization-dependent and depolarization-independent contraction. Histamine H_1 receptors, serotonin, angiotensin II and vasopressin receptors are coupled similarly to evoke contraction. (a) Small arterial resistance vessels and the portal vein express abundant L-type Ca^{2+} channels. Electrical depolarization activates the Ca^{2+} channels, leading to contraction. (b) In large arteries, contraction is often independent of membrane potential; it is mediated by receptor-operated TRPC channels and by Ca^{2+} release from the sarcoplasmic reticulum store (SR), followed by Ca^{2+} sensitization. PIP_2, phosphatidyl inositol bisphosphate; i, current; MLCK, myosin light chain kinase.

G_q protein into $G_q\alpha$ and $G_q\beta\gamma$ components, which activate the membrane-bound enzyme phospholipase C β (PLCβ). The PLCβ catalyses the breakdown of a membrane lipid, phosphoinositol bisphosphate, into cytosolic inositol trisphosphate (IP$_3$) and lipid-soluble diacylglycerol (DAG) (Figure 12.6). The DAG activates the ROCs, leading to extracellular Ca^{2+} influx

and contraction. Note that this 'pharmacomechanical' contraction does not require membrane depolarization – although the ROC-conducted current can cause a small, incidental depolarization (Figure 12.2c). **Depolarization-independent contraction** is typical of **large arteries**, which have relatively few voltage-operated L-type Ca^{2+} channels.

The i_{cat} **TRP channel** is a cation-conducting channel, related to ROCs, that contributes to **noradrenaline-induced electrical excitation in arterioles**. The receptor–Gq–PLCβ–DAG pathway activates the TRP channel, which conducts an inward current of cations, i_{cat} (Ca^{2+}, Na^+). Current i_{cat}, along with a chloride current (see below), creates an excitatory junction potential, which can trigger an action potential in arteriolar VSM (Figure 12.6a).

Constitutive TRP channel activity provides a low, background permeability in unstimulated vessels, resulting from background levels of DAG. The DAG is generated by phospholipase D acting on the membrane lipid, phosphatidylcholine. The resulting small, inward cation current contributes to the relatively depolarized state of resting VSM.

TRP protein, or Transient Receptor Potential protein, was discovered in mutant *Drosophila* fruit flies with photoreceptors that respond only transiently to light. The mammalian TRP channel comprises a ring of four TRP proteins, each with six transmembrane helices, similar to K_v (Figure 3.12, middle) but lacking the S4 arginine charges that confer voltage sensitivity. There are 28 different mammalian TRP proteins, and they can form homo- or heterotetrameric channels (a mix of TRP species) – so TRP channels are very diverse, and include ROCs, cat-SOCs and SACs (Table 12.2).

The **store-operated channels** in VSM are cation-conducting TRP channels of low selectivity (cat-SOCs), unlike the highly Ca^{2+}-selective CRAC store-operated channel (Section 9.3). The cat-SOC is activated when IP_3, generated by the receptor-G_q–PLCβ pathway, releases the endoplasmic reticulum store. Receptor activation thus leads to contraction through both ROC and cat-SOC activation.

Stretch-activated channels (SACs) are mechanosensitive TRP channels that are activated by stretch of the vessel wall. They contribute to a contractile response of blood vessels to stretch, called the myogenic response, which is the basis of autoregulation (Sections 13.2 and 13.6).

Chloride channels contribute to agonist-induced electrical excitation

Electrically excitable myocytes express not only i_{cat} TRP channels but also chloride-conducting channels activated by cytosolic Ca^{2+} (Cl_{Ca}, Figure 12.6a). VSM intracellular Cl^- concentration is unusually high, ~54 mM (Table 12.1), due to the activity of $Na^+K^+2Cl^-$ co-transporters and Cl^-–HCO_3^-

exchangers (Figure 12.5). The resulting Cl^- equilibrium potential is -20 mV (Table 12.1). Consequently, when the Cl^- channels open, the basal membrane potential of -50 mV drives Cl^- ion out of the cell (cf. Cl^- influx in neurons), depolarizing it towards the Cl^- equilibrium potential. The Cl^- current, along with i_{cat}, generates the agonist-evoked **excitatory junction potential** (see below). A few Cl^- channels may also be open in the basal state, contributing to the relatively depolarized basal potential.

Vascular myocytes thus express a bewildering armory of diversely activated ion-conducting channels. The next section draws the threads together to show how receptor activation leads, via ion channel activation, to myocyte contraction.

12.5 From sympathetic stimulation to contractile response

The single most important physiological regulator of vascular tone is the sympathetic vasoconstrictor system, which innervates nearly all arteries and arterioles. The sympathetic fibres release **noradrenaline** (Section 14.1), which activates myocyte $α_1$-adrenoceptors (synonym, $α_1$-adrenoreceptor). Many other vasoconstrictor agonists, such as angiotensin II, vasopressin, serotonin, thromboxane and endothelin, activate G-protein-coupled receptors that trigger broadly similar pathways to the α-adrenoceptor.

Sympathetic junctional varicosities release noradrenaline and ATP

The terminal part of a sympathetic axon runs along the adventitia–media border and has a string of swellings, ~1000 per fibre, called **junctional varicosities** (Figures 1.11 and 14.2). There are up to six varicosities per myocyte, and the distance from varicosity to nearest myocyte is ~75 nm. Each varicosity contains ~500 small, dense-cored vesicles grouped near the membrane and a smaller number of large vesicles. The vesicles contain a variable mixture of noradrenaline and ATP, which are released when an action potential arrives.

Transmitter release is quantal

When a sympathetic action potential reaches a varicosity, the depolarization activates N-type calcium channels in the varicosity membrane, raising intraneural $[Ca^{2+}]$. The Ca^{2+} triggers the discharge of a single vesicle into the junctional cleft.

Neurotransmitter is thus released as a discrete, standard-size packet or **quantum**. Only ~1 in every 100 action potentials succeeds, however, in releasing a quantum from a given varicosity. The released noradrenaline diffuses rapidly across the short neuromuscular gap and binds to adrenoceptors on the vascular myocyte. The ATP binds to vascular P_{2X} purinergic receptors.

Adrenoceptors differ in type, agonist affinity, coupling and effect

Adrenoceptors are not linked directly to the ion channels that they regulate, but act via metabolic pathways. Such receptors are said to be '**metabotropic**'. There are two main classes of adrenoceptor, the α- and β-adrenoceptor. Both are G-protein-coupled receptors, but they are linked to different intracellular pathways, so that α-adrenoceptors elicit vasoconstriction and β-adrenoceptors elicit vasodilatation. In most, but not all, tissues, α-adrenoceptors predominate. The α- and β-adrenoceptors are further subdivided as follows.

- **Alpha₁-receptors** are abundant in most systemic blood vessels. They have a greater affinity for noradrenaline than adrenaline. The activated receptor triggers the G_q–PLCβ–IP_3–DAG cascade (Figures 12.6 and 12.7), which increases sarcolemmal conductance to cations and chloride ions. The resulting depolarization leads to vasoconstriction (see below).

- **Alpha₂-receptors** are abundant in cutaneous blood vessels and junctional varicosities

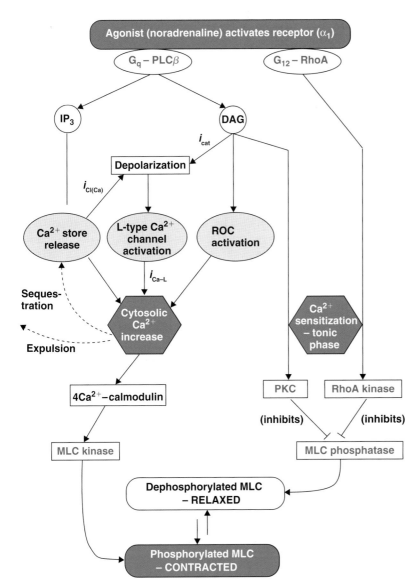

Figure 12.7 Pathways mediating noradrenaline-induced vasoconstriction. Relative importance of various pathways varies with vessel type, tissue and agonist. Abbreviations as in Figure 12.6.

(Figure 14.2). The α_2-receptor has a greater affinity for adrenaline than noradrenaline. The receptor is coupled to a different G protein to the α_1-receptor, namely G_i. It therefore acts through a different intracellular pathway. G_i protein inhibits a vasodilator pathway, the adenylyl cyclase–cAMP pathway (Section 12.7). The net effect is a fall in K_{ATP} channel conductance, leading to depolarization and vasoconstriction.

- **Beta$_1$-adrenoceptors** are found in the cardiac pacemaker and myocardium. The β_1-receptor has a greater affinity for noradrenaline than adrenaline. It is coupled to G_s-protein, which stimulates the adenylyl cyclase–cAMP pathway, leading to an increase in heart rate and contractility (Figure 4.9).
- **Beta$_2$-adrenoceptors** are abundant in the arterial vessels of myocardium, skeletal muscle and liver, while in other blood vessels they are outnumbered by α_1-receptors. The β_2-receptor has a greater affinity for adrenaline than noradrenaline. Like β_1, β_2 is coupled to G_s-protein, which stimulates the adenylyl cyclase–cAMP pathway. This leads to vasodilatation (Section 12.7).

To summarize, noradrenaline is more potent than adrenaline in activating α_1 and β_1-receptors. Adrenaline is more potent than noradrenaline in activating α_2 and β_2-receptors. The rest of this section concentrates on the pathways activated by the ubiquitous, physiologically most important receptor, the α_1-adrenoceptor.

α_1-adrenoceptors activate the phospholipase C–IP$_3$–DAG pathway

The α_1-adrenoceptor is coupled to the trimeric membrane GTPase, **G_q protein**. The activated receptor splits the trimer into its component subunits, $G_q\alpha$ and $G_q\beta\gamma$. These activate the membrane-bound enzymes **phospholipase C β1** and **β2** respectively (Figures 12.6 and 12.7). Phospholipase C splits a membrane phospholipid, phosphatidyl inositol bisphosphate (PIP$_2$), into two messenger molecules, inositol trisphosphate and diacylglycerol.

Inositol trisphosphate (IP$_3$) activates Ca^{2+}-release channels on the sarcoplasmic reticulum, releasing the Ca^{2+} store. The consequences depend on SR distribution. If the SR is scanty and close to the sarcolemma, the increase in free Ca^{2+} may be confined largely to the subsarcolemmal space, activating calcium-activated chloride channels. The resulting depolarizing current, $i_{Cl(Ca)}$, contributes to a slow-rising excitatory junction potential (see

below). If the SR is extensive, as in large artery myocytes, store discharge contributes to a rise in global cytosolic Ca^{2+} concentration, leading to contraction.

Diacylglycerol (DAG), the other messenger product, activates i_{cat} TRP channels. The depolarizing current i_{cat}, along with $i_{Cl(Ca)}$, creates a slow-rising, excitatory junction potential. DAG and Ca^{2+} also activate protein kinase C, which contributes to Ca^{2+} sensitization (see below).

α_1-adrenoceptors can evoke membrane depolarization

The release of both noradrenaline and ATP by sympathetic fibres evokes a complex electrical and mechanical response. To simplify matters, let us consider first the effect of a pulse of noradrenaline alone, delivered by a micropipette to an isolated vascular myocyte (Figure 12.8). The α_1-adrenoceptor activation is followed by a 0.1–1.0 second delay, as the G_q–PLCβ–DAG/IP$_3$–Ca^{2+} pathway grinds into action. Then a slow depolarization develops, the **slow excitatory junction potential** or **slow EJP**. The slow EJP is generated by i_{cat} (DAG-activated TRP channels) and $i_{Cl(Ca)}$ (Ca^{2+}-activated chloride channels) (Figure 12.6a). If the EJP is big enough and the myocyte has abundant VSCCs (e.g. arteriolar myocytes), an action potential ensues; VSCCs activated by the EJP cause more depolarization, activating more VSCCs, and so on (positive feedback). The rapidly increasing inward current i_{Ca-L} generates the upstroke of the action potential (Figure 12.8). The action potential is of variable amplitude and lasts 10–100 ms. The attendant transient

Figure 12.8 Response of an action potential-generating vascular myocyte to a brief pulse of noradrenaline from a micropipette (cf. sympathetic vesicle, Figure 12.9). VSCC, voltage-sensitive channel permeable to Ca^{2+}. (Courtesy of Professor WA Large, Department of Pharmacology, St. George's Hospital Medical School, London.)

increase in cytosolic $[Ca^{2+}]$ causes a brief, twitch contraction. Repolarization is brought about by a K^+ efflux through K_v, K_{Ca} and K_{ir} channels.

Contraction may/may not depend on membrane depolarization

Although α_1–adrenoceptor activation can trigger contraction through action potentials, as above, it can also cause contraction through depolarization-independent pathways. Depending on the mix of ion channels in a particular vessel, contraction can be triggered in three ways:

- **Contraction induced by action potentials** (Figure 12.2a and b). In some arterioles, small arteries and certain veins, VSCCs are so abundant that strong sympathetic stimulation triggers VSCC-based action potentials. Extracellular Ca^{2+} influx during the action potential raises intracellular Ca^{2+}, causing a twitch contraction. This has been called electromechanical coupling.
- **Contraction induced by graded, sustained depolarization** (Figure 12.1). In many blood vessels, noradrenaline evokes a graded, sustained depolarization, but no action potentials. The depolarization is brought about by i_{cat} and $i_{Cl(Ca)}$, which are activated via the G_q–PLCβ–IP$_3$/DAG pathway (Figure 12.6a). The depolarization activates VSCCs, leading to a sustained contraction. This is again electromechanical coupling.
- **Contraction unrelated to membrane potential** (Figures 12.2c and 12.6b). In large arteries, the myocytes often have abundant ROCs but few VSCCs. Noradrenaline raises the cytosolic Ca^{2+} partly through DAG-activated ROCs and partly through IP$_3$-mediated stored release. The contraction is not evoked by membrane depolarization – though the ROC current may cause a small, coincidental depolarization. This type of activation has been called pharmacomechanical coupling.

Sympathetic stimulation can evoke fast and slow EJPs, and both depolarization-dependent and depolarization-independent contraction

Having considered how noradrenaline alone affects vascular myocytes, we can return to the more complex case of sympathetic stimulation, which releases both noradrenaline and ATP. Sympathetic stimulation can evoke both depolarization-independent and depolarization-dependent contraction in the same

myocyte. This is illustrated by the response of a small arterial vessel to moderate sympathetic stimulation (Figure 12.9a). When the local sympathetic fibres are stimulated briefly, the myocyte electrical response has two components. After a very short latency, ~15 ms, there is a small, rapidly rising depolarization of -10 mV that is short-lived (1 s) – the **fast excitatory junction potential** (fast EJP). This is followed by a slow-rising, longer-lasting depolarization, similar to the **slow EJP** evoked by noradrenaline (Figure 12.8). What causes the two electrical responses?

The **fast EJP** is abolished by inhibitors of the purinergic (ATP) receptor, P$_{2X}$, so it must be triggered by sympathetic ATP (for proof, see Figure 14.3). Unlike the metabotropic adrenoceptor, the P$_{2X}$ receptor is an '**ionotropic**' receptor; that is to say, the receptor is directly linked to a cation-conducting channel, which is part of the same macromolecule (a **ligand-gated** channel).

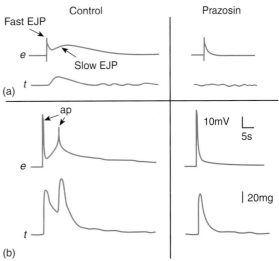

(a)

(b)

Figure 12.9 Simultaneous records of contractile tension (t) and membrane potential (e) recorded by an intracellular microelectrode in a rat tail artery. The perivascular nerves were stimulated by a single external pulse in each frame in the absence (*left*) or presence (*right*) of an α-adrenoceptor blocker, prazosin. (a) Medium intensity stimulation produced a fast excitatory junction potential (fast EJP, ATP-mediated) and a slow EJP (noradrenaline-mediated). Contraction preceded the slow EJP and was blocked by prazosin (depolarization-independent contraction). (b) Stimulation at higher intensity evoked larger fast and slow EJPs, each of which triggered an action potential (ap), with associated twitch contractions (depolarization-dependent contractions). Only the slower potentials and contraction were blocked by prazosin (From Cheung DW. *Pfluger's Archiv* 1984; **400**: 335–7, with kind permission from Springer Science and Business Media.)

Channel activation is therefore very fast. The activated channel conducts a small depolarizing current of Ca^{2+} and Na^+ into the myocyte. The **slow EJP** is abolished by α_1-adrenoceptor blockers, such as prazosin, so it is clearly triggered by noradrenaline (Figure 12.9, top right). It is generated by i_{cat} and $i_{Cl(Ca)}$, as described earlier (Figure 12.6a).

The **mechanical response** in Figure 12.9a, a slow contraction, is puzzling on close inspection. It cannot be caused by the slow EJP, because the contraction starts before the slow EJP. Nor can the contraction be caused by the fast EJP, since prazosin abolishes the contraction but not the fast EJP (Figure 12.9a, top right). The slow contraction is in fact an example of **depolarization-independent contraction**, due to ROC activation by α_1-adrenoceptors.

At a higher intensity of sympathetic stimulation, the fast EJP becomes larger and activates sufficient VSCCs to trigger an action potential and twitch contraction (Figure 12.9b). The slow depolarization becomes larger too, triggering another action potential, which produces a twitch superimposed on the underlying slow contraction. The twitches are examples of **depolarization-dependent contraction**, while the underlying slow contraction reflects depolarization-independent contraction. Both processes can occur in the same myocyte. It should be noted, however, that the electrical response to sympathetic stimulation varies greatly from vessel to vessel; not all vessels respond as above, although the pattern is a common one.

Intracellular free Ca^{2+} shows two phases during a vasoconstriction

If the vessel wall is loaded with a Ca^{2+}-sensitive fluorescent dye, it is found that the cytosolic free Ca^{2+} concentration exhibits two distinct phases following stimulation. In the **initial, transient phase** there is a rapid increase in cytosolic Ca^{2+} concentration, from $\sim 0.1\,\mu M$ to $\sim 1\,\mu M$. This occurs synchronously in all the myocytes throughout the vessel wall, and is followed almost immediately by a rise in tension (Figure 12.4a). In the **second, tonic phase**, starting 30–60 s later, the average cytosolic $[Ca^{2+}]$ in the vessel wall retreats to a lower but still suprabasal level; yet the force of contraction is well maintained. During the second phase individual myocytes may exhibit intermittent, asynchronous Ca^{2+} waves (Figure 12.4a), especially in small artery myocytes with a low contractile tone; the second phase Ca^{2+} tend to be more stable in vessels with a high basal tone. The pathways responsible for the two phases are as follows.

The initial phase is due to Ca^{2+} store release and extracellular Ca^{2+} influx

The initial large increase in myocyte free Ca^{2+} results from the release of stored Ca^{2+} from the SR, particularly in large arteries, aided by an influx of extracellular Ca^{2+}, particularly in small arteries and arterioles (Figure 12.7). In large arteries, Ca^{2+} store release accounts for most of the initial cytosolic Ca^{2+} transient, because the SR is well developed. Store discharge is triggered chiefly by receptor-induced IP_3 production. Store replenishment is brought about by an influx of extracellular Ca^{2+} ions through the store-operated TRP channels in the adjacent sarcolemma (capacitative Ca^{2+} entry). In smaller, resistance arteries/arterioles, extracellular Ca^{2+} influx is more important, because small resistance vessels tend to have scanty SR but abundant VSCCs. The VSCCs are activated by depolarization, which is brought about by i_{cat} and $i_{Cl(Ca)}$. Extracellular Ca^{2+} influx through the activated VSCCs, and also through ROCs, raises the cytosolic Ca^{2+} concentration.

To summarize the initial 30–60 s phase of vasoconstriction, the agonist–receptor complex activates the $PLC\beta$–IP_3–DAG pathway. IP_3 releases stored Ca^{2+}, which raises cytosolic Ca^{2+} and activates depolarizing current $i_{Cl(Ca)}$. The DAG activates depolarizing current i_{cat}. The depolarization by i_{cat} and $i_{Cl(Ca)}$ increases the open-state probability of sarcolemmal VSCCs, admitting extracellular Ca^{2+}. DAG also activates sarcolemmal ROCs, that admit extracellular Ca^{2+}. A $4Ca^{2+}$–calmodulin complex then activates MLCK, which phosphorylates the myosin light chains, enabling the myosin heads to form crossbridges with the actin filament. Crossbridge flexion then generates shortening and tension.

The second phase is sustained by extracellular Ca^{2+} influx and Ca^{2+} sensitization

During the tonic phase, the mean cytosolic Ca^{2+} concentration, averaged across the whole tunica media, drops below the transient peak value; and in some vessels the individual myocytes develop intermittent Ca^{2+} waves (Figure 12.4a). Each Ca^{2+} wave is generated by SR store discharge by IP_3. Since the sarcolemmal pumps expel some Ca^{2+} during each wave, extracellular Ca^{2+} influx through VSCCs and cat-SOCs is needed to recharge the stores. The importance of extracellular Ca^{2+} influx during tonic contraction is demonstrated by the relaxation induced by nifedipine and cat-SOC blockers.

During the tonic phase vasoconstriction is well maintained despite a fall in mean cytosolic $[Ca^{2+}]$ (Figure 12.4a). Therefore, some additional mechanism must come into play. This mechanism is Ca^{2+} **sensitization** – that is to say, a given level of Ca^{2+} has an increased contractile effect during the tonic phase.

Tonic Ca^{2+} sensitization is mediated by rhoA kinase and PKC

Ca^{2+} sensitization is brought about by kinases that are activated by the G protein-coupled receptors (Figure 12.7). Kinases are a large family of enzymes that phosphorylate other proteins to change their activity. The kinase chiefly responsible for Ca^{2+} sensitization is **rhoA kinase**. Agonist–receptor complexes coupled to G_{12} protein activate **rhoA**,

a monomeric GTPase that activates rhoA kinase. RhoA kinase inhibits myosin light chain phosphatase, the enzyme responsible for dephosphorylating the myosin head and turning off the myosin motor. This shifts the dynamic balance between MLC kinase and MLC phosphatase in favour of phosphorylation, despite a fall in Ca^{2+}–calmodulin.

Ca^{2+} sensitization is also promoted in some vessels by **protein kinase C-α** (PKCα), which is activated by DAG and cytosolic Ca^{2+} (Figure 12.6b). PKC activates CPI–17 protein, which, like rhoA kinase, inhibits myosin light chain phosphatase. PKC also triggers a MAP kinase pathway that phosphorylates **caldesmon**, a regulatory protein on the actin filament, facilitating crossbridge formation. This may explain why adrenergic-stimulated tone is maintained in some vessels despite a fall in myosin light chain phosphorylation.

12.6 Vasomotion (rhythmic contractions)

Most arteries and veins exhibit a stable vascular tone, but many arterioles (e.g. skeletal muscle, skin, Figure 15.10c), along with terminal pial arteries and the portal vein (Figure 12.2a), exhibit rhythmic contractions called vasomotion. Arteriolar vasomotion may help reduce net capillary filtration rate (Section 11.6). Vasomotion occurs several times per minute, and is brought about by co-ordinated, synchronous oscillations in cytosolic $[Ca^{2+}]$ throughout the tunica media (cf. asynchronous oscillations in the myocytes of tonically contracted vessels). The oscillations are due primarily to the cyclical release of the SR Ca^{2+} store by IP_3, boosted by VSCCs that are activated as $i_{Cl(Ca)}$ depolarizes the myocyte. The relaxation phase is due to Ca^{2+} sequestration by the SR pumps and repolarization by the calcium-activated BK current. Synchronization between the myocytes is probably mediated by the homocellular gap junctions, and in some cases the myoendothelial gap junctions, since vasomotion is endothelium-dependent in some vessels. In the portal vein, a different mechanism seems to operate; spontaneous myocyte depolarization triggers action potentials, which open VSCCs and cause the Ca^{2+} oscillation.

12.7 Physiological vasodilator mechanisms

The account so far has concentrated on vascular contraction. But a major function of blood vessels, especially resistance vessels, is to dilate, so as to raise

---

Regulation of vascular myocyte tone

- Active vascular tension (tone) is sustained. Tone is regulated by the sympathetic neuroeffector noradrenaline, circulating hormones (adrenaline, angiotensin II, vasopressin) and local factors (e.g. NO, EDHF, endothelin, hypoxia, histamine and other autacoids).
- Tone depends primarily on cytosolic $[Ca^{2+}]$. Ca^{2+}–calmodulin complex activates myosin light chain (MLC) kinase, which phosphorylates myosin heads to cause crossbridge formation. Conversely, if $[Ca^{2+}]$ falls, dephosphorylation by constitutively active MLC phosphatase causes relaxation.
- Agonists (e.g. noradrenaline) that activate G_q-protein-coupled receptors (e.g. α_1-adrenoceptor) can raise cytosolic $[Ca^{2+}]$ in three ways.
  - (i) G_q-activated PLCβ generates IP_3, which releases the Ca^{2+} store and activates store-operated Ca^{2+} channels (cat-SOCs).
  - (ii) PLCβ generates DAG, which activates receptor-operated Ca^{2+} channels (ROCs).
  - (iii) IP_3 and DAG trigger depolarizing currents that activate voltage-sensitive L-type Ca^{2+} channels (VSCCs).
- Tone is also regulated by rhoA kinase and protein kinase C, which sensitize the cell to Ca^{2+} by inhibiting MLC phosphatase.
- Vascular relaxation is brought about by reducing the free cytosolic $[Ca^{2+}]$ and/or Ca^{2+} desensitization. Free $[Ca^{2+}]$ can be reduced by hyperpolarization-induced closure of VSCCs (e.g. metabolic hyperaemia, EDHF), or by cAMP-activated protein kinase A (e.g. adrenaline-activated β_2 adrenoceptors), or by cGMP-activated protein kinase G (e.g. NO, penile erection).

blood flow to exercising muscle, myocardium, etc. Vasodilatation is not an active process; it is simply a reduction of tonic contractile tension, i.e. a relaxation, and it can be brought about by four mechanisms:

- hyperpolarization
- the adenylyl cyclase–cAMP–protein kinase A (PKA) pathway
- the guanylyl cyclase–cGMP–protein kinase G (PKG) pathway
- desensitization to Ca^{2+}.

The first three mechanisms produce vasodilatation by **reducing the cytosolic Ca^{2+} concentration**, which reduces MLC kinase activity. This allows the constitutive background MLC phosphatase activity to predominate and turn off the myosin motor. The fourth vasodilator mechanism, **desensensitization to Ca^{2+}**, produces vascular relaxation despite little fall in cytosolic Ca^{2+} concentration.

Hyperpolarization mediates vasodilatation by extracellular K^+, EDHF, hypoxia and neuropeptides

Hyperpolarization closes VSCCs, leading to a fall in cytosolic free $[Ca^{2+}]$ and vasodilatation (Figure 12.1). Examples are as follows.

- **Skeletal muscle contraction, myocardial contraction and brain activity** raise the K^+ ion concentration in the local interstitial fluid. Extravascular K^+ increases vascular K_{ir} activity (Section 12.4), leading to hyperpolarization and vasodilatation. This is one of several mechanisms that match blood flow to tissue metabolic activity (metabolic hyperaemia, Section 13.4).
- **Endothelium-derived hyperpolarization factors** (EDHF) elicit vasodilatation through myocyte hyperpolarization. The identity of EDHF (e.g. K^+, epoxyeicosatrienoic acid) was reviewed in Section 9.5. In feed arteries, conducted vasodilatation is due to the conduction of endothelial hyperpolarization into myocytes through myoendothelial gap junctions (Section 13.7).
- **Hypoxia**, if severe, can activate myocyte K_{ATP} channels (Section 12.4), leading to hyperpolarization, reduced cytosolic $[Ca^{2+}]$ and hypoxic vasodilatation. In many arteries, however, Ca^{2+} desensitization is the main mechanism underlying hypoxic vasodilatation, and there is little reduction in cytosolic $[Ca^{2+}]$.

- **Sensory nerve neuropeptides**, such as calcitonin-gene-related peptide and vasoactive intestinal polypeptide, are released during inflammation, and contribute to the vasodilatation of inflammation by causing hyperpolarization (Section 14.4).
- **K_{ATP}-activating drugs**, such as diazoxide, pinacidil and cromakalim, elicit vasodilatation through myocyte hyperpolarization.

cAMP–PKA-mediated vasodilatation is triggered by adrenaline β_2-receptors

Circulating adrenaline dilates the resistance vessels of skeletal muscle, myocardium and liver, because vascular β_2-adrenoceptors are strongly expressed in these tissues. (In most other tissues, α_1 density exceeds β_2 density, so adrenaline causes vasoconstriction.) The β_2-adrenoceptor is coupled to the trimeric membrane GTPase G_s, which activates membrane-bound adenylyl cyclase (Figure 12.10). Many other physiological vasodilators likewise activate G_s-coupled receptors, including **adenosine** (A_{2A} receptor), **prostacyclin** (EP_4 receptor), **histamine** (H_2 receptor), **vasoactive intestinal polypeptide** and **calcitonin-gene related peptide**. The activation of adenylyl (or adenylate) cyclase by any of these G_s-coupled receptors catalyses the conversion of ATP to cyclic adenosine monophosphate, cAMP. cAMP activates the phosphorylating enzyme **protein kinase A**. Protein kinase A (PKA) induces vascular relaxation by multiple actions (Figure 12.10).

- PKA phosphorylates **phospholamban**, a protein that normally acts as a brake on the Ca^{2+}–ATPase pump. Phosphorylation reduces this braking effect. PKA therefore stimulates SR and sarcolemma **Ca^{2+} pump activity**, leading to a fall in cytosolic free Ca^{2+}.
- PKA also phosphorylates **K_{ir}, K_{ATP} and K_{Ca} channels**, increasing their open state probability. The resulting hyperpolarization closes VSCCs and thus reduces extracellular Ca^{2+} influx.
- PKA phosphorylates and thereby **inhibits MLCK**. This reduces myosin activation at a given Ca^{2+} concentration, i.e. it reduces Ca^{2+} sensitivity.

The PKA activator, cAMP, is continuously degraded by the enzyme **phosphodiesterase type III** (Figure 12.10). Drugs that inhibit phosphodiesterase III, such as milrinone and cilostazol, raise intracellular cAMP, leading to vasodilatation.

Figure 12.10 Pathways by which adrenaline-activated β_2-adrenoceptors bring about vasodilatation. Adenosine A_{2A} receptors, histamine H_2 receptors, VIP and CGRP receptors are likewise coupled to adenylyl (adenylate) cyclase, leading to vasodilatation. Adenylyl cyclase can be activated directly by the drug forskolin. AMP, adenosine monophosphate; PDE III, phosphodiesterase III. Other abbreviations, see text. (After Ushio-Fukai M *et al. Journal of Physiology* 1993; **462**: 679–96, with permission from Wiley-Blackwell.)

cGMP–PKG-mediated vasodilatation is induced by nitric oxide

Nitric oxide (NO), nitrodilator drugs such as glyceryl trinitrate (commonly used to relieve angina), and the hormone atrial natriuretic peptide cause vasodilatation by raising the intracellular concentration of **cyclic guanosine monophosphate** (cGMP). NO activates guanylyl (guanylate) cyclase, which catalyses the production of cGMP from guanosine trisphosphate (Section 9.4, Figure 9.10). The cGMP activates **protein kinase G**, which has similar actions to PKA; it phosphorylates phospholamban to disinhibit the Ca^{2+}–ATPase pumps, leading to Ca^{2+} sequestration and Ca^{2+} expulsion; and

it reduces Ca^{2+} sensitization. In this way NO contributes to flow-induced vasodilatation, inflammatory vasodilatation, endotoxin shock and sexual erection (Chapter 13). The treatment of erectile dysfunction by the cGMP-boosting drug **sildenafil** (**Viagra**) is covered in Section 13.3.

Desensitization to Ca^{2+} occurs in hypoxic arteries

In many arteries hypoxia causes vasodilatation despite little fall in cytosolic free Ca^{2+} concentration (Figure 13.5). The vasodilatation is brought about by reduced myosin phosphorylation, possibly through the inhibition of rhoA kinase (Figure 12.7).

SUMMARY

- Vascular smooth muscle (VSM) comprises circumferential, spindle-shaped myocytes. Gap junctions provide an electrical connection between the myocytes, and between myocyte and endothelium. The contractile machinery comprises interdigitating thick myosin filaments and thin actin filaments. The latter are anchored to cytoplasmic dense bodies and sarcolemmal dense bands.

- Contraction is driven primarily by cytosolic $[Ca^{2+}]$, which forms a Ca^{2+}–calmodulin complex that activates **myosin light chain kinase** (MLCK). MLCK phosphorylates myosin heads, which then form myosin–actin crossbridges, causing contraction. The long duration of the crossbridges (latch state) maintains vascular tone with relatively little energy expenditure. When MLCK activity is reduced, dephosphorylation by **myosin light chain phosphatase** leads to relaxation.

■ Sarcolemmal **K^+ channels** conduct an outward current that generates a basal potential of about $-50\,mV$. Inward-rectifier K_{ir}, ATP-sensitive K_{ATP}, voltage-sensitive K_v and Ca-activated K_{Ca} (BK) channels all contribute. An inward cation current through constitutively active TRP channels contributes to the relatively depolarized basal potential.

■ Sarcolemmal **voltage-sensitive L-type Ca^{2+} channels** (VSCCs) exhibit an increase in open probability with membrane depolarization, leading to extracellular Ca^{2+} influx and contraction. **Depolarization-dependent contraction** is prominent in small, arterial resistance vessels, because they strongly express VSCCs.

■ **Sympathetic fibre activity** causes resistance vessels contraction. Fibre varicosities release ATP and noradrenaline, which evoke VSM **fast and slow excitatory junction potentials** (depolarizations) respectively. Noradrenaline α_1-adrenoceptors are G_q-coupled to PLCβ, which generates IP$_3$ and DAG. DAG activates cation-conducting TRP channels (current i_{cat}); IP$_3$ releases stored Ca^{2+} to activate Cl^- channels (current $i_{Cl(Ca)}$). Depolarization by i_{cat} and $i_{Cl(Ca)}$ creates the slow EJP. If the EJPs are large and VSCCs are abundant, as in arterioles, VSCC activation generates a **Ca^{2+}-mediated action potential** and twitch.

■ **Depolarization-independent contraction** can occur in large arteries. When a G_q-protein-coupled receptor, such as α_1 or H_1, activates the PLCβ–IP$_3$–DAG pathway, the IP$_3$ releases the sarcoplasmic reticulum **Ca^{2+} store** (substantial in large arteries), while DAG activates **receptor-operated cation channels** (ROCs) that conduct extracellular Ca^{2+} into the cell.

■ During prolonged vasoconstriction, an initial, transient phase of high cytosolic $[Ca^{2+}]$ due to store release is followed by a sustained phase of lower but still elevated $[Ca^{2+}]$. The contraction is maintained by (i) continuing **Ca^{2+} influx** through VSCCs, ROCs and SOCs (store-operated channels); and (ii) increased sensitivity to Ca^{2+}. **Ca^{2+} sensitization** is brought about by the inhibition of myosin light chain phosphatase by rhoA kinase and protein kinase C.

■ Some arterioles undergo rhythmic contractions (**vasomotion**), caused by regular, spontaneous waves of Ca^{2+} discharge from the sarcoplasmic reticulum store.

■ **Vasodilatation** is usually brought about by a **fall in cytosolic $[Ca^{2+}]$**, which deactivates MLCK, allowing myosin phosphatase to predominate and turn off the myosin motor. In addition, **desensitization to Ca^{2+}** can contribute to vasodilatation. Cytosolic $[Ca^{2+}]$ can be reduced by the following three mechanisms.

■ **Hyperpolarization** reduces VSCC open probability, leading to vasodilatation. In active skeletal muscle, myocardium and brain, increased interstitial $[K^+]$ raises the K_{ir} channel open probability, leading to hyperpolarization. This contributes to metabolic hyperaemia. Endothelium-derived hyperpolarizing factors (K^+, EET) likewise cause myocyte hyperpolarization and vasodilatation, as do some neuropeptides. Severe hypoxia activates K_{ATP} channels, leading to hyperpolarization and vasodilatation.

■ **cAMP-PKA**. G_s-coupled receptors, such as β_2-adrenoceptors, adenosine A_{2A} and histamine H_2 receptors, activate the adenylate cyclase–cAMP–protein kinase A pathway. PKA stimulates Ca^{2+}–ATPase pumps to reduce cytosolic $[Ca^{2+}]$; it phosphorylates K^+ channels to cause hyperpolarization, leading to VSCC closure; and it inactivates MLCK. This is how adrenaline causes vasodilatation in myocardium and skeletal muscle.

■ **cGMP-PKG**. Nitric oxide, nitrodilator drugs and atrial natriuretic peptide activate the guanylate cyclase–cGMP–protein kinase G pathway. PKG has similar effects to protein kinase A. NO mediates flow-induced dilatation, the vasodilatation of inflammation and sexual erection.

Further reading

Reviews and chapters

Albert A, Large WA. Signal transduction pathways and gating mechanisms of native TRP-like cation channels in vascular myocytes. *Journal of Physiology* 2006; **570**: 45–51.

Bény J-L, Koenigsberg M, Sauser R. Role of myoendothelial communications in arterial vasomotion. *American Journal of Physiology* 2006; **291**: H2036–8.

Cohen AW, Hnasko R, Schubert W, Lisanti MP. Role of caveolae and caveolins in health and disease. *Physiological Reviews* 2004; **84**: 1341–79.

Haddock RE, Hill CE (2005) Rhythmicity in arterial smooth muscle. *Journal of Physiology* 2005; **566**: 645–56. (Vasomotion)

Hirst GDS, Edwards FR. Sympathetic neuroeffector transmission in arteries and arterioles. *Physiological Reviews* 1989; **69**: 546–604.

Ledoux J, Werner ME, Brayden JE, Nelson MT. Calcium-activated potassium channels and the regulation of vascular tone. *Physiology* 2006; **21**: 69–79.

Li P-L, Lee HC, Nelson MT, Meininger GA, Van Breemen C. Novel Ca^{2+} signalling mechanisms in vascular myocytes: Symposium overview. *Acta Physiologica Scandinavica* 2003; **179**: 339–52.

Jackson WF. Potassium channels in the peripheral microcirculation. *Microcirculation* 2005; **12**: 113–27.

Mulvany MJ, Alkjaer C, Arner A, Hellstrand P. Vascular smooth muscle (symposium). *Acta Physiologica Scandinavica* 1998; **164**: 339–644.

O'Donnell ME, Owen NE. Regulation of ion pumps and carriers in vascular smooth muscle. *Physiological Reviews* 1994; **74**: 683–722.

Quayle JM, Nelson MT, Standen NB. ATP-sensitive and inwardly rectifying potassium channels in smooth muscle. *Physiological Reviews* 1997; **77**: 1165–216.

Somlyo AP, Somlyo AV. Ca^{2+} sensitivity of smooth muscle and non-muscle myosin II: Modulation by G proteins, kinases and myosin phosphatase. *Physiological Reviews* 2003; **83**: 1325–58.

Taggart MJ. Smooth muscle excitation–contraction coupling: A role for caveolae and caveolins? *News in Physiological Science* 2001; **16**: 61–5.

Wier WG, Morgan KG. α_1-Adrenergic signaling mechanisms in contraction of resistance arteries. *Reviews of Physiology, Biochemistry and Pharmacology* 2003; **150**: 91–139.

Research papers

See www.hodderplus.com/cardiovascularphysiology for a full list of Research papers for this chapter.

CHAPTER 13

Control of blood vessels: I. Intrinsic control

Learning objectives

After reading this chapter you should be able to:

- Sketch the myogenic response of arterioles to a pressure change and explain its importance (13.2).
- List the chief roles of nitric oxide in the circulation (13.3).
- State the role of metabolic hyperaemia and name the putative mediators (13.4).
- Give thumbnail sketches of the autacoids histamine, bradykinin, serotonin, PAF, prostacyclin and thromboxane (13.5).
- Illustrate 'autoregulation' by drawing a plot of blood flow versus perfusion pressure. Draw a second curve to show how autoregulation is affected by metabolic hyperaemia (13.6).
- Explain how dilatation is co-ordinated along the arterial tree in exercise (13.7).
- Outline how post-ischaemic hyperaemia arises (13.8).
- Explain the basis of ischaemia–reperfusion injury (13.9).

13.1 Overview of vascular control and its roles

The tension exerted by vascular smooth muscle is called the vascular 'tone'. Vascular tone regulates the calibre of the resistance vessel, and hence the blood flow through it. An increase in tone causes vasoconstriction and reduces local flow. Conversely, a fall in tone causes vasodilatation, by allowing the blood pressure to distend the relaxed vessel. Vascular tone is thus an essential prerequisite for vasodilatation (loss of tone), and basal vascular tone is high in tissues capable of substantially increasing their blood flow (hyperaemia), e.g. skeletal muscle.

Arterial vessels maintain some vascular tone even when the tonic sympathetic vasoconstrictor nerve activity is blocked. This is called **basal tone**. Basal tone is generally low in veins. Basal tone is the result of tonic vasoconstrictor influences (constitutively active myocyte TRP channels, myogenic response,

endothelin), partially offset by tonic vasodilator influences (nitric oxide, EDHF). Vascular tone *in vivo* is generally supra-basal due to the tonic vasoconstrictor activity of sympathetic fibres.

Before we delve further into the processes that regulate vascular tone, let us first summarize its many roles, drawing together key points from earlier chapters.

Vascular tone regulates regional blood flow, arterial blood pressure, capillary filtration rate and central venous pressure

- **Regional blood flow** through a tissue is altered through changes in resistance vessel radius, r. A small change in r has a huge effect on resistance to flow, due to the r^4 term in Poiseuille's law (Section 8.7). This allows tissues to alter their blood flow over a huge range. In skin, skeletal muscle and exocrine glands the **flow can be**

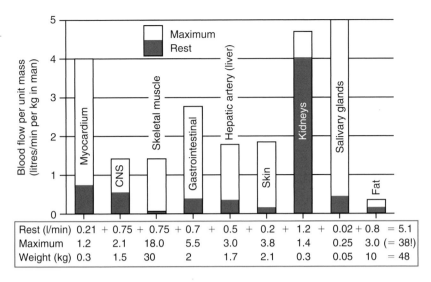

Figure 13.1 Wide range of blood flow from rest to maximal in tissues of a 70 kg human. Maximal flow through all organs simultaneously can never be achieved, because at 38 litres/min it exceeds maximum cardiac output. CNS, central nervous system. (Data from Mellander S, Johansson B. *Pharmacological Reviews* 1968; **20**: 117–96, by permission.)

	Myocardium	CNS	Skeletal muscle	Gastrointestinal	Hepatic artery (liver)	Skin	Kidneys	Salivary glands	Fat	
Rest (l/min)	0.21 +	0.75 +	0.75 +	0.7 +	0.5 +	0.2 +	1.2 +	0.02 +	0.8	= 5.1
Maximum	1.2	2.1	18.0	5.5	3.0	3.8	1.4	0.25	3.0	(= 38!)
Weight (kg)	0.3	1.5	30	2	1.7	2.1	0.3	0.05	10	= 48

increased 20-fold by vasodilatation, to meet the demands of temperature regulation, exercise and liquid secretion, respectively (Figure 13.1). Indeed the maximal tissue blood flows are so huge that they could never be achieved simultaneously, because the total flow would then exceed the maximum output of the heart.

- **Arterial blood pressure** is the product of total peripheral resistance and cardiac output (Section 8.5). The continual adjustment of resistance vessel tone helps control arterial pressure during normal activities, such as standing up. During hypovolaemic emergencies such as haemorrhage, vasoconstriction helps to maintain the blood pressure.
- **Capillary recruitment** and **capillary pressure** are regulated by local arteriolar tone. Vasodilatation in exercising muscle improves perfusion homogeneity and perfused capillary surface area, boosting solute exchange (Figures 10.14). Arteriolar tone also regulates capillary pressure, and therefore fluid exchange and plasma volume (Figure 11.4).
- **Central venous pressure** is regulated by the tone of the peripheral veins and venules. Peripheral venoconstriction displaces blood into the central veins, thus raising the cardiac filling pressure and stroke volume (Starling's law of the heart, Section 6.6).

From the above résumé we see that changes in vascular tone act both at a **local** level to regulate tissue perfusion, nutrient and water exchange; and at the level of the **whole animal** to regulate arterial blood pressure, plasma volume, central venous pressure and stroke volume.

Vascular tone is controlled by intrinsic and extrinsic mechanisms

The processes that regulate vascular tone fall into two classes: intrinsic and extrinsic (Figure 13.2). Intrinsic regulation is regulation by factors located entirely within an organ or tissue. Extrinsic regulation is regulation by factors from outside the organ. **Intrinsic regulatory mechanisms** include:

- **the Bayliss myogenic response** to arterial pressure;
- **endothelial secretions** (nitric oxide, EDHF, prostacyclin, endothelin);
- **vasoactive metabolites** generated by active tissues, e.g. adenosine;
- **autacoids** (vasoactive paracrine secretions such as histamine); and
- **temperature**, which is chiefly important in the skin (Chapter 15).

Many major responses are mediated purely by intrinsic regulation, notably **flow autoregulation**, **functional and reactive hyperaemia**, **inflammatory vasodilatation** and **arterial vasospasm**.

Extrinsic regulation is brought about by:

- **vasomotor nerves**, mainly sympathetic; and
- **vasoactive hormones** such as adrenaline, angiotensin II and vasopressin.

The control hierarchy

Vascular regulation involves a hierarchy of control processes. The lowest level is intrinsic regulation by the Bayliss myogenic response. The middle level is the modulation of the myogenic response by

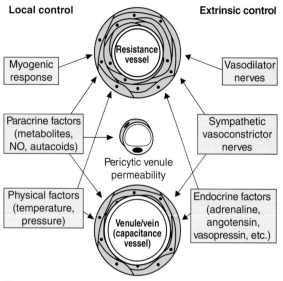

Figure 13.2 Overview of vascular control.

Figure 13.3 Change in diameter of isolated rat cerebral artery upon raising luminal pressure P. Initial passive stretch is followed by active contraction – the Bayliss myogenic response. This is abolished by the L-type Ca^{2+} channel blocker, nimodipine. Wall tension T, calculated from Laplace's law (eqn. 8.8), is increased and provides a sustained stimulus. (Based on McCarron JG, Crichton CA, Langton PD, MacKenzie A, Smith GL. *Journal of Physiology* 1997; **498**: 371–9, with permission from Wiley-Blackwell; and Carlson BE, Secomb TW. *Microcirculation* 2005; **12**: 327–38, with permission from Taylor & Francis Group.)

endothelial secretions, vasoactive metabolites and autacoids. These two levels of control provide for local tissues needs, e.g. constancy of renal perfusion (myogenic response), hyperaemia of exercising muscles (vasoactive metabolites). The highest level of control is exercised by the extrinsic factors (Chapter 14), which modify or override the intrinsic controls to meet the needs of the whole animal, as in the sympathetic-mediated peripheral vasoconstriction during a haemorrhage.

13.2 Myogenic response to blood pressure changes

Arterial vessels respond actively to changes in transmural pressure, as follows.

Arterial vessels contract when blood pressure is raised – the Bayliss myogenic response

The myogenic response was first described by Sir William Bayliss, brother-in-law of Ernest Starling, in 1902. When blood pressure is raised acutely in an artery or arteriole, the pressure at first distends the vessel. Within seconds, however, most systemic arterioles and arteries react and undergo a well-sustained contraction – the myogenic response (Figure 13.3). Conversely, a fall in pressure triggers a fall in vascular tone and vasodilatation. The myogenic response is important because (i) it contributes to basal tone and (ii) it stabilizes tissue blood flow and capillary filtration pressure if arterial pressure changes (autoregulation, Section 13.6). The myogenic response is well developed in the brain, kidney and myocardium, but not skin.

The myogenic response is mediated by depolarization and Ca^{2+}

When an arterial myocyte is stretched, it depolarizes to around $-40\,mV$. This activates L-type Ca^{2+} channels, leading to a rise in cytosolic free $[Ca^{2+}]$ and contraction. The depolarization is attributed to stretch-activated channels, namely TRP cation channels, volume-regulated chloride channels and ENaC-like channels (epithelial Na^+ channels), because the myogenic response is impaired by gadolinium (TRP-channel blocker), chloride channel blockers and amiloride (ENaC blocker), as well as Ca^{2+} channel blockers (Figure 13.3).

The above pathway drives the initial myogenic vasoconstriction. Over longer periods, Ca^{2+} sensitization by protein kinase C and rhoA kinase helps maintain the response (Figure 12.7). The depolarization is sustained by reduced K_{Ca} channel activity, elicited by the vasoconstrictor 20-HETE (20-hydroxy-eicosa-tetra-enoic acid). 20-HETE is produced from arachidonic acid by the enzyme P450 ω-hydroxylase.

When a vessel narrows due to the myogenic response, the endothelial shear stress increases, stimulating the endothelium to produce more nitric oxide and EDHF. These vasodilators help prevent excessive myogenic constriction.

Wall tension sustains the myogenic response

A puzzling feature of the myogenic response is that the vessel wall is only stretched temporarily, at the start. During the tonic contraction the vessel circumference and myocyte lengths are actually smaller than at the outset, yet the response is well maintained (Figure 13.3). However the wall **tension** is increased, due to the rise in pressure (Laplace's law, Section 8.7). It is thought, therefore, that the response is mediated by tension, acting on the membrane ion channels and on membrane integrins linked to protein kinases.

External pressure impairs flow and can cause pressure ulcers

When pressure is applied to the outside of a blood vessel, the vessel is compressed and blood flow falls. This happens to the intramural coronary arteries during systole, temporarily impairing myocardial perfusion (Figure 15.5). Similarly, blood flow to skeletal muscle is impaired during a contraction, because intra-muscle pressure can reach 270–570 mmHg (Figure 13.8). Sitting, kneeling and lying compresses blood vessels in the skin. If this is prolonged, as in elderly bedridden or paralysed patients, the resulting impairment of skin nutrition can cause horrific ulcers over the buttocks and heels, called **pressure ulcers** (**bed sores**). These can be avoided by good nursing care, namely regularly turning the patient to relieve the cutaneous compression.

13.3 Regulation by endothelium

Endothelium produces the vasoconstrictor endothelin and the vasodilators nitric oxide (NO), endothelium-derived hyperpolarizing factor (EDHF) and prostacyclin (PGI_2). These are paracrine agents, acting locally on neighbouring myocytes. Their production and roles were covered in Sections 9.4 and 9.5; here we concentrate on vascular regulation by NO and endothelin.

The chief roles of NO in vascular control are:

- continuous modulation of **basal tone**
- reduction of basal tone in **pregnancy**
- **flow-induced vasodilatation** of conduit arteries to muscle in exercise
- vasodilatation mediated by **cholinergic parasympathetic fibres**
- vasodilatation of **sexual erection**
- vasodilatation during **inflammation** and **endotoxic shock**.

Shear-stimulated NO production modulates basal vascular tone

The chief, normal stimulus for endothelial NO production is the **shear stress** exerted by the bloodstream, which drives ~60–80% of tonic NO formation. Other stimuli include circulating **insulin** and **oestrogen**. Shear stress, not flow, is clearly the stimulus, because raising the blood viscosity (and hence shear stress) evokes vasodilatation when flow is held constant. Shear stress is sensed by the endothelial glycocalyx, which activates the PI_3 kinase–PKB pathway (Figure 9.10). This increases the activity of endothelial NO synthase, **eNOS**. Since NO causes local vasodilatation, it reduces shear stress. Shear-dependent NO production thus results in a negative feedback loop that helps to stabilize endothelial shear stress.

NO is evidently produced continuously and influences human peripheral resistance, because the synthesis inhibitor L-NMMA reduces blood flow in the forearm (Figure 13.4). NOS inhibitors also approximately halve the renal blood flow, a greater effect than in most other tissues. Human vascular tone is thus the result of a balance between tonic relaxation mediated by NO (also EDHF and prostacyclin) and tonic vasoconstriction mediated by constitutive TRP channel activity, the myogenic response, endothelin, sympathetic vasomotor activity and circulating hormones.

During **pregnancy** high oestrogen levels stimulate NO production, leading to a generalized vasorelaxation. Along with the expansion of the uterine and placental vascular beds by angiogenesis, this greatly reduces peripheral resistance. Consequently, blood pressure falls, despite a 50% increase in cardiac output.

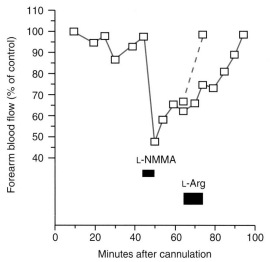

Figure 13.4 Role of nitric oxide (NO) in regulating vascular resistance of human forearm. An inhibitor of NO production, N-monomethyl-L-arginine (L-NMMA), was infused into the brachial artery. The 50% reduction in flow indicates that there is normally a tonic production of the vasodilator NO. Inhibition was reversed by the NO substrate, L-arginine (broken line). (After Vallance P, Collier J, Moncada S. *The Lancet* 1989; **ii**: 997–1000, with permission from Elsevier.)

Shear-stimulated NO production causes large-artery dilatation during exercise

When fluid is pumped through an isolated, large artery, raising the flow causes vasodilatation. This flow-induced dilatation is mediated by shear stress, and can be blocked by inhibitors of NO secretion. Flow-induced dilatation occurs in small arteries too, where EDHF may contribute to the response. Flow-induced vasodilatation can be demonstrated in human arteries *in vivo* during exercise. For example, the diameter of the human brachial artery increases by ≥10% during forearm exercise. At the onset of the exercise the small resistance vessels inside the active muscle dilate first (metabolic vasodilatation, Section 13.4), lowering the vascular resistance. This raises the blood flow through the conduit artery supplying the muscle. The resulting rise in artery shear stress stimulates NO secretion. Thus the conduit artery dilates, even though it is a considerable distance from the intra-muscle vasodilator metabolites.

The pressure profiles in Figures 1.10 and 8.16 show that conduit artery resistance is only a tiny fraction of the resting vascular resistance. So is the dilatation of a large artery of any real value during exercise? The answer is 'Yes', for two reasons. First, dilatation attenuates the rise in endothelial shear stress in the big vessels. Second, once resistance vessel dilatation in the exercising muscle has reduced the downstream resistance to a low level, the upstream conduit artery resistance becomes a significant fraction of the total vascular resistance. This would limit the increase in blood flow, were it not for the flow-induced artery vasodilatation. Endothelial NO thus **couples conduit artery resistance to arteriolar resistance**.

Neural NO mediates the vasodilatation of sexual erection

Penile erection is brought about by the dilatation of helicine arteries and smooth muscle in the corpus cavernosum; clitoral erection has a similar basis. The dilatation is triggered by nitridergic parasympathetic nerves, i.e. nerve fibres that contain a neural isoform of nitric oxide synthase, **nNOS**, and generate NO (Section 14.2). The NO produces vasodilatation through the guanylyl cyclase–cGMP–PKG pathway (Figure 9.10). Male impotence can be treated by inhibitors of the cGMP-degrading enzyme **phosphodiesterase type 5**, such as sildenafil (Viagra), which raises vascular cGMP and thereby amplify the erectile effect of nitridergic fibre activity.

Endothelial NO contributes to the vasodilatation of inflammation

The familiar redness and heat of an inflamed tissue are caused by vasodilatation. The vasodilatation is due partly to increased NO production. Several inflammatory autacoids, including bradykinin, thrombin and substance P, produce vasodilatation by activating **eNOS**. In addition, the inflammatory cytokines induce the synthesis of a third isoform, inducible nitric oxide synthase, **iNOS**.

Inducible NOS contributes to endotoxin shock

Endotoxin shock is a severe, intractable form of hypotension caused by bacterial infection. Endotoxin is a bacterial lipopolysaccharide that stimulates circulating monocytes and tissue macrophages to secrete cytokines, such as interferon-γ. Over several hours the cytokines induce the transcription-translation of an isoform of NOS called inducible nitric oxide synthase, **iNOS** (NOS-II). iNOS differs from constitutively expressed eNOS in that it is a cytosolic enzyme (cf. caveolin-bound eNOS); it does not require activation by Ca^{2+}–calmodulin; and it produces NO at a much faster rate than eNOS. The induction of iNOS in vascular myocytes, macrophages and endothelial cells contributes to a generalized vasodilatation and hypotension. Disappointingly, the treatment of endotoxin shock with iNOS inhibitors has not significantly improved survival rates, to date.

Nitrate drugs act through NO release

Drugs, such as glyceryl trinitrate, sodium nitroprusside and isosorbide dinitrate, have long been used as vasodilators to treat cardiac angina. It is now appreciated that the nitrodilators act by mimicking endothelial NO. They are very effective as venodilators and large artery dilators. Their therapeutic benefit is due partly to the reduction of central venous pressure by peripheral venodilatation, and partly to the reduction of systolic blood pressure through arterial relaxation (increased compliance) and reduced wave reflection (Section 8.4). Both changes reduces the cardiac stroke work and hence O_2 demand.

Endothelin contributes to basal tone and pathological conditions

Endothelium also constitutively secretes a vasoconstrictor peptide, endothelin. Endothelin ET_A and ET_B receptors on arterial and venous myocytes activate the PLC–DAG pathway, which activates TRPC non-selective cation channels and thereby raises the cytosolic free $[Ca^{2+}]$ (Figure 12.6b). Due to the prolonged binding of endothelin, the vasoconstriction and venoconstriction last 2–3 hours.

Physiological role

Although plasma endothelin levels are low, the $ET_{A/B}$-receptor antagonist **bosentan** causes a small fall in blood pressure. Similarly, phospharamidon, an inhibitor of endothelin production, causes dilatation in the human forearm and rat coronary artery. These observations show that endothelin makes a small contribution to the basal tone of resistance vessels.

Pathological roles

Hypoxia stimulates endothelin production, so plasma levels increase with altitude and may contribute to **high-altitude pulmonary hypertension**. Plasma endothelin is also raised in **pre-eclamptic toxaemia**, the acute hypertension of pregnancy. Endothelin makes a small contribution to essential hypertension (Chapter 18). In **heart failure**, a raised plasma endothelin also contributes to the characteristic renal and peripheral vasoconstriction.

Consequently, bosentan significantly increases peripheral blood flow, dilates veins and reduces blood pressure in heart failure patients. **Subarachnoid haemorrhage**, **ischaemic stroke**s and **brain trauma** raise the endothelin content of cerebrospinal fluid, contributing to the **cerebral vasospasm** associated with these conditions. Cerebral vasospasm is ameliorated by bosentan.

13.4 Regulation by metabolic vasoactive factors

As the celebrated eighteenth century anatomist John Hunter pointed out, 'Blood flow goes where it is needed'. When the metabolic activity of **myocardium, skeletal muscle** or **cerebral neurons** increases, the blood flow to the active region increases substantially, within seconds (Figures 13.1, 13.7 and 13.8). This metabolism-driven increase in blood flow is called **functional hyperaemia** or **metabolic hyperaemia** or **metabolic vasodilatation**. Metabolic hyperaemia is graded, so oxygen delivery increases in proportion to oxygen demand (Figure 15.4). The hyperaemia is caused by vasodilator substances released from the active cells, as indicated by experiments in which the fluid bathing stimulated cardiac myocytes acquires a vasodilator capacity, in proportion to stimulation intensity. The metabolic vasodilators act locally on the resistance vessels within the active tissue, with the more distal, smallest resistance vessels showing greater sensitivity than the more proximal, larger vessels (Figure 13.9). Despite a century of research, however, we still do not know for certain which agents account for metabolic hyperaemia. Potassium ions, H^+ ions (acidosis), hypoxia, adenosine, ATP, phosphate ions, hyperosmolarity and hydrogen peroxide all increase in the interstitium with increased tissue activity, and each has a vasodilator effect. Their relative importance seems to depend on the time point and the particular tissue. Potassium ions and CO_2, for example, are particularly important regulators of cerebral vessels, while potassium and adenosine seem important in striated muscle.

Interstitial K^+

When muscles contract or cerebral neuron activity increases, the outward, repolarizing current of the action potential transfers intracellular K^+ into the extracellular space. In the early stage of exercise, interstitial $[K^+]$ can more than double in an active skeletal muscle, from 4 mM to 9 mM. This stimulates the hyperpolarizing $3Na^+–2K^+$ pumps of vascular myocytes and increases their K_{ir} channel activity (Section 12.4). The resulting hyperpolarization leads to vasodilatation (Section 12.7). Rises in interstitial $[K^+]$ are most pronounced at early time-points, then decay as the tissue approaches a new steady state, especially in the brain. Therefore, interstitial $[K^+]$ may contribute more to the rapid-onset, initial phase of metabolic hyperaemia (first few seconds) than the later, sustained phase.

Acidosis

Increased metabolic activity causes local tissue acidosis, due to the generation of more CO_2 (forming carbonic acid in solution) and lactic acid. Acidosis causes vasodilatation (Figure 12.1), as discovered by WH Gaskell in 1880. **Cerebral blood vessels** are particularly sensitive to CO_2, so arterial pCO_2 is an important regulator of cerebral blood flow (Figure 15.13). Vessels in skeletal muscle and myocardium, however, respond only weakly, so acidosis probably contributes relatively little to exercise hyperaemia. Acidosis causes vasorelaxation via hyperpolarization and endothelial NO release (Appendix 2).

Hypoxia

Hypoxia can affect blood vessels locally and/or via reflexes. This section describes the local effect; hypoxia-induced reflexes are covered in Chapter 18. Hypoxia affects systemic and pulmonary vessels differently, as follows.

Hypoxia dilates systemic resistance vessels

The partial pressure of O_2 in arterial blood, P_{aO_2}, is normally 100 mmHg or 13 kPa. When blood with a P_{aO_2} of <40 mmHg (<5 kPa) is perfused through skeletal muscles, myocardium or the brain, the arterioles dilate (Figure 13.5). Hypoxia thus has a local vasodilator effect, and the increase in blood flow helps offset the low O_2 content. Even isolated vascular myocytes exhibit hypoxic relaxation, so it is not endothelium or NO dependent. Hypoxic vasodilatation is mediated by multiple mechanisms, which differ between vessel (Appendix 2). In some vessels, hypoxia activates K_{ATP} and possibly K_{ir} channels, leading to a hyperpolarization-mediated fall in $[Ca^{2+}]$ and relaxation (Figure 12.1). But in other vessels $[Ca^{2+}]$ remains almost unchanged – instead, Ca^{2+} sensitivity falls (Figure 13.5). Desensitization

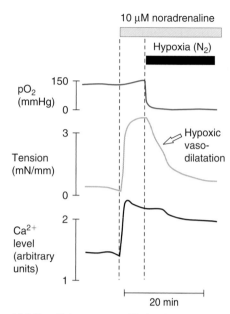

Figure 13.5 Vasodilator response of isolated rat mesenteric artery to acute hypoxia. Since vasodilatation is a loss of tone, tone was first established using noradrenaline. Hypoxic vasodilatation of this vessels involves little to no fall in Ca^{2+}, and is due to a fall in sensitivity to Ca^{2+}. In some arteries, hypoxia reduces intracellular free Ca^{2+}, due to a hyperpolarization-mediated closure of L-type Ca^{2+} channels. (Adapted from Bruce J, Taggart M, Austin C. *Microvascular Research* 2004; **68**: 303–312, with permission from Elsevier.)

is probably due to hypoxic inhibition of rhoA kinase, leading to reduced myosin light chain phosphorylation (Figure 12.7).

Although hypoxia causes vasodilatation, the arterioles are perfused with blood of normal oxygen content in exercising muscle or myocardium. Since O_2 permeates the arteriole wall freely, the vascular myocytes are unlikely to be hypoxic, except during a sustained muscle contraction (which impairs perfusion). The skeletal muscle fibres, by contrast, become hypoxic as their O_2 consumption rises, leading to the formation of the vasodilator **adenosine** (see below).

Hypoxia constricts pulmonary vessels and large systemic arteries

Although hypoxia dilates systemic arterioles, it constricts pulmonary blood vessels. Hypoxic pulmonary vasoconstriction is a normal, physiologically beneficial response (Section 15.5), though it can cause problems at high altitude. Hypoxia can also trigger vasospasm in large systemic arteries, such as coronary arteries, due partly to the release of noradrenaline from the hypoxic sympathetic fibres (Appendix 2, 'Hypoxia').

Adenosine

The vasodilator adenosine may account for ~20–40% of the sustained phase of metabolic hyperaemia in exercising skeletal muscle, and contributes to myocardial hyperaemia too. Adenosine is formed in active myocardium and skeletal muscles by the dephosphorylation of extracellular adenosine monophosphate (AMP) by AMP $5'$-nucleotidase, an ecto-enzyme (outward facing enzyme). AMP, a breakdown product of ATP, is released into the extracellular fluid in increasing amounts during exercise or systemic hypoxia. Adenosine binds to vascular myocyte A_{2A} receptors, which are coupled to the Gs–adenylyl cyclase–cAMP vasodilator pathway (Figure 12.10; also Appendix 2).

A good correlation has been reported between myocardial metabolic rate, coronary blood flow and coronary venous adenosine content. Experimental degradation of the myocardial adenosine, by infusing adenosine deaminase, approximately halves the metabolic hyperaemia. Similarly, the metabolic hyperaemia of skeletal muscle or brain is substantially attenuated by perfusion with the adenosine receptor blocker phenyltheophylline. Considerable hyperaemia always persists, however, so adenosine is clearly not the sole factor mediating metabolic hyperaemia.

By contrast, adenosine A_1 receptors in the kidney are coupled to G_i protein, so adenosine triggers vasoconstriction in renal afferent arterioles. This is part of a feedback system to stabilize glomerular filtration rate (tubuloglomerular feedback).

Phosphate ions and hyperosmolarity

A rise in interstitial phosphate or osmolarity elicits vasodilatation, and both changes occur during exercise. **Inorganic phosphate ions** are released into the interstitial fluid of active muscle following the breakdown of creatine phosphate and ATP. This change, in combination with the accumulating K^+ ions and lactate (30 mM lactate in intense exercise, cf. 0.6 mM normally), raises the **osmolarity** of the interstitial fluid during the early stages of exercise. As a result, the osmolarity of the venous blood from active muscle increases by 4–40 milliosmoles per litre.

Hydrogen peroxide

Hydrogen peroxide (H_2O_2) is a freely permeable, hyperpolarizing vasodilator. It is generated by mitochondrial superoxide dismutase from superoxide, O_2^-. Mitochondrial production of superoxide increases as O_2 consumption increases. A good correlation between H_2O_2 production and the degree of metabolic hyperaemia has been reported in myocardium and skeletal muscle.

To summarize, no one metabolic vasodilator can explain the rapid onset and sustained nature of metabolic hyperaemia. Many factors seem to contribute, and a full 'accountancy' still eludes us, despite more than a century of research.

Mechanisms of action of individual vasodilators

Some readers will wish to know more about how each metabolic vasodilator acts. Others may feel that their heads are spinning enough already! Multiple pathways are generally involved, and brief accounts are provided in the Appendix 2 under the same headings as above.

13.5 Regulation by autacoids

Autacoids (auto, self; akos, remedy) are organic, paracrine vasoactive chemicals, i.e. agents produced locally, released locally and acting locally on nearby vascular myocytes. Autacoids are involved mainly in pathological events, such as inflammation and bleeding. They include histamine, bradykinin, serotonin (5-hydroxytryptamine), prostaglandins, thromboxane, leukotrienes and PAF (platelet activating factor). The following 'thumbnail sketches' describe the principal autacoids.

Histamine

Histamine is formed by the decarboxylation of the amino acid histidine. It is stored in granules in basophilic leukocytes and tissue mast cells, particularly in tissues that interface with the environment, i.e. skin, lungs and gut. Histamine is one of the chemical mediators of **inflammation**, being released in response to trauma and allergic reactions (urticaria, anaphylaxis, asthma). Histamine H_1 receptors on postcapillary venules are coupled to the G_q–PLC pathway, leading to increased venular permeability (Figure 11.30). H_2 receptors on arteriolar myocytes are coupled to the G_s–adenylyl cyclase pathway, leading to vasodilatation (Figure 12.10). Histamine thus dilates arterioles and increases venular permeability – the characteristic features of inflammation. Cutaneous histamine elicits the itchy, prickling sensation of mild inflammation, and also the Lewis triple response (Section 14.4). The culprits, the H_1 receptors, can be blocked by the 'antihistamine' mepyramine.

Bradykinin

Bradykinin is a nonapeptide, cleaved from its parent plasma protein, kininogen, by the enzyme kallikrein. Kallikrein is activated during **inflammation**. Bradykinin, like histamine, elicits vasodilatation and venular hyperpermeability, thereby contributing to the hyperaemia and swelling of inflammation. Bradykinin is also the most potent **pain** producing autacoid. Endothelium constitutively expresses bradykinin B_2 receptors, which are G_q- or G_i-coupled; B_1 receptors are induced by inflammation. Receptor activation stimulates the endothelium to produce NO in some tissues, prostacyclin in others, and possibly EDHF in human skin. These agents then act locally to cause vasodilatation.

Serotonin (5-hydroxytryptamine, 5-HT)

Serotonin is synthesized by tryptophan hydoxylase from the amino acid tryptophan in intestinal enterochromaffin cells, endothelium, some central neurons and stinging nettles. Circulating serotonin also accumulates inside platelets at a high concentration. There are at least seven types of serotonin HT receptor. The principle effects are vasoconstriction, venular hyperpermeability and pain.

- **Platelet serotonin.** When the circulation is breached, platelets encounter collagen, which causes the platelets to release their serotonin into the serum (hence the name serotonin). Arterial myocyte $5HT_{2A}$ receptors are coupled to the PLC–IP_3 pathway (Figure 12.6), so an intense vasospasm ensues, slowing or arresting the bleeding. This beneficial mechanism can cause harm, however, in atheromatous coronary arteries. If the surface of the atheromatous plaque splits, exposing collagen, platelets are activated inappropriately, and the released serotonin, along with thromboxane and PAF (see below), cause **coronary vasospasm** and angina.
- **Enterochromaffin (argentaffin) cells** in the intestinal mucosa contain ~90% of all serotonin. Here serotonin helps regulate intestinal motility. The argentaffin cells occasionally give rise to a **carcinoid tumour**, which releases large quantities of serotonin into the circulation. This causes attacks of hypertension and diarrhoea.
- **Central neuron serotonin.** Serotonin is a central neurotransmitter, and the serotonin antagonist, lysergic acid diamine (LSD), is hallucinogenic. Serotonin is also found in neurons

close to large intracranial blood vessels and in perivascular nerve fibres. Its release following a cerebral haemorrhage activates $5HT_{1D}$ receptors on the cerebral blood vessels, leading to **cerebral artery vasospasm** and hence cerebral infarction (haemorrhagic stroke). Conversely, excessive cerebral vasodilatation, which can cause vascular headaches and migraine (Section 15.4), can be treated with the selective $5HT_{1D}$ agonist **sumatriptan**.

- **Pulmonary hypertension.** Pulmonary arterial hypertension is a chronic, little understood condition that leads to right ventricular failure. There is growing evidence that some forms of this condition are due to the proliferation of pulmonary arterial myocytes under the influences of serotonin.

Prostaglandins and thromboxane (eicosanoids, prostanoids)

Prostaglandins and thromboxane are vasoactive agents synthesized from a 20-carbon unsaturated fatty acid in the cell membrane, **arachidonic acid** (AA). Since AA is an eicosa-tetra-enoic acid (eicosa-, 20 carbon chain; tetra-, four double bonds), these agents are called 'eicosanoids'. The rate limiting step in eicosanoid production is usually the formation of AA from membrane phospholipids by phospholipase A_2. The downstream pathway from AA to both prostaglandins and thromboxane involves the constitutively expressed enzyme **cyclo-oxygenase 1** (COX1) and, in inflamed tissues, COX2. Anti-inflammatory **steroids** inhibit COX production. **Non-steroidal anti-inflammatory drugs** (NSAIDs – aspirin, ibuprofen, indomethacin) are COX1-2 inhibitors.

Prostaglandins are synthesized by vascular endothelium, fibroblasts, macrophages and leukocytes. The F series, PGFs, are mainly vasoconstrictors. The important E series (e.g. PGE_2) and prostacyclin (PGI_2) are **vasodilators** (Figure 9.8). They contribute to **reactive hyperaemia** (see later), **sweating-related cutaneous vasodilatation**, and to the **vasodilatation and oedema of inflammation**, for example in arthritis. Although not inflammatory by themselves, PGE_2 and PGI_2 potentiate the inflammatory action of histamine and bradykinin and sensitize the nociceptive C fibres ('pain' receptors) – hence the effectiveness of NSAIDs in reducing the inflammatory swelling and pain of arthritis. PGI_2, which is produced continuously by endothelium, also inhibits platelet aggregation and is thus **antithrombotic** (Section 9.5).

Thromboxane A$_2$ is synthesized by COX in platelets. It is a powerful vasoconstrictor and thrombotic agent. Following a bleed, the shed platelets release both thromboxane and serotonin, and the ensuing vasoconstriction helps stop the bleeding. Since coronary atheroma sometimes activates platelets inappropriately (see 'Serotonin'), the resulting shower of thromboxane and serotonin can cause **coronary artery vasospasm** and angina at rest. Thromboxane also has a key role in **thrombosis**, the formation of an organized blood clot inside a vessel; released thromboxane mediates the aggregation of platelets, which is the first step in thrombosis. Since low-dose **aspirin** inhibits platelet COX and reduces the thromboxane content, it helps protect against thrombosis. Low-dose aspirin does not much affect endothelial COX, so the production of the anti-aggregation factor PGI$_2$ continues, tipping the balance against thrombosis. Low-dose aspirin is therefore prescribed prophylactically for patients with coronary atheroma.

Leukotrienes

Leukotrienes are vasoactive ecosanoids produced from AA by the action of 5-lipoxygenase (LOX, cf. COX) in leukocytes. They contribute to the **inflammatory response** by causing leukocyte margination-emigration and venular hyperpermeability, e.g. the bronchial inflammation of asthma. Their gap-inducing action on venules is 1000-fold more potent than that of histamine. Leukotrienes can also cause vasoconstriction or dilatation, depending on the tissue.

Platelet activating factor (PAF)

PAF is a vasoactive lipid generated by activated inflammatory cells, such as polymorphonuclear leukocytes and macrophages. It is produced from acyl-PAF by phospholipase A$_2$. Although its name stems from its ability to promote platelet aggregation, PAF actually exerts many of its major effects on smooth muscle. It causes bronchoconstriction in asthmatics, and may also contribute to the vasospasm of atheromatous coronary arteries. PAF also contributes to the venular hyperpermeability of **inflammation (Figure 11.28).

13.6 Autoregulation of blood flow

The intrinsic mechanisms described above – the myogenic response, endothelial secretions, vasodilator metabolites and autacoids – account for several major circulatory responses without any help from extrinsic nerves or hormones. The most important of these intrinsic responses are the **autoregulation of flow**, **metabolic hyperaemia** and **post-ischaemic (reactive) hyperaemia**, as follows.

Autoregulation keeps blood flow almost constant when pressure changes

The relation between perfusion pressure and blood flow in myocardium, brain, kidney, skeletal muscle and intestine is a remarkable one, because changes in perfusion pressure over the physiological range have little effect on the steady state blood flow. In other words, a plot of flow versus pressure is almost flat over the physiological pressure range – a phenomenon called autoregulation (Figures 13.6a, 13.7 and 8.21). At first acquaintance this seems to defy the laws of physics, which state that flow is proportional to perfusion pressure (Sections 1.5 and 8.7); but such laws do not take into account the active responses of contractile resistance vessels. A rise in arterial pressure does indeed raise flow initially; but within 30–60 seconds the arterioles respond by contracting. This increases the vascular resistance and reduces the flow to close to its former level. Conversely, a fall in arterial pressure evokes vasodilatation, which reduces the resistance and restores the flow. Active changes in vascular calibre thus hold flow almost constant in the steady state. Autoregulation nevertheless operates over a limited pressure range, and severe hypotension will cause a fall in cerebral, myocardial and renal perfusion. Autoregulation is absent in the pulmonary circulation (as is to be expected!) and in the cutaneous circulation.

The usefulness of autoregulation is that, within its upper and lower limits, it protects organ perfusion against minute-to-minute fluctuations in arterial blood pressure. In the **brain**, autoregulation maintains blood flow during the hypotension caused by spinal anaesthesia. In the **myocardium**, it helps maintain blood flow downstream of a stenosed, atheromatous coronary artery, where pressure is reduced. In the **kidney** it stabilizes the glomerular filtration rate by maintaining a constant renal perfusion and glomerular capillary pressure. The latter point bring us to the second, less well recognised function of autoregulation, namely the stabilization of capillary pressure.

Autoregulation stabilizes capillary pressure

Autoregulation stabilizes not only tissue perfusion but also the capillary blood pressure and fluid

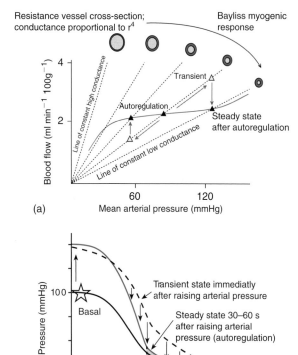

Figure 13.6 Autoregulation of (a) blood flow and (b) capillary pressure in isolated, perfused skeletal muscle. (a) Raising or lowering blood pressure transiently raises or lowers blood flow as dictated by Poiseuille's law (lines of constant conductance; grey arrows). The myogenic response then actively changes the resistance vessel radius, producing a new isoconductance line and restoring flow to close to its former level in the steady state (vertical grey arrows). (b) Dashed lines show the transient state immediately after changing perfusion pressure from a control level of 100 mmHg (star), before autoregulation has had time to kick in. Over the next 30–60 s arteriolar contraction/dilatation readjusts the flow and capillary pressure to a steady-state value similar to before (solid red curve). ((a) Drawn partly from data of Jones RD, Berne RM. *Circulation Research* 1964; **14**: 126.)

turnover (Figure 13.6b). When an isolated skeletal muscle is perfused by a pump, elevation of the pump pressure from 30 to 170 mmHg causes only a 2 mmHg rise in capillary pressure. This is because the autoregulatory contraction of the arterioles raises the pre- to postcapillary resistance ratio R_A/R_V; and capillary pressure is inversely related to R_A/R_V (Figure 11.4). The bigger pressure drop across the increased resistance R_A prevents capillary blood pressure from increasing substantially when arterial pressure is raised. This protects tissues against oedema when arterial pressure is high. Capillary pressure autoregulation is crucial in the renal

glomeruli, where it ensures a virtually **constant glomerular filtration rate** for waste-product elimination.

Autoregulation is due mainly to the myogenic response

The mechanisms underlying autoregulation are the myogenic response (Figure 13.3), vasodilator washout and, in the kidney, tubuloglomerular feedback. Vasodilator washout is the removal of vasodilator metabolites from the tissue by a transiently increased blood flow when arterial pressure rises. Indirect evidence indicates that the **myogenic mechanism** predominates in the brain, intestine, liver and spleen, and contributes to renal autoregulation. For example, autoregulation in the brain and kidney is severely impaired by blocking the formation of 20-HETE, the vasoconstrictor involved in sustaining the myogenic response.

In the kidney, the myogenic response accounts for roughly half of the autoregulation. A specialized, local mechanism called **tubuloglomerular feedback** accounts for the other half. If glomerular blood pressure increases, increased capillary filtration delivers more fluid and salt into the renal tubule. The NaCl is sensed by macula densa cells in the ascending loop of Henle, which lie adjacent to

Figure 13.7 Distinct effects of perfusion pressure and metabolic activity on coronary blood flow in dog. Dashed lines are theoretical pressure–flow lines at constant conductance; the steepest line has the highest conductance. At any given metabolic rate, i.e. heart rate (HR), blood flow increases relatively little with perfusion pressure, due to a shift to a lower conductance line as pressure is raised. This is autoregulation. At any given perfusion pressure, flow increases with metabolic rate (heart rate). This is metabolic hyperaemia. (Data from Laird. In: Holland A, Noble M (eds). *Cardiac Metabolism*. Chichester: Wiley, 1983: 257–78.)

the glomerulus in a complex called the **juxtaglomerular apparatus**. Macula densa activation leads, via adenosine and mesangial A_1 receptors, to contraction of the adjacent afferent arteriole, reducing glomerular capillary blood pressure to its former level.

Autoregulated flow can be changed, by metabolic factors and sympathetic activity

Autoregulation does not mean that the blood flow is unchangeable; it means that the flow is insensitive to physiological changes in arterial pressure. Changes in metabolic or sympathetic activity can still alter the blood flow, by resetting the autoregulation to operate at a different level of flow. Figure 13.7 illustrates how **autoregulation and changes in blood flow can coexist**. An increase in cardiac work increases the coronary blood flow (metabolic hyperaemia), but the pressure–flow relation remains relatively flat at each work intensity. In other words, the metabolic vasodilators reset autoregulation to operate at a higher, but still autoregulated, flow.

13.7 Metabolic (functional) hyperaemia

In skeletal muscle, myocardium and brain, the blood flow increases almost linearly with the metabolic rate of the tissue, so that blood flow in the steady state is almost directly proportional to the oxygen consumption (Figures 13.7 and 15.4). This beautiful and striking coupling of supply to demand is called metabolic hyperaemia (alias functional hyperaemia, active hyperaemia, metabolic vasodilatation). In the initial few seconds of muscle hyperaemia the vasodilatation may be due to myogenic relaxation in response to intermittent compression by the contracting muscle. In the later, sustained phase, the coupling is probably brought about by the metabolic vasodilators described in Section 13.4, namely **interstitial K^+ ions**, **acidosis, adenosine, ATP, phosphate, hyperosmolarity** and **hydrogen peroxide**. Most of these agents not only act directly on resistance vessels but also inhibit noradrenaline release from sympathetic fibres (neuromodulation, Figure 14.2). Studies using inhibitors of eNOS and COX indicate that **NO and prostaglandins** too contribute to skeletal muscle hyperaemia, by ~20–33%. In limbs with ischaemic arterial disease, bradykinin also contributes. These multiple factors can increase the muscle blood flow more than 20-fold during heavy exercise (Figure 13.1).

It is worth emphasizing that **metabolic hyperaemia is mediated entirely by intrinsic factors, not vasodilator nerves**. Also, much confusion can be avoided by noting that metabolic hyperaemia, which is an increase in flow and a form of automatic regulation, should not be called autoregulation, which is a constancy of flow in the face of pressure changes. The coexistence of these two very different phenomena is illustrated in Figure 13.7.

Muscle blood flow oscillates during rhythmic exercise

During rhythmic exercise the mean blood flow through the exercising muscle increases, but the flow actually falls during each contraction phase, because the vessels inside the contracting muscle are compressed (Figure 13.8). The pressure exerted on the outside of the vessels in contracting human skeletal muscle can reach 270–570 mmHg. Similarly, myocardial blood flow falls sharply at the onset of systole (Figure 15.5). Most of the hyperaemia in skeletal and myocardial muscle occurs during the relaxation phases. Muscle myoglobin holds a small reserve of O_2 for use during the poorly perfused contraction phase.

The onset-related O_2 debt is repaid by post-exercise hyperaemia

As indicated earlier, the hyperaemia of exercise develops in two phases. There is a moderate increase in blood flow within seconds (Figure 13.8), but the full, sustained response takes a minute or so to develop. Since the muscle's demand for more O_2

Figure 13.8 Oscillating increase in blood flow (metabolic hyperaemia) in human femoral artery during rhythmic quadriceps exercise. Flow was measured by the Doppler ultrasound method. Note the relatively slow initial phase of the hyperaemia, creating an oxygen debt. The post-exercise period of hyperaemia repays the nutritional debt. (From Walloe L, Wesche J. *Journal of Physiology* 1988; **405**: 257–73, with permission from Wiley-Blackwell.)

increases instantly upon contraction, the blood flow and O_2 supply fail to match demand during the first minute or so, and the muscle must draw on its reserve of high-energy creatine phosphate instead. This metabolic deficit, or 'oxygen debt', has to be repaid at some point by extra O_2 consumption. The O_2 debt may cease to grow once the blood flow has reached a steady state, where blood flow is directly proportional to O_2 consumption. When the exercise stops, the hyperaemia does not cease instantly but decays gradually over many minutes (Figure 13.11). This is called **post-exercise hyperaemia**. The post-exercise hyperaemia quickly repays the metabolic debt, and persists for several minutes longer, helping restore muscle pH and temperature to baseline.

Hyperaemia is impaired by static, isometric exercise

During static, isometric exercise, such as holding a heavy weight, the increase in blood flow through the muscle is much less pronounced than during dynamic exercise. This is because the sustained increase in intra-muscle pressure limits the dilatation of the resistance vessels. Consequently, blood flow fails to match O_2 consumption and a large O_2 debt accumulates rapidly. This leads to the anaerobic production of lactic acid and rapid muscle fatigue.

Figure 13.9 Differential control of the arterial tree. Metabolic vasodilators dominate the terminal arterioles. Sympathetic vasoconstrictor nerves dominate the more proximal resistance vessels. Ascending (conducted) vasodilatation involves endothelial electrical transmission up the arterial tree to feed arteries. Flow-induced vasodilatation, mediated by nitric oxide, is important in the conduit and proximal feed arteries. (Adapted from Brown MD. In: Jordan D, Marshall J (eds). *Cardiovascular Regulation*. London: Portland Press, 1995: 113–26, © Portland Press Ltd.)

The whole arterial tree undergoes co-ordinated dilatation

The arterial tree supplying a skeletal muscle is shown in Figure 13.9. The resistance of the main conduit artery and its chief branches, the feed arteries, is relatively small under resting conditions, namely <30% of that of the narrow resistance vessels. During metabolic hyperaemia the resistance of the resistance vessels can fall to 1/20th of normal. Under these conditions, the resistance of the conduit and feed arteries would seriously limit the increase in blood flow, unless these arteries likewise dilated. Happily, the metabolic vasodilatation of the resistance vessel triggers mechanisms that dilate the local conduit and feed arteries (see below). Thus a co-ordinated dilatation of arterioles, terminal arteries, feed arteries and conduit arteries contributes to the exercise hyperaemia.

Since the conduit and feed arteries are generally located outside the active muscle, they are beyond the reach of the metabolic factors that mediate resistance vessel dilatation. So how are they induced to dilate? The mechanisms are:

- **metabolic vasodilatation** of the terminal arteries and arterioles, i.e. resistance vessels;
- **ascending (conducted) vasodilatation** of small feed arteries; and
- **flow-induced vasodilatation** of the large, conduit artery.

The graded sensitivity of each type of vessel to these mechanisms is illustrated in Figure 13.9.

Feed arteries exhibit ascending (conducted) vasodilatation, mediated by endothelium

A feed artery is a vessel of diameter up to 0.5 mm located between the terminal resistance arteries and the main arterial supply vessel, the conduit artery (e.g. a branch of the brachial artery). Feed arteries exhibit the strange property of ascending or conducted vasodilatation. That is to say, when the intramuscle arteriolar network is dilated by vasoactive metabolites, or in a laboratory setting by a vasodilator such as bradykinin or acetylcholine, the dilatation spreads rapidly up the arterial system in a proximal direction. As a result, feed arteries several millimetres upstream dilate within 30 seconds or so, even though they may be outside the muscle. Ascending vasodilatation can be blocked by creating a ring of damaged endothelium, indicating

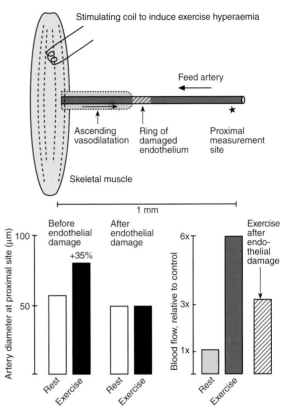

Figure 13.10 Ascending or conducted vasodilatation in a feed artery following contractions of a hamster muscle. Metabolic hyperaemia caused a six-fold increase in blood flow. After destruction of the ring of endothelium, the ascending dilatation halted at the ring and the metabolic hyperaemia fell by 47%. (Adapted from Segal SS, Jacobs TL. *Journal of Physiology* 2001; **536**: 937–46, with permission from Wiley-Blackwell.)

that it depends on **endothelial conduction** (Figure 13.10). Fast-conducted and slow-conducted mechanisms are responsible, as follows.

Fast-conducted, electromechanical response. Metabolic vasodilators in the active tissue cause hyperpolarization of the local endothelial cells (EC), partly by raising intracellular Ca^{2+}, which activates small- and intermediate-conductance K_{Ca} channels (SK, IK – Section 9.3), and partly by adenosine-mediated activation of the K_{ATP} channels of EC. EC hyperpolarization is rapidly conducted proximally through EC homocellular gap junctions (Figure 9.7), at several mm/s, and is transmitted to the vascular myocytes of feed arteries through **myoendothelial gap junctions** (Figures 1.11, 9.1, 9.7). The endothelium-dependent vascular hyperpolarization causes closure of the vascular myocyte L-type Ca^{2+} channels and hence vasodilatation of the proximal, feed artery.

Slow-conducted, pharmacomechanical response. The endothelial Ca^{2+} release evoked by the agonists triggers an ascending wave of Ca^{2+} release, that passes slowly from endothelial cell to endothelial cell. The ascending EC Ca^{2+} wave causes an ascending wave of endothelial nitric oxide and prostacyclin production, which helps maintain the proximal vasodilatation.

Conduit arteries undergo flow-induced dilatation, mediated by NO

The human brachial artery can dilate by $\geqslant 10\%$ during forearm exercise. As the resistance vessels undergo metabolic vasodilatation, blood flow through the conduit artery increases. This increases the shear stress on the arterial endothelium, stimulating the production of NO, which dilates the conduit artery. Thus the widening of the conduit artery is automatically triggered by the downstream metabolic hyperaemia.

Summary of increased blood flow to exercising muscle

An increase in tissue metabolic activity elicits a co-ordinated dilatation of the arterial system supplying that tissue. The primary event is dilatation of local arterioles within the tissue by locally released vasoactive agents such as adenosine, K^+, H^+, phosphate, hyperosmolarity and H_2O_2. The peripheral, metabolic vasodilatation triggers conducted vasodilatation of the feed arteries (mediated by endothelial hyperpolarization) and flow-induced vasodilatation of conduit arteries (mediated by endothelial NO). Both the latter changes are necessary for the full expression of the hyperaemia. Indeed, one study showed that blocking the ascending vasodilatation reduced exercise hyperaemia by 50%.

13.8 Post-ischaemic (reactive) hyperaemia

The arterial blood supply to a tissue may sometimes be impeded by external compression, either naturally (e.g. brachial artery compression when the arm is rested over the back of a chair) or by sphygmomanometry or surgery. The blood flow may fall to a level where it no longer supplies the tissue's O_2 requirement, a condition called **ischaemia**. When the compression is removed, the

Figure 13.11 Forearm blood flow measured in a medical student by venous occlusion plethysmography. Release of a brachial artery occlusion cuff that had cut off blood flow for 120 seconds resulted in post-ischaemic hyperaemia (red line). Black line shows post-exercise hyperaemia following 30 seconds of strenuous forearm exercise; blood flow remains elevated for longer after exercise. Insets show typical forearm volume traces during these plethysmographic measurements. See Figure 8.5 for venous occlusion plethysmography.

tissue blood flow is initially many times faster than normal, followed by a period of exponential decay (Figure 13.11). This is called post-ischaemic or reactive hyperaemia. It is obvious in the skin, which flushes a bright pink after a period of compression, and it occurs in most other tissues too. Its value lies in rapidly restoring the supply of O_2 and nutrients to ischaemic tissue, and washing out accumulated waste products.

The mechanisms of reactive hyperaemia remains incompletely understood. After short arterial occlusions, $<30\,s$, reactive hyperaemia is probably due chiefly to the **myogenic response;** the upstream arterial occlusion reduces pressure in the resistance vessels, causing them to dilate myogenically. After longer occlusions, **vasodilator metabolites** may accumulate. A 3-min occlusion produces maximal vasodilatation in human limbs, and release is followed by a maximal hyperaemia that decays exponentially over $\sim 60\,s$. Even longer occlusions cause a prolonged, post-ischaemic plateau at maximal hyperaemia, before the exponential decay phase sets in. Local anaesthetics substantially reduce cutaneous reactive hyperaemia, implicating the release of sensory nerve **vasodilator neuropeptides** in the response (Section 14.4). The hyperaemia is also reduced in some tissues by the COX inhibitor indomethacin, implicating **prostaglandins** in the response. Nitric oxide appears to play a minor, sometimes negligible role.

13.9 Ischaemia–reperfusion injury

Surgeons sometimes arrest the blood supply to peripheral tissues for an hour or more, for example during limb orthopaedic surgery, aortic aneurysm repair and organ transplantation (kidney, heart–lung, liver). When the clamped artery is released, it is often found that, instead of the brisk reactive hyperaemia that follows a few minutes of occlusion, the hyperaemia is weak and the blood flow falls to abnormally low levels within minutes – the **no-reflow phenomenon**. Moreover, the tissues show biochemical and structural signs of cellular damage soon after the flow is restarted. This is called **ischaemia-reperfusion injury**, and is most marked in the intestine, liver and heart. It can also affect the survival of the rim of tissue around a myocardial or cerebral infarct.

Ischaemia–reperfusion injury is to a large extent caused by the restored blood supply, surprisingly. For example, 3 hours of ischaemia followed by an hour of reperfusion produces more tissue damage than does 4 hours of ischaemia. What component of the blood causes the damage? Reperfusion with leukocyte-free blood attenuates reperfusion injury; and reperfusion with hypoxic blood likewise attenuates the injury. Both white cells and O_2 thus contribute to reperfusion injury. A third factor, particularly in the heart, is post-ischaemic Ca^{2+} overload (Section 6.12).

Leukocyte adhesion contributes to reperfusion injury

In laboratory experiments, antibodies against the leukocyte–endothelial adhesion molecules attenuate the reperfusion injury. During a period of prolonged ischaemia, microvascular endothelial cells begin to express selectins and other surface adhesion molecules. When leukocytes arrive in the restored bloodstream, they adhere to the sticky endothelium (Figure 9.11). Since leukocytes are ~100 times stiffer than red cells, the adherent cells physically obstruct microvascular perfusion. The situation is further exacerbated by ischaemic swelling of the endothelial cells. The result is the no-reflow phenomenon. Adherent leukocytes also contribute actively to the tissue injury. They release leukotrienes and PAF, which cause inflammation; they release elastase, a potent tissue protease; and they generate superoxide anions, which damage the tissues.

Free oxygen radicals too contribute to reperfusion injury

Oxygen in the restored bloodstream contributes greatly to the tissue injury. On reaching the ischaemic tissue, some oxygen molecules are converted into free radicals – highly reactive particles with an unpaired electron in the outer shell. The free oxygen radicals are superoxide O_2^- •, the hydroxyl radical OH • and, via a reaction with NO, peroxynitrite $ONOO^-$. The free radicals react with lipids and amino acids to damage cell membranes and enzymes.

The free oxygen radicals come from two sources during reperfusion. One is the adherent, activated leukocyte. Leukocytes contains the enzyme **NADPH oxidase**, (nicotinamide adenine dinucleotide phosphate oxidase), which generates superoxide radicals. The normal role of the radicals is to kill pathogens, but in reperfusion injury the tissue itself is damaged.

The other source of the radicals is tissue **xanthine dehydrogenase**, an enzyme that is abundant in the myocardium and intestinal mucosa. Intestinal villi in particular have a high concentration of xanthine dehydrogenase and are very sensitive to reperfusion injury. During the ischaemic period a Ca^{2+}-triggered protease converts the xanthine dehydrogenase into **xanthine oxidase**. At the same time the substrate for this enzyme, hypoxanthine, is generated by the breakdown of adenosine, itself the breakdown product of ATP. When reperfused O_2 reaches the metabolically altered tissue, the hypoxanthine is oxidized to xanthine by the xanthine oxidase, and in the course of this reaction harmless molecular O_2 is converted into superoxide O_2^- • and hydrogen peroxide H_2O_2. Reperfusion thus generates a burst of toxic radicals.

Reperfusion injury can be attenuated by **superoxide dismutase**, a scavenger of free oxygen radicals – confirming their role in reperfusion injury. Reperfusion injury can also be attenuated in many tissues by **allopurinol**, an inhibitor of xanthine oxidase. During coronary bypass surgery, allopurinol can be given prior to reperfusion to improve ventricular function after reperfusion.

Cytosolic Ca^{2+} overload contributes to myocardial reperfusion injury

Reperfusion injury in the heart is further exacerbated by the overloading of the cardiac myocytes with Ca^{2+} during the ischaemic period. This is described under 'The paradox of myocardial ischaemia–reperfusion injury' in Section 6.12.

SUMMARY

- Though complex in detail, the control of blood vessels can be conceptualized as a hierarchy of three control systems, each of which can override and modify the lower one.

- The **lowest level of control** is the **Bayliss myogenic response**, namely vascular contraction in response to an increase in blood pressure. The myogenic response contributes to basal tone in resistance vessels and to **autoregulation**. Autoregulation is the maintenance of a near-constant blood flow and capillary pressure when arterial pressure changes. Autoregulation is well developed in the brain, myocardium and kidneys.

- A **second level of control** is superimposed by **local vasoactive agents**. Agents released when tissue metabolic rate increases, such as adenosine, CO_2, lactate, K^+, phosphate, osmolarity and H_2O_2, dilate the local arterioles. The resulting **metabolic hyperaemia** couples tissue perfusion to local O_2 consumption, particularly in the brain, myocardium and skeletal muscle. **Ascending (conducted) vasodilatation** of the feed arteries ensures upstream vessels do not limit the hyperaemia. **Flow-induced vasodilatation** of the conduit artery, mediated by NO, ensures that the main artery in turn does not limit flow to the feed arteries.

- A short period of reduced perfusion (seconds–minutes) evokes **post-ischaemic (reactive) hyperaemia**, due to the myogenic response and metabolite accumulation. Longer periods of ischaemia (an hour) may be followed by **poor reflow** and **reperfusion injury**, caused by leukocyte adhesion, toxic oxygen radical generation, and (in myocardium) cytosolic Ca^{2+} overload.

- **Endothelial nitric oxide** exerts a tonic vasodilator influence on basal tone, especially in pregnancy. NO mediates flow-induced vasodilatation in conduit arteries, and the vasodilator action of bradykinin, substance P and acetylcholine. Inducible NO synthase contributes to endotoxin hypotension. Nitridergic parasympathetic fibres induce the dilatation that drives genital erection.

- **Autacoids** are paracrine, vasoactive agents such as histamine, bradykinin, serotonin, prostaglandins, thromboxane, leukotrienes and PAF. Autacoids modify local vascular tone, chiefly in pathological situations such as inflammation (vasodilatation by histamine, bradykinin, prostaglandins) and bleeding (vasoconstriction by serotonin, thromboxane).

- The **third level of control** is the neuroendocrine system, which brings the vasculature under central and reflex control for the benefit of the organism as a whole (Chapter 14).

Further reading

Reviews and chapters

Berry CE, Hare JM. Xanthine oxidoreductase and cardiovascular disease: Molecular mechanisms and pathophysiological implications. *Journal of Physiology* 2004; **555**: 589–606. (Ischaemia–reperfusion injury)

Canty JM, Iyer VS. Hydrogen peroxide and metabolic coronary flow regulation. *Journal of the American College of Cardiology* 2007; **50**: 1279–81.

Clifford PS, Hellsten Y. Vasodilatory mechanisms in contracting skeletal muscle. *Journal of Applied Physiology* 2004; **97**: 393–403.

Granger DN, Korthuis RJ. Physiological mechanisms of postischemic tissue injury. *Annual Review of Physiology* 1995; **57**: 311–32.

Gustafsson F, Holstein-Rathlou N-H. Conducted vasomotor responses in arterioles: Characteristics, mechanisms and physiological significance. *Acta Physiologica Scandinavica* 1999; **167**: 11–21.

Hill MA, Davis MJ. Coupling a change in intraluminal pressure to vascular smooth muscle depolarization: Still stretching for an explanation. *American Journal of Physiology* 2007; **292**: H2570–2. (Bayliss myogenic response mechanisms)

Marshall JM. The integrated response to hypoxia: From circulation to cells. *Experimental Physiology* 1999; **84**: 449–70.

Melkumyants AM, Balashov SA, Khayutin VM. Control of arterial lumen by shear stress on endothelium. *News in Physiological Sciences* 1995; **10**: 204–10.

Moncada S, Higgs EA. The discovery of nitric oxide and its role in vascular biology. *British Journal of Pharmacology* 2006; **147** (Suppl. 1): S193–201.

Roman RJ. P-450 metabolites of arachidonic acid in the control of cardiovascular function. *Physiological Reviews* 2002; **82**: 131–85.

Schubert R, Lidington D, Bolz SS. The emerging role of Ca^{2+} sensitivity regulation in promoting myogenic vaso-constriction. *Cardiovascular Research* 2008; **77**: 8–18.

Research papers

See www.hodderplus.com/cardiovascularphysiology for a full list of Research papers for this chapter.

CHAPTER 14

Control of blood vessels: II. Extrinsic control by nerves and hormones

Learning objectives

After reading this chapter you should be able to:

- Sketch the sympathetic pathway from brainstem to blood vessel and adrenal medulla (14.1).
- Name the neurotransmitters and receptors mediating sympathetic vasomotor neurotransmission (14.1).
- List the chief functions of sympathetic vasoconstrictor nerves (14.1).
- State the distribution, roles and neurotransmitters of parasympathetic vasodilator nerves (14.2) and sympathetic vasodilator nerves (14.3).
- Explain the meaning of 'sensory axon reflex' (14.4).
- Contrast the cardiovascular effects of intravenous adrenaline and noradrenaline (14.6).
- Outline the formation, action and regulation of angiotensin II, vasopressin and atrial natriuretic peptide (14.7–14.9).
- State the importance and main mechanisms of venous control (14.10).

The previous chapter focused on the **intrinsic regulation** of vascular tone by mechanisms originating from within the tissue itself, such as metabolic hyperaemia in exercising muscle and myocardium. Local mechanisms, however, serve local needs. To serve the needs of the whole organism, such as blood pressure homeostasis or the sentient control of a specific organ (e.g. erectile tissue), the central nervous system superimposes a sentient control system, acting through vasomotor nerves and hormones. Since neural and hormonal control is imposed from outside the tissue itself, this is called **extrinsic regulation**. Extrinsic regulation is in general the motor, efferent limb of a vascular reflex. The sensory, afferent limbs of the reflexes are described in Chapter 16.

Extrinsic regulation involves three kinds of autonomic vasomotor nerve:

- sympathetic vasoconstrictor nerves
- parasympathetic vasodilator nerves
- sympathetic vasodilator nerves.

Note that the labels 'vasoconstrictor' and 'vasodilator' refer to the effect of an increase in nerve activity. It is important to remember that **a reduction in vasoconstrictor fibre activity causes vasodilatation**; vasodilatation does not necessarily require vasodilator fibres. The flushed skin of warm hands is an example of vasodilatation brought about by reduced sympathetic vasoconstrictor activity. Of the various autonomic vasomotor nerves, the sympathetic vasoconstrictor fibres are the most widespread and most important physiologically. Students accustomed to associating sympathetic activity with alarm and dilatation should note that **the vast majority of sympathetic vasomotor fibres are vasoconstrictor fibres**.

14.1 Sympathetic vasoconstrictor nerves

The sympathetic system comprises bulbospinal, preganglionic and postganglionic fibres

The sympathetic vasoconstrictor system consists of a three-neuron pathway that starts in the brainstem medulla. Medullary pre-sympathetic neurons send **bulbospinal fibres** (axons) down the spinal cord (Figure 14.1). The bulbospinal fibres synapse with sympathetic preganglionic neurons in the intermediolateral columns of grey matter, located in thoracicolumbar segments T1 to L3.

Preganglionic cholinergic fibres activate nicotinic receptors in sympathetic ganglia

The tonically active excitatory and inhibitory bulbospinal fibres, plus local spinal inputs, regulate the output of the preganglionic spinal neurons. Their axons, the sympathetic preganglionic fibres, travel through the ventral roots of the spinal nerves and **white rami communicantes** to enter the prevertebral right and left **sympathetic chains** (Figure 4.5).

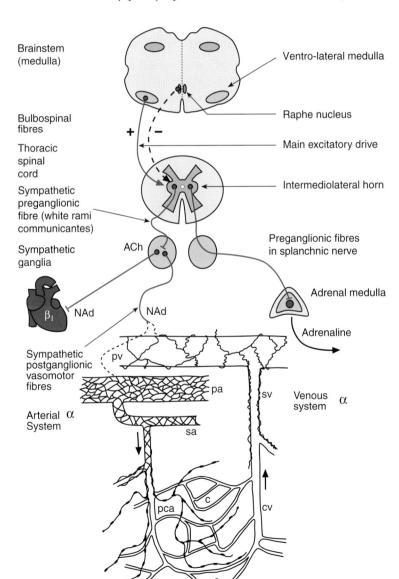

Figure 14.1 Sympathetic innervation of cardiovascular system. Alpha and β refer to predominant adrenoceptor. NAd, noradrenaline; ACh, acetylcholine. One descending tract (bulbospinal tract) excites the sympathetic intermediolateral cells; other bulbospinal fibres inhibit the cell. pa and pv, primary, conduit artery and vein to an organ, respectively; sa and sv, small artery and vein, respectively; pca, precapillary arteriole; c, capillary; cv, collecting venule. (Adapted from Furness JB, Marshall JM. *Journal of Physiology* 1974; **239**: 75–88, with permission from Wiley-Blackwell.)

The axons may travel up or down the sympathetic chain for several segments before synapsing with postganglionic neurons; and some do not synapse until they reach the adrenal medulla or a more distant ganglion (coeliac, hypogastric). The preganglionic fibres are mostly cholinergic and the **postganglionic receptors are nicotinic**. They are blocked by hexamethonium and stimulated by **smoking**, which thus causes vasoconstriction and blood pressure elevation. Smoking-induced vasoconstriction is compounded by reduced nitric oxide availability (Concept box 14.1).

CONCEPT BOX 14.1

Smoking and the vascular system

- The stimulation of nicotinic receptors on postganglionic neurons increases sympathetic vasoconstrictor activity.
- Smoking-activated leukocytes generate free radicals in oxidative bursts. NO reacts with the free oxygen radicals. This forms harmful peroxynitrite and reduces beneficial NO levels.
- Raised sympathetic activity coupled with reduced nitric oxide availability cause smoking-induced vasoconstriction.
- Smoking-induced vasoconstriction raises blood pressure and reduces coronary and cutaneous blood flow.
- Low levels of NO and prostacyclin facilitate platelet aggregation, atheroma progression and thrombosis.
- The walls of arterioles are thickened, probably due to the hypertension and to the loss of the inhibitory effect of NO on myocyte proliferation.

Postganglionic noradrenergic fibres innervate blood vessels

Sympathetic postganglionic neurons send non-myelinated axons through the **grey rami communicantes** into the ventral roots of the spinal nerves, for distribution in mixed peripheral nerves. Some fibres also course directly over the major vessels. Postganglionic fibres terminate in branches that run along the outer border of the tunica media, penetrating it only in veins. Most small arteries and terminal resistance arteries are richly innervated, whereas arterioles are poorly innervated (Figure 14.1), being controlled chiefly by intrinsic mechanisms (Figure 13.9). The venous innervation is similar but less dense, and skeletal muscle veins have almost no sympathetic innervation.

Terminal varicosities release packets (quanta) of noradrenaline

The terminal axon resembles a string of beads (Figure 1.11). Each bead, or **varicosity**, contains numerous **dense-cored vesicles** (Figure 14.2). Each vesicle is filled with concentrated noradrenaline (norepinephrine in the American literature) at up to 1 molar, and also ATP. The noradrenaline is synthesized from the amino acid tyrosine via two intermediate products, DOPA (*di*hydroxy-*p*henyl*a*lanine) and dopamine. Out of the thousands or so varicosities per axon, only a small proportion release a vesicle as an action potential sweeps along the axon; so only a small fraction of the stored noradrenaline is released per action potential.

Vesicle release, or **exocytosis**, is triggered by a rise in cytosolic $[Ca^{2+}]$ as the action potential actives axonal N-type Ca^{2+} channels. The Ca^{2+}

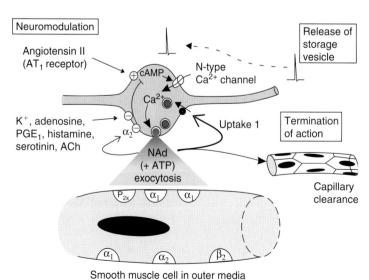

Smooth muscle cell in outer media

Figure 14.2 Sympathetic neuromuscular transmission. Noradrenaline (NAd) binds to post-junctional α_1-receptors; α_2-receptors are generally more remote from the junction. Pre-junctional α_2-receptors, and receptors for many intrinsic vasodilators, inhibit cAMP production to attenuate Ca^{2+} channel opening and vesicle release (negative sign). Angiotensin receptors promote more transmitter release per action potential (positive sign). ATP is a co-transmitter in some sympathetic fibres. Not to scale (varicosity 2 μm long × 1 μm wide, axon 0.1–0.5 μm wide, myocyte 4 μm wide centrally).

activates a protein on the vesicle membrane, synaptobrevin. If the vesicle is close to the surface membrane, the synaptobrevin binds to the membrane protein syntaxin. This 'docking' process allows the two membranes to fuse and release the vesicle contents. **Guanethidine** blocks exocytosis by acting as a local anaesthetic on sympathetic terminals, and was formerly used to treat hypertension. Conversely, **amphetamines** have a sympathomimetic effect, because they displace noradrenaline from the vesicle into the cytosol, from where it escapes into the extracellular fluid.

Noradrenaline activates vascular α-adrenoceptors and contraction

The released noradrenaline diffuses rapidly across the junctional gap and binds to α-adrenoceptors on the vascular myocyte membrane, leading to vascular contraction (Figure 12.9). Adrenoceptor classification is summarized in Table 14.1. Alpha$_1$-receptors are found on most blood vessels. They activates G_q protein, leading to vasoconstriction through depolarization-dependent and/or depolarization-independent pathways (Figure 12.6). Alpha$_2$-receptors are G_i-coupled and more limited in distribution. They occur as pre-junctional receptors on sympathetic varicosities, and as post-junctional receptors on resistance vessels in human skin and limbs, additional to the ubiquitous α_1-receptors. Alpha$_1$ and α_2 contribute roughly equally to sympathetic-mediated vascular resistance in resting human limbs. The α_2-receptor is important in the response of skin blood vessel to temperature (Section 15.3).

Noradrenaline is removed quickly after release

The action of noradrenaline is terminated by three processes. (i) Around 80% of the noradrenaline is

Table 14.1 Pharmacology of cardiovascular adrenergic transmission

Receptor	Subtype	Principal location and effect	Agonists: relative potency	Antagonists	Therapeutic use of antagonists
α		Vascular myocytes: vasoconstriction	Noradrenaline (NA) and adrenaline (Ad) NA > Ad	Phentolamine, phenoxybenzamine Ergotamine	Raynaud's vasospasm Acute hypertension (phaeochromocytoma) Migraine
	α_1	Post-junctional receptor on most vessels. Vasoconstriction via G_q, PLC, ↑ IP_3 and DAG	NA > Ad, Phenylephrine	Prazosin, doxazosin, terazosin	Essential hypertension
	α_2	1. Autoreceptor of sympathetic varicosity: inhibits NA release. 2. Abundant post-junctional receptor in human skin vessels and muscle distal arterioles. Vasoconstriction via G_i, ↓ cAMP	Ad > NA Clonidine	Yohimbine, rauwolscine	–
β		1. SA node and myocardium: ↑ heart rate and contractility 2. Arterioles of heart, skeletal muscle and liver; vasodilatation	NA, Ad Isoprenaline	Propranolol, oxprenolol, alprenolol	Angina (↓ cardiac work) Hypertension
	β_1	SA node and myocardium: ↑ heart rate and contractility via G_s, adenylyl cyclase, ↑cAMP	NA > Ad Dobutamine (use; acute cardiac failure)	Atenolol, metroprolol, practolol (toxic)	Angina (↓ cardiac work) Hypertension (↓ cardiac output) Arrhythmias
	β_2	Arterioles of heart, skeletal muscle, liver Also bronchiole smooth muscle. Dilatation via G_s, ↑cAMP	Ad > NA Salbutamol, terbutaline		

transported back into the varicosity by a Na^+–Cl^-–amine co-transporter called **Uptake 1**, driven by the Na^+ gradient. Uptake 1 can be blocked by **reserpine**, a former anti-hypertensive drug that causes noradrenaline depletion. Mood enhancers such as **cocaine** and **tricyclic antidepressants** (e.g. desipramine) likewise inhibit Uptake 1, and the attendant rise in extracellular noradrenaline in the heart can cause a tachycardia or arrhythmia. (ii) Significant amounts of noradrenaline also diffuse into the capillary bloodstream. This sympathetic '**spillover**' accounts for much of the circulating plasma noradrenaline in humans. (iii) Smaller amounts of transmitter are degraded by a post-junctional, intracellular enzyme, catechol-O-methyltransferase.

Noradrenaline release is modulated by local metabolites and agonists

The amount of noradrenaline that is released depends not only on impulse frequency but also on the chemical environment of the varicosity – a process known as **neuromodulation** (Figure 14.2). Metabolic vasodilators such as adenosine, H^+ and K^+ ions depress noradrenaline release, thereby enhancing their vasodilator effect. Most vasodilator autacoids have a similar action. Noradrenaline itself binds to pre-junctional α_2-receptors (autoreceptors) to inhibit further exocytosis and thus prevent excessive discharge of vesicles. The α_2-receptors, being coupled to inhibitory G_i protein, lower the varicosity cAMP level, which leads to a fall in axonal N-type Ca^{2+} channel opening. By contrast, the hormone **angiotensin II facilitates noradrenaline exocytosis** and thereby amplifies its own direct vasoconstrictor effect.

ATP and neuropeptide Y contribute to sympathetic neuromuscular transmission

The α-adrenoceptor blockers phentolamine and phenoxybenzamine completely abolish the sympathetic vasoconstrictor response in most veins and the pulmonary artery. In many systemic arteries, however, the inhibition is only partial. This led to the discovery of co-transmitters in the sympathetic varicosity, namely the purine ATP and the peptide neuropeptide Y (Table 14.2). The contribution of co-transmitters varies from tissue to tissue.

ATP is co-released with noradrenaline in some large and small arteries. The ATP stimulates post-junctional P_{2X} purinergic receptors. These '**ionotropic**' receptors are physically part of an ion channel protein (unlike '**metabotropic**' α-receptors, which activate enzyme cascades). Ligand binding to the P_{2X} receptor activates a cation conductance, partially selective for Ca^{2+} over Na^+. The cation current causes a fast, brief depolarization of the myocyte – the fast excitatory junction potentials in Figures 14.3 and 12.9).

Neuropeptide Y (NPY) is synthesized in the postganglionic cell body and transported slowly along the axon to the sympathetic terminals in skeletal muscle, kidney, salivary gland, spleen and

Table 14.2 Main co-transmitters in perivascular nerve fibres[a]

Main co-transmitters	
Sympathetic vasoconstrictor fibre	Noradrenaline (NA)
	Adenosine triphosphate (ATP)
	Neuropeptide Y (NPY)
Parasympathetic dilator fibre	Acetylcholine (ACh)
	Vasoactive intestinal polypeptide (VIP)
	Nitric oxide (NO)
Sensory dilator fibre (C-fibre)	Substance P (SP)
	Calcitonin-gene related peptide (CGRP)
	ATP

[a]The ratio of transmitter substances within the fibre varies from tissue to tissue.
(From Burnstock G. *Acta Physiologica Scandinavica* 1988; **133** (Suppl. 571): 53–7.)

Control (a)
Fast EJP
Slow EJP
Phentolamine 6 min (b)
α, β-methylene ATP + Phentolamine (c)
5 mV
10 s

Figure 14.3 Evidence for co-transmission by noradrenaline and ATP in sympathetic fibres innervating rat tail artery. (a) Myocyte intracellular potential during repeated sympathetic stimulation (dots), showing fast excitatory junction potentials (fast EJP, spike) on top of a slower depolarization (slow EJP, baseline under spikes). NB The spikes are not action potentials, as is evident from the voltage scale. (b) Phentolamine, an α-adrenoceptor blocker, abolishes the slow EJP. (c) Desensitization of purinergic receptors by α, β-methylene ATP abolishes the fast EJPs. (After Sneddon P, Burnstock G. *European Journal of Pharmacology* 1984; **106**: 149–52, with permission from Elsevier.)

nasal mucosa. It may be stored in large dense-cored vesicles along with noradrenaline. It is co-released chiefly by the high frequency sympathetic activity associated with stress; the high frequency raises the neural $[Ca^{2+}]$ sufficiently to dock the NPY-containing vesicles with the varicosity membrane. NPY produces a slower, more prolonged depolarization than ATP and sensitizes the post-junctional membrane to noradrenaline (neuromodulatory effect).

Sympathetic fibres are tonically active

Sympathetic vasoconstrictor fibres are continuously active, though the average frequency is low in resting humans (0.5–1 impulses/second) and even maximal activity average only 8–10 impulses/second. Activity is uneven; it occurs in bursts in muscle and is irregular in skin. Nevertheless, the tonic activity contributes substantially to resting vascular tone, so **a fall in sympathetic vasomotor activity or pharmacological blockade causes vasodilatation**. Sympathetic blockade increases the blood flow to resting skeletal muscle two- to three-fold – though this is far from maximal flow, owing to the persistence of basal tone.

Sympathetic drive to one tissue is independent of that to another tissue

Sympathetic drive to each tissue (skin, muscle, kidney, etc.) appears to be controlled by distinct groups of neurons in the ventrolateral medulla (organotopic organization). Their responsiveness falls into three main classes: barosensitive, thermosensitive and glucosensitive. The barosensitive sympathetic pathway innervates muscle, kidneys, viscera, etc. and is controlled predominantly by blood pressure sensors (baroreceptors, Chapter 16). Thermosensitive sympathetic vasoconstrictor fibres innervate mainly the skin, and are regulated predominantly by hypothalamic core temperature sensors and emotion. Glucosensitive sympathetic fibres innervate the adrenal medulla, and are activated by hypoglycaemia and exercise. They stimulate adrenaline release.

Although a generalized activation of all sympathetic vasomotor fibres occurs in certain circumstances, e.g. during a haemorrhage, this is often not the case. For example, during the human **alerting response** to stress, sympathetic vasoconstrictor drive to the skin is increased (causing blanching), while at the same time the vasoconstrictor drive to skeletal muscle is reduced (causing vasodilatation). Activation of the sympathetic system is thus not

an 'all-or-none' affair; it is finely graded and is adjusted regionally according to need.

Reduced sympathetic activity elicits vasodilatation

Although it is natural to think of vasoconstriction as the primary role of vasoconstrictor nerves, vasodilatation by reduced sympathetic activity is important too. Indeed, it was flushing of the rabbit ear on cutting the nervous innervation that led the celebrated French physiologist, Claude Bernard, to discover the sympathetic vasomotor system in 1851. Two examples of vasodilatation in humans through reduced sympathetic activity are as follows.

- If blood pressure rises acutely, the baroreceptor reflex evokes a widespread fall in sympathetic activity (Section 16.2). The resulting vasodilatation helps to bring blood pressure back towards normal.
- When body temperature rises during exercise, the hypothalamic temperature-regulating centre evokes a fall in vasoconstrictor nerve activity to the skin, and the ensuing cutaneous vasodilatation helps to bring the temperature back down (Section 15.3).

Increased sympathetic activity raises peripheral resistance, reduces local blood flow and boosts central blood volume

The principal effects of an increase in sympathetic vasomotor activity in a given tissue are as follows:

- **Tissue blood flow** is reduced by contraction of the local resistance vessels (Figure 14.4, label c).
- **Tissue blood volume** is reduced by contraction of the local veins (Figure 14.5). This can squeeze 28 ml blood/kg out of the intestinal tract and liver, and 15 ml/kg from skin, into central veins. Skeletal muscle veins lack an effective innervation, but 7.5 ml/kg can nevertheless be expelled as local venous pressure is lowered by the contraction of upstream resistance vessels (Figure 14.4, label a).
- **Capillary pressure** is reduced by the resistance vessel contraction, as explained in Figure 11.11b. This allows interstitial fluid to be absorbed into the plasma compartment by osmosis in accordance with the Starling principle (Figure 14.4, label b).
- **Total peripheral resistance** (TPR) is raised in proportion to the amount of tissue involved and the severity of the vasoconstriction. A global

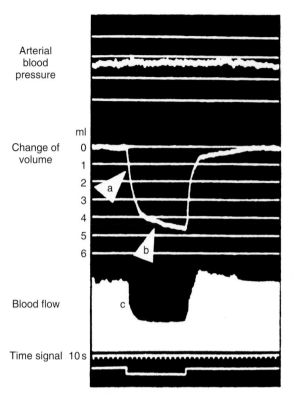

Figure 14.4 Three effects of sympathetic stimulation in cat hindquarters (2 impulses/s, square signal). Arrow 'a' shows fall in volume of blood, caused by reduced diameter of capacitance vessels (secondary to a fall in venous pressure following resistance vessel contraction – veins in skeletal muscle have little direct innervation). Arrow 'b' shows a slower fall in tissue volume due to the osmotic absorption of interstitial fluid by capillaries, as capillary pressure is reduced by resistance vessel contraction. Label 'c' shows fall in blood flow caused by resistance vessel contraction. (From Mellander S. *Acta Physiologica Scandinavica* 1960; **50** (Suppl.): 176, with permission from Wiley-Blackwell.)

Figure 14.5 Active splanchnic venoconstriction mediated by increases in sympathetic activity in a dog. Sympathetic activity was raised reflexly by step reductions in pressure in an isolated carotid sinus, while measuring splanchnic arterial inflow and venous outflow. Each transient excess of outflow over inflow marks an episode of venoconstriction. ΔV, displaced blood volume. Aortic pressure rises due to the reflex, sympathetically mediated rise in peripheral resistance. (After Hainsworth R, Karim F. *Journal of Physiology* 1976; **262**: 659–77, with permission from Wiley-Blackwell.)

increase in sympathetic outflow to multiple tissues, e.g. on standing up, raises TPR substantially. This helps to restore a fallen arterial blood pressure, since arterial pressure = cardiac output × TPR. Indeed, the **regulation of blood pressure through the adjustment of TPR** is a major function of the sympathetic vasomotor system, both normally and in pathophysiological situations. To this end, sympathetic activity is regulated by reflexes initiated by arterial pressure receptors (Chapter 16).

A global increase in sympathetic outflow is a major part of the body's defence against hypovolaemia (low blood volume, e.g. haemorrhage). The reduced peripheral blood flow, displacement of blood from peripheral to central veins, interstitial fluid absorption and increase in TPR are a life-preserving package of responses, since they help preserve the cardiac output and arterial pressure (Section 18.2).

Sympathetic activity contributes to regular oscillations in blood pressure

The sympathetic drive to skeletal muscle waxes and wanes over the respiratory cycle. Left ventricle output likewise oscillates with respiration, falling during inspiration (Section 2.5, 'splitting of second sound'). These oscillations cause the mean arterial pressure to fall by a few mmHg during inspiration and rise during expiration (**Traube–Hering waves**, Section 8.5, 12–14 cycles/min). Human blood pressure may also oscillate at a slower frequency than the breathing cycle, ~6 cycles/min. These are called **Mayer waves**. Mayer waves are attributed to cyclic changes in sympathetic vasomotor tone, driven by a resonance in the baroreceptor reflex.

14.2 Parasympathetic vasodilator nerves

In a **few, specialized tissues** the arteries and resistance vessels are innervated by vasodilator fibres **as well as** the ubiquitous sympathetic vasoconstrictor fibres. Vasodilator fibres are found in the parasympathetic, sympathetic and sensory systems. This section deals with the first of these.

The parasympathetic system comprises long preganglionic fibres and short postganglionic fibres

Parasympathetic vasodilator fibres have a more restricted distribution than sympathetic vasoconstrictor fibres, and are not tonically active; they are only activated when organ function demands a rise in blood flow.

Parasympathetic **preganglionic fibres** are much longer than their sympathetic counterparts; they extend all the way from the central nervous system to the innervated tissue. They emerge from the central nervous system in two 'outflows', one carried by the **cranial nerves** (e.g. vagus) and the other by the **sacral spinal nerves**. The cranial outflow innervates the cerebral and coronary arteries, salivary glands, exocrine pancreas and gastrointestinal mucosa. The sacral outflow innervates the genitalia, bladder and colon. Skin and muscle do not have a parasympathetic innervation.

In the end-organ the long, preganglionic fibres synapse with short, **postganglionic neurons**. The short postganglionic axons innervate the resistance vessels. Like sympathetic terminals, the axons have multiple varicosities containing vesicles of neuroeffector. Parasympathetic vesicles are small and clear, and contain acetylcholine.

Parasympathetic vasodilatation is mediated by acetylcholine and NANC transmitters

Parasympathetic postganglionic terminals release the classic neurotransmitter **acetylcholine**, which elicits vasodilatation (Figures 9.8, top left and 14.6a). Acetylcholine activates muscarinic M_3 receptor on the vessel endothelium, triggering the endothelial G_q–PLC–Ca^{2+} pathway to stimulate endothelial nitric oxide production (Figure 9.10). The nitric oxide diffuses into the myocytes to cause relaxation. By contrast, acetylcholine causes contraction in de-endothelialized vessels (Figure 9.8, top right). This is because myocytes too express muscarinic M_3 receptors, which raise $[Ca^{2+}]$ via the G_q–PLC pathway. The endothelial effect predominates in intact vessels.

The muscarinic receptor blocker, **atropine**, inhibits parasympathetic vasodilatation; but the inhibition is often incomplete (Figure 14.6d). This is because the parasympathetic fibres in some tissues also release **non-adrenergic, non-cholinergic (NANC) transmitters**. The NANC transmitters are **vasoactive intestinal polypeptide** (VIP), **substance P** (another neuropeptide) and **nitric**

oxide. Nitric oxide is generated by 'nitridergic' parasympathetic terminals fibres in erectile tissue and possibly cerebral, temporal, mesenteric and coronary arteries.

Salivary and pancreatic vasodilatation underpins fluid secretion

Blood flow to the submandibular **salivary gland** increases ten-fold when the parasympathetic fibres of the chorda tympani nerve are activated. The increase in perfusion supplies the water needed for salivation, since a salivary gland can secrete its own weight in fluid in just 1 min. The vasodilatation is mediated partly by acetylcholine and partly by VIP and substance P. In the **pancreas**, VIP seems to be the main parasympathetic transmitter, rather than acetylcholine. Such fibres are said to be 'peptidergic'. In the **intestinal submucosa**, the postganglionic transmitter is mainly acetylcholine, acting via endothelial NO production (since the vasodilatation is largely blocked by L-NMMA, an inhibitor of endothelial nitric oxide synthase).

Parasympathetic vasodilatation brings about genital erection

Sacral parasympathetic fibres form the nervi erigentes, which innervate the blood vessels of the genital erectile tissue, i.e. the penis and clitoris – so

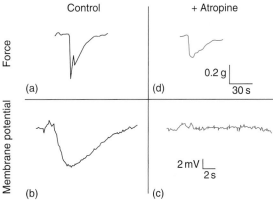

Figure 14.6 Parasympathetic-mediated vasodilatation of rabbit lingual artery; noradrenergic fibres blocked by guanethidine. (a) Mechanical response to perivascular fibre stimulation, showing arterial dilatation. (b) Corresponding membrane potential, showing slow hyperpolarization of a myocyte (baseline −51 mV). (c) Total abolition of electrical response by atropine, proving that the electrical response is purely cholinergic. (d) The dilatation, however, was only partly blocked by atropine, indicating the release of a non-cholinergic vasodilator too, probably vasoactive intestinal polypeptide. (From Brayden JE, Large WA. *British Journal of Pharmacology* 1986; **89**: 163–71, with permission from Wiley-Blackwell.)

these vasomotor nerves are truly essential to the continuation of the species! In the penis an artery in the centre of each corpus cavernosum gives rise to helicine resistance arteries, which feed blood into the cavernous venous sinuses. Parasympathetic activity profoundly dilates the resistance arteries, causing the corpora to swell. Since the swelling compresses the outflow veins against the outer coat of the corpora, the tunica albugenia, the usual balance of resistances is reversed – the resistance to inflow becomes smaller than the resistance to outflow. The venous sinuses of the corpora cavernosa therefore fill with blood at a high pressure, creating distension and erection. A fall in sympathetic vasoconstrictor drive reinforces the dilatation. In the absence of sexual excitement, detumescence is maintained by sympathetic α-adrenergic tone in the penile arteries and corpus smooth muscle.

Parasympathetic-induced erection is not blocked by atropine, but is blocked by inhibitors of nitric oxide synthase. This shows that the parasympathetic fibres are chiefly **nitridergic** rather than cholinergic. The axons contain nitric oxide synthase and secrete NO upon electrical stimulation. **Sildenafil (Viagra)**, a successful treatment for human erectile dysfunction, amplifies the biochemical effect of the NO–cGMP pathway by inhibiting **phosphodiesterase type 5**, the enzyme that normally degrades cGMP (Figure 9.10). A common side effect is vascular headache due to cerebral artery dilatation.

Parasympathetic **VIP** too may contribute to erectile vasodilatation, since VIP is present in penile parasympathetic fibres and appears in penile venous blood following pelvic fibre stimulation.

14.3 Sympathetic vasodilator nerves

As emphasized repeatedly, most sympathetic vasomotor fibres are noradrenergic and cause vasoconstriction. In certain species and tissues, however, there is a limited distribution of sympathetic **cholinergic** (acetylcholine-releasing) fibres that cause vasodilatation.

Sympathetic cholinergic fibres mediate sweating and cutaneous vasodilatation

Human sweat glands are innervated by sympathetic cholinergic fibres (sudomotor fibres), which elicit cutaneous vasodilatation as well as sweating. The fibres release acetylcholine, which stimulates the vascular endothelium to produce prostacyclin (via COX1) and EDHF, along with a little nitric oxide (Section 9.5). Since the sudomotor-mediated vasodilatation is only partially inhibited by atropine, additional NANC transmitters must also contribute to the dilatation. VIP seems to be one such factor, being demonstrable in vasomotor fibres close to the sweat glands.

In non-primate muscle, sympathetic cholinergic fibres mediate the vasodilatation of the alerting response

In the cat, dog, goat and sheep, but not primates, the small arteries of skeletal muscle are innervated by sympathetic cholinergic vasodilator nerves, stimulation of which increases muscle blood flow. The sympathetic cholinergic fibres are controlled by the forebrain and are not tonically active, unlike the sympathetic vasoconstrictor fibres (Table 14.3). They play no part in the baroreflex control of blood pressure and are activated solely as part of the **alerting response**, which is a co-ordinated set of cardiac and vascular changes evoked by mental stress, fear, danger (Section 16.8). The cholinergic vasodilatation increases the muscle blood flow in anticipation of exercise, but fails to increase the microvascular permeability–surface area product – probably because cholinergic fibres innervate chiefly the arteries of diameter 0.1–0.2 mm rather than arterioles. Metabolic hyperaemia, by contrast, has its

Table 14.3 Contrasting organisation of sympathetic vasoconstrictor and vasodilator nervous systems

Feature	Sympathetic vasoconstrictor fibre	Sympathetic vasodilator fibre
Main neuroeffector	Noradrenaline (and ATP)	Acetylcholine (and VIP)
Distribution	Most organs and tissue	Only sweat glands in humans. Skeletal muscle in non-primates
Tonically active?	Yes	No
Central control	Brainstem	Forebrain
Involvement in baroreceptor reflex	Major role	Negligible
Role in blood pressure homeostasis	Very important	Unimportant
Duration of effect	Mostly well sustained	Transient

greatest effect on arterioles (Figure 13.9), recruits capillaries and thus raises the permeability–surface area product as well as blood flow. It cannot be emphasized too strongly that **local metabolic factors cause the functional hyperaemia associated with normal, non-emotional exercise**, not sympathetic vasodilator nerves.

In human muscle, adrenaline and other mechanisms mediate the vasodilatation of the alerting response

Acute mental stress, such as mental arithmetic, evokes vasodilatation in human forearm muscles (Figure 14.7), though not in the calf. This alerting response was formerly attributed to a sympathetic cholinergic innervation, but more recent observation indicate otherwise, as follows. (i) Primates as a group lack a sympathetic cholinergic innervation to the muscle vasculature (cf. skin vasculature). (ii) Electrode recordings show that the sympathetic activity in human muscle is reduced, not increased, by stress. (iii) Axillary

nerve block does not prevent the human forearm vasodilator response to stress. Beta-adrenoceptor blockers, however, significantly attenuate the human response, indicating that it is due in part to circulating **adrenaline**. Plasma adrenaline concentration doubles during the alerting response, due to the sympathetic stimulation of the adrenal medulla. An additional factor is a **reduction in sympathetic vasoconstrictor activity** to the muscle, though this alone is insufficient to explain the large increase in flow. (The finding in some, but not all, studies that atropine, a blocker of acetylcholine muscarinic receptors, attenuates human stress-induced vasodilatation remains a puzzle.)

14.4 Nociceptive C-fibre mediated vasodilatation

Antidromic stimulation of sensory C fibres causes cutaneous vasodilatation

The curious ability of sensory nerves to cause cutaneous vasodilatation was discovered by William Bayliss early in the twentieth century. He stimulated the dorsal root of a spinal nerve antidromically, sending action potentials in the 'wrong' direction down the sensory nerves, and found that this caused cutaneous vasodilatation. Antidromic activity probably contributes to the characteristic segmental cutaneous hyperaemia of **shingles**, a dorsal root infection by herpes zoster (a reactivated form of latent varicella zoster, the chickenpox virus).

C-fibre-mediated vasodilatation is part of the Lewis triple response

The motor function of nociceptive (harm-sensing) sensory fibres, i.e. the C-fibres, was revealed further in the Lewis triple response, described in 1927. Sir Thomas Lewis noted that the reaction of human skin to a mild trauma such as a scratch has three components.

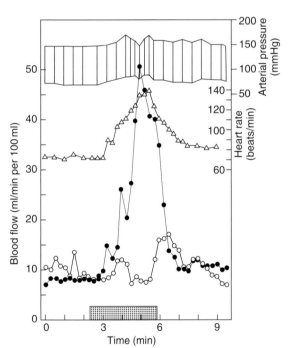

Figure 14.7 A classic demonstration of the human altering response. Closed circles, forearm blood flow, mainly to muscle; open circles, hand blood flow, mainly to skin; triangles, heart rate. During the time represented by the rectangle, the experimenters made the subject believe that he was bleeding badly through a leak in the apparatus (!). The increase in forearm flow is comparable with that in severe exercise, and greatly exceeds the maximum flow produced by the withdrawal of sympathetic vasoconstrictor tone. (From Blair DA, Glover WE, Greenfield ADM, Roddie LC. *Journal of Physiology* 1959; **148**: 633–47, with permission from Wiley-Blackwell.)

- **Local redness** along the line of the scratch is caused by local vasodilatation, resulting probably from the release of K^+ ions and inflammatory autacoids by activated cells.
- **Local swelling** along the line of the scratch (a wheal) is caused by inflammatory oedema resulting from microvascular damage (Section 11.11).
- **The spreading flare** is an area of redness that gradually extends laterally from the line of trauma for 2–3 cm. Humans and rats exhibit this response, but many other species do not.

Remarkably, the flare must be mediated by sensory fibres, because it abolished by sensory denervation or by local anaesthetics such as lignocaine (Figure 14.8). Since the flare spreads too quickly to be explained by autacoid diffusion, Lewis suggested that it is mediated by a C-fibre **sensory axon reflex**, as follows.

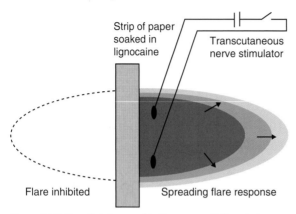

Figure 14.8 Vasodilatation mediated by sensory C-fibres in human skin, seen *en face*. Nociceptive C-fibres were stimulated by transcutaneous electrical stimulation. The spreading flare was recorded by a laser Doppler imager. The flare is abolished by the sensory anaesthetic lignocaine. (Based on Schmelz M, Petersen LJ. *News in Physiological Sciences* 2001; **16**: 33–7, with permission from American Physiological Society.)

The C-fibre sensory axon reflex causes the spreading flare

The flare is mediated by nociceptive (harm-sensing) C-fibres. Trauma triggers C-fibre action potentials, which not only propagates centrally but also passes down an axon side branch, travelling antidromically to blood vessels up to a centimetre away (Figure 14.9). Arrival of the action potential in the axon branch terminal causes it to release vasodilator neuropeptides. These include **substance P**, which activates endothelial NK_1 receptors to stimulate NO production; and **calcitonin-gene related peptide** (CGRP), which activates the vascular myocyte cAMP pathway (Figure 12.10). CGRP is extremely potent and its effect lasts many hours. **Mast cell histamine** too is implicated, at least in rat skin and some human dermatogical conditions. Many substance P-containing fibres terminate on mast cells, which express NK_1 receptors. Receptor activation causes the mast cell to release its histamine granules, exacerbating the vasodilatation.

C-fibre antidromic activity can lead to neurogenic inflammation

Antidromic stimulation of C-fibres not only causes vasodilatation but also venular hyperpermeability,

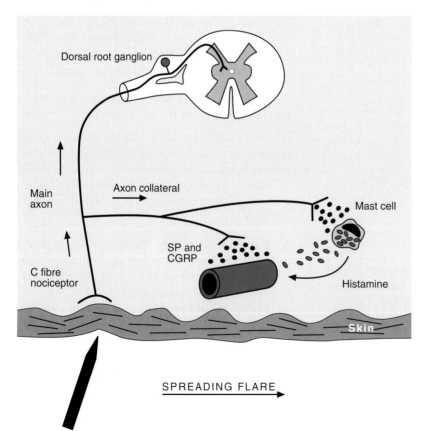

Figure 14.9 The sensory axon reflex and spreading flare response to a scratch. Vasodilatation is due to the release of substance P (SP) and CGRP from nociceptive C-fibre axon branches. In rat skin and possibly some human dermatological conditions, collateral endings near mast cells also trigger histamine granule release, which augments the flare. (After Foreman JC. *Allergy* 1987; **42**: 1–11 with permission from Wiley-Blackwell.)

due to the action of substance P and histamine on venular endothelium (Section 11.11). The resulting plasma exudation and high-protein oedema is called neurogenic inflammation. Neurogenic inflammation is readily elicited in rat skin and synovial joints. Healthy human skin is not very susceptible to neurogenic inflammation, but becomes susceptible when sensitized by dermatological disorders.

14.5 Hormonal control of the circulation

Many hormones influence the heart and circulation. Hormones such as adrenaline, vasopressin and angiotensin are in general less important than autonomic nerves for physiological, acute cardiovascular regulation, but become major regulators in pathological situations such as haemorrhagic hypovolaemia or transplanted hearts. The main cardiovascular hormones, **adrenaline**, **vasopressin**, **angiotensin** and **atrial natriuretic peptide**, are described in Sections 14.6–14.9. Except for adrenaline, they also regulate renal tubular function to control extracellular fluid volume. Other hormones with significant cardiovascular effects, such as **insulin**, **thyroxine, oestrogen** and **relaxin**, are described briefly in this section.

Insulin

Insulin stimulates endothelium to produce NO, so insulin has vasodilator and antithrombotic actions. It also inhibits vascular smooth muscle growth and migration. These important, anti-atheroma effects are reduced in diabetics, who either lack insulin or are resistant to it. This may contribute to the high incidence of atheroma, ischaemic heart disease and limb ischaemia in diabetics. Diabetes is a major risk factor for these conditions.

Thyroxine

Thyroxine induces cardiac myocytes to express a high density of β_1-adrenoceptors, and thereby enhances contractility. Hyperthyroidism increases basal metabolic rate, which leads to a generalized vasodilatation, fall in total peripheral resistance, tachycardia and rise in stroke volume.

Oestrogen

The ovarian follicle hormone 17β-oestradiol causes vasodilatation in many tissues, including the female genitourinary system (uterus, vagina, kidneys), mammary glands, heart and skin. Its acute vasodilator, action is mediated partly by the activation of endothelial nitric oxide synthase via the protein kinase B pathway (Figure 9.10) and partly through activation of vascular myocyte BK_{Ca} channels. During pregnancy, high levels of oestrogen cause a characteristic fall in blood pressure by mid-term. Oestrogen reduces the incidence of coronary artery disease in pre-menopausal women, probably by a genomic upregulation of nitric oxide synthase and prostacyclin production.

Relaxin

Relaxin is a peptide hormone secreted by the ovarian corpus luteum during pregnancy and parturition. It causes vasodilatation in the uterus, mammary gland and heart, and acts by attenuating endothelin-mediated vasoconstriction.

14.6 Adrenaline and noradrenaline

The adrenal gland is situated at the upper pole of the kidney. Its outer part, the cortex, secretes the steroid hormones cortisol and aldosterone. It inner part, the medulla (10% of the gland) comprises chromaffin cells that secrete the catecholamines adrenaline (epinephrine) and noradrenaline (norepinephrine). Noradrenaline is methylated by N-methyltransferase to form adrenaline, which accounts for ~80% of catecholamine secretion in humans. In diving mammals, by contrast, noradrenaline is the chief product, contributing to muscle vasoconstriction during dives.

The adrenal vasculature is organized as a **cortico-medullary portal system**; see Section 1.8 for portal systems. This carries cortisol-rich blood from the cortex to many chromaffin cells in the medulla, where the high cortisol concentration induces N-methyltransferase expression and hence adrenaline production. Other chromaffin cells are supplied directly via medullary arteries, express less N-methyltransferase and secrete noradrenaline.

Although the human medulla secretes mainly adrenaline, the basal plasma adrenaline concentration (0.1–0.5 nM) is lower than the noradrenaline concentration (0.5–3.0 nM). The relatively high circulating noradrenaline is due mainly to **spillage** from the tonically active, sympathetic vasomotor terminals (Figure 14.2), so it is often used as a measure of sympathetic activity. For example, plasma noradrenaline approximately doubles on standing up due to increased sympathetic activity, while plasma adrenaline changes little. The circulating **half-life** of the catecholamines is only a few minutes, so the circulating concentration can be adjusted rapidly. The catecholamines are taken up by non-neural tissue for **degradation** by catechol-O-methyltransferase, and by nerve endings for degradation by mono-amine oxidase.

Adrenaline secretion is stimulated by sympathetic preganglionic fibres in stress situations

During embryogenesis the medullary chromaffin cells develop from postganglionic sympathetic neurons. This accounts for their innervation by preganglionic sympathetic fibres in the splanchnic nerve (Figure 14.1). Sympathetic activity thus regulates adrenaline secretion. Secretion is stimulated in response to four main stresses, namely:

- **exercise**
- **alerting** (the alerting response to fear–flight–fight situations)
- **hypotension** and
- **hypoglycaemia**.

During exercise the plasma adrenaline concentration can reach 5 nM, and noradrenaline 10 nM. The latter is due partly to spillover from the increased sympathetic activity.

Adrenaline has both metabolic and cardiovascular effects

The cardiovascular effects of adrenaline at physiological concentrations are relatively minor compared with those of the autonomic nerves and intrinsic regulators. Consequently, the **metabolic effects of adrenaline are as important as its cardiovascular effects**, albeit not our main concern here. Adrenaline stimulates **glycogenolysis** in skeletal muscle and **lipolysis** in adipose tissue, thereby releasing glucose into the bloodstream. Adrenaline also has the following cardiovascular effects.

- **Cardiac contractility and heart rate are raised** via the activation of the cardiac β_1-adrenoceptors (Section 4.5).
- **Arterial and venous constrictions** are induced in tissues with a predominance of vascular α-adrenoceptors, such as the **skin and intestines**. The ingrained belief of many students that adrenaline always causes vasodilatation is untrue.
- **Vasodilatation in myocardium, skeletal muscle and liver** is due to their abundance of β_2-adrenoceptors, along with the high affinity of adrenaline for this class of receptor

(Table 14.1). The β_2-adrenoceptor is coupled to the vasodilator G_s – adenylyl cyclase – cAMP pathway (Figure 12.10). If the β-receptors are blocked by propranolol, adrenaline causes vasoconstriction even in skeletal muscle, because it also activates α-receptors. Noradrenaline vasoconstricts muscle, because it has a higher affinity for α-receptors than β-receptors.

Since myocardial vasodilatation improves coronary perfusion, adrenaline is often injected as an emergency measure during a **cardiac arrest** – though it appears to have relatively little effect on the outcome.

Adrenaline and noradrenaline have different net effects on the circulation

As explained above, adrenaline and noradrenaline at physiological concentrations have opposite effects on skeletal muscle, which is the most abundant tissue in the body (~40% by weight). Consequently, their effects on the systemic circulation differ substantially (Figure 14.10).

Intravenous noradrenaline causes a widespread systemic vasoconstriction, which **greatly increases the total peripheral resistance** and arterial blood pressure. The raised pressure triggers a baroreceptor reflex, which reduces the sympathetic drive to the heart and increases the parasympathetic drive. This more than offsets the direct stimulatory effect of

Figure 14.10 Contrasting effects of intravenous adrenaline and noradrenaline in man. Dashed red line is mean blood pressure. For explanation, see text. An initial transient drop in blood pressure during adrenaline infusion is not shown on this time scale. (From classic monograph, Barcroft H, Swan HJC. *Sympathetic Control of Human Blood Vessels*. London: Edward Arnold, 1953, by permission.)

noradrenaline on the pacemaker and myocardium, resulting in a fall in heart rate and cardiac output.

Intravenous adrenaline, by contrast, **reduces the total peripheral resistance**, because the vasodilatation in skeletal muscle outweighs the vasoconstriction in other tissues. Mean blood pressure changes little (Figure 14.10). Consequently, the stimulation of the heart by adrenaline is not opposed by the baroreflex, and cardiac output increases markedly.

A rare tumour of the medullary chromaffin cells, the **phaeochromocytoma**, secretes a mixture of catecholamines and causes hypertension. The latter can be treated with α-antagonists such as phentolamine.

14.7 Vasopressin (antidiuretic hormone)

Vasopressin is a vasoconstrictor nonapeptide that is synthesized by the magnocellular (big) neurons of the supraoptic and paraventricular nuclei of the hypothalamus (Figure 14.11). The vasopressin is transported along the neuron axon, which passes

down the pituitary stalk into the posterior pituitary gland. The arrival of action potentials stimulates Ca^{2+}-dependent secretion of the vasopressin from the axon terminals into the bloodstream. The half-life of vasopressin in the bloodstream is only ~5 min, so the circulating level can be rapidly adjusted. Vasopressin secretion is regulated by two kinds of sensory input – one from central osmoreceptors and the other from cardiovascular pressure receptors.

Osmoreceptors regulate diuresis via vasopressin

Osmoreceptors are neurons in the anterolateral hypothalamus that are sensitive to plasma osmolarity. They are located in the organum vasculosus lamina terminalis and subfornicular organ which, appropriately, lack a blood–brain barrier; the capillary endothelium is fenestrated at these sites. The osmoreceptors are excited by a rise in plasma osmolarity above 280–285 mOs, e.g. during dehydration. Cholinergic axons extend from the osmoreceptors to synapse with the nearby magnocellular neurons,

Figure 14.11 Regulation of vasopressin secretion; relative contribution of arterial baroreceptors and low pressure atrial receptors varies between species. ABP, arterial blood pressure, regulated by resistance vessel tone; AP, atrial pressure, regulated by renal control of extracellular fluid volume; OVLT, organum vasculosus lamina terminalis; SFO, subfornicular organ; SON, supraoptic nucleus; PVN, paraventricular nucleus; CVLM, caudal ventrolateral medulla. Inset shows sensitivity to plasma osmolarity and increase caused by blood loss.

stimulating them to secret vasopressin. Since a 2% rise in plasma osmolarity has the same stimulatory effect as a 10% fall in blood volume, vasopressin secretion is more sensitive to plasma osmolarity than blood volume. The osmoreceptors also project to **parvocellular (small) neurons** in the paraventricular nucleus, which influence sympathetic activity; consequently, water deprivation increases peripheral vasoconstrictor sympathetic activity, as well as vasopressin levels.

The main role of vasopressin at its normal, low plasma concentrations is to regulate the amount of water excreted by the kidneys, in order to stabilize the plasma volume and osmolarity. This is reflected in its alternative name, 'anti-diuretic hormone' (diuresis is urine production). Vasopressin stimulate high affinity V_2 receptors on the renal collecting ducts, leading to increased water reabsorption and the prevention of dehydration. At physiological osmolarity, ~294 mOs, the circulating vasopressin concentration is near the middle of the renal dose–response range, so water excretion can be adjusted up or down by changes in circulating vasopressin.

Cardiovascular pressure receptors stimulate vasopressin secretion during hypovolaemia

Vasopressin secretion is also stimulated by **a fall in blood volume and blood pressure**, for example during a haemorrhage or severe dehydration. Pressure receptors in the heart and arteries, described in Chapter 16, send information about the central blood volume and arterial pressure to the brainstem. From here, the information is relayed to the magnocellular neurons via an inhibitory synapse. As a result of the inhibitory step, a fall in cardiovascular receptor traffic leads to a rise in vasopressin secretion (Figure 14.11). Once the blood volume falls by more than 10%, vasopressin secretion increases steeply. The vasopressin causes peripheral vasoconstriction – though this requires a higher circulating concentration than the anti-diuretic action, because the vascular V_1 receptors have a lower affinity than the renal duct V_2 receptors. The low affinity vascular V_1 receptors are coupled to the G_q–PLC pathway that leads to vasoconstriction (Figure 12.6).

Vasopressin-induced vasoconstriction helps to support the arterial blood pressure in hypovolaemic patients, and contributes to the characteristic pallor of their skin. In cerebral and coronary vessels, however, vasopressin stimulates the endothelium, leading to NO-mediated vasodilatation. Vasopressin thus redistributes the limited cardiac output of hypovolaemia in favour of the brain and heart. At the same time, urine production is reduced to a minimum to conserve body fluid. If vasopressin is absent, as in **diabetes insipidus** and Brattleboro rats, the blood pressure is abnormally depressed during dehydration or haemorrhage.

Nausea is a further, potent stimulus for vasopressin secretion. During nausea and vomiting the vasopressin level can reach 50 times that required for antidiuresis. The resulting vasoconstriction contributes to the characteristic grey pallor of nausea. The vasoconstrictor action of injected vasopressin can also be used in an emergency to reduce the bleeding from oesophageal varices, a common feature of portal hypertension.

14.8 Renin–angiotensin–aldosterone system (RAAS)

Angiotensin II is a vasoconstrictor peptide, production of which increases when blood pressure falls. Its role is to help maintain the extracellular fluid volume and arterial blood pressure. It achieves this through three principal actions. (1) Angiotensin II stimulates **aldosterone** secretion by the adrenal cortex. Aldosterone promotes renal salt and water retention to maintain the extracellular fluid and plasma volume, and is essential to life. (2) Angiotensin II causes a generalized **vasoconstriction**, partly by direct action and partly by boosting sympathetic activity. This raises peripheral resistance and blood pressure. (3) Angiotensin II stimulates the sensation of **thirst**, and hence fluid intake.

The half-life of angiotensin II in the circulation is ~20 min, and it is inactivated by the liver. Circulating angiotensin levels are normally low, and angiotensin inhibitors cause only a small fall in blood pressure in healthy humans. In patients with clinical hypertension, however, angiotensin inhibitors reduce blood pressure markedly. In general, angiotensin becomes important in pathological situations, namely hypovolaemia, cardiac failure and clinical hypertension.

Angiotensin II production is mediated by renin and endothelial ACE

Angiotensin production is initiated by the secretion of **renin** (pronounced ree-nin) into the renal bloodstream (Figure 14.12). Renin is a proteolytic enzyme that is synthesized, stored and secreted by specialized cells in the wall of renal afferent arterioles, called **juxtaglomerular (JG) cells**

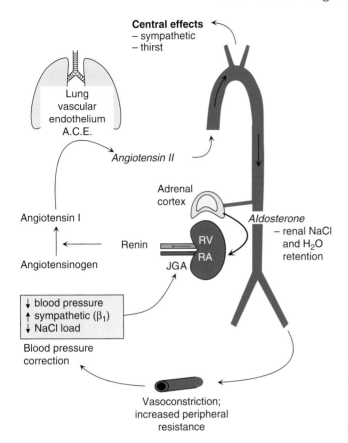

Figure 14.12 Renin–angiotensin–aldosterone system. JGA, juxtaglomerular apparatus, RA and RV, renal artery and vein. Central effects are stimulation of sympathetic outflow, reduction in sensitivity of baroreceptor reflex and stimulation of thirst.

('juxta'-glomerular, close to glomeruli). Renin attacks a plasma α_2-globulin, angiotensinogen, to cleave off a decapeptide called angiotensin I. Angiotensin I has little activity, but it is cleaved further by an ecto(outside)-enzyme on the surface of endothelial cells, **angiotensin converting enzyme (ACE)**, to generate an active octapeptide, angiotensin II. This process takes place mainly in the lungs, because this is the first major expanse of endothelium encountered by venous angiotensin I. **ACE inhibitors** such as captopril, enalapril and ramiprilat block the formation of angiotensin II; but as ACE normally degrades circulating bradykinin too, ACE inhibitors also raise circulating bradykinin levels, with unwanted side effects. These can be avoided by using the **angiotensin II receptor blocker**, losartan. Cleavage of one more amino acid from some angiotensin II molecules by aminopeptidase forms a hepta-peptide, angiotensin III.

Angiotensin II supports blood pressure via aldosterone secretion

At normal, physiological concentrations angiotensin II and III help stimulate the secretion of the steroidal hormone **aldosterone** by the outermost adrenal cortex (zona glomerulosa). Over the course of an hour or so, aldosterone stimulates the renal distal convoluted tubules to increase the rate of Na^+ reabsorption, in exchange for K^+ and H^+. The response is slow because it requires the synthesis and insertion of Na^+–K^+ pumps into the basal membrane and epithelial Na^+ channels (ENaC) into the apical membrane of the tubule cells. The Na^+ reabsorbed from the tubular fluid draws water with it by osmosis. In this way, the RAAS maintains the plasma volume and therefore arterial blood pressure. Failure of the adrenal cortex to secrete aldosterone leads to severe hypotension and hyperkalaemia – a potentially fatal condition called **Addison's disease**. Conversely, an adrenal tumour may secrete excessive amounts of aldosterone, leading to salt and water retention and hypertension (**Conn's syndrome**).

Angiotensin II also supports blood pressure through direct vasoconstriction

Angiotensin II binds to AT_1 receptors on vascular myocytes. Since AT_1 receptors are coupled to the

G_q–PLC–diacyl glycerol pathway, they trigger depolarization-independent and depolarization-dependent contraction (Figures 12.6 and 12.7). This tonic, vasoconstrictor action of angiotensin II contributes to the peripheral resistance, and thus to blood pressure maintenance – though the contribution is quite modest at basal concentrations. Angiotensin II makes a much greater contribution, however, at the raised concentrations found in **hypovolaemia, clinical shock, cardiac failure** and **hypertension**. In hypovolaemia, shock and cardiac failure, angiotensin II causes pronounced vasoconstriction of skin, splanchnic and renal vessels. In clinical shock and renal artery stenosis, angiotensin contracts the renal **glomerular efferent arterioles** (Figure 1.5), which helps maintain the glomerular capillary pressure and filtration rate. Many, but not all, patients with essential hypertension have raised renin and angiotensin II levels, so **ACE inhibitors** (captopril, enalapril, ramiprilat) and **AT$_1$ blockers** (losartan) are valuable anti-hypertension drugs.

Angiotensin II also increases cardiac contractility during hypovolaemia and shock, partly by enhancing the plateau Ca^{2+} current, and partly by stimulating sympathetic activity, as described next.

Angiotensin II also supports blood pressure by peripheral and central sympathetic amplification and by eliciting thirst

Angiotensin II raises the peripheral resistance not only by direct vasoconstrictor action but also by interacting with the brainstem, sympathetic ganglia and sympathetic terminals to boost sympathetic-induced vasoconstriction. Angiotensin II diffuses into the area postrema of the brainstem, where the blood–brain barrier is deficient. The area postrema is rich in angiotensin receptors and their activation **increases the sympathetic preganglionic outflow**. AT$_1$ receptors on the postganglionic neurons of the **sympathetic ganglia** further facilitate the generation of sympathetic action potentials. **Sympathetic terminal varicosities** likewise have AT$_1$ receptors, activation of which facilitates the release of noradrenaline by sympathetic action potentials (neuromodulation, Figure 14.2). In cardiac failure, raised angiotensin II levels contribute to the increased sympathetic activity, fluid retention (via aldosterone) and high cardiac filling pressures (Section 18.5).

In addition to its pro-sympathetic actions, angiotensin III acts on the hypothalamus to stimulate the sensation of **thirst**, a common symptom in patients with hypovolaemia. Fluid intake helps restores plasma volume in such patients.

Negative feedback loops regulate RAAS

The concentration of circulating angiotensin II depends on the rate at which renal JG cells secrete renin. Renin exocytosis is controlled by multiple factors, which create negative feedback loops to support arterial blood pressure during hypovolaemia, as follows.

- **Hypotension** activates the RAAS directly, because the JG cells of afferent arterioles are inhibited by stretch. In patients with **renal artery stenosis**, the low pressure beyond the stenosis activates the RAAS inappropriately, causing hypertension.

- The increased **renal sympathetic activity** and circulating adrenaline during hypotension stimulate β_1-adrenoceptors on JG cells. The resulting rise in intracellular cAMP stimulates renin secretion and thus helps to correct the hypotension.

- **A fall in NaCl concentration at the macula densa** stimulates renin production. The macula densa is a NaCl-sensitive group of cells in the renal tubule (ascending loop of Henle) directly adjacent to the JG cells, forming the **juxtaglomerular apparatus**. Hypotension and increased sympathetic activity reduce the glomerular filtration rate, which reduces the amount of NaCl reaching the macula densa. This stimulates the macula densa, leading to RAAS activation. The resulting rise in aldosterone stimulates the distal tubules to reabsorb more Na^+ and water, to maintain extracellular fluid volume.

- **Atrial natriuretic peptide** and angiotensin II both inhibit the secretion of renin. The natriuretic effect of atrial natriuretic peptide is partly due to RAAS inhibition.

14.9 Natriuretic peptides

Natriuretic peptides (NPs), as the name implies, stimulate renal salt excretion. They act as a counterweight to the salt-retaining RAAS, and have an anti-hypertensive action. Thus the inactivation of NP receptors by gene-targeting in mice results in hypertension. Natriuretic peptides come in three flavours: ANP (atrial natriuretic peptide), BNP (brain type, which is also produced by some atrial and ventricular cells) and CNP (endothelial cell type). ANP is the chief circulating form normally, but ventricular BNP secretion increases greatly in heart failure. ANP and BNP are secreted by specialized cardiac myocytes in response to high cardiac filling pressures, and their multiple actions help reduce plasma volume, return the filling pressure to normal and reduce arterial pressure. The actions are as follows.

- NPs cause a **moderate dilatation** of resistance vessels.
- NPs **increase renal salt and water excretion (natriuresis and diuresis)** through three mechanisms. (i) Afferent arteriole dilatation raises the glomerular filtration rate. (ii) Na^+ reabsorption in the proximal and distal tubules is inhibited. (iii) Renin and aldosterone secretion are inhibited.
- The lowering of plasma volume by NPs is greater than can be accounted for by the rather moderate diuresis. This is because NPs also cause **fluid transfer from the plasma to the interstitial compartment**. This is due partly to precapillary vasodilatation, which raises the capillary filtration pressure, and partly to an increase in venular permeability, up to two-fold.

NPs bring about the above effects by binding to NP receptors on vascular myocytes, endothelium and tubular epithelium. The NP receptor is a transmembrane protein with guanylyl cyclase activity in its cytoplasmic section. Consequently, the activated receptor raises the intracellular cGMP level, which induces vasodilatation (Section 12.7) and venular hyperpermeability (Figure 11.30).

Plasma ANP concentration is normally extremely low. Even when increased two- to four-fold, for example by central venous pressure elevation during whole-body immersion in water, there is little consistent change in renal excretion. In heart failure, however, circulating natriuretic peptide level can increase 10- to 30-fold, and ventricle-derived BNP 200-fold. This probably helps to mitigate the accumulation of extracellular fluid in heart failure (Chapter 18). BNP can be used as a biochemical index of heart failure, and high levels correlate with a poor prognosis.

14.10 Special features of venous control

The venous system has been called 'the Cinderella of the circulation' because it is often neglected. The control of peripheral veins (capacitance vessels) is important, however, because peripheral venous tone regulates the distribution of blood between peripheral vessels and the thorax, and thereby **regulates cardiac filling pressure** and stroke volume.

Differentiation of the venous system

The venous system has four distinctive compartments functionally (Figure 14.13). The **central, thoracic compartment**, consisting of the great veins, right heart and pulmonary vessels, is essentially passive. The central blood volume determines the cardiac filling pressure, which influences the stroke volume (Starling's law of the heart). The three **peripheral compartments** have differing characteristics as follows.

Splanchnic veins

The veins of the gastrointestinal tract, liver and spleen contain ~20% of the total blood volume at rest. They are innervated by sympathetic constrictor nerves and express α-adrenoceptors. During exercise or hypotension, increases in sympathetic activity and adrenaline stimulate splanchnic vein contraction (Figure 14.5). This displaces blood into the central veins and helps to maintain the cardiac filling pressure at times of circulatory stress.

Skeletal muscle veins

The veins inside skeletal muscles are poorly innervated. Their volume is influenced chiefly by the muscle pump and posture (gravity). Although direct sympathetic control of these veins is almost non-existent, their volume is nevertheless affected indirectly by sympathetic vasomotor activity, because arteriolar constriction reduces venular pressure. This causes the venous system to recoil elastically and displace blood centrally (Figure 14.4, label a).

Cutaneous veins

The veins of the skin are richly innervated by sympathetic noradrenergic fibres. High core temperatures reduce cutaneous sympathetic activity, leading to venodilatation and a flushed appearance. Conversely, during cold weather or clinical hypotension, cutaneous sympathetic activity increases, leading to venoconstriction and blanching of the skin. Cutaneous sympathetic activity is also increased by emotional stress, deep inspiration and exercise (Figure 14.14).

Comparison of venous and arteriolar control

Veins and resistance vessels respond in similar ways to many stimuli; in the skin, for example, both

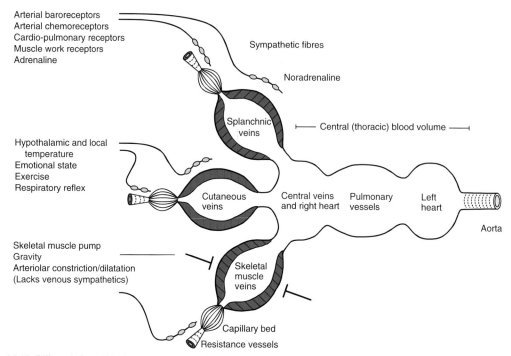

Figure 14.13 Differentiation within the venous system. Changes in central blood volume and cardiac filling pressure are brought about by contraction of peripheral veins, especially splanchnic veins. Factors regulating the different venous beds are listed on the left.

Figure 14.14 Sympathetic control of human cutaneous veins. Blood flow was arrested by a sphygmomanometer cuff. A rise in the pressure of stationary blood trapped in the veins signals venoconstriction. LBNP, lower body negative pressure. (After Rowell LB. *Human Circulation Regulation during Physical Stress.* New York: Oxford University Press, 1986, with permission from Oxford University Press.)

constrict during hypotension. There are also differences in behaviour, however, as follows.

- Most venules and veins have **little basal tone** in the absence of sympathetic activity (though the portal vein is actively contractile in many species).
- Veins generally show **little myogenic response** to stretch (though there are exceptions).
- Veins and arterioles may respond differently to agonists, due to differences in receptor expression.

Angiotensin II, for example, has little direct effect on veins but a powerful effect on arterioles. (Angiotensin II does, however, contribute to the intense venoconstriction of patients in cardiac failure, acting indirectly by sympathetic potentiation.) **Glyceryl trinitrate** has a greater dilator effect on veins than on arterioles, and its efficacy in relieving angina is due partly to the reduction of cardiac filling pressure, and therefore cardiac work, following venodilatation.

SUMMARY

- Vascular tone is regulated by a three-tier hierarchy of interacting controls. The lowest level of control is the Bayliss myogenic response, which provides autoregulation. The next level of control involves intrinsic (locally produced) vasoactive agents, e.g. endothelial secretions, metabolic vasodilators, autacoids. The highest level of control is the **neuroendocrine system**, which brings the vasculature under central control for the benefit of the organism as a whole.

- **Sympathetic vasoconstrictor fibres** to the skin, muscle, kidney and gut are tonically active. Their terminal varicosities release noradrenaline to activate α-adrenoceptors, which raise vascular tone. Sympathetic drive to resistance vessels is varied in order to stabilize arterial blood pressure, regulate tissue perfusion and adjust fluid partitioning between plasma and interstitium. Sympathetic drive to splanchnic and cutaneous veins is varied in order to maintain central blood volume and cardiac filling pressure. Sympathetic drive is regulated by bulbospinal fibres descending from the brainstem to the thoracic preganglionic neurons.

- **Parasympathetic vasodilator fibres** travel in the cranial and sacral outflows. The cranial outflow innervates the salivary glands, pancreas and gut, and evokes secretory hyperaemia. The sacral outflow innervates the genitalia (erectile tissue), bladder and colon. The main parasympathetic effectors are acetylcholine, VIP and NO.

- **Nociceptive C-fibres** in the skin cause the spreading flare component of the Lewis triple response to trauma. This is an axon reflex, mediated by substance P, CGRP and mast cell histamine. C-fibres also mediate neurogenic inflammation.

- **Hormonal control** by adrenaline, angiotensin II and vasopressin supports blood pressure, especially under stressful conditions such as hypovolaemic shock.

- **Adrenaline** is secreted by the adrenal medulla in response to exercise, the alerting response, hypotension and hypoglycaemia. Secretion is triggered by preganglionic sympathetic activity. Adrenaline promotes glucose release into the bloodstream; helps to raise cardiac output; causes β-adrenoceptor-mediated vasodilatation in skeletal muscle and myocardium; and α-adrenoceptor-mediated vasoconstriction in the skin, intestinal tract and other tissues.

- **Angiotensin II** is formed in the lungs by the action of endothelial ACE on angiotensin I. The latter is generated in renal plasma by the enzyme renin. Renin is secreted by renal juxtaglomerular cells in response to low blood pressure, renal sympathetic activity and a low NaCl load. Angiotensin II stimulates aldosterone secretion; and it causes vasoconstriction both directly and by enhancing sympathetic activity. Angiotensin thus supports plasma volume and blood pressure.

- **Vasopressin** (anti-diuretic hormone) is produced by hypothalamic magnocellular neurons and is released from the posterior pituitary. Secretion is stimulated by hypertonicity (central osmoreceptors) and hypotension (cardiovascular receptors). The vasoconstrictor action supports blood pressure during hypovolaemic shock.

- **Atrial natriuretic peptide** is secreted by the atria in response to distension. It reduces plasma volume by a mild diuretic action and by enhancing microvascular filtration through vasodilatation and increased permeability. Levels are high in heart failure.

Further reading

Reviews and chapters

Brock JA, Cunnane TC. (1993) Neurotransmitter release mechanisms at the sympathetic neuroeffector junction. *Experimental Physiology* 1993; **78**: 591–614.

Burnstock G. ATP as a neurotransmitter. *Trends in Pharmacological Sciences* 2006; **27**: 166–76.

Elser M, Jennings G, Lambert G, Meredith I, Horne M, Eisenhofer G. Overflow of catecholamine neurotransmitters to the circulation: source, fate and functions. *Physiological Reviews* 1990; **70**: 963–82.

Fitzsimons JT. Angiotensin, thirst and sodium appetite. *Physiological Reviews* 1998; **78**: 583–686.

Folkow B, Nilsson H. Transmitter release at adrenergic nerve endings: Total exocytosis or fractional release? *News in Physiological Sciences* 1997; **12**: 32–6.

Hainsworth R. The importance of vascular capacitance in cardiovascular control. *News in Physiological Sciences* 1991; **5**: 250–4.

Holmes CL, Landry DW, Granton JT. Vasopressin and the cardiovascular system part 2. *Critical Care* 2004; **8**: 15–23.

Huang A, Kaley G. Gender-specific regulation of cardiovascular function: oestrogen as key player. *Microcirculation* 2004; **11**: 9–38.

Jänig W. Pre- and postganglionic vasoconstrictor neurons. *Annual Reviews of Physiology* 1988; **50**: 525–39.

Lehr H-A. Microcirculatory dysfunction induced by cigarette smoking. *Microcirculation* 2000; **7**: 367–84.

Lundberg JM, Pernow J, Lacroix JS. Neuropeptide Y: Sympathetic cotransmitter and modulator? *News in Physiological Sciences* 1989; **4**: 13–17.

Marshall JM. The venous vessels within skeletal muscle. *News in Physiological Sciences* 1991; **6**: 11–15.

Mather K, Anderson TJ, Verma S. Insulin action in the vasculature: Physiology and pathophysiology. *Journal of Vascular Research* 2001; **38**: 415–22.

Monos E, Berczi V, Nadasy G. Local control of veins: Biomechanical, metabolic and humoral aspects. *Physiological Reviews* 1995; **75**: 611–66.

Persson PB, Skalweit A, Thiele BJ. Controlling the release and production of renin. *Acta Physiologica Scandinavica* 2004; **181**: 375–81.

Potter LR, Abbey-Hosch S, Dickey DM. Natriuretic peptides, their receptors, and cyclic guanosine monophosphate-dependent signaling functions. *Endocrine Reviews* 2006; **27**: 47–72.

Simonsen U, Garcia-Sacristan A, Prieto D. Penile arteries and erection. *Journal of Vascular Research* 2002; **39**: 283–303

Schmelz M, Petersen LJ. Neurogenic inflammation in human and rodent skin. *News in Physiological Sciences* 2001; **16**: 33–7.

Wallin BG, Fagius J. Peripheral sympathetic neural activity in conscious humans. *Annual Reviews in Physiology* 1988; **50**: 565–76.

Wiers WG, Morgan KG. α_1-adrenergic signaling mechanisms in contraction of resistance arteries. *Reviews of Physiology, Biochemistry and Pharmacology* 2003; **150**: 91–139.

Research papers

See www.hodderplus.com/cardiovascularphysiology for a full list of Research papers for this chapter.

CHAPTER 15

Specialization in individual circulations

Learning objectives

In this chapter, the learning objectives and summary are combined as a Key features box after each section.

Very many factors regulate vascular tone (Chapters 12–14). Their relative importance varies, however, from organ to organ, as explained in this chapter. Carbon dioxide, for example, is a major regulator of cerebral but not cutaneous blood flow. This chapter also explains how the different circulations exhibit specializations that underpin the particular function of a tissue. A major function of skin, for example, is to regulate body temperature, so its circulation exhibits specializations for heat exchange. The five special circulations described here – myocardium, skeletal muscle, skin, brain and lung – were chosen partly for their clinical importance and partly for their contrasting characteristics. The splanchnic circulation is described briefly under 'Feeding and digestion' in Section 17.5. The same, unifying approach is adopted for each system as follows.

- **Special tasks** imposed on the circulation by the tissue's particular functions are outlined first.
- **Adaptations** that help the circulation accomplish its special tasks are considered under the headings 'Structural adaptation' and 'Functional adaptation'.
- **Vascular problems** specific to the particular organ/tissue are described.
- Finally, **techniques** for assessing each circulation are outlined.

15.1 Coronary circulation

> Coronary blood flow, resting human
> 70–$80 \, \mathrm{ml \, min^{-1} \, 100 \, g^{-1}}$
> Coronary blood flow during heavy exercise (maximal cardiac work)
> 300–$400 \, \mathrm{ml \, min^{-1} \, 100 \, g^{-1}}$

The right and left coronary arteries arise from the aorta immediately above the aortic valve cusps, in dilatations called the sinuses of Valsalva (Figures 1.4, 1.6). Branches of the **left coronary artery** supply mainly the left ventricle and interventricular septum; the **right coronary artery** supplies mainly the right ventricle, although the distribution is variable (Figure 15.1). About 95% of the coronary venous blood returns through the **coronary sinus** into the right atrium (Figure 1.4). The rest drains into the cardiac chambers through the anterior coronary and Thebesian veins. Some **Thebesian veins** drain into the left side of the heart, contributing to the slight deoxygenation of arterial blood (saturation $\sim$97%). The coronary circulation is the shortest in the body, with a mean transit time of only 6–8 s in a resting human.

Special tasks

- The coronary circulation must deliver O_2 at a high rate to match the basal myocardial demand

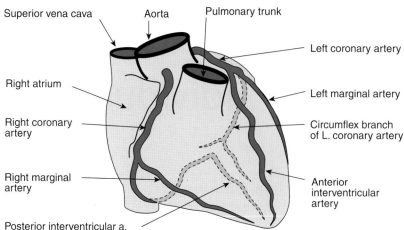

Figure 15.1 Human coronary arteries, anterior view.

Figure 15.2 Capillaries density (number/area) in skeletal and cardiac muscle, on same scale. Each tissue has ~1 capillary (red circle) per muscle fibre; but myocardial fibres are smaller, so myocardial capillary density is greater and diffusion distance correspondingly shorter. Open circles in skeletal muscle are capillaries not perfused with blood at any given moment in resting muscle. (From Renkin EM. In: Marhetti G, Taccardi B (eds). *International Symposium on Coronary Circulation*. Basel: Karger, 1967: 18–30.)

($\sim 8\,\mathrm{ml\,O_2\,min^{-1}\,100\,g^{-1}}$ in a resting human), which is $20\times$ that of resting skeletal muscle.

- During exercise the coronary circulation must increase O_2 delivery to match the increase in cardiac work ($\geqslant 5\times$), i.e. coronary blood flow must be coupled to cardiac work.

Structural adaptation

Myocardial capillary density is very high – roughly one capillary per myocyte (3000–$5000\,\mathrm{mm^{-2}}$ section, Figure 15.2). This creates a large endothelial surface area and reduces the maximum diffusion distance to $\sim 9\,\mu\mathrm{m}$ (myocytes being $18\,\mu\mathrm{m}$ wide), thereby facilitating O_2 and nutrient transfer to the myocytes. **Myoglobin** ($3.4\,\mathrm{g/l}$) facilitates O_2 transport within the cardiac myocytes (Section 10.11).

Exercise training increases the coronary artery width and the number of arterioles and capillaries, to keep pace with the increase in ventricular mass.

Functional adaptations

High basal flow and O_2 extraction

To satisfy the high metabolic demand, coronary blood flow per gram of tissue is about ten times the whole-body average. Endothelial **nitric oxide** production helps maintain this high flow, since flow is reduced by 60% by eNOS inhibitors. Despite the high flow, myocardium has to extract 65–75% of the O_2 to meet its needs (cf. whole-body average 25% at rest). This reduces the blood O_2 content from $195\,\mathrm{ml/l}$ (arterial) to 50–$70\,\mathrm{ml/l}$ (coronary sinus) (Figure 15.3). During heavy exercise the extraction can rise to 90%. **Fatty acid** extraction is likewise high (40–70%), but **glucose** extraction is usually low (2–3%), showing that fatty acids are the preferred substrate of myocardium.

Metabolic hyperaemia is the dominant form of vascular regulation

The extra O_2 required at high cardiac work rates is supplied mainly by increases in coronary blood flow rather than extraction, since extraction is already high at basal work rates. The coupling between coronary blood flow and myocardial work is remarkable; flow increases almost linearly with cardiac O_2 consumption at light to moderate work rates (Figure 15.4), while at high work rates O_2 extraction rises too. This is a classic example of metabolic hyperaemia (Section 13.7).

The elegant coupling between supply and demand is achieved by the myocardium releasing vasodilator substances in proportion to its work rate. However, as one investigator put it, the nature of the

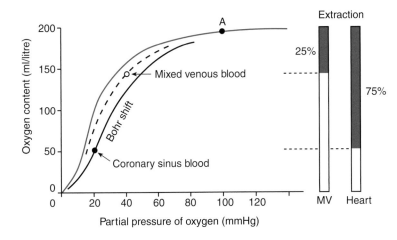

Figure 15.3 O_2 dissociation curves of arterial blood (P_{CO_2} 40 mmHg), mixed venous blood (P_{CO_2} 46 mmHg) and coronary sinus blood (P_{CO_2} 58 mmHg). CO_2 shifts the dissociation curve to the right (Bohr shift), which enhances myocardial O_2 unloading. A, arterial values. Mixed venous blood refers to resting human.

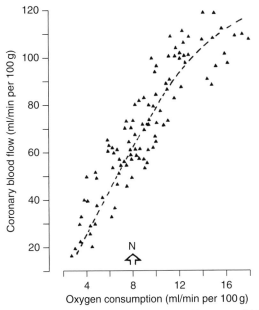

Figure 15.4 Effect of cardiac work, as measured by myocardial O_2 consumption, on coronary blood flow in dog. N, normal resting level. Cardiac work was altered by adrenaline or blood withdrawal. (From Berne RM, Rubio R. In: Berne RM, Sperekalis N (eds). *Handbook of Physiology, Cardiovascular System*, Vol. 1, The Heart. Bethesda, MD: American Physiological Society, 1979: 873–952, by permission.)

vasodilators remains a well-sought but carefully guarded secret of nature. One contender is **adenosine**, generated by the breakdown of ATP (Section 13.4). Adenosine binds to vascular A_{2A} receptors, activating the G_s–adenylyl cyclase–cAMP vasodilator pathway (Figure 12.10). However, the effects of adenosine inhibitors on myocardial hyperaemia have proved variable, ranging from little to a ~50% reduction. Other factors such as increases in **H_2O_2 production, interstitial K^+ and H^+** also contribute to resistance vessel dilatation. Upstream dilatation of the coronary arteries is mediated by

nitric oxide, produced by the shear-stimulated endothelium (Figure 13.9).

Autoregulation too is well developed in the coronary circulation (Figure 13.7). This stabilizes myocardial perfusion when blood pressure fluctuates, and can prevent under-perfusion, down to ~50 mmHg. When myocardial work increases, the metabolic vasodilators **re-set** autoregulation to operate at a higher flow.

Sympathetic vasomotor activity maintains high vascular tone at rest

Sympathetic vasoconstrictor fibres innervate myocardial arteries and arterioles, and the tonic α-adrenoceptor activation contributes to coronary vascular tone and resistance. During exercise cardiac sympathetic activity increases, and β_1-adrenoceptor-mediated tachycardia and increased contractility raise the cardiac work rate. The latter elicits a metabolic vasodilatation, which overcomes the concomitant α-adrenoceptor-mediated vasoconstriction. Thus sympathetic activity normally raises rather than reduces myocardial blood flow.

Adrenaline causes coronary vasodilatation

Adrenaline levels increase during the alerting response, exercise and hypovolaemia. This activates β_1-adrenoceptor on cardiac myocytes, raising cardiac work, and activates β_2-adrenoceptors on coronary vascular myocytes, causing vasodilatation (Figure 12.10). Adrenaline thus increases coronary blood flow. The increase can precede exercise (feed-forward), before the more powerful metabolic hyperaemia is triggered.

Ischaemic vasodilatation limits damage by coronary artery disease

Myocardial ischaemia elicits marked vasodilatation, due partly to the breakdown of ATP to adenosine,

Figure 15.5 Blood flow in left coronary artery of conscious dog, recorded by electromagnetic flow meter. Note the sharp curtailment of flow at the onset of systole (arrow). Most coronary flow occurs during diastole (shaded area). Time lines 0.1 s. (After Khouris EM, Gregg DE, Rayford CR. *Circulation Research* 1965; **17**: 427–37.)

a powerful coronary vasodilator. Also, the fall in ATP/ADP ratio activates K_{ATP} channels in the vascular smooth muscle, leading to hyperpolarization and further vasodilatation (Table 12.2). Ischaemic vasodilatation, downstream from a coronary artery stenosis, helps to maintain the resting coronary flow in angina patients (Concept box 15.2). Also, ischaemic vasodilatation at the margins of an infarct helps to limit its extent.

Special problems

Systole obstructs coronary blood flow

About two-thirds of the coronary arterial system is intramural, i.e. inside the myocardium. Intramural vessels are compressed during systole, especially during the isovolumetric contraction phase, when coronary blood pressure is at its minimum (~80 mmHg) and stress within the left ventricle wall is maximal (~240 mmHg). At this point, coronary artery flow stops briefly or even reverses (Figure 15.5). Full flow is only restored in diastole. About **80% of coronary blood flow occurs during diastole** at basal heart rates, so coronary perfusion is driven chiefly by **diastolic blood pressure**, not systolic pressure. The timing of the reflected pulse wave, by augmenting either diastolic or systolic pressure, affects the ratio of coronary perfusion to cardiac work (Figure 8.10). The beneficial effect of β-blockers in heart failure is partly due to the bradycardic lengthening of diastole, and hence the interval of good perfusion.

In **aortic valve stenosis**, the high resistance to ejection further increases the systolic stress within the left ventricle wall, especially during exercise. This exacerbates the systolic impairment of myocardial perfusion, leading to angina-like chest pain and collapse during exercise; see Clinical case, 'The elderly man with a murmur'.

Human coronary arteries are functional end-arteries prone to atheroma

Coronary arteries are a common site for atheroma (atherosclerosis). Section 9.10 outlined the pathology of atheroma, Concept box 15.1 shows the risk factors, and Table 17.4 highlights the distinction from arteriosclerosis. Briefly, atheroma is a cholesterol-rich, subintimal plaque that narrows the coronary artery lumen, limiting blood flow and causing ischaemic pain (angina) during exercise. Atheroma may also trigger arterial thrombosis (the formation of an organized blood clot), which blocks a coronary artery and causes myocardial infarction.

The narrowing of even one branch of a coronary artery is serious, because human coronary arteries are **functional end-arteries**, i.e. they have ineffective anastomoses. This is not so in all species; dogs have relatively good arterio-arterial anastomoses, and are less prone to myocardial infarction (Figure 15.6, top). Although humans have some arterio-arterial anastomoses between distal branches of the coronary tree, they are only 20–350 μm wide and transmit relatively little flow. Consequently, an

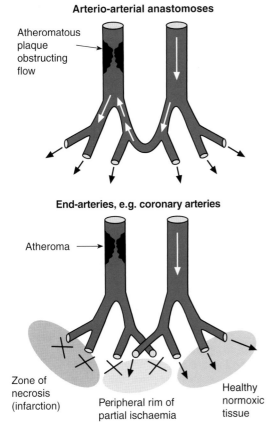

Arterio-arterial anastomoses

Atheromatous plaque obstructing flow

End-arteries, e.g. coronary arteries

Atheroma

Zone of necrosis (infarction)

Peripheral rim of partial ischaemia

Healthy normoxic tissue

Figure 15.6 Arterio-arterial anastomoses affect susceptibility to infarction following arterial obstruction. (*Lower panel*) Human, baboon, rabbit and pig coronary arteries are functional end-arteries. Acute ligation of a major vessel in the pig heart reduces perfusion to 0.6% in the downstream territory. (*Upper panel*) Dog coronary circulation has better arterio-arterial anastomoses. Acute ligation of a major canine coronary artery reduces myocardial perfusion less severely, to ~16%.

upstream obstruction reduces distal tissue perfusion to a few percent of normal, causing myocardial ischaemia (Figure 15.6, bottom).

Acute coronary obstruction by a thrombus causes myocardial infarction (a heart attack)

The sudden obstruction of an atheromatous coronary artery by thrombosis is the commonest cause of death in the West. The downstream zone of ischaemic myocardium is called a myocardial **infarct** (Figure 1.2). Here, the accumulation of interstitial K^+, H^+, adenosine and other factors stimulates nociceptors (Section 16.3). This causes a band of **crushing chest pain**, often radiating into the arms and neck. Contractility is impaired (Section 6.12), causing **acute cardiac failure**. **Sympathetic activity** increases due to the pain and clinical shock. **Arrhythmias** are common

(Sections 3.9, 4.7 and 5.8). The pathophysiological changes are brought together in Figure 6.22. Residual coronary blood flow is often so low that myocytes begin to die after a few hours (**necrosis**). The region affected (e.g. inferior, posterior) depends on which branch of the coronary artery is obstructed. Subendocardium (inner tissue) is often affected more than subepicardium, because systolic wall stress is greater in the subendocardium, curtailing subendocardial perfusion at low blood pressures.

Diagnosis is based on the characteristic history, ECG changes (Figure 5.11b), leakage of myocardial intracellular enzymes into the bloodstream (Section 6.14), echocardiography and nuclear imaging. **Treatment** includes:

- supplementary oxygen;
- morphine, to reduce the pain and the pro-arrhythmogenic sympathetic activity;
- fibrinolytic agents, such as streptokinase, to dissolve the thrombus;
- low-dose aspirin, to inhibit further platelet clotting;
- β-adrenoceptor blockers, to reduce cardiac work and the risk of subsequent arrhythmias. ACE inhibitors too reduce cardiac work.
- statins to lower blood lipids.

Chronic coronary stenosis causes angina

Arteries normally offer negligible resistance to flow compared with arterioles. Even severe atheromatous stenosis of the artery, if it develops slowly, may have little effect on flow during rest, because the rise in proximal resistance is offset by a fall in distal resistance. This is brought about partly by **distal arteriogenesis** (proliferation and widening of small, distal arterial vessels under the influence of growth factors), and partly by **distal vasodilatation**, due to vasodilator metabolite accumulation (Section 13.4) and the myogenic response to the reduced distal pressure (Sections 13.2 and 13.6).

The above compensations often maintain an adequate perfusion at rest. During **exercise**, however, the fixed resistance of the stenosed artery prevents flow from increasing sufficiently to meet the increase in myocardial O_2 demand. Even if the distal resistance vessels undergo maximal metabolic and ischaemic vasodilatation, the **proximal stenosis** now dominates the total resistance to flow; for a worked example, see Concept box 15.2. Exercise therefore precipitates local myocardial ischaemia, leading to nociceptors activation and a crushing chest pain, reversible on rest, called angina pectoris. Correspondingly, the **exercise ECG test** shows

CONCEPT BOX 15.2

Exercise-induced angina

- Resistances in series summate. If a healthy coronary artery has a resistance of 1 unit and coronary resistance vessels have a resistance of 19 units, the total resistance is 20 units.

- During exercise, metabolic vasodilatation of the myocardial resistance vessels reduces their resistance, e.g. to 4 units. Total resistance of the healthy coronary circulation is now 5 units. Myocardial blood flow increases four-fold (20/5), meeting the increased O_2 demand.

- Consider a severely stenosed coronary artery, of resistance 10 units, in a resting subject. Distal arteriogenesis and dilatation reduces the distal coronary resistance from 19 to, say, 10 units. Total resting vascular resistance is still 20 units, so **resting** flow is normal.

- When the patient **exercises**, the reserve dilatation of coronary resistance vessels reduces the distal resistance further, e.g. to 3 units. But total resistance, 13 units, is now dominated by the stenosis. Myocardial blood flow increases only about one and a half fold (20/13). This fails to meet the increased O_2 demand, leading to ischaemia and angina during exercise.

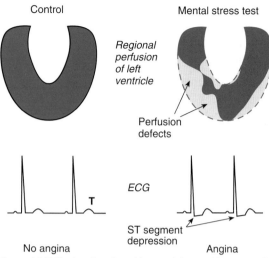

Figure 15.7 Nuclear imaging of human left ventricle myocardial perfusion, based on ^{82}Rb isotope uptake from bloodstream. Being adjacent to K^+ in the Atomic Table, rubidium is taken up by healthy myocardium. Control: uniform perfusion and normal ECG with patient relaxed. Stress test (mental arithmetic) in this patient caused angina, areas of defective myocardial perfusion (cold spots) and ST segment depression (ischaemia), due to increased cardiac work and sympathetic coronary vasoconstriction. Exercise test shows similar changes. In angina cases, cold spots resolve on rest; in infarct patients, they persist. Thallium-201 may be used rather than rubidium. (Redrawn from Deanfield JE, Shea M, Kensett M *et al. Lancet* 1984; **2**: 1001–5, with permission from Elsevier.)

test shows a corresponding, reversible ST-segment depression (Figure 15.7). As the eminent anatomist John Hunter once remarked in relation to his own stress-induced angina, 'My life is at the mercy of any rascal who chooses to annoy me'; and Hunter did indeed die during a stressful medical committee meeting. Severe **cold** can likewise trigger a reflex sympathetic constriction of ischaemic coronary vessels, triggering angina or exacerbating exercise-induced angina.

Three forms of angina are recognized. **Stable angina** is exercise-induced angina that is predictable for a given level of exercise. **Unstable angina** is exercise-induced angina occurring at progressively lower levels of exertion. **Variant angina** (resting angina, Prinzmetal angina) is less common and occurs at rest. It is caused by an episode of coronary artery **vasospasm**, i.e. intense, prolonged contraction of the atheromatous artery. Vasospasm usually occurs downstream of an atheromatous plaque, due to the release of serotonin and thromboxane from atheroma-activated platelets. Thus variant angina is precipitated by reduced myocardial O_2 supply, whereas exercise-induced angina is precipitated by increased myocardial O_2 demand.

acute ST segment depression during exercise, resolved by rest (Figures 5.11a).

Other triggers for angina include mental stress and cold. **Mental stress** increases coronary sympathetic vasomotor activity, leading to the contraction of atheromatous coronary arteries. The resulting regional ischaemia causes angina. The **stress ECG**

Treatment is based on physiological principles. Emotional stress must be avoided and the following pharmacological and surgical therapies are available.

- **Nitrodilator drugs** offer rapid relief and/or prevention. **Glyceryl trinitrate** dilates systemic veins and conduit arteries, but not the stenosed artery. It has relatively little effect on arterioles and peripheral resistance. The venodilatation reduces cardiac filling pressure (preload). Conduit artery relaxation reduces the pulse wave velocity, which delays the wave reflection and thereby reduces systolic pressure (afterload) (Figure 8.10). The fall in preload and afterload reduces cardiac work and therefore O_2 demand. Nitrodilators may also dilate coronary collateral vessels that bypass the stenosis. **Nicorandil** is both a nitrodilator and activator of K_{ATP} channels (hyperpolarization), causing venodilatation; the fall in cardiac work helps prevent angina.
- **β-adrenergic blockers**, such as propranolol (non-selective), atenolol and metoprolol (β_1 selective), reduce myocardial O_2 demand by reducing heart rate and cardiac contractility. A rate of $60\,min^{-1}$ usually prevents angina attacks. **Ca^{2+} channel blockers** (nifedipine, amlodipine) likewise reduce cardiac work and O_2 demand. The new chronotropic drug, **ivabradine**, inhibits the pacemaker depolarizing current i_f to reduce heart rate and hence O_2 demand. Such drugs are taken prophylactically by patients with frequent, severe angina.
- **Predisposing factors** (Concept box 15.1) should be treated, e.g. **statins** to reduce hypercholesterolaemia.
- **Low-dose aspirin** reduces platelet aggregation and is taken as a prophylaxis against progression to thrombosis.
- **Angioplasty** is the surgical dilatation of a localised proximal stenosis by a balloon-tipped catheter. A small tube, or **stent**, is then inserted to maintain patency. **Coronary bypass** is a more invasive procedure for severe cases, in which a stenosed length of artery is replaced with a segment of saphenous vein or internal mammary artery.

Assessment of human coronary circulation

Coronary sinus thermodilution measures coronary blood flow quantitatively, as described in

The Coronary Circulation

Special tasks
- Maintain a high basal rate of O_2 supply
- Increase the O_2 supply in proportion to cardiac work rate

Functional adaptations
- High O_2 extraction (>60% at rest)
- Metabolic vasodilatation dominates regulation
- Good autoregulation
- Vascular β_2-adrenoceptors, so adrenaline causes vasodilatation

Special problems
- Flow during systole is obstructed by systolic wall stress; aggravated by aortic stenosis
- Functional end-arteries in man, so thrombosis → infarction (heart attack)
- Chronic stenosis by atheroma → exercise-induced angina
- Sympathetic vasoconstrictor activity plus atheroma → stress-induced angina
- Coronary artery vasospasm downstream of atheroma → variant (resting) angina

Assessment in man
- Coronary angiography locates the stenosed segment(s)
- Coronary sinus thermal dilution method measures absolute flow
- Isotope imaging shows distribution of perfusion
- Exercise/stress ECG assesses latent ischaemia (ST depression during test)

KEY FEATURES BOX 15.1

Section 7.2. **Coronary angiography** is used to locate atheromatous obstructions, often as a guide to vascular surgery. The artery is perfused with a radio-opaque contrast medium, which is imaged by X-ray. **Electron beam computed tomography** (EBCT) images the dense calcification associated with atheroma, and is highly predictive of future ischaemic heart disease. **Gamma scans** (nuclear imaging) assess the distribution of myocardial perfusion (Figure 15.7). A gamma-emitting isotope such as thallium or rubidium is infused into the circulation and its appearance in myocardium is imaged by a gamma-camera. Due to the similarity to K^+, thallium and rubidium are pumped into the myocytes by the Na^+–K^+ pump. Regions with inadequate perfusion are revealed by patches of defective uptake.

15.2 Skeletal muscle circulation

> Flow, rest, postural (tonic) muscle
> $15 \, ml \, min^{-1} \, 100 \, g^{-1}$
> Flow, rest, phasic muscle $3–5 \, ml \, min^{-1} \, 100 \, g^{-1}$
> Max. flow, phasic exercise, sedentary subject
> $250 \, ml \, min^{-1} \, 100 \, g^{-1}$
> Max. flow, phasic exercise, endurance athlete
> $400 \, ml \, min^{-1} \, 100 \, g^{-1}$

The skeletal muscle and coronary circulations have much in common, notably the important role of metabolic hyperaemia in each; but there are also important differences, such as the major contribution of the skeletal muscle circulation to the reflex regulation of blood pressure.

Special tasks

- During exercise the muscle circulation must increase the O_2 and glucose delivery to match the increase in work, i.e. blood flow must be coupled to exercise intensity.
- Since skeletal muscle constitutes ~40% of the body mass, its vascular resistance has a major effect on total peripheral resistance, and must help regulate arterial blood pressure.

Structural adaptations

Muscle capillary density is adapted to the particular muscle's function. **Postural muscles** (e.g. soleus) tend to be continuously active, with tonically active, slow oxidative (red) fibres, so they have a higher capillary density than phasic muscles. **Phasic muscles** (e.g. forearm, gastrocnemius) consist chiefly of fast, glycolytic white fibres. **Endurance training** stimulates capillary angiogenesis via growth factors. The number of capillaries per muscle fibre increases in proportion to the mitochondria per fibre. The arterial vessels likewise adapt, in order to conduct a staggering maximal blood flow of $400 \, ml \, min^{-1}$ $(100 \, g)^{-1}$ in endurance-trained muscles.

Functional adaptations

Vascular tone is high at rest

Vascular tone is a prerequisite for dilatation, since dilatation is simply a loss of tone. The high tone of the resistance vessels in resting muscle is evident from the 50- to 100-fold increase in vascular conductance in active muscle. The basal tone is mainly non-neural in origin, since sympathetic denervation merely doubles vascular conductance.

Muscle vascular resistance helps regulate blood pressure

The arterial vessels of human muscle are richly innervated by tonically active, sympathetic vasoconstrictor fibres. Proximal vessels (feed arteries to first-order arterioles) express predominantly α_1-adrenoceptors, while the more distal second- and third-order arterioles express α_2-adrenoceptors. **Muscle sympathetic activity** is regulated by a reflex from **baroreceptors** that sense blood pressure (Chapter 16); the baroreflex raises sympathetic activity when blood pressure falls (e.g. orthostasis, hypovolaemia). Activity reaches its maximum after a severe haemorrhage (mean $6–10 \, s^{-1}$). The attendant rise in vascular resistance reduces muscle blood flow to about one-fifth of normal and helps maintain the arterial blood pressure.

During **exercise** the resistance vessels dilate, but tonic sympathetic vasoconstrictor activity continues to modulate the tone of the α_1-adrenoceptor-rich feed arteries and proximal resistance vessels, guided by the baroreflex. This prevents an excessive fall in total peripheral resistance; unrestrained vasodilatation in a large mass of intensively used muscle (e.g. cross-country skiing) would otherwise cause arterial hypotension. The dilated terminal arterioles, with abundant α_2-receptors, become unresponsive to sympathetic activity during exercise hyperaemia (**functional sympatholysis**).

Metabolic vasodilatation increases blood flow in active muscle

Muscle blood flow begins to increase within ~1 s of starting exercise and reaches a sustained level in ~40 s (Figure 13.8). In phasic muscle the increase can reach 50-fold and account for 80–90% of the cardiac output (cf. 18% at rest). Indeed, if all the muscles of the body dilated maximally at the same time, demand would exceed the heart's output capacity. The hyperaemia is due almost entirely to the fall in muscle vascular resistance, not the small rise in arterial pressure associated with exercise. The sustained phase is brought about by **metabolic vasodilatation** of the resistance vessels, accompanied by a permissive **ascending dilatation** of feed arteries and **flow-induced dilatation** of conduit arteries (Figure 13.9). The rapid, initial phase is due partly to the venous muscle pump (see below) and partly to the myogenic response to compression, while by 4 s the K^+ ions released by the contracting muscle begin to contribute.

As in the myocardium, O_2 supply is tightly coupled to demand; blood flow increases in almost direct proportion to muscle metabolic rate. The identity of the metabolic vasodilators remains controversial. Over the first few minutes, muscle K^+ efflux during action potential repolarization raises the local **interstitial [K^+]** in proportion to exercise intensity. Interstitial [K^+] can reach 11 mM in exhausting exercise, sufficient to produce near maximal vasodilatation in some muscles. This, along with increases in interstitial **osmolarity** (by 20–30 mOs), **inorganic phosphate**, **adenosine** and **acid** (released by contracting muscle), probably accounts for much of the early hyperaemia. Nitric oxide and prostaglandins too make a moderate contribution.

As exercise continues, the elevated interstitial K^+ and osmolarity decay, though not to basal levels, so other factors must sustain the vasodilatation. Interstitial **adenosine** concentration increases in proportion to exercise intensity, and some studies using blockers indicate that adenosine accounts for up to 40% of the sustained vasodilatation. Mitochondrial production of the vasodilator **H_2O_2** likewise increases as O_2 consumption increases.

The skeletal muscle circulation has two further special adaptations, namely β_2-adrenoceptor-mediated vasodilatation to **adrenaline** (Section 14.6) and, in non-primates only, sympathetic cholinergic activation during the alerting response (Section 14.3).

Capillary recruitment improves solute exchange in active muscle

In resting muscle the terminal arterioles contract intermittently and asynchronously (vasomotion). As a result, only a half to a third of muscle capillaries is well perfused at any one instant (Figure 15.2, left panel). During metabolic hyperaemia, arteriolar dilatation increases the fraction of capillaries that is well perfused with blood (capillary recruitment, Figure 10.14). This raises the effective **surface area** for gas exchange and shortens the extravascular **diffusion distance**.

O_2 extraction rises; O_2 debt and lactate accumulate

The diffusion gradient in resting muscle (arterial P_{O_2} 100 mmHg, intracellular P_{O_2} ~20 mmHg) drives the extraction of 25–30% of the O_2 from the perfusing blood. During exercise, muscle intracellular P_{O_2} falls, so O_2 extraction increases, and can reach 80–90% (Figure 10.16). In severe exercise the intracellular P_{O_2} falls so low that the muscle fibre switches to anaerobic glycolysis, generating **lactic acid**. Interstitial lactic acid helps stimulate muscle metaboreceptors, which drive the exercise pressor

reflex (Section 16.6). Plasma lactate rises from 0.5 mM at rest (plasma pH 7.4) to $\leqslant$20 mM in extreme exercise (pH 6.9). The amount of lactate formed is a biochemical index of the deficit in muscle O_2 supply – the 'oxygen debt', which can reach several litres. When the exercise terminates, blood flow remains raised for several minutes (Figures 13.8 and 13.11). This **post-exercise hyperaemia** resupplies the muscle with O_2 and washes out the accumulated lactic acid. The circulating lactate is taken up by the heart as a primary substrate, and also by the liver for resynthesis into glycogen.

The venous muscle pump enhances perfusion during rhythmic exercise

Exercise hyperaemia is due primarily to a rise in vascular conductance, but perfusion is also enhanced modestly in rhythmic exercise by the intermittent compression of deep veins, particularly in the calf. In a stationary, standing adult, gravity raises the arterial and venous pressures in the calf equally, by ~70 mmHg, to 165 mmHg and 80 mmHg, respectively (Figure 15.8). The pressure difference driving blood through the resting calf muscle is therefore $(165 - 80) = 85$ mmHg. During walking, running or cycling, the calf muscle pump reduces the venous pressure to ~35 mmHg (Figure 8.26), which increases the pressure difference to 130 mmHg, a 50% rise. This contributes to the immediate onset of exercise hyperaemia, over a time interval that is too brief to invoke metabolic vasodilators (Figure 13.8).

Special problems

Muscle contraction compresses intra-muscle blood vessels

When a muscle contracts at >30–70% maximum force, the internal stress compresses the intra-muscle

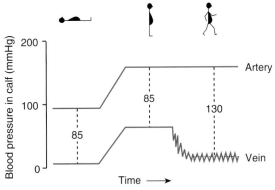

Figure 15.8 Effect of posture and muscle pump on absolute pressures and on the difference in pressure driving blood through calf.

vessels. Consequently, perfusion oscillates during rhythmic exercise (Figure 13.8). During a sustained contraction, perfusion is markedly impaired. The O_2 stored as oxymyoglobin is only sufficient for 5–10 s of muscle contraction, so the muscle quickly becomes hypoxic and switches to anaerobic glycolysis, producing lactate. This leads to rapid fatigue, a scenario familiar to anyone who has carried a heavy suitcase any distance.

Active muscle swells, due to increased capillary filtration

Increased fluid translocation across the capillary bed of an exercising muscle causes the muscle to swell, creating the 'pumped' muscle of intense exercise.

The forces responsible are described in Section 11.9. During whole-body exercise, the fluid translocation into active muscle can reduce the plasma volume by 10–15%.

Intermittent claudication is due to ischaemic leg artery disease

The major arteries of the leg are common sites for atheroma, particularly in diabetic patients and smokers, leading to chronic stenosis. Similar arguments apply as in Concept box 15.2 (heart). At first, ischaemic leg pain occur only on walking, and is relieved by rest (intermittent claudication). Severe cases progress to chronic pain at rest, **arterial ulcers** and **gangrene**, at which point amputation becomes necessary.

Measurement of human muscle perfusion

The soft tissue of a human limb consists mainly of skeletal muscle. Limb blood flow can be measured by **venous occlusion plethysmography** (Figures 8.5 and 13.11) or **Doppler velocimetry** of the principal artery (Figure 13.8). The **ankle–brachial pressure index**, ABPI, assesses artery patency (Section 8.5). Local capillary perfusion rate can be estimated by the **Kety radioisotope clearance method** (Figure 8.6).

15.3 Cutaneous circulation

Blood flow, thermoneutral (27°C)
$10–20\,\mathrm{ml\,min^{-1}\,100\,g^{-1}}$
Minimal blood flow $1\,\mathrm{ml\,min^{-1}\,100\,g^{-1}}$
Maximum blood flow $150–200\,\mathrm{ml\,min^{-1}\,100\,g^{-1}}$

The skin is the organ of temperature regulation in humans, with a blood flow that can change >100-fold. Adult skin surface area is ~1.8 m², weight 2–3 kg and thickness 1–2 mm (epidermis plus dermis). The epidermis is avascular, but the dermis is well vascularized (Figure 15.9). Unlike muscle and myocardium, skin has a relatively constant, low metabolic rate, so its O_2 needs are satisfied by a low blood flow, aided by the direct diffusion of O_2 into the superficial ~100 µm epidermis. Temperature, not metabolic rate, is the principal factor regulating skin blood flow.

Special tasks

Cutaneous blood flow must regulate core temperature

The temperature of the human core (brain, thorax, abdominal organs) is held constant at 37.0–37.5°C

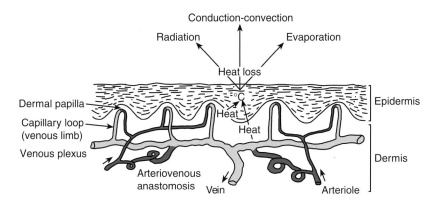

Figure 15.9 Dermal vascular arrangement and heat flux in a human extremity, e.g. fingers, ear lobe (acral skin). Non-acral skin of limbs and trunk lacks arteriovenous anastomoses. Red cell volume and oxygenation in subpapillary venous plexus influence skin colour.

by adjusting cutaneous heat loss to match core heat production. The main heat-dissipating surface is the skin in humans, and the tongue in many furry mammals. In a thermoneutral environment, namely 27–28°C for a naked human, the skin temperature is ~33°C. Heat is dissipated by three processes: radiation, conduction–convection and evaporation (Figure 15.9).

- The rate of heat loss by **radiation** is proportional to the difference between ambient temperature and skin temperature. The latter depends on the rate at which cutaneous blood flow delivers heat.

- During **conduction–convection**, warm skin heats up the adjacent air by conduction, and the warmed air is removed by convection (air currents). Conductive heat loss increases with skin temperature, so this form of heat loss is again dependent on cutaneous blood flow.

- The **evaporation of sweat** consumes 2.4 kJ heat energy per gram (latent heat of evaporation), and both the water and the heat are delivered to the skin by the bloodstream.

Cutaneous blood flow is thus the key factor regulating heat loss by all three physical processes. The skin itself is **poikilothermic**, not homeothermic; its temperature varies widely, with extremes of 0°C and 45°C possible for short periods without tissue damage.

Cutaneous vessels must participate in defence against the environment

The other major role of skin is to provide a defence against the environment. The vasculature contributes to this through the Lewis triple response to trauma.

In addition, emotion-related changes in human skin colour contribute to **non-verbal communication**.

Structural adaptations

Arteriovenous anastomoses (AVAs) abound in the extremities

Acral or glabrous skin is specialized skin with numerous, direct connections between dermal arterioles and venules, called arteriovenous anastomoses or AVAs (Figure 15.9). AVAs are coiled, muscular-walled vessels, ~35 μm wide, discovered originally in the rabbit ear by RT Grant in 1930. In humans they occur in exposed regions with a high surface area/volume ratio (fingers, toes, palm and sole, lips, nose, pinna of ear). AVAs have little basal tone and are controlled almost exclusively by sympathetic vasoconstrictor fibres, whose activity is influenced by the **hypothalamic temperature-regulating centre**. AVAs also respond directly to ambient temperature, being dilated by heat and constricted by cold.

In a thermoneutral environment the sympathetic drive to acral skin is high, so the AVAs are contracted and conduct little blood. By contrast, basal sympathetic drive to the skin of the limbs and trunk is low. Thus sympathectomy or a local nerve block causes greater cutaneous hyperaemia in the extremities than proximally. When the core temperature exceeds 37.5°C, the hypothalamus reduces the vasoconstrictor drive to the AVAs, allowing them to dilate. This creates a low-resistance shunt into the dermal venous plexus, raising the cutaneous blood flow and heat delivery (Figure 15.9). Since heat readily crosses the vein wall, skin temperature rises and heat loss increases. Conversely, under cold conditions the AVAs are constricted to conserve heat. It is worth reiterating that the **dilatation** of AVAs **increases heat loss**, since the contrary is still taught in some school biology textbooks. The following 'aide-memoire' might well have been sung by the mud-loving hippopotamus in Flanders and Swan's famous comic song:

> A – V – A's, let 'em flood,
> There's nothing quite like them
> For cooling the blood.
> So dilate them widely,
> Let's lose heat right blithely –
> But close them up tightly
> When chill is the mud.

Venous–arterial countercurrent exchanger in limbs conserves heat

The flippers of whales and the feet of wading birds possess an elaborate countercurrent heat-conserving mechanism. The cooled blood returning from the cold extremity drains into deep veins that ramify around the main artery. Heat passes from the warm arterial blood into the cool venous blood, so the extremity receives pre-cooled arterial blood, which reduces heat loss to the environment. This also occurs in human limbs to a minor degree.

Functional adaptations

Cutaneous blood flow is affected by both **ambient** and **core** temperature.

Cutaneous vascular tone is inversely related to ambient temperature

Cutaneous arterioles, venules and small veins dilate in response to local warming and contract in response to cooling, down to 10–15°C (Figure 15.10a). **Skin colour** is affected by the volume and O_2 content of blood in the dermal venous plexus, so warmth causes flushing (increased flow of well-oxygenated blood into the dilated venular plexus) and cold causes pallor. Warmth-induced vasodilatation promotes heat loss, while cold-induced vasoconstriction promotes heat conservation, thereby contributing to core temperature homeostasis. The mechanisms mediating the local heat and cold responses differ, as follows.

Heat-induced vasodilatation is due in part to increased eNOS activity. Also, at >30°C, sensory C-fibres release substance P and CGRP (Figure 14.9). Consequently heat-induced flushing is blocked by local anaesthesia.

Cold-induced vasoconstriction is greatly attenuated by α_2-adrenoceptor blockers (yohimbine, rauwolscine) and by sympathetic inhibition, showing that it depends on tonic sympathetic activity and α_2-**adrenoceptors**, which are expressed by cutaneous vascular myocytes. Cold induces the insertion of more α_2-adrenoceptors from the myocyte Golgi apparatus into the plasma membrane, raising the apparent affinity for the sympathetic transmitter noradrenaline. Also, eNOS activity declines. These changes lead to cold-induced vasoconstriction.

The immersion of one hand in cold water elicits a small contralateral **reflex vasoconstriction** in the opposite hand. This is due partly to a spinal sympathetic reflex and partly to cooled blood affecting the hypothalamic temperature sensors. **Facial cold** causes a peripheral vasoconstriction and a rise in systolic pressure, due partly to increased wave reflection. This can aggravate angina and may contribute to the well-documented rise in heart attacks and deaths in cold weather.

Severe ambient cold causes paradoxical cold vasodilatation

When a hand is placed in water at 10°C or lower, the initial cold-induced vasoconstriction gives way to dilatation after 5–10 min (paradoxical cold vasodilatation), with flushing and pain relief (Figure 15.10c). This occurs in regions rich in AVAs, and contributes to the cold, red noses and hands seen in frosty weather. The phenomenon is attributed to the paralysis of noradrenergic neurotransmission by the cold and the release of vasodilators such as prostacyclin. Cold-induced vasodilatation is well developed in Arctic Indians and Norwegian fishermen, and helps prevent skin damage during prolonged cold exposure. If the exposure persists, vasoconstriction recurs after a while. During prolonged exposure the skin oscillates between periods of vasoconstriction and vasodilatation at 15–20 min intervals. This is called the **hunting reaction**.

Core temperature strongly influences cutaneous sympathetic vasomotor activity

A rise in core temperature (e.g. during exercise) is sensed by **warmth receptors** in the anterior hypothalamus, which project to pre-sympathetic neurons in the brainstem. These evoke changes in the sympathetic vasomotor and sudomotor drive to the skin, resulting in cutaneous vasodilatation and sweating (Figures 15.10b and 15.11). The 'thermosensitive' sympathetic pathway (responsive also to emotion) is mediated by different neurons to the 'barosensitive' sympathetic pathway regulating blood pressure (Chapter 16); cutaneous arterioles have a relatively sparse innervation by the latter. In **acral skin**, the thermoregulatory vasodilatation is brought about mainly by **reduced sympathetic vasoconstrictor** drive to the AVAs. In **non-acral skin** (limbs, trunk, scalp), the dilatation is closely associated with sweating and is due mainly to **increased sympathetic cholinergic vasodilator**

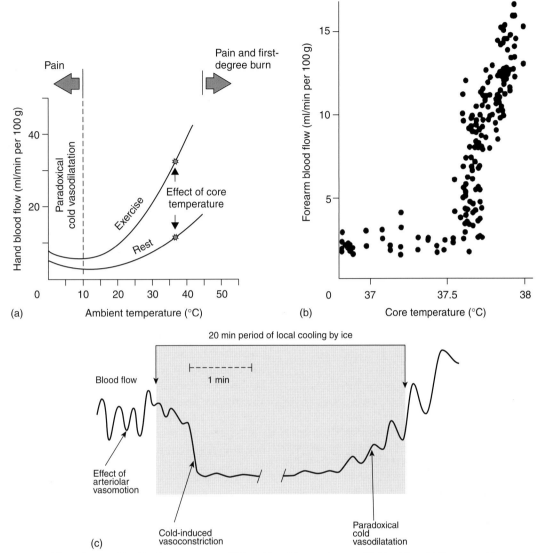

Figure 15.10 Effect of external (ambient) temperature and internal (core) temperature on skin blood flow. (a) Response of immersed hand to water temperature, when internal heat load is low (rest) or high (exercise). Note the paradoxical cold vasodilatation at <10°C. (b) Response of forearm blood flow, measured by plethysmography, to rise in core temperature induced by leg exercise. The hyperaemia is due to cutaneous vasodilatation; flow in the muscles actually fell (xenon clearance method). (c) Cold-induced vasoconstriction in human calf skin recorded by laser Doppler fluxmeter, changing to paradoxical cold vasodilatation after 10–20 min. The oscillation in arteriolar tone at normal temperature is an example of vasomotion. (a) After Greenfield ADM. In: Hamilton WF, Dow P (eds). *Handbook of Physiology, Cardiovascular System*, Vol. III, Part II, Peripheral Circulation. Bethesda, MD: American Physiological Society, 1963: 1325–52; (b) from Johnson JM, Rowell JB. *Journal of Applied Physiology* 1975; **39**: 920–4, with permission of the American Physiological Society; (c) based on Van den Brande P, De Coninck A, Lievens P (1997) *International Journal of Microcirculation* **17**: 55–60.

activity, being inhibited by local nerve block (Figure 15.11) or botulinum toxin, an inhibitor of cholinergic vesicle release. Pharmacological inhibitor studies indicate that the neuroeffector is partly acetylcholine, partly VIP (vasoactive intestinal polypeptide) and partly NO. Both VIP and nNOS (neural isoform of nitric oxide synthase) are present in cutaneous cholinergic nerves and in sweat glands.

The above response is finely **graded** and spans a massive flow range (Figure 15.10b). During **cold stress** the entire skin perfusion can fall to just 20 ml/min, which allows the full insulating action of the subcutaneous fat to protect the core temperature. During **heat stress**, adult human skin perfusion can reach 7–8 l/min. This necessitates a major increase in the cardiac output, to ~13 l/min, of which more than half goes to the skin. A compensatory vasoconstriction in the splanchnic, renal and skeletal muscle circulations helps maintain arterial blood pressure.

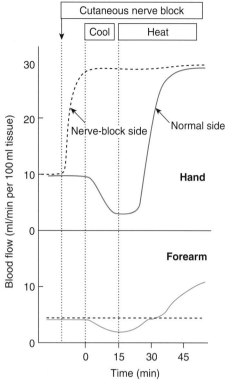

Figure 15.11 Contrast between cutaneous vascular control in hand and arm. Dashed line shows marked effect in hand, but not forearm, of sympathetic fibre block by local anaesthetic. Core temperature was then cooled, followed by heating, by placing legs in cold/hot water (upper limbs at room temperature). Results shows that, in the hand, sympathetic restraint of arteriovenous flow is great at thermoneutrality, and heat-mediated dilatation is due chiefly to abolition of this restraint. In more proximal skin (arm) sympathetic-induced tone is slight and vasodilatation depends on increased sympathetic cholinergic fibre activity. (After Roddie IC. In: Shepherd JT, Abboud FM (eds). *Handbook of Physiology, Cardiovascular System*, Vol. III, Part 1, Peripheral Circulation. Bethesda, MD: American Physiological Society, 1983: 285–317.)

The cutaneous circulation helps regulate arterial and central venous pressure

If blood pressure falls, e.g. during hypovolaemia, acute cardiac failure and other cases of clinical shock, there is an intense cutaneous venoconstriction and arteriolar constriction, causing the characteristic **pale, cold skin of patients in clinical shock**. The constriction is driven by angiotensin, vasopressin, adrenaline and increased sympathetic vasoconstrictor activity. The increase in cutaneous vascular resistance helps to support arterial pressure, while the venoconstriction helps to support central venous pressure. The importance of cutaneous vasoconstriction was noted during World War I; wounded men who were rescued quickly and warmed in blankets (producing cutaneous dilatation) survived haemorrhage less well than the men

who could not be reached for some time and retained their reflex cutaneous vasoconstriction.

Exercise evokes an initial, sympathetic-mediated cutaneous vasoconstriction, but this changes to dilatation when core temperature rises. Stimuli that elicit the **alerting (defence) response**, such as mental arithmetic, cause a transient cutaneous venous and arteriolar constriction (Figure 14.14). **Deep inspiration** has the same effect.

Orthostasis elicits the cutaneous veni-arteriolar response

Lowering a limb below heart level (dependency) causes a marked vasoconstriction of cutaneous resistance vessels (Figures 8.6 and 11.5). Indeed, cutaneous perfusion in the dependent foot falls by two thirds. This response to dependency helps to maintain central arterial pressure during standing, and to minimize dependent oedema formation. The arteriolar contraction is somehow triggered by the dependency-induced venous congestion – the **veni-arteriolar response**; but the link is poorly understood. The Bayliss myogenic response may contribute, but in addition local nerve fibres seem to be involved, since the response is abolished by local anaesthetics. The former view that the veni-arteriolar response is a 'sympathetic axon reflex' is now questioned, because the response is not prevented by a blocking dose of the α-antagonist phentolamine.

The cutaneous circulation as the mirror of the soul?

Poets and playwrights have long emphasized the way skin colour responds to emotional state. Skin colour is strongly affected by vascular tone, because pinkness/pallor depends on the mass and oxygenation of red cells in the subpapillary venous plexus. We blush with embarrassment (vasodilatation) and blanch with fear or stress (vasoconstriction elicited by the alerting response).★

★Juliet was evidently a blusher. Her nurse, announcing Romeo's desire to marry her, remarked:

> There stays a husband to make you a wife:
> Now comes the wanton blood up in your cheeks,
> They'll be in scarlet straight at any news.
> (Romeo and Juliet, Act 2, Sc. 5)

The defence or alerting response has the opposite effect. When Salisbury tells King Richard of his army's desertion, the King pales, crying:

> But now the blood of twenty thousand men
> Did triumph in my face, and they are fled;
> And, till so much blood thither comes again,
> Have I not reason to look pale and dead?
> (Richard II, Act 3, Sc. 2)

Blushing is poorly understood because it is difficult to produce on demand. Folkow and Neil, in their classic textbook *The Circulation*, recall how they were unable to make a habitual blusher blush in a laboratory setting, either by insults or rude jokes, but when they disconnected their equipment and thanked the subject, she blushed violently. Blushing is often associated with emotional sweating and is probably mediated by sympathetic cholinergic fibres innervating the face, neck and upper chest. Emotional stimuli can also evoke hyperaemia in the gastric and colonic mucosa.

Trauma increases skin blood flow

The cutaneous vascular response to trauma is summarized by the **Lewis triple response** (Figures 14.8 and 14.9). Both blood flow and capillary permeability increase, thereby boosting the delivery of white cells and immunoglobulins to the injured site.

Special problems

Compression leads to pressure ulcers

Skin gets sat on and leaned on for long periods, causing vascular compression. **Pressure-induced vasodilatation** (dilatation evoked by innocuous external pressure) delays the onset of ischaemia; and skin tolerates ischaemia better than most tissues. Pressure-induced vasodilatation may be mediated by vasoactive peptides (e.g. CGRP) released by skin sensory fibres, since it is blocked by local anaesthetics. If the compression is maintained, increasing discomfort normally triggers a shift in position. This relieves the compression and allows **reactive (post-ischaemic) hyperaemia** to increase cutaneous perfusion for a while. The associated flush is obvious in white-skinned humans. For mechanisms, see Section 13.8.

In patients who are elderly, enfeebled, paraplegic or comatose, there is little or no voluntary shifting of position to relieve skin compression. If major pressure areas such as the heels and buttocks are not relieved by regularly turning the patient, the skin undergoes ischaemic necrosis over days–weeks, resulting in deep **pressure ulcers** (**bed sores**). The elderly are particularly prone to bed sores because the skin becomes thin and frail with ageing. A low incidence of bed sores in a geriatric ward is a sign of good nursing care.

Cutaneous vasodilatation contributes to fainting and heat exhaustion in hot weather

The dilatation of cutaneous veins in hot weather reduces central venous pressure, which predisposes the subject to **postural fainting**. The classic example is the guardsman who faints while standing to attention on a hot day. Resistance vessel vasodilatation increases capillary filtration pressure, leading to **tissue swelling** – hence the common experience that a ring often feels tight on the finger during hot weather. Heavy exercise in a hot environment can lead to **heat exhaustion**. The combination of

---

KEY FEATURES BOX 15.3

The Cutaneous Circulation

Special tasks
- Regulate body temperature
- Respond to traumatic breaches of the integument

Structural adaptations
- Arteriovenous anastomoses in acral skin (fingers, palms, toes, lips, nose, ears) dilate to dissipate heat

Functional adaptations
- Sympathetic nerves, not metabolic hyperaemia, are the dominant control system
- Core temperature receptors in hypothalamus control sympathetic vasoconstrictor fibres to acral skin (AVAs) and sympathetic vasodilator fibres to non-acral skin
- Ambient cold causes veno- and vasoconstriction (α_2-mediated), followed by paradoxical cold vasodilatation. Heat causes dilatation
- Cutaneous veno- and vasoconstriction driven by the baroreflex support the circulation during hypotension or acute cardiac failure
- The veni-arteriolar response reduces the perfusion of dependent skin
- Stress causes vasoconstriction, embarrassment vasodilatation.
- The Lewis triple response enhances perfusion and immunoglobulin escape in damaged skin
- Reactive hyperaemia restores nutrition rapidly after compression

Special problems
- Prolonged compression → pressure ulcers ('bed sores')
- Heat → tissue swelling and venodilatation, aggravating postural hypotension, which may cause fainting. Heat-induced cutaneous dilatation plus strenuous exercise → heat exhaustion
- Ambient cold → sustained, damaging vasoconstriction in fingers of Raynaud's patients

Assessment in man
- Laser Doppler probe assesses red cell flux
- Kety's isotope clearance method measures local dermal perfusion

cutaneous vasodilatation (for heat loss) and muscle vasodilatation reduces the peripheral resistance profoundly, while plasma volume and cardiac filling pressure are lowered by sweating, fluid filtration into the exercising muscle and cutaneous venodilatation. The resulting fall in cardiac output, combined with the excessive fall in peripheral resistance, leads to arterial hypotension and collapse (heat exhaustion).

Cold triggers Raynaud's disease

During cold weather, paradoxical cold vasodilatation normally prevents any tissue damage. In **Raynaud's disease**, however, the vessels of the fingers show an exaggerated, sustained vasoconstriction to cold, usually in women. This leads to severe blanching, numbness, tingling or pain in the finger tips, and local tissue ischaemia.

In severe **eczema and psoriasis**, the skin's normal vasoconstrictor response to cold is prevented by inflammatory vasodilatation. Temperature regulation becomes unstable and occasionally necessitates hospitalization.

Measurement of human cutaneous blood flow

- The **laser–Doppler 'flowmeter'** (really a cell flux meter) provides a rapid, semi-quantitative measure of red cell flux in a patch of superficial dermis.
- **Thermography**, the imaging of surface temperature by an infrared camera, has been used as an indirect index of flow; but epidermal temperature depends on ambient temperature and skin thickness as well as blood flow.
- **Venous occlusion plethysmography** (Figure 8.5) can be adapted to a single digit, where most of the blood flow is cutaneous.
- **Kety's isotope clearance technique** measures nutritive flow (Figure 8.6).

15.4 Cerebral circulation

Mean blood flow, whole brain
$55 \, \text{ml} \, \text{min}^{-1} \, 100 \, \text{g}^{-1}$
Basal blood flow, grey matter
$100 \, \text{ml} \, \text{min}^{-1} \, 100 \, \text{g}^{-1}$

The human brain (~1.5 kg) forms only 2% of the body mass. Nevertheless, it receives 14% of the resting cardiac output and accounts for nearly 20% of resting O_2 consumption. Most of the blood goes to the neuron-rich grey matter (40% of brain mass) and a smaller proportion to the white matter (chiefly myelinated axon tracts). The cerebral arterioles are unusually short and thin walled, so large cerebral arteries account for an unusually high fraction of the vascular resistance (40–50%) and have a rich autonomic innervation.

Special tasks

Maximum security of O₂ supply

Grey matter has a very high rate of oxidative metabolism, $\sim 7 \, \text{ml} \, O_2 \, \text{min}^{-1} \, 100 \, \text{g}^{-1}$, which raises jugular venous blood temperature by ~0.3°C. Due to its high O_2 demand, grey matter is exquisitely sensitive to hypoxia; consciousness is lost after a few seconds of cerebral ischaemia, and irreversible neuronal damage follows within ~4 min. The primary task of the cerebral circulation, therefore, is to maintain O_2 delivery at all costs.

Local cerebral perfusion must adapt to changes in neuronal activity

Many mental functions are well localized, such as visual interpretation in the occipital cortex. Increased local neuronal activity raises the local metabolic rate, as shown by increased uptake of radiolabelled glucose and O_2. For example, illumination of the retina raises the metabolic rate of the occipital visual cortex. The cerebral vessels must therefore adjust blood flow locally, so as to match the varying local demand for O_2.

Structural adaptations

The circle of Willis helps safeguard the arterial supply

The **basilar** and **internal carotid arteries** enter the cranial cavity and anastomose to form a circle around the optic chiasma, the circle of Willis (Figure 15.12). (The young assistant employed by Thomas Willis to draw the circle later designed St Paul's Cathedral in London, being one Christopher Wren.) **Anterior, middle** and **posterior cerebral arteries** arise from the circle of Willis. This arrangement helps preserve cerebral perfusion if a carotid artery is obstructed, at least in the young; in elderly subjects the anastomoses are less effective. The main cerebral arteries divide into **pial arteries** that run over the surface of the brain. Pial artery pressure is unusually low, ~50% of systemic pressure, because the distal/proximal resistance ratio is low. Pial arteries give off fine arteries that penetrate the parenchyma and divide into short arterioles.

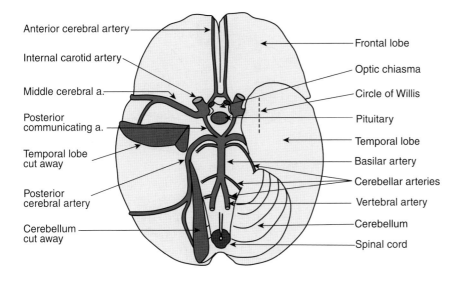

Figure 15.12 Circle of Willis and main cerebral arteries in man, viewed from the underside of the brain. The blood reaches the circle of Willis via the basilar artery and two internal carotid arteries.

A high capillary density optimizes O$_2$ transport

Grey matter contains ~3000–4000 capillaries per mm^2 cross section, similar to myocardium. This creates a large surface area for O$_2$ diffusion and reduces the extravascular diffusion distance to ≤10 μm. Cerebral capillaries have exceptionally tight endothelial junctions, which create a blood–brain barrier for lipid-insoluble solutes (see later).

Functional adaptations

Cerebral blood flow is regulated chiefly by intrinsic mechanisms, namely autoregulation and functional hyperaemia, rather than vasomotor nerves and hormones.

Grey matter has a very high basal blood flow

Blood flow to the grey matter is a very high, ~100 ml min^{-1} 100 g^{-1} – over ten times the whole body average. Fractional O$_2$ extraction, ~35%, is likewise above average.

Cerebral perfusion pressure is safeguarded by brainstem regulation of other circulations

As in any tissue, blood flow depends on vascular conductance and arterial pressure. Unlike other tissues, however, the brain can safeguard its blood supply by strangling the blood supply to other, less vital tissues, while sparing itself – a selfish organ, but wisely so! When necessary (e.g. acute hypovolaemia, clinical shock), the perfusion of the peripheral tissues, except myocardium, is restricted via sympathetic-mediated vasoconstriction, to maintain arterial blood pressure and hence cerebral perfusion. The brain also has control over the cardiac output via the autonomic nerves.

Figure 15.13 Autoregulation of cerebral perfusion at normal arterial P_{CO_2} (solid line); star marks normal operating point. Over the autoregulated range flow changes by only 6% per 10 mmHg pressure change. A raised arterial CO$_2$ causes cerebral vasodilatation (upper dashed line); a low CO$_2$, usually due to hyperventilation, causes vasoconstriction, leading to dizziness. Local sympathetic stimulation affects flow significantly only when arterial pressure is high (lower dashed line). (After Heistad DD, Kontos HA. In: Shepherd JT, Abboud FM (eds). *Handbook of Physiology, Cardiovascular System*, Vol. III, Part 1, Peripheral Circulation. Bethesda, MD: American Physiological Society, 1983: 137–81, by permission.)

Cerebral autoregulation maintains perfusion during hypotension

A further safeguard against under-perfusion is provided by autoregulation, which is very well developed in the brain (Figure 15.13). If arterial blood pressure falls, cerebral resistance vessels dilate to maintain perfusion. Below the limit of ~60 mmHg, however, cerebral blood flow declines steeply. Hypotension of this severity therefore leads to mental confusion and syncope. The upper limit of autoregulation is ~150–160 mmHg.

Cerebral vessels are dilated by arterial CO_2 and hypoxia

Cerebral resistance vessels are unusually sensitive to arterial CO_2 (Figure 15.13). **Hypercapnia** causes cerebral vasodilatation, which helps to maintain O_2 supply during asphyxia. The vasodilatation is partly mediated by endothelial NO and partly by a fall in vascular myocyte pH due to the carbonic acid. Conversely, **hypocapnia** causes cerebral vasoconstriction. If the arterial P_{CO_2} is reduced to 15 mmHg by hyperventilation (normal P_{CO_2} 40 mmHg), vasoconstriction halves the cerebral blood flow, and can be observed in the retina, which is embryologically an extension of the brain. Thus **panic hyperventilation** in adults, or hyperventilation for fun by children, can reduce cerebral perfusion sufficiently to cause disturbed vision, dizziness and even fainting. The traditional remedy is to breath in and out of a paper bag (not plastic), so that expired CO_2 is re-breathed.

Local hypoxia causes cerebral vasodilatation, due partly to adenosine formation. **Systemic hypoxia**, however, stimulates ventilation, and the resulting hypocapnia causes a counteracting cerebral vasoconstriction. As a result of these two opposite effects, systemic hypoxia has only a minor effect on human cerebral blood flow.

Regional neuronal activity evokes regional metabolic hyperaemia

Shining a light into one eye increases the local blood flow and temperature in the corresponding occipital cortex and lateral geniculate body. Cerebral vessels thus display excellent functional/active/metabolic hyperaemia. Increased mental activity evokes hyperaemia in many other regions too (Figure 15.14). The functional hyperaemia is mediated partly by **interstitial [K$^+$]**, which is raised initially by the outward, repolarizing K^+ currents of active neurons (Figure 15.15). The rise in K^+ is not well maintained, however. Sustaining factors include interstitial adenosine and astrocyte activation. Interstitial **adenosine**, a powerful cerebral vasodilator, increases rapidly in response to electrical stimulation and hypoxaemia, and is well sustained. **Astrocytes** are located between the neurons and blood vessels, and are thought to be stimulated by active neurons. As Ca^{2+} rises in the stimulated astrocytes, they release vasodilators such as eicosatrienoic acids (EETs, Section 9.5) close to the vessel. This results in the vasodilatation of both local resistance vessels and upstream, pial vessels (**neurovascular coupling**).

(a) Control, resting

(b) Movement of contralateral hand

(c) Reasoning test

Figure 15.14 Functional/metabolic hyperaemia in human cortex shown by xenon-133 imaging. Red areas show raised flow, 20% above mean. (a) Frontal lobe hyperaemia in resting, pensive subject. (b) Hyperaemia of the hand area of the upper motor, premotor and sensory cortex during voluntary movement of the contralateral hand. (c) Hyperaemia in precentral and postcentral areas during a reasoning test. (Data from Ingvar DH. *Brain Research* 1976; **107**: 188–97; and Lassen NA, Ingvar DH, Skinhoj E. *Scientific American* 1978; **239**: 50–9.)

Extracerebral arteries are innervated by both sensory and motor fibres

Intracerebral arterioles are poorly innervated, but the cerebral arteries on the brain surface are innervated by nociceptive C-fibres, parasympathetic vasodilator fibres and sympathetic vasoconstrictor fibres.

Perivascular nociceptive C-fibres are abundant and probably mediate the pain of **vascular headaches**, including the severe pains of meningitis, migraine and strokes. These sensory fibres also

Figure 15.15 Effect of neuronal activity on rat cerebellar blood flow (CeBF), monitored by laser Doppler; an example of metabolic hyperaemia. Concomitant interstitial K^+ concentration $[K^+]_o$ was monitored by an ion-sensitive electrode. Neurons were activated by remote electrical stimulation of parallel fibre system at frequency indicated in Hertz. (From Caesar K, Akgören N, Mathiesen C, Lauritzen M. *Journal of Physiology* 1999; **520**: 281–92, by permission.)

have a motor function, for they contain the vasodilator neurotransmitters **calcitonin gene-related peptide** (CGRP) and **substance P**, which in the skin are involved in several vasodilator responses (Section 14.4). C-fibre-mediated vasodilatation probably contributes to the hyperaemia of meningitis, seizures and the headache phase of migraine.

Parasympathetic vasodilator fibres contain acetylcholine and VIP, and may likewise contribute to the vasodilatation of vascular headaches.

Sympathetic vasoconstrictor fibres release noradrenaline and neuropeptide Y, but the noradrenaline has only a weak effect, because cerebral vessels express few α-adrenoceptors. **Neuropeptide Y** is abundant in cerebral sympathetic varicosities and probably accounts for much of the evoked vasoconstriction. Even so, the maximal effect of sympathetic stimulation in humans is only a 37% rise in cerebral vascular resistance (cf. 500% in skeletal muscle). Its chief role may be to protect the blood–brain barrier against disruption by sudden rises in arterial pressure.

Cerebral capillaries form a tight blood–brain barrier

Lipid-soluble molecules, such as O_2, CO_2 and general anaesthetics, diffuse freely across cerebral capillaries, whereas lipid-insoluble solutes, such as plasma salts, L-glucose, mannitol, catecholamines and angiotensin, fail to permeate the cerebral capillary wall in most regions of the brain (cf. free permeation in most tissues). This 'blood–brain barrier' to lipophobic solutes was discovered through the simple observation that an intravenous injection of an ionic dye stains almost every tissue in the body except the nervous system and testis.

The **functions** of the blood–brain barrier are:

- to protect the delicate neuronal circuits from interference by circulating solutes such as catecholamines, which are also neurotransmitters;
- to maintain a tight control of pH and K^+ concentration in the cerebrospinal and interstitial fluid; and
- to prevent the washout of synaptic neurotransmitters from the brain parenchyma.

As J Barcroft eloquently remarked in his book, *Architecture of Physiological Function*, 'To look for high intellectual development in a milieu whose properties have not become stabilized is to seek music among the crashings of a rudimentary wireless, or ripple patterns on the surface of the stormy Atlantic.'

The blood–brain barrier is created by specialized endothelial cell junctions (Section 10.8). Multiple junctional strands, composed of cadherin-10, claudin-1, occludin and ZO-1/2, form an unbroken seal between the cells (Figure 9.3). Also the caveola–vesicle system is very scanty. These structural specializations are probably induced by the astrocytes, the 'feet' of which envelop over 80% of the abluminal surface of a brain capillary.

In certain, specific locations, the blood–brain barrier is **physiologically defective**. Here plasma solutes can gain access to intracerebral receptors. In the **circumventricular region**, fenestrated capillaries allow sodium chloride access to the osmoreceptors of the laminae terminalis and subfornicular organ, and angiotensin II access to the subfornicular thirst centre. In the **area postrema** of the lateral medulla, angiotensin II accesses pre-sympathetic neurons, and circulating emetics access the vomiting centre. **Pathological breakdown** of the normal barrier is described under 'Special problems'.

Cerebral endothelium expresses special carriers to transport metabolites and K^+

The main neuronal energy source is D-**glucose** (dextrose, $C_6H_{12}O_6$), as demonstrated by the neuronal O_2/glucose consumption ratio of almost 6/1. Unlike the impermeant stereo-isomer L-glucose, D-glucose crosses the blood–brain barrier rapidly by **facilitated diffusion**. The D-glucose binds reversibly to a specific carrier protein in the endothelial cell membrane, GLUT-1. Consequently, uptake exhibits typical carrier-based phenomena, such as saturation and stereospecificity. Transport is nevertheless passive, being driven by the glucose concentration gradient created by neuronal consumption. Cerebral endothelium also expresses carriers for **adenosine, metabolic acids** (lactate, pyruvate), **neutral amino acids** (e.g. phenylalanine), **anionic amino acids** (e.g. glutamate) and **cationic amino acids** (e.g. arginine).

There is also **active K^+ transport** across cerebral endothelium. When interstitial $[K^+]$ is raised by neuronal electrical activity, a Na^+–K^+ ATPase in the abluminal endothelial membrane expels K^+ ions from the interstitium. Interstitial K^+ homeostasis is of course vital for the neuron resting potential. This active role of cerebral endothelium is supported by five to six times as many mitochondria as in muscle endothelium.

Special non-lymphatic pathways drain fluid from the brain

The brain lacks a lymphatic system. Instead, the cerebral interstitial fluid communicates with the cerebrospinal fluid (CSF), which drains through two specialized pathways. (i) The **arachnoid granulations** in the walls of the cranial venous sinuses transmit CSF directly into the venous system. (ii) Some CSF flows along the sheath of the olfactory nerve, exiting the skull through the perforated cribriform plate. This fluid is then absorbed by the **olfactory mucosa lymphatics**.

Special problems

Blood–brain barrier breakdown

Disorganization of the endothelial junctional protein causes barrier breakdown in numerous pathological conditions, including severe, acute hypertension, cerebral haemorrhage, ischaemia (strokes), hypoxia (high altitude exposure) and inflammation (meningitis, multiple sclerosis). The attendant rise in paracellular permeability leads to cerebral oedema, which impairs brain function and can induce fits (e.g. eclamptic toxaemia of pregnancy). These changes can be ameliorated by glucocorticoids and blockers of inflammatory mediator receptors.

Standing up can cause transient cerebral hypoperfusion and dizziness

The pull of gravity during orthostasis (upright position) has no direct effect on cerebral blood flow, because the cerebral circulation becomes an inverted U-tube siphon; the effect of gravity on the carotid and vertebral arteries is offset by the its effect on the jugular and vertebral veins and CSF (Figures 8.2 and 8.25, bottom panel). Standing up does, however, reduce cerebral perfusion transiently through a fall in cardiac output. Venous pooling in the legs lowers the central venous pressure and hence cardiac output (Starling's law), which causes

a transient postural hypotension. Although this is quickly corrected by the baroreflex (Chapter 16), it can reduce cerebral perfusion sufficiently to cause a passing dizziness or even fainting (postural syncope, Section 17.1). The internal jugular vein collapses above heart level during orthostasis, because gravity reduces its internal pressure to below atmospheric pressure (Figure 8.20). Consequently, much of the venous drainage is shunted into the vertebral venous plexus.

Space-occupying lesions elicit Cushing's reflex

Unlike other organs, the brain is confined within a rigid case, the cranium. Consequently, a large space-occupying lesion, such as a cerebral tumour or haemorrhage, raises the intracranial pressure and displaces the brainstem down into the foramen magnum, the opening in the base of the skull that admits the spinal cord. The brainstem contains the vasomotor control centres, and compression triggers an increase in their activity. This raises peripheral sympathetic vasomotor activity and hence the arterial blood pressure (**Cushing's reflex**). The raised blood pressure helps to maintain cerebral perfusion despite the raised intracranial pressure and it also evokes a bradycardia through the baroreflex. The combination of **bradycardia** and **acute hypertension is** recognized by neurologists as the hallmark of a large, space-occupying lesion.

Carotid/cerebral artery atheroma causes thrombo-embolic strokes

Around 80% of strokes (cerebral infarcts) are caused by a **thrombus** forming on an atheromatous plaque in the internal carotid artery or a major cerebral vessel, and/or by **embolism**, the lodging of a detached thrombus at a downstream vascular narrowing. An internal carotid thrombus often embolizes into the middle cerebral artery, due to their close anatomical relation (Figure 15.12). Thrombo-embolism causes characteristic patterns of neurological deficit, due to the infarction of the grey matter in the artery's territory. For example, obstruction of the left middle cerebral artery (generally the dominant side, containing the language centres) causes a right-sided hemiplegia and sensory loss plus aphasia, i.e. loss of language-related skills (speech, comprehension, reading, writing).

Arterial vasospasm causes haemorrhagic strokes

Around 20% of strokes are caused by a haemorrhage. **Subarachnoid haemorrhage** is bleeding on the surface of the brain, under the arachnoid membrane. This accounts for ~10% of cerebrovascular cases, and is often caused by the rupture of a saccular ('berry') aneurysm in the circle of Willis. **Intracerebral haemorrhage** is bleeding within the brain parenchyma. It is often caused by the rupture of microaneurysms (Charcot–Bouchard aneurysms) in patients with hypertension. The haemorrhage may trigger **cerebral artery vasospasm**, which reduces perfusion sufficiently to cause a stroke. Factors contributing to the vasospasm include **serotonin** from shed platelets and perivascular nerves, **neuropeptide Y** from sympathetic varicosities, **endothelin-1** and **Ca^{2+} sensitization**. The vasospasm is usually treated with the Ca^{2+}-channel blocker nimodipine, which has some selectivity for cerebral vessels. ET$_A$ receptor antagonists too ameliorate the vasospasm.

Cerebral vasodilatation contributes to migraine headaches

Migraine headache is preceded, in ~20% of cases, by a **visual prodroma** – flickering wavy lines in the visual field. This used to be attributed to vascular contraction in the visual pathway; but it now seems that it may be due to a neuronal phenomenon, cortical spreading depression. The ensuing severe **headache** is associated with dilatation of the large extracerebral vessels, such as the middle cerebral artery, and perivascular inflammation. The vascular headache is mediated by perivascular nociceptive C-fibres and the dilatation is attributed to the **release of substance P and CGRP** from the perivascular fibres (jugular venous CGRP rises), coupled with local **depletion of the vasoconstrictor serotonin** (urinary serotonin metabolite excretion rises). Cerebral vessels express serotonin 5HT$_{1D}$ receptors, and the agonist **sumatriptan** is an effective treatment for migraine headaches.

The other major nociceptor-rich intracranial structure, besides the major arteries, is the dura mater, which contributes to the severe headache of meningitis.

Measurement of human cerebral blood flow

- **Carotid angiography** (arteriography) is the X-ray imaging of the major cerebral arteries during the infusion of radio-opaque contrast medium into the internal carotid artery. This assesses cerebral vessel patency, aneurysms, and the anatomical course deviations caused by tumours.
- **Transcranial Doppler velocimetry** assesses flow in the major cerebral arteries.

The Cerebral Circulation

KEY FEATURES BOX 15.4

Special tasks
- Maintain a high O$_2$ delivery to O$_2$-hungry, hypoxia-intolerant grey matter
- Increase regional O$_2$ supply in response to regional activity
- Maintain a tightly regulated neuronal environment

Structural adaptations
- Anastomosis of major arteries forms circle of Willis
- High capillary density facilitates gas exchange
- Tight endothelial junctions form blood–brain barrier

Functional adaptations
- High basal blood flow due to low arteriolar resistance
- Brain controls rest of circulation through baroreflex to safeguard its own perfusion pressure. Cerebral vessels are 'excused' from the baroreflex and have only a weak sympathetic innervation
- Good autoregulation of flow if blood pressure falls
- Strong vasodilatation to CO$_2$ and asphyxia
- Well-developed regional metabolic hyperaemia in response to neuronal activity, mediated by interstitial K$^+$, adenosine and astrocyte neurovascular coupling
- Blood–brain barrier creates a well-regulated neuronal environment, with specific carriers for facilitated diffusion of D-glucose and amino acids

Special problems
- Blood–brain barrier breakdown (paracellular junction leakage) → cerebral oedema in severe hypertension, cerebral haemorrhage, strokes, high altitude hypoxia, inflammatory disorders
- Postural syncope if baroreflex impaired
- Space-occupying lesions (tumours, haemorrhage) → bulbar ischaemia and Cushing's reflex
- Atheroma of carotid/cerebral arteries → thrombo-embolic strokes
- Subarachnoid/intracerebral aneurysm bleeding → vascular spasm → haemorrhagic strokes
- Vascular dilatation → headaches, migraine

Assessment in man
- Carotid angiography
- Transcranial Dopplerimetry
- Xenon-133 and SPECT imaging

- **SPECT imaging** (single photon emission compound tomography) assesses regional perfusion by imaging the brain with a gamma-camera after the intra-arterial injection of a lipophilic, high energy gamma-emitting isotope.

15.5 Pulmonary circulation

> Blood flow (cardiac output), resting human
>   4–6 litre min^{-1}
> Maximum flow, exercising non-athlete
>   20–25 litre min^{-1}

The pulmonary circulation differs markedly from the above systemic circulations.

- Pressures are low and flows high, due to the low pulmonary vascular resistance.
- Autoregulation of flow is absent and basal tone is low.
- Sympathetic vasomotor nerves have no major role.
- Metabolic vasodilatation has no role; alveolar perfusion vastly exceeds metabolic demand.
- Pulmonary hypertension readily causes failure of the thin-walled right ventricle (~3 mm).

The metabolic needs of the alveoli are grossly oversupplied by the pulmonary blood flow, and the bronchi are supplied with systemic, arterial blood through a separate **bronchial circulation**. Some bronchial venous blood drains into the pulmonary veins (Figure 1.5). This, coupled with Thebesian vein drainage into the left heart, reduces the arterial O_2 saturation to ~97%.

Special tasks

Since the role of the lungs is gas exchange, the pulmonary circulation must (i) allow blood to equilibrate with the gas phase; and (ii) perfuse each alveolus in proportion to its ventilation, i.e. local blood flow must match local gas supply. A secondary task of pulmonary endothelium is the enzymatic modification of circulating peptides, such as angiotensin I and bradykinin.

Structural adaptations

Dense capillary packing and ultra-short diffusion distance produce efficient gas exchange

The density of capillaries in the alveolar wall is extraordinary; blood flows over the alveolar surface almost as a continuous sheet, because there is so little tissue separating adjacent capillaries (Figure 15.16). Moreover the endothelium–epithelium layer separating the plasma and alveolar gas is extremely thin, ~0.3 μm. The short diffusion distance and massive capillary surface area (90–126 m^2 for the two human lungs) allow very high O_2 transfer rates. Consequently, O_2 transfer is limited chiefly

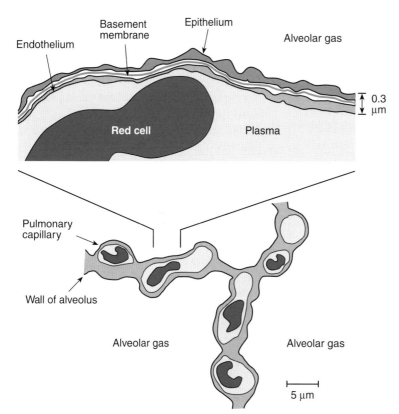

Figure 15.16 Ultrastructure of alveolar wall and pulmonary capillaries, based on electron micrographs. Note high ratio of blood to tissue and extreme thinness of membrane separating plasma from alveolar gas, ~0.3 μm.

Table 15.1 Typical pressures in human pulmonary circulation

	Pulmonary artery (mmHg)			Pulmonary capillary (mmHg)[a]	Pulmonary vein (mmHg)
	Systolic	Diastolic	Mean		
Rest					
Supine	25	12	17[b]	13	9
Upright	22	9	14	9	5
Heavy exercise					
Upright[c]	40	24	30	18	6

[a]Pulmonary capillary pressure is midway between arterial and venous pressures because the pulmonary pre- to postcapillary resistance ratio R_A/R_V is ~1 (cf. 4 in systemic circulation); see Pappenheimer–Soto-Rivera equation, Figure 11.4.
[b]Pulmonary hypertension is a resting mean pulmonary arterial pressure of $\geqslant 25$ mmHg.
[c]Submaximal treadmill exercise, cardiac output 17.5 l/min, O_2 consumption 2.35 l/min.
Sources: Nichols WW, O'Rourke MF (eds). *McDonald's Blood Flow in Arteries*, 5th edn. London: Arnold, 2005: 307–20; Stickland MK, Welsh RC, Haykowsky MJ *et al. Journal of Physiology* 2004; **561**: 321–9; Caro *et al. The Mechanics of the Circulation*. Oxford University Press, 1978.

by the blood flow, i.e. by cardiac output (**flow limited exchange**, Section 10.10).

Numerous short arterioles create a low resistance to flow

Pulmonary arteries and arterioles are shorter and thinner walled than their systemic counterparts, so they offer less hydraulic resistance. Consequently, a small pressure gradient and thin right ventricle wall (~3 mm) suffice to drive pulmonary perfusion (Table 15.1). Due to the low arteriolar resistance, pulmonary capillary pressure is pulsatile and the pre/postcapillary resistance ratio, which determines capillary pressure (Figure 11.4), is ~1, in contrast to ~4 in systemic circulations. A ratio of 1 means that pulmonary capillary pressure is midway between the arterial and venous pressures. The low pulmonary capillary pressures (9–18 mmHg) prevent stress damage to the extremely thin alveolar membrane.

Functional adaptations

Blood gases equilibrate despite short transit times

The volume of blood in the pulmonary capillaries of a resting human is ~100 ml, and the blood flow is ~5000 ml min^{-1} (cardiac output). Blood therefore traverses the pulmonary capillaries in 100/5000 min, or ~1 s – the mean **transit time**. Although the transit time is very short, 1 s is more than long enough for the blood gases to equilibrate with the alveolar gas (as in curves 1–3 of Figure 10.13a).

During **exercise** the increased right ventricular output shortens the transit time. It also raises pulmonary pressure (Figure 15.17), which distends the vessels and increases pulmonary capillary volume by about one and a half fold. Since transit time is volume/flow, the increase in volume helps limit the

shortening of the transit time to ~0.3 s. The blood still equilibrates with the alveolar gas, or very nearly so, during the shortened time in the pulmonary capillary. Since equilibration is achieved by the end of the capillary bed, gas exchange is **flow-limited** (Section 10.10) and the **uptake of O_2 is directly proportional to the pulmonary blood flow** (Fick's principle, Section 7.1).

Endurance athletes generate exceptionally high cardiac outputs during extreme performance, and this causes a marked fall in arterial P_{O_2} and oxygen saturation. The same is true of racehorses, though not all mammals. Non-athletes too display a small fall in saturation during heavy exercise (Figure 15.17). A likely explanation is that the pulmonary transit time becomes so short that full gaseous equilibration is no longer achieved (**diffusion-limited exchange**, curve 4 of Figure 10.13a). An additional, possibly minor factor may be the opening up of pulmonary arteriovenous shunts that bypass the capillaries.

Hypoxic pulmonary vasoconstriction optimizes local ventilation/perfusion ratios

In the systemic circulation local hypoxia causes vasodilatation (Section 13.4), but in the pulmonary circulation it causes vasoconstriction (hypoxic pulmonary vasoconstriction, HPV). The role of HPV is to preserve an optimum, uniform alveolar ventilation/perfusion ratio, $\dot{V}/\dot{Q}$, throughout the lungs, in normal and pathological states. For efficient oxygenation, each alveolus requires the same $\dot{V}/\dot{Q}$ ratio, namely 0.8 at rest (alveolar ventilation 4 l/min, cardiac output 5 l/min). HPV helps to maintain this ratio throughout the lung in supine humans. (Changes during orthostasis are considered

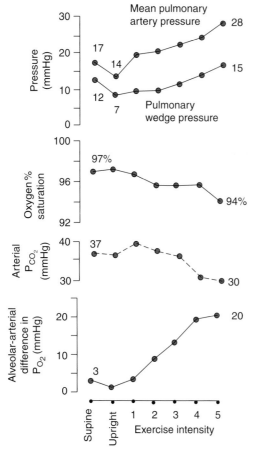

Figure 15.17 Effect of orthostasis (standing) and exercise on pulmonary blood pressures and arterial O_2 saturation in healthy non-athletes; wedge pressure is a clinical measure of venular pressure (see text). Orthostasis reduces pulmonary blood pressure, exercise increases it. High intensity exercise reduced arterial saturation, despite the hyperventilation revealed by the fall in arterial P_{CO_2}. The desaturation is attributed to reduced transit time (diffusion limitation), ventilation/perfusion mismatch and arteriovenous shunt vessels, which have been demonstrated in human lungs *post mortem*. (Data from Stickland *et al. Journal of Physiology* 2004; **561**: 321–9.)

The controversial, multiple mechanisms that underlie HPV are summarized in Appendix 2, 'Hypoxia and vascular tone'.

Pulmonary vascular pressure–volume and pressure–flow relations are passive, lacking autoregulation

Due to its great vascularity and distensibility, the pulmonary circulation contains **12–16% of the total blood volume** in a supine human, i. e. $\sim$600 ml. On standing, venous pooling in the legs reduces pulmonary blood volume by $\sim$20% and pulmonary pressures by 3–4 mmHg (Table 15.1 and Figure 15.17). The pulmonary blood volume can be increased transiently to $\sim$1 litre by a forced inspiration, because inspiration reduces intrathoracic pressure. Pulmonary blood volume can be reduced to $\sim$300 ml by a forced expiration, because expiration raises intrathoracic pressure (Valsalva manoeuvre, Section 17.2).

Pulmonary vascular resistance is about one-sixth of the systemic resistance, so resting pulmonary arterial pressure is only 22–25 mmHg systolic, 9–12 mmHg diastolic (Table 15.1). The pressure–flow relation in an isolated, perfused lung is typical of passive, slightly distensible tubes; the curve steepens slightly with pressure because vascular distension increases vascular conductance (Figure 15.19a). This contrasts with the highly autoregulated relations in brain, myocardium and kidney; autoregulation would be counterproductive in the lungs, since it would prevent pulmonary flow from increasing with pressure.

Exercise increases pulmonary artery pressure and flow

During exercise the increased right ventricular output raises the pulmonary artery pressure (Figure 15.17 and Table 15.1). In **young adults** performing supine exercise, pulmonary blood flow increases almost linearly with pressure gradient (pulmonary artery pressure minus left atrial pressure) (Figure 15.19b, middle line). In **endurance-trained athletes** the pressure–flow relation is steeper, because the 'trained' pulmonary vessels have a higher conductance, i.e. they transmit more flow per unit pressure (Figure 15.19b, left). Conversely, at **high altitude** the pressure–flow relation becomes flatter, because chronic HPV reduces vascular conductance (Figure 15.19b, right).

Increased pulmonary pressure during exercise improves apical perfusion and O_2 transfer capacity

In standing/sitting humans the lung apices are not well perfused at rest, due to the effect of gravity

under 'Special problems'.) If a group of alveoli is under-ventilated and therefore hypoxic, perhaps due to a slight airway narrowing or mucus, the resistance vessels supplying that region undergo HPV (Figure 15.18). This reduces the local alveolar blood flow $\dot{Q}$ to match the reduced local alveolar ventilation $\dot{V}$, and diverts blood away from hypoxic alveoli, so that relatively little under-oxygenated blood is added to arterial blood. Thus, although pulmonary HPV is the opposite response to the hypoxic vasodilatation of systemic vessels, both responses are well adapted to the local needs.

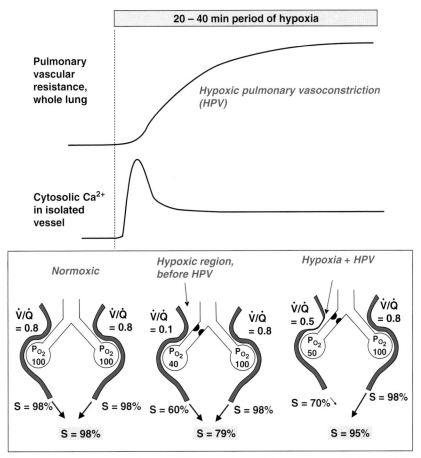

Figure 15.18 (*Top*) Hypoxic pulmonary vasoconstriction (HPV) in a perfused whole lung exposed to hypoxia. (*Middle*) Corresponding change in vascular myocyte cytosolic Ca^{2+} in an isolated rat pulmonary artery exposed to hypoxia. (*Bottom*) Effect of local alveolar hypoxia and HPV on gas exchange. HPV prevents extremely low ventilation/perfusion ratios, $\dot{V}/\dot{Q}$, and thus preserves the O_2 saturation (*S*) of mixed arterial blood. P_{O_2} in mmHg; arrow size indicates flow magnitude. (Based on Robertson TP, Aaronson PI, Ward JPT. *American Journal of Physiology* 1995; **268**: H301–7, with permission from the American Physiological Society.)

(Figure 15.20). During exercise the rise in pulmonary artery pressure greatly improves apical perfusion, boosting the O_2 transfer capacity of the lungs. Mean pulmonary artery pressure reaches ~30 mmHg during strenuous upright exercise, cf. ~14 mmHg at rest.

Low capillary pressure reduces alveolar membrane stress and fluid filtration

As noted earlier, **pulmonary capillary pressure** is only ~9 mmHg at heart level in the upright position. This reduces the tension in the alveolar-endothelial membrane to a low level, obviating rupture of this ultra-thin membrane. Although the capillary pressure is much lower than plasma colloid osmotic pressure, pulmonary capillaries are nevertheless in a state of filtration (Figure 11.12, lowest point), because lung interstitial fluid has a high colloid osmotic pressure (Table 11.2).

Capillary filtrate is prevented from accumulating within the alveoli and airways by epithelial ion channels and pumps, and is cleared as **lung lymph**. Airway epithelial cells express amiloride-sensitive, Na^+-conducting channels (**ENaC**) on the luminal surface and $\mathbf{Na^+}$–$\mathbf{K^+}$ **pumps** on the basolateral surface. As Na^+ is absorbed from the airways through these channels, water follows it by osmosis. Mice lacking functional ENaC die from pulmonary oedema soon after birth. (In the fetus, by contrast, a chloride pump into the airways causes water to flow into the airways; the switch to Na^+-driven water absorption occurs at birth.)

Pulmonary oedema is a life-threatening excess of interstitial fluid, arising from left ventricular failure, mitral stenosis, high altitude exposure or sepsis. Its clinical manifestations are cough, dyspnoea, crepitations (airways crackles), and in the worst cases pink, frothy sputum, with arterial desaturation.

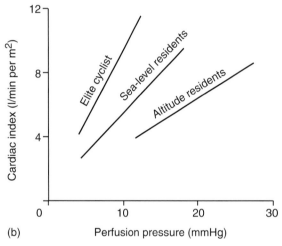

(b)   Perfusion pressure (mmHg)

Figure 15.19 Pressure–flow relations in pulmonary circulation. (a) Isolated cat lung perfused with plasma, with venous pressure (P_v) set to zero or 12 cmH$_2$O and airway pressure to 4 cmH$_2$O. Dashed lines are lines of constant conductance; actual pulmonary conductance increases as arterial pressure rises. Consequently, a 4× increase in right cardiac output requires less than a 4× increase in pressure. (b) Human curves during supine exercise. 'Perfusion pressure' is pulmonary artery pressure minus left atrial pressure; airway pressure is atmospheric. ((a) From Banister RJ, Torrance RW. *Quarterly Journal of Experimental Physiology* 1960; **45**: 352–7, with permission from Wiley-Blackwell; (b) from Grover RF *et al.* Pulmonary circulation. In: Shepherd JT, Abboud FM (eds). *Handbook of Physiology, Cardiovascular System*, Vol III, Peripheral Circulation. Bethesda, MD: American Physiological Society, 1983: 103–36, by permission.)

Causes included alveolar-endothelial barrier breakdown, impaired epithelial Na$^+$ clearance (e.g. high altitude hypoxia) and haemodynamic abnormalities (raised pulmonary capillary pressure, cardiogenic oedema). Left atrial pressure elevation to >20 mmHg raises capillary pressure sufficiently to

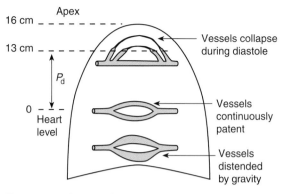

Figure 15.20 Gradient of perfusion in human lung in upright position at rest. Scale shows vertical distance above heart. Diastolic artery pressure P_d is 13 cmH$_2$O (~9 mmHg) at heart level, falling to zero (atmospheric) 13 cm above heart. Vessels higher than this are perfused only during systole. Perfusion was measured by external gamma counting following an injection of radioisotope into the right heart.

generate pulmonary oedema; smaller increases are within the safety margin against oedema (Section 11.10), but nevertheless cause **dyspnoea** (difficulty in breathing). Dyspnoea results from distension of the lung vasculature by a raised pulmonary venous pressure (**pulmonary congestion**), which makes the lungs stiff and difficult to inflate.

Pulmonary endothelium modifies circulating vasoactive agents

As blood passes through the lungs, it is exposed to 90–126 m^2 of endothelium. This huge surface area facilitates the chemical modification of circulating vasoactive substances by endothelial ecto-enzymes. Angiotensin-converting enzyme (ACE) converts angiotensin I to angiotensin II and degrades circulating bradykinin. Many other vasoactive substances (serotonin, prostaglandin E, leukotrienes) are also removed by lung endothelium.

Special problems

Orthostasis causes a vertical perfusion gradient

When humans adopt an upright position, the distribution of pulmonary blood flow is distorted by gravity. Mean pulmonary arterial pressure is ~14–15 mmHg at heart level (Table 15.1), but gravity raises this to ~21 mmHg in the lung bases, and reduces it to ~3 mmHg in the apices. The high pressure at the base distends the vessels there, raising their vascular conductance and hence the basal perfusion (Figure 15.20). Conversely, vessels at the apex collapse during diastole, because these vessels are ~16 cm above heart level, whereas diastolic pressure is only 13 cmH$_2$O (9 mmHg, Table 15.1). The apex is therefore perfused only during systole at rest (Figure 15.20), and the **mean flow through the apex is about one-tenth of the flow through the base**. As noted earlier, efficient gas exchange requires a uniform alveolar $\dot{V}/\dot{Q}$ of ~0.8 throughout the lung. Although alveolar ventilation $\dot{V}$ is likewise greater at the base than apex, the ventilation gradient does not fully compensate for the even bigger gradient of flow, $\dot{Q}$. A standing human, therefore, has a higher $\dot{V}/\dot{Q}$ at the apex than the base. This $\dot{V}/\dot{Q}$ mismatch slightly impairs the efficiency of blood oxygenation during orthostasis.

Pulmonary arterial hypertension leads to right ventricular failure

Although HPV is valuable in minimizing local $\dot{V}/\dot{Q}$ mismatch, it can be deleterious when the whole lung becomes hypoxic, as happens when low-altitude dwellers move to high altitude. The chronic hypoxia raises the pulmonary vascular resistance, which causes chronic pulmonary arterial hypertension, defined as a resting mean of $\geq 25\,mmHg$. Because the wall of the right ventricle is only ~3 mm thick, its ability to withstand a chronic increase in afterload is poor. Consequently, hypoxic chronic pulmonary hypertension can lead to right ventricular failure in mountaineers. Pulmonary arterial hypertension also occurs at low altitudes, where its aetiology is poorly understood. There is evidence that some cases are due to the proliferation of pulmonary arterial myocytes under the influences of serotonin.

Pulmonary embolism impairs right ventricular output

A venous thrombus in a deep leg vein (often arising during a period of immobility) or pelvic veins (e.g. after surgery) may become detached (embolize). The embolus is washed through the right heart into the pulmonary artery, until it jams in a branch. This raises pulmonary vascular resistance, hence pulmonary arterial pressure and right ventricular afterload. A rise in arterial pressure reduces stroke volume (Figure 6.11b, loop 3). Embolism thus causes a sharp fall in right ventricular output, which in turn reduces left ventricular output, leading to collapse.

High stresses in the thin alveolar-endothelial membrane may rupture it

The blood–gas barrier is extremely thin, ~0.3 μm, so the tensile force per unit thickness of membrane (stress) is substantial, even though capillary pressure is low. The stress is probably carried mainly by type IV collagen in the basement membrane, which

is only ~50 nm thick in places (Figure 15.16). If the stress is raised by pulmonary capillary hypertension, as in patients with **mitral valve stenosis**, the membrane may break down in places, causing **pulmonary oedema** and, in severe cases, **alveolar**

The Pulmonary Circulation

Special tasks
- Respiratory gas exchange
- Enzymatic modification of circulating peptides, notably angiotensin I to II

Structural adaptations
- Extremely high capillary density and extremely short diffusion distance
- Short arterioles of low resistance allow large flow (right ventricular output) under a low pressure head

Functional adaptations
- Transit time of 0.3–1.0 s is long enough to allow blood–alveolar gas equilibration
- Hypoxic pulmonary vasoconstriction matches local alveolar blood perfusion to local ventilation
- Flow increases in proportion to pressure; no autoregulation
- Low capillary pressure reduces membrane stress and fluid filtration
- Endothelial enzymes modify/degrade circulating vasoactive peptides

Special problems
- Apices not well perfused in orthostasis, but this improves during exercise
- At extreme flows (athletes) capillary transit time of <0.3 s causes arterial under-oxygenation
- Chronic hypoxia causes chronic vasoconstriction. The resulting pulmonary arterial hypertension can lead to right heart failure, as can other forms of pulmonary arterial hypertension
- Pulmonary embolism can cause a sudden fall in cardiac output and collapse
- Ultra-thin alveolar/endothelial membrane (0.3 μm). In mitral stenosis, pulmonary capillary hypertension raises membrane stress and leads to leakage

Assessment in man
- Fick principle based on O_2 uptake measures pulmonary blood flow (cardiac output)
- Indicator and thermal dilution methods likewise measure pulmonary blood flow
- Pulmonary wedge pressure indicates pulmonary venular pressure

KEY FEATURES BOX 15.5

haemorrhage. This occurs most dramatically in thoroughbred racehorses. Racehorses are capable of extremely high cardiac outputs, >300 l/min, which raises the pulmonary arterial pressure to 120 mmHg and left atrial pressure to 70 mmHg! This can lead to race-induced pulmonary haemorrhage. In strenuous human exercise, fortunately, the rise in pulmonary pressure is considerably more modest (Table 15.1).

Assessment in man

The measurement of pulmonary blood flow is, of course, the measurement of right ventricle cardiac output. This can be measured by the **Fick principle**, **indicator dilution method** and **thermal dilution method** (Chapter 7). Pulmonary microvascular pressure is estimated clinically by advancing a catheter through the pulmonary artery until the tip wedges in a narrow arterial vessel, blocking the downstream flow. The pressure of the stationary distal column of blood, the **pulmonary wedge pressure**, equals that in the nearest distal perfused vessel, usually a venule.

Further reading

Reviews and chapters

Coronary circulation

Duncker DJ, Bache RJ. Regulation of coronary blood flow during exercise. *Physiological Reviews* 2008; **88**: 1009–86.

Helisch A, Schaper W. Arteriogenesis: The development and growth of collateral arteries. *Microcirculation* 2003; **10**: 83–97.

Kuo L. Coronary vasodilatation and K$_{ATP}$ channels; independence from NO. *News in Physiological Sciences* 1997; **12**: 246–7.

Mary DASG. Reflex effects on the coronary circulation. *Experimental Physiology* 1992; **77**: 243–70.

Nichols WW, O'Rourke MF (eds). The coronary circulation. In: *McDonald's Blood Flow in Arteries*, 5th edn. London: Arnold, 2005: 321–38.

Skeletal muscle circulation

Joyner MJ. Exercise hyperaemia: Are there any answers yet? *Journal of Physiology* 2007; **583**: 817. (Introduction to a series of symposium articles).

Joyner MJ. Feeding the sleeping giant: Muscle blood flow during whole body exercise. *Journal of Physiology* 2004; **558**: 1.

Intaglietta M, Johnson PC (eds). Functional capillary density: Active and passive determinants. *International Journal of Microcirculation* 1995; **15**: 213–76.

Marshall JM. The roles of adenosine and related substances in exercise hyperaemia. *Journal of Physiology* 2007; **583**: 835–45.

Rowell LB. *Human Cardiovascular Control*. New York: Oxford University Press, 1993.

Shepherd JT. Circulation to skeletal muscle. In: Shepherd JT, Abboud FM (eds). *Handbook of Physiology, Cardiovascular System*, Volume III, Part 1, Peripheral Circulation. Bethesda, MD: American Physiological Society, 1983: 319–70.

Wittenberg BA, Wittenberg JB. Transport of oxygen in muscle. *Annual Review of Physiology* 1989; **51**: 857–78.

Cutaneous circulation

Braverman IM. Ultrastructure and organization of the cutaneous microvasculature in normal and pathological states. *Journal of Investigative Dermatology* 1989; **93** (Suppl.): 2S–9S.

Johnson JM. How does skin blood flow get so high? *Journal of Physiology* 2006; **577**: 768.

Johnson JM. Mechanisms of vasoconstriction with direct skin cooling in humans. *American Journal of Physiology* 2007; **292**: H1690–1.

Roddie LC. Circulation to skin and adipose tissue. In: Shepherd JT, Abboud FM (eds). *Handbook of Physiology, Cardiovascular System*, Volume III, Part 1, Peripheral Circulation. Bethesda, MD: American Physiological Society, 1983: 285–317.

Cerebral circulation

Bradbury MWB. The blood–brain barrier. *Experimental Physiology* 1993; **78**: 453–72.

Duelli R, Kuschinsky W. Brain glucose transporters: Relationship to local energy demand. *News in Physiological Sciences* 2001; **16**: 71–6.

Faraci FM, Heistad DD. Regulation of the cerebral circulation: role of endothelium and potassium channels. *Physiological Reviews* 1998; **78**: 53–74.

Goadsby PJ. Vasoactive peptides in migraine and cluster headaches. In: Edvinsson L, Uddman R (eds). *Vascular Innervation and Receptor Mechanisms*. New York: Academic Press, 1993: 415–24.

Heistad DD. What's new in the cerebral microcirculation? *Microcirculation* 2001; **8**: 365–75.

Juul R, Edvinsson L. Perivascular peptides in subarachnoid haemorrhage. In: Edvinsson L, Uddman R (eds). *Vascular Innervation and Receptor Mechanisms*. New York: Academic Press, 1993: 399–414.

Saez JC. Astrocytes as connexin-dependent signaling cells for local blood flow regulation. *American Journal of Physiology* 2008; **294**: H586–7.

Pulmonary circulation

Aaronson PI, Robertson TP, Knock Ga *et al.* Hypoxic pulmonary vasoconstriction: mechanisms and controversies. *Journal of Physiology* 2006; **570**: 53–8.

Bahkle YS. Pharmacokinetic and metabolic properties of the lung. *British Journal of Anaesthesia* 1990; **65**: 79.

Butler J. The bronchial circulation. *News in Physiological Sciences* 1991; **6**: 21–5.

Leach RM, Treacher DF. Clinical aspects of hypoxic pulmonary vasoconstriction. In Control of the Pulmonary Circulation. Physiological Society Symposium. *Experimental Physiology* 1995; **80**: 865–75.

Lumb A (ed.). *Nunn's Applied Respiration Physiology*, 6th edn. Oxford: Elsevier, 2005.

Maina JN, West JB. Thin and strong! The bioengineering dilemma in the structural and functional design of the blood–gas barrier. *Physiological Reviews* 2005; **85**: 811–44.

Nichols WW, O'Rourke MF. The pulmonary circulation. In: Nichols WM, O'Rourke MF (eds). *McDonald's Blood Flow in Arteries*, 5th edn. London: Arnold, 2005: 307–20.

Olver RE, Walters DV, Wilson S. Developmental regulation of lung liquid transport. *Annual Review of Physiology* 2004; **66**: 77–101.

Research papers

See www.hodderplus.com/cardiovascularphysiology for a full list of Research papers for this chapter.

CHAPTER 16

Cardiovascular receptors, reflexes and central control

Learning objectives

After reading this chapter you should be able to:

- Outline the locations and properties of arterial baroreceptors (16.1).
- State the reflex effects of baroreceptors and their role in hypovolaemia (16.2).
- Outline the properties and roles of veno-atrial stretch receptors (16.3, 16.4).
- State the neural origin of ischaemic cardiac pain (16.3).
- Outline the reflex responses to a rise in CVP and fluid volume in humans (16.4).
- Explain the role of the kidneys in long-term blood pressure regulation (16.5).
- Outline the location and role of peripheral arterial chemoreceptors (16.6).
- State the cardiovascular reflex evoked by lung stretch receptors (16.6).
- Outline the role of muscle work receptors during exercise (16.6).
- List the roles of the medulla oblongata in cardiovascular control (16.7).
- Define the alerting response and central command (16.8).
- Explain how inspiration affects vagal outflow to the pacemaker (16.9).

The activity of the cardiovascular sympathetic and parasympathetic nerves is controlled by the brain; and the brain is guided by sensory information coming from neural receptors both inside and outside the circulation. (The term 'receptor' in this context means a sensory nerve ending, not a drug-binding molecule.) The afferent, sensory fibres, central relays and efferent, motor fibres together form cardiovascular reflex arcs (Figure 16.1). Key **sensors** include pressure receptors in the walls of specific systemic arteries (arterial baroreceptors), and pressure receptors in the heart (cardiopulmonary receptors). Their afferent fibres transmit information about arterial blood pressure and cardiac filling to the **brainstem**, where the information is integrated with information from muscle receptors, arterial chemoreceptors and other sensors. The integration

of information and computation of an appropriate response involves much up-and-down traffic between the brainstem, hypothalamus, cerebellum and cortex. **Pre-sympathetic and parasympathetic outflows** from the brainstem are then adjusted to initiate an appropriate cardiovascular response.

The reflexes are often, but not invariably, directed at stabilizing blood pressure. For example, the reflex response to a rise in blood pressure is a bradycardia and peripheral vasodilatation, which restore blood pressure to its original level (a **depressor reflex**). This is an example of **negative feedback** – a change in the sensed variable (blood pressure) triggers an inhibitory response that returns the variable towards its control value, or **set point**. Other reflexes, such as those from arterial and muscle chemoreceptors, are

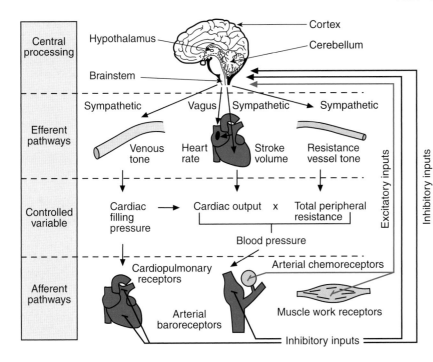

Figure 16.1 Overview of neural reflex control of the circulation; 'inhibitory' and 'excitatory' refer to net effect on cardiac output and blood pressure. Inhibitory reflexes are depressor, excitatory reflexes are pressor.

excitatory, i.e. they raise rather than stabilize pressure (**pressor reflexes**). The brain can also initiate non-reflex changes. For example, at the start of exercise a signal from the cerebral cortex, called **central command**, increases the heart rate almost instantly. This process is termed **feedforward** (cf. feedback).

16.1 Arterial baroreceptors

The prefix 'baro-' means pressure. A baroreceptor is a sprayed sensory fibre ending, packed with mitochondria and connected to a myelinated or non-myelinated afferent axon. Baroreceptors occur in the adventitia of arteries at two main locations: the carotid sinus and aortic arch (Figure 16.2).

The **carotid sinus** is a thin-walled dilatation at the origin of the internal carotid artery. Afferent fibres from the carotid sinus baroreceptors form the carotid sinus nerve. This joins the **glossopharyngeal nerve** (IXth cranial nerve) to reach the petrous ganglion, where the parent neurons are located. Like all afferent neurons the petrous neurons are bipolar. Their central axons continue up the glossopharyngeal nerve to the brainstem and terminate in the **nucleus tractus solitarius**.

Aortic baroreceptors are found mainly on the transverse arch of the aorta. Their fibres form the aortic or 'depressor' nerve in some species, then ascend in the **vagus** (Xth cranial nerve) to the sensory neurons of the nodose ganglion. The central axons again terminate in the nucleus tractus

solitarius of the brainstem. **Coronary arteries** too possess baroreceptors, at least in dogs, and the coronary baroreflex is of similar potency to the carotid sinus baroreflex.

Baroreceptors are stretch receptors

The baroreceptors are mechanoreceptors that respond to stretch. A rise in arterial pressure stretches the artery wall, which deforms and excites the receptor terminals. The wall of the carotid sinus is relatively thin, and the sinus diameter changes by ~15% with each pulse. If distension is prevented by a plaster cast, the baroreceptors no longer respond to changes in blood pressure.

Baroreceptors exhibit static and dynamic sensitivity

Arterial baroreceptors respond not only to the magnitude of the pressure (static sensitivity) but also to its rate of change (dynamic sensitivity). If the carotid sinus is distended rapidly in an experiment, an individual baroreceptor fibre first fires off a volley of action potentials at a high frequency (**dynamic response** to the pressure change), then the firing frequency declines (**adaptation**) until it stabilizes at a lower, but still raised, frequency that signals the new pressure level (**static response**) (Figure 16.3, fibre 1). The adaptation may be due to mechanical creep of the receptor within its stretched environment, and/or ion channel adaptation.

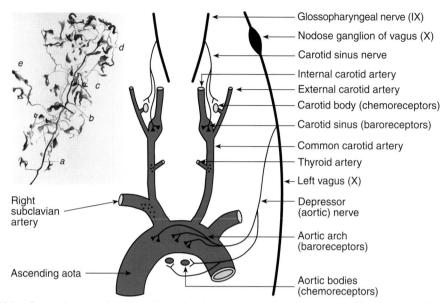

Figure 16.2 Main reflexogenic zones of arterial system; minor baroreceptor regions shown as dots. Right vagus not shown. (*Inset*) Single baroreceptor ending in human carotid sinus. (From Abraham A. *Microscopic Innervation of the Heart and Blood Vessels in Vertebrates Including Man.* Oxford: Pergamon Press, 1969, with permission from Elsevier.)

Figure 16.3 Firing characteristics of baroreceptor afferents. *Fibres 1 and 2.* Action potentials in myelinated afferents of cat carotid sinus when non-pulsatile arterial pressure (AP) is raised (fibre 1) or reduced (fibre 2). *Fibre 3.* Single baroreceptor fibre from rabbit aorta responding to a normal, pulsatile pressure. There are four impulses per pulse when pulse pressure is high (arrow) and three when it is lower. Time intervals 0.1 s. (Fibres 1 and 2 after Landgren S. *Acta Physiologica Scandinavica* 1952; **26**: 1–34, with permission from Wiley-Blackwell; fibre 3 from Downing SE. *Journal of Physiology* 1960; **150**: 210–13, with permission from Wiley-Blackwell.)

Conversely, when pressure is reduced, the baroreceptor fibre transiently falls silent (dynamic 'off' response), then resumes activity at a new, lower rate (static 'off' response) (Figure 16.3, fibre 2). As a result of its dynamic sensitivity, a baroreceptor fibre *in vivo* characteristically fires a burst of action potentials in systole and falls silent in diastole (Figure 16.3, fibre 3).

A-fibres have lower thresholds and are more sensitive than C-fibres

There are two kinds of arterial baroreceptor, the A-fibre and the C-fibre. The distinction is based on myelination, conduction velocity and threshold. The **threshold** of a baroreceptor is the lowest pressure that triggers an action potential in its axon.

A-fibres are large-diameter, fast-conducting, myelinated fibres with low thresholds, in the range 30–90 mmHg (Figure 16.4a). A-fibres are active at normal blood pressure and fire a burst of impulses with each arterial pulse. A-fibres are less numerous than C-fibres.

C-fibres are the more abundant, small-diameter, slow-conducting, unmyelinated fibres with high thresholds, in the range 70–140 mmHg. Only a quarter or so of the C-fibres are active at normal blood pressures. The active fibres fire in phase with the pulse, but at a low frequency.

The mean discharge frequency in a baroreceptor fibre increases with mean blood pressure, above threshold. The steepness of the relation is called the **sensitivity** of the fibre. A-fibres are two to three times more sensitive than C-fibres in the middle of their respective operating ranges (Figure 16.4a). A-fibres can also achieve higher discharge frequencies than C-fibres.

C-fibres are important at high blood pressures, when A-fibre activity saturates

When blood pressure reaches a high level, the A-fibre activity reaches a maximum frequency (**saturation**), whereas the C-fibres remain responsive to pressure at these levels (Figure 16.4a). Therefore, C-fibres of high threshold are important for signalling graded information about high blood pressures. The A-fibres are important for signalling changes around normal blood pressure, aided by ~25% of the C-fibres with low enough thresholds.

Recruitment extends the signalling range of multi-fibre nerves

The carotid sinus nerve and aortic nerve contain large numbers of A- and C-fibres. When blood pressure rises, not only does the discharge frequency increase in previously active fibre, but also previously silent fibres of high threshold begin to fire (**recruitment**). Due to recruitment, the multi-fibre nerve has a wider operating range than a single fibre, and can keep the brainstem informed about a wider range of pressures (Figure 16.4b).

Baroreceptors signal pulse pressure as well as mean pressure

Carotid baroreceptors signal not only the mean pressure but also the size of the oscillation about the mean, i.e. the pulse pressure. The greater the oscillation in pressure about a given mean, the greater the average baroreceptor activity (Figure 16.4b).

Figure 16.4 Effect of arterial blood pressure on baroreceptor traffic and reflex change in systemic blood pressure in anaesthetized dogs. (a) Response of a single A-fibre and C-fibre to increasing pressure. (b) Average discharge rate in multi-fibre carotid sinus nerve: pulsatile pressures evoke higher activity. (c) Raising pressure in a vascularly isolated, perfused baroreceptor region triggers a reflex fall in systemic arterial blood pressure, mediated by bradycardia and peripheral vasodilatation. Pulsatility strengthens this depressor reflex. (From (a) Coleridge HM, Coleridge JCG, Schultz HD. *Journal of Physiology* 1987; **394**: 291–313; (b) Korner PI. *Physiological Reviews* 1971; **51**: 312–67, with permission from the American Physiological Society; and (c) Angell-James JE, De Burgh Daly M. *Journal of Physiology* 1970; **209**: 257–93, with permission from Wiley-Blackwell.)

Consequently, a pulsating pressure has a greater reflex effect than a steady pressure (Figure 16.4c). The difference is due partly to the dynamic sensitivity of the receptors, partly to recruitment of extra fibres during each systole, and partly to the gradual adaptation of brainstem neurons to a steady signal. The signalling of pulse pressure is particularly important during **orthostasis** and **moderate haemorrhage**, when there is a fall in pulse pressure (due to the fall in cardiac stroke volume), but often little fall in mean arterial pressure (Figure 18.2).

Carotid sinus and aortic baroreceptors have similar properties

Carotid sinus A-fibres have slightly lower thresholds than aortic arch A-fibres, but otherwise the receptors and reflexes elicited by the two reflexogenic zones are broadly similar. Both regions have strong reflex effects on human heart rate, but the aortic baroreceptors have a stronger effect on vasomotor nerve activity. What, then, are the reflexes elicited by baroreceptors?

16.2 The baroreflex

The baroreflex adjusts the cardiac output and peripheral vascular tone to stabilize the arterial blood pressure. The reflex response to an acute rise in arterial blood pressure is described first, then the medically important response to a fall in pressure, such as occurs during hypovolaemia.

Acute pressure elevation triggers a depressor reflex

In 1886 Ludwig and Cyon noted that electrical stimulation of the aortic nerve causes a reflex fall in heart rate and blood pressure – the depressor reflex. Hering discovered later that stimulation of the carotid sinus nerve elicits the same reflex (Figure 16.5). In normal life, an acute rise in arterial pressure increases the baroreceptor traffic, which is conveyed by the vagi and glossopharyngeal nerves to the brainstem, where it activates polysynaptic central pathways. These **enhance the vagal parasympathetic output** to the heart and **inhibits the sympathetic output** to the heart and systemic vasculature (Figure 16.6), with the following effects.

- A fall in sympathetic vasomotor activity causes **peripheral vasodilatation**, which **reduces total peripheral resistance**. Human sympathetic

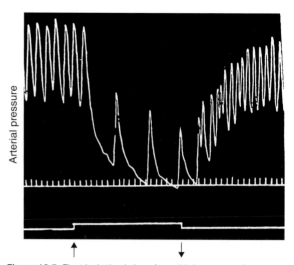

Figure 16.5 Electrical stimulation of carotid sinus nerve of dog elicits reflex hypotension and bradycardia. This is the classic smoked-drum record of Hering, who discovered the carotid baroreflex in 1923. Time intervals 0.2 s. (From Hering. *Die Karotissinusreflexe auf Herz und Gefässe*. Dresden: T. Steinkopf, 1927.)

Figure 16.6 Effect of raising arterial pressure (*bottom trace*) in the artificially perfused carotid arteries and aorta of a rat. Cardiac vagal activity increased, cardiac sympathetic fibre activity decreased and heart rate slowed. Peripheral sympathetic vasoconstrictor activity decreased (sympathetic chain, level T12). (Adapted from Simms AE, Paton JFR, Pickering AE. *Journal of Physiology* 2007; **579**: 473–86, with permission from Wiley-Blackwell.)

vasomotor activity ceases entirely if blood pressure is raised rapidly to >150/90 mmHg.
- A fall in cardiac sympathetic activity and rise in vagal parasympathetic activity cause **bradycardia** and **reduced myocardial contractility**, which together reduce the cardiac output.

Since mean blood pressure equals cardiac output × peripheral resistance, the above changes return the raised arterial pressure towards normal (Figure 16.1). The baroreflex is thus a buffer against acute changes in blood pressure. The buffering process is rapid; the latency between baroreceptor stimulation and the onset of bradycardia is only 0.5 s, and the latency for vascular dilatation is ~1.5 s.

Knowledge of the carotid sinus reflex can occasionally be put to practical use in patients experiencing a supraventricular tachycardia. **Massage of the carotid sinus** region, which is located just below the angle of the jaw, stimulates the baroreceptors. The resulting reflex increase in parasympathetic drive to the heart can sometimes halt the tachycardia.

Hypovolaemia triggers multiple compensatory reflexes

Acute hypovolaemia is a fall in blood volume, a common cause of which is a serious haemorrhage (Section 18.2). Since this is a common emergency in nature, the reflex responses are important for survival, both clinically and in evolutionary terms. Hypovolaemia reduces the cardiac stroke volume and arterial pulse pressure, and in severe cases it also reduces mean arterial blood pressure. The fall in baroreceptor traffic triggers the following reflex responses.

- Increased cardiac sympathetic activity and reduced vagal parasympathetic activity cause a **tachycardia** and **increased myocardial contractility**. These changes help restore the depressed cardiac output.
- Increased sympathetic vasomotor activity causes **vasoconstriction of peripheral resistance vessels**. The resulting rise in total peripheral resistance helps to maintain the mean arterial pressure. In humans the splanchnic circulation, kidneys and forearm muscles participate strongly in the carotid sinus reflex, the skin to a lesser degree.
- Increased sympathetic vasomotor activity also causes **splanchnic venoconstriction**, which displaces blood from the gut and liver into the central veins (Figures 14.5 and 14.13). Blood is also displaced from the poorly innervated skeletal muscle veins, because arteriolar contraction reduces local venous pressure (Figure 14.4) and because circulating adrenaline, vasopressin and angiotensin cause widespread venoconstriction. The displaced venous blood helps to restore the **central venous pressure** and hence stroke volume (Starling's law).
- Increased sympathetic splanchnic nerve activity stimulates **adrenaline secretion** by the adrenal medulla. Adrenaline stimulates the heart and enhances glycogenolysis.

- The sympathetic-induced contraction of pre-capillary resistance vessels reduces the capillary pressure. This initiates a gradual **osmotic absorption of interstitial fluid**, which partially restores the depleted plasma volume (Figures 11.4 and 11.11b).
- Increased renal sympathetic activity activates the **renin–angiotensin–aldosterone system** (Figure 14.12). The circulating angiotensin II contributes to the generalized vasoconstriction. The aldosterone promotes renal salt and water retention, which helps correct the hypovolaemia in the long term.
- Baroreceptor unloading (fall in activity) in primates evokes a reflex rise in **vasopressin (ADH) secretion** from the posterior pituitary gland (Figure 14.11). Vasopressin causes an antidiuresis and adds to the peripheral vasoconstriction.

The baroreflex evoked by acute hypovolaemia thus stimulates the heart, raises peripheral resistance, attenuates the fall in central venous pressure, partially restores plasma volume and promotes renal fluid retention (Section 18.2). Together these responses support the arterial blood pressure and cerebral perfusion. It is estimated that the rise in peripheral resistance accounts for about three-quarters of the initial blood pressure recovery.

The baroreflex 'gain' and 'setting' can be changed

In animal studies the operating characteristics of the baroreflex can be assessed by measuring the changes in heart rate and systemic blood pressure when a vascularly isolated baroreceptor region is distended (Figure 16.4c). In humans the baroreflex is assessed by measuring the change in heart rate when arterial blood pressure is raised by intravenous phenylephrine, a vasoconstrictor drug; or by measuring both arterial pressure and heart rate when the carotid sinus is distended by external suction. Using these techniques, a stimulus–response curve can be plotted to determine the gain and setting of the baroreflex (Figure 16.7). '**Gain**' (**sensitivity**) is the maximum slope of the response curve. Gain is reduced by ageing and chronic hypertension, because the distensibility of the artery wall declines. **Set point** is the pressure that the reflex strives to maintain. This can be altered by neural interactions in the central nervous system (central resetting) or by physical changes around the receptor (peripheral resetting), as follows.

Figure 16.7 Resetting of human baroreflex during cycling (red line). Carotid sinus was distended by a suction collar around the neck to evaluate the reflex. 'X' shows increase in set point during exercise; sensitivity (slope) was unchanged. After partial neuromuscular blockade by curare, a greater central command was needed to achieve the same level of exercise, and this reset the curve further. This shows that central command contributes to exercise resetting. (Based on Gallagher KM, Fadel, PJ, Strømstad M *et al. Journal of Physiology* 2001; **533**: 861–70, with permission from Wiley-Blackwell.)

Central resetting

During **exercise**, impulses from the higher regions of the brain (central command), and from afferents in the active muscle, reset the baroreflex to operate around a higher pressure (Figure 16.7, middle curve). If the muscle afferent input is blocked by epidural anaesthesia, quadriceps exercise induced by electrical stimulation (no central command) no longer resets the baroreflex. The degree of resetting is proportional to the work intensity. This allows arterial pressure to rise without evoking a reflex inhibition of heart rate. The baroreflex is nevertheless active throughout the exercise period, striving to maintain the blood pressure at its new set point.

A different form of central modulation occurs with every breath and accounts for **sinus arrhythmia**, the tachycardia associated with each inspiration in humans (Figure 5.4a). The brainstem neurons that drive inspiration also inhibit the cardiac vagal motor neurons, rendering them briefly unresponsive to the baroreceptor input (Figure 16.17). The resulting fall in vagal activity causes a tachycardia during each inspiration.

Peripheral resetting

If blood pressure is raised for a substantial period, the baroreceptor threshold shifts to a new, higher pressure over hours and days. This causes a right-ward shift of the stimulus–response curve and reinstates the receptors on a steep part of the stimulus–response curve, where they operate most effectively – though the resetting is not perfect. Peripheral resetting has the advantage of **extending the range** over which the reflex can operate effectively. Its **disadvantage** is that the baroreceptors cannot inform the brain reliably about absolute blood pressure over extended periods; after peripheral resetting a high pressure may produce little more baroreceptor traffic than an earlier lower pressure.

The ambiguity of baroreceptor information over extended periods is exacerbated by sympathetic fibres that innervate the carotid sinus and enhance its baroreceptor activity. Because the baroreceptors fail to provide unambiguous information about absolute blood pressure, it is thought that they are not sufficient, unaided, to control blood pressure in the long term. The major role of arterial baroreceptors appears to be the short-term stabilization of blood pressure over seconds–minutes.

The baroreflex provides short-term homeostasis of blood pressure

When an experimental animal is deprived of its baroreceptor input, its arterial pressure becomes very unstable from minute to minute. For example, in a normal dog walking up a 21-degree incline, the blood pressure rises by only ~10 mmHg; but when the dog is deprived of the baroreflex, the same exercise raises the blood pressure by 50 mmHg (Figure 16.8). The major role of the baroreflex is thus to buffer short-term fluctuations in arterial pressure.

When the baroreceptor nerves of a dog are first cut, the animal becomes very hypertensive for the first few days, but the time-averaged blood pressure then settles down to a level only ~11 mmHg above normal – albeit with fluctuations around the mean over a wider range than normal (Figure 16.9a). The fact that the average blood pressure settles down to a near-normal level indicates that additional factors help regulate blood pressure in the long term. Nevertheless, the small rise in time-averaged pressure indicates that arterial baroreceptors do make some long-term contribution to blood pressure regulation, despite partial resetting.

16.3 Receptors in the heart and pulmonary arteries

The heart and pulmonary artery are richly innervated by afferent fibres, ~80% of which are small-diameter, unmyelinated fibres (Figure 16.10).

Figure 16.8 A dog walking up an increasingly steep slope normally experiences only a small rise in arterial pressure (mean increase 12 mmHg). After elimination of the carotid sinus and aortic arch reflexes, exercise caused much bigger increases in pressure (mean 51 mmHg). (Data from Walgenbach SC, Donald DE. *Circulation Research* 1983; **52**: 253–62.)

Figure 16.9 Contribution of baroreceptors to arterial pressure level and stability. (a) In normal dog, range of arterial pressure over time was narrow (control). A few days after chronic arterial baroreceptor denervation, mean pressure was only moderately raised, but the fluctuations about the mean increased markedly, i.e. pressure was less stable. (b) After denervation of the cardiopulmonary receptors (CP) as well as arterial baroreceptors, there was a marked rise in mean pressure, as well as pressure instability. ((a) From Cowley AW, Liard JF, Guyton AC. *Circulation Research* 1973; **32**: 564–78; (b) Persson PB, Ehmke H, Kirchheim HR. *News in Physiological Sciences* 1989; **4**: 56–9, by permission.)

The cardiopulmonary afferents fall into four main categories:

1 **Ventricular chemosensors** mediate cardiac pain and make up most of the non-myelinated afferents. They travel in the cardiac sympathetic nerves and vagi, which are 'mixed nerves', i.e. they carry both motor and sensory fibres.

2 **Myelinated veno-atrial mechanoreceptors** are mechanoreceptors distributed around the right and left veno-atrial junctions, served by myelinated vagal afferent fibres. They signal central blood volume.

3 **Non-myelinated cardiac mechanoreceptors** are mechanoreceptors in the ventricles, atria and pulmonary artery served by non-myelinated fibres. They travel in both the vagus and the cardiac sympathetic nerves.

4 **Coronary artery baroreceptors** function much like other arterial baroreceptors and travel in the vagi. Their reflex potency is several times greater than that of left ventricular mechanoreceptors.

Cardiac de-afferentation studies show that the cardiopulmonary afferents have a net tonic inhibitory effect on heart rate and peripheral vascular tone, similar to arterial baroreceptors. Thus the non-selective stimulation of the cardiac receptors by intracoronary injections of veratridine causes a reflex bradycardia, vasodilatation and hypotension (Bezold–Jarisch response). This kind of mass,

Figure 16.10 Distribution of cardiopulmonary afferent endings. Squares, myelinated veno-atrial stretch receptors; circles, unmyelinated mechanoreceptors; stars, arterial baroreceptors; triangles, nociceptive chemosensors; RA and LA, right and left atria, respectively; PA, pulmonary artery. Recordings of veno-atrial receptor activity in dogs shown on left. (Based on Kappagoda CT, Linden RJ, Sivananthan N. *Journal of Physiology* 1979; **291**: 393–412, with permission from Wiley-Blackwell.)

unphysiological stimulation, however, obscures the fact that the different receptors can elicit different reflexes.

Ventricular chemosensitive fibres mediate ischaemic heart pain

Most unmyelinated, left ventricular fibre endings are chemosensitive. They can be activated by adenosine, bradykinin, prostaglandins, histamine, 5-hydroxytryptamine, platelet-released thromboxane, lactic acid, K^+ ions and reactive oxygen species. These are substances released by ischaemic myocytes. The axons, mainly C-fibres and some Aδ fibres, travel in the cardiac sympathetic nerves and vagi. The chemosensitive sympathetic fibres are known to mediate the pain of angina and heart attacks, since surgical interruption of the pathway relieves chronic ischaemic cardiac pain in >80% of cases. The sympathetic afferents ascend the spinal cord in the cervical spinothalamic tract, where there is **convergence** with somatic afferents – that is to say, a neuron receives inputs from both the cardiac nociceptors and somatic afferents. This is probably why cardiac pain seems to emanate from the chest wall, shoulders and arms (**referred pain**). The excitatory reflex effect is an **increase in sympathetic activity** (which is pro-arrhythmogenic), tachycardia and a rise in blood pressure.

Myelinated veno-atrial stretch receptors monitor atrial filling

Veno-atrial fibres are normally the most active of the non-coronary afferents in animals; human data are lacking. The receptors are branched, endocardial sprays, resembling arterial baroreceptors, served by large, myelinated vagal afferent fibres. Activity is pulsatile, coinciding with atrial systole (A wave, type A pattern) or atrial filling (V wave, type B pattern) (Figure 16.10). An increase in **cardiac blood volume** stretches the veno-atrial receptors and increases the discharge frequency. Veno-atrial receptors thus transmit information about central venous pressure and cardiac filling. When stimulated experimentally, by inflating a small balloon at the veno-atrial junction, two reflexes are elicited, namely tachycardia and diuresis (increased urine production).

The **tachycardia** is mediated, unusually, by a selective increase in sympathetic drive to the pacemaker with no fall in vagal parasympathetic activity. The tachycardia shifts blood from the congested venous system into the arterial system. The '**Bainbridge effect**', discovered in 1915, is a tachycardia induced by the rapid infusion of a large volume of saline into the venous system. The response is mediated partly by the veno-atrial stretch receptors and partly by pacemaker distension.

The **diuresis** and natriuresis (increased salt excretion) establish a negative feedback loop that helps to regulate the plasma volume and hence atrial distension. The diuresis is brought about partly by a fall in sympathetic nerve activity specifically to the kidneys (not other tissues), causing renal vasodilatation; and partly by changes in the circulating levels of vasopressin (anti-diuretic hormone), angiotensin, aldosterone and atrial natriuretic peptide.

Unmyelinated cardiac mechanoreceptors signal over-distension

A minority of small-diameter, unmyelinated cardiac fibres are mechanoreceptors, located in the left ventricle and atria. The activity of the unmyelinated left ventricular mechanoreceptors is weak unless the heart is distended. Similarly, unmyelinated atrial mechanoreceptors fire only when atrial filling is at its highest, e.g. during the V wave of inspiration. Like the baroreceptors, the unmyelinated cardiac mechanoreceptors elicit a depressor reflex, i.e. bradycardia and peripheral vasodilatation. In laboratory animals, the reflex is weak and probably of little importance, but the situation may be different in humans, as described next.

16.4 Reflexes from cardiac receptors in humans

Most of our knowledge of cardiac mechanoreceptors and reflexes comes of necessity from laboratory animals. In humans, cardiac transplantation involves some afferent denervation, and reflex studies in these patients indicate that humans too possesses **central volume receptors** (atrial stretch receptors and left ventricular mechanoreceptors).

Cardiac volume receptors reflexly regulate peripheral vascular tone in humans

Raising the legs above heart level increases intrathoracic venous pressure and central blood volume, with little rise in arterial pressure. This elicits a graded reflex vasodilatation in the skin and skeletal muscle (Figure 16.11). Conversely, if central blood volume is reduced by applying suction to the lower body in a sealed container, there is reflex vasoconstriction in the muscle and splanchnic circulations, a rise in circulating noradrenaline and stimulation of the renin–angiotensin–aldosterone system (RAAS). This occurs even when the lower body negative pressure is so mild that arterial pressure does not

Figure 16.11 Reflex vasodilatation in human forearm muscle evoked by a rise in intrathoracic blood volume. (a) Intrathoracic blood volume increased by raising legs. (b) Legs raised but pneumatic cuff around thigh at 180 mmHg prevented translocation of blood into thorax; no change in forearm perfusion. (c) Legs and lower trunk elevated, to raise central venous pressure further (*inset*). This increased the reflex vasodilatation. (d) Pneumatic cuff around neck inflated to 30 mmHg to reduce carotid sinus distension; very little reflex change in forearm blood flow. (From Roddie IC, Shepherd JT, Whelan RF. *Journal of Physiology* 1957; **139**: 369, with permission from Wiley-Blackwell.)

change detectably, thus excluding the baroreflex. Moreover, the reflex is greatly attenuated in **cardiac transplant patients with denervated ventricles**, indicating that human left ventricular mechanoreceptors may be important in the reflex regulation of peripheral vascular tone (cf. minor role in laboratory animals).

Cardiac and arterial receptors reflexly influence the renal regulation of extracellular fluid volume

Plasma is the only component of extracellular fluid whose volume and pressure are sensed, and the cardiovascular sensors initiate reflexes to maintain a normal extracellular fluid volume. The cardiopulmonary stretch receptors and arterial baroreceptors can be stimulated experimentally by immersing a human feet-down in water; the water pressure displaces ~700 ml blood into the thorax (Figure 8.24), which distends the heart by ~180 ml in diastole and raises arterial blood pressure by ~10 mmHg. These stimuli elicit a substantial diuresis, which helps reduce the raised filling pressures and arterial pressure. The diuresis is mediated by **renal vasodilatation** (selective inhibition of renal sympathetic activity), reduced **vasopressin**, reduced **RAAS** activation and increased **atrial natriuretic peptide**. Similarly, astronauts subjected to zero gravity experience a redistribution of venous blood from legs to thorax, provoking a reflex diuresis. When the astronaut returns to earth, the reduced plasma volume, coupled with a weakened baroreflex, causes orthostatic intolerance (postural hypotension). It is clear from these examples that cardiovascular receptors influence renal fluid excretion, so as to maintain a normal cardiac filling pressure and arterial pressure. This link is important for the long-term regulation of blood pressure, as described next.

16.5 Long-term regulation of arterial blood pressure: the kidney link

As indicated earlier, the arterial baroreflex is primarily a short-term buffer of arterial blood pressure, effective over seconds–minutes. The preservation of a normal, time-averaged blood pressure over longer periods – days and weeks – also requires the maintenance of a normal blood volume, because blood volume influences cardiac filling pressure and output (Starling's law), and hence arterial blood pressure (eqn 8.5). Blood comprises mainly red cells and plasma, both of which are influenced by the kidneys. Consequently, **the kidneys are crucial to long-term blood pressure regulation**. For example, when renal function is manipulated in a dog so as to raise the extracellular salt mass, the plasma volume and time-averaged arterial blood pressure likewise increase (Figure 16.12).

To regulate **red cell mass**, the kidneys secrete a haemopoietic hormone, **haemopoietin**. To regulate **plasma volume**, the kidneys adjust the rate of **excretion of salt**, via RAAS (Figure 14.12). Extracellular water mass closely matches extracellular sodium mass (Figure 16.12a), because the osmoreceptor–vasopressin system preserves isotonicity (Figure 14.11). Plasma is, of course, part of the extracellular fluid compartment. In **Addison's disease**, where adrenal failure reduces the concentration of circulating aldosterone, sodium loss results in a reduced extracellular fluid volume, leading to life-threatening hypotension.

Through what mechanisms is the kidney informed of the state of the circulation? The mechanisms fall into two classes. (1) Cardiac stretch receptors and arterial baroreceptors monitor central blood volume and arterial blood pressure, and reflexly regulate the secretion of **hormones** controlling renal function. (2) Arterial pressure also

Figure 16.12 Effect of changes in renal retention of salt and water on long-term arterial blood pressure (mean over 24 h), in dogs. Renal perfusion pressure was altered experimentally, independently of upper aortic blood pressure, to evoke changes in circulating renin–angiotensin–aldosterone, and hence in salt and water retention. (*Upper panel*) Water retention was closely coupled to salt retention (mainly Na^+, some K^+). (*Lower panel*) The rise in arterial blood pressure was closely coupled to the rise in body water, presumably via the Frank–Starling mechanism. (Data redrawn from Seeliger, Wronski, Ladwig *et al. Clinical and Experimental Pharmacology and Physiology* 2005; **32**: 394–9, with permission from Wiley-Blackwell.)

affects renal excretion directly, by a process termed **pressure natriuresis**.

Cardiovascular pressure receptors reflexly regulate hormones that act on the nephron

The circulating levels of all the hormones controlling renal salt and water excretion are influenced by cardiovascular receptors, as follows.

The **renin–angiotensin–aldosterone system**, which promotes salt and water retention, is inhibited by a rise in arterial pressure, partly through renal afferent arteriole sensors and partly through a baroreflex-mediated fall in renal sympathetic activity (Figure 14.12). RAAS inhibition results in natriuresis and diuresis, which reduces extracellular fluid volume and returns the raised blood pressure to normal. Conversely, if blood pressure falls, RAAS activation promotes salt and water retention, leading to the restoration of the depressed blood pressure.

Antidiuretic hormone (ADH, vasopressin), which promotes water retention, is secreted when plasma osmolarity rises (Figure 14.11). This ensures that water excretion matches sodium excretion, keeping the plasma isotonic. ADH secretion is also stimulated by a fall in central blood volume and arterial pressure, via reduced arterial baroreceptor traffic in primates, or reduced veno–atrial receptor traffic in other species. The resulting fluid retention helps restore the reduced extracellular fluid volume and blood pressure to normal.

Atrial natriuretic peptide, which promotes salt excretion and diuresis, is released in response to atrial distension. This links renal function directly to central blood volume. The effect of ANP at physiological concentrations, however, is weak (Section 14.9).

Pressure natriuresis; a rise in renal arterial pressure directly increases salt and water excretion

Pressure natriuresis is an increase in renal salt and water excretion in response to a rise in renal arterial pressure. A rise in renal arterial pressure has little effect on glomerular capillary pressure or filtration rate, because these parameters are subject to excellent autoregulation. The proposed mechanism is, therefore, that the pressure rises in the renal medullary capillaries, which are thought to be less well autoregulated. A rise in medullary capillary pressure increases the renal interstitial fluid pressure, which impairs the reabsorption of tubular fluid. Thus a diuresis and natriuresis follows. There is controversy over the importance of pressure natriuresis relative to the powerful RAAS.

Cardiac and arterial receptors together underpin long-term pressure homeostasis

To summarize, **cardiac mechanoreceptors** and **arterial baroreceptors** regulate the levels of circulating angiotensin, aldosterone, vasopressin and atrial natriuretic peptide, which in turn regulate renal salt and water excretion, and hence plasma volume. Thus the cardiovascular receptors and their central pathways, aided by renal pressure natriuresis, are important for the long-term regulation of mean blood pressure. If the input from one group of receptors alone is interrupted, blood pressure rises only a little in the long term (Figure 16.9a). This is fortunate for patients with transplanted hearts, who lose their ventricular mechanoreceptor input but have little problem regulating their blood pressure. Evidently one group of receptors can largely compensate for lack of the other group. (This illustrates the Comroe principle – if a job is

Regulation of arterial blood pressure

- Mean arterial pressure is determined by total peripheral resistance and cardiac output. The arterial baroreflex adjusts both determinants, to stabilize the arterial pressure over seconds–minutes.
- A rise in arterial pressure stimulates the arterial baroreceptors. This evokes a reflex fall in sympathetic outflow and rise in cardiac vagal parasympathetic outflow. The ensuing peripheral vasodilatation and bradycardia lower the raised arterial pressure, returning it to its set point (depressor reflex).
- Conversely, hypovolaemia unloads the baroreceptors, leading to a reflex rise in sympathetic outflow, which helps maintain blood pressure.
- The set point of the baroreflex can be raised by central command and muscle afferents (metaboreceptors). This raises blood pressure during exercise.
- In the longer term, blood pressure homeostasis depends on the renal regulation of extracellular fluid volume. Renal excretion is enslaved to blood pressure through two kinds of mechanism. (a) The circulating level of excretion-regulating hormones (vasopressin, angiotensin II, aldosterone, atrial natriuretic peptide) is controlled by cardiovascular receptors. (b) Pressure natriuresis causes an increase in salt and water excretion when renal artery pressure rises.

CONCEPT BOX 1.1

worth doing, the body has more than one way of doing it!) If both the cardiac and arterial receptors are denervated, there is a sustained elevation of renin–angiotensin–aldosterone levels and sustained hypertension (Figure 16.9b).

16.6 Excitatory inputs: muscle work receptors, arterial chemoreceptors, lung stretch receptors

As well as depressor reflexes to stabilize the arterial blood pressure, there are excitatory reflexes that help stimulate the cardiovascular system during challenges such as exercise and hypoxia. Excitatory reflexes raise the blood pressure (pressor reflexes) and are initiated by several classes of sensory receptor:

- muscle work receptors (metaboreceptors and mechanoreceptors)
- arterial chemoreceptors
- lung stretch receptors
- the external senses.

Work receptors in skeletal muscle help drive the exercise pressor response and tachycardia

During exercise the arterial blood pressure rises (the exercise pressor response) and the heart rate increases. These changes are driven partly by 'central command' from the cerebral cortex, and partly by a reflex from work-activated receptors in skeletal muscle – that is to say, nerve endings activated by muscle contraction (excluding muscle spindles, which do not contribute to cardiovascular control). There are two types of work receptor, the mechanoreceptor and the chemosensitive metaboreceptor.

Muscle mechanoreceptors are stimulated by local pressure and muscle contraction, and are served mainly by small, myelinated axons (group III). They chiefly influence heart rate. The reflex effect is to **inhibit cardiac vagal tone**, which helps increase heart rate quickly in the first few seconds of exercise, complementing the central command (Figure 16.13).

Muscle metaboreceptors are chemosensitive endings of unmyelinated group IV axons (mainly). They reflexly **increase sympathetic vasomotor activity** and thus contribute to the exercise pressor response. They also boost cardiac contractility at high levels of activation. The human muscle metaboreflex was demonstrated in a simple, ingenious experiment by Alam and Smirk, in 1937 (Figure 16.14). The subject performed forearm exercise and, just before the end of the exercise, a pneumatic cuff was inflated around the upper arm, to trap local chemical stimulants in the forearm. The exercise pressor response (though not the tachycardia) was then partly maintained after the active exercise finished, and only subsided fully when the cuff was released.

Metaboreceptors are activated by numerous chemicals released by contracting muscle fibres (ATP, K^+, $H_2PO_4^-$, prostaglandin PGE_2, bradykinin, 20-HETE and, to a lesser degree, adenosine and lactic acid acting on acid-sensing ion channels, ASIC). These agents accumulate to higher levels during **isometric (static) exercise** than dynamic exercise, because an isometric contraction restricts local blood flow (Section 15.2). Consequently, the metaboreceptors act as **sensors of under-perfusion**, i.e. they sense a mismatch between O_2 supply and demand, and they cause blood pressure to rise much higher during isometric exercise than during dynamic exercise (Figure 17.6). The reflex, sympathetic-mediated peripheral vasoconstriction raises arterial blood pressure without impeding flow in the active muscle itself, because metabolic vasodilatation

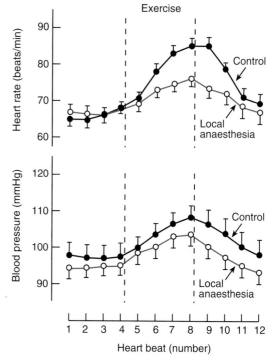

Figure 16.13 Evidence that a reflex from muscle work receptors (mechanoreceptors and metaboreceptors) contributes to exercise tachycardia and the exercise pressor response in humans. The response to 4 s of maximal voluntary handgrip was attenuated when muscle afferent traffic was blocked by local anaesthesia of the axillary and radial nerves, leaving motor function unimpaired. Note the rapidity with which the heart responds at the onset of exercise. (From Lassen A, Mitchell JH, Reeves DR, Rogers HB, Secher J. *Journal of Physiology* 1989; **409**: 333–41, with permission from Wiley-Blackwell.)

Figure 16.14 Evidence that human muscle metaboreceptors contribute to the exercise pressor response. Isometric handgrip raises blood pressure. If blood is then trapped in the exercised arm by inflating a brachial cuff to supra-systolic pressure, the exercise pressor response is partly maintained, until the cuff is released. (Data from Rusch NJ, Shepherd JT, Webb RC, Vanhoutte PM. *Circulation Research* 1981; **48** (Suppl. 1): 118–25, by permission.)

predominates locally (Section 15.2). The rise in arterial pressure is particularly advantageous in isometric exercise, because it helps counteract the maintained compression of the intramuscular blood vessel by contracted muscle. In this way, the pressor reflex can maintain muscle perfusion at isometric contractions up to 50% of maximum voluntary contraction. More forceful contractions, however, impede the local perfusion.

In human studies both metaboreceptors and mechanoreceptors can be blocked by a local anaesthetic, while preserving motor axon function. This markedly reduces both the exercise pressor response and the tachycardia, but does not abolish them completely (Figure 16.13). The exercise pressor response is exaggerating heart failure and chronic hypertension.

The arterial chemoreflex supports blood pressure during asphyxia and clinical shock

Arterial chemoreceptors monitor respiratory gas levels, being stimulated by arterial hypoxaemia (low P_{O_2}), hypercapnia (high P_{CO_2}), acidosis and hyperkalaemia. They are located mainly in the **carotid bodies** (not the carotid sinus) and the **aortic bodies** – small, highly vascularized nodules adjacent to the carotid sinus and aorta (Figure 16.2). The carotid bodies have such an extremely high blood flow, $\sim 20\,ml\,g^{-1}\,min^{-1}$, that the venous blood has near-arterial gas levels. The aortic bodies have a somewhat lower blood flow and their chemoreceptors can be stimulated by hypotension and anaemia, as well as blood chemistry changes. The chemoreceptor afferent fibres travel in the IXth and Xth cranial nerves (glossopharyngeal and vagus), along with the baroreceptor afferents.

The arterial chemoreceptors normally regulate alveolar ventilation, but they also drive important circulatory reflexes during **asphyxia** (hypoxia plus hypercapnia) and **clinical shock**. The arterial chemoreflex elicits the following cardiovascular changes.

- **Peripheral resistance increases**, due to a reflex increase in peripheral sympathetic vasomotor drive to skeletal muscle, renal and splanchnic vascular beds.
- **Splanchnic veins constrict**, due to a reflex increase in sympathetic activity. This helps support central venous pressure and hence stroke volume.
- **Blood pressure rises**, due to the above two effects.
- **Tachycardia** is an indirect consequence of the increased breathing. If the chemoreceptors are stimulated during artificial ventilation at a fixed rate, the chemoreflex actually elicits a moderate **bradycardia**. When a subject breathes spontaneously, however, the chemoreflex stimulates deeper, more rapid breathing, and this stimulates stretch receptors within the lungs. These evoke a **lung inflation reflex** (see below), which causes a marked tachycardia, overriding the moderate chemoreflex bradycardia.

The cardiovascular effects of the arterial chemoreflex are particularly important in the following situations.

1. **Asphyxia** (concomitant hypoxaemia and hypercapnia) stimulates arterial chemoreceptors very strongly, causing a reflex rise in sympathetic activity and blood pressure. The latter, along with the hypercapnic vasodilatation of the cerebral circulation, raises cerebral perfusion and hence O_2 delivery (Figure 15.13). In **obstructive sleep apnoea**, repeated episodes of airway blockage trigger chemoreflex-mediated episodes of nocturnal hypertension.

2. **Clinical shock** is a syndrome (group of signs and symptoms, Section 18.2) resulting from hypovolaemia (e.g. severe haemorrhage), hypotension and circulatory failure. Carotid and aortic body perfusion falls during clinical shock, with particularly marked effects on the less vascular aortic bodies. The chemoreceptors are excited by the resulting 'stagnant hypoxia', and by the arterial metabolic acidosis of clinical shock (Figure 18.3). The chemoreflex drives the **rapid breathing** of patients in hypotensive shock, and raises sympathetic vasomotor activity to increase **peripheral resistance** and support arterial blood pressure. This is particularly **important when blood pressure falls below the operating range of the baroreflex**. Most baroreceptor fibres fall silent below $\sim 70\,mmHg$, whereas arterial chemoreceptor activity continues to increase at pressure below 70 mmHg. The importance of the chemoreflex during severe haemorrhage has been confirmed experimentally in dogs; cutting the chemoreceptor nerves caused a sharp fall in blood pressure and large increase in mortality rate.

3. **The diving reflex.** The important contribution of arterial chemoreceptors to the bradycardia and peripheral vasoconstriction of diving is described in Section 17.6.

Lung stretch receptors cause reflex tachycardia

The lung mechanoreceptors are excited by inspiration. Their afferent fibres inhibit the cardiac vagal

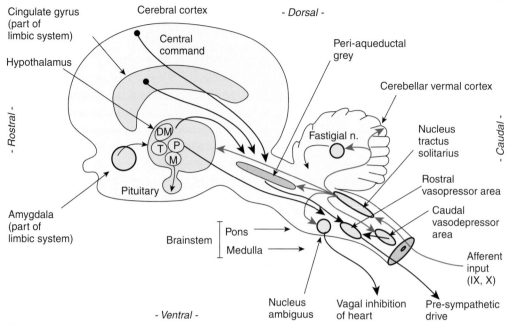

Figure 16.15 Longitudinal pathways mediating cardiovascular regulation in cat brain. DM, dorsomedial nucleus and perifornicular hypothalamus (alerting response); M, magnocellular neurons of supraoptic and paraventricular hypothalamic nuclei (synthesize vasopressin); P, parvocellular neurons of paraventricular nucleus (modulate sympathetic activity); T, temperature-regulating centre, anterior hypothalamus.

parasympathetic neurons in the brainstem and thus cause a reflex tachycardia, for example during **asphyxia**. The lung mechanoreceptor reflex is powerfully reinforced by inspiratory neurons in the brainstem, which likewise inhibit the cardiac vagal neurons. Consequently, each inspiration is associated with both reflex and central inhibition of the cardiac vagal neurons. This causes **sinus arrhythmia**, a regular increase in human heart rate during the inspiration phase of breathing (Figure 5.4a). A sudden, deep inspiration also elicits a reflex vaso- and venoconstriction in human skin, called the **inspiratory gasp reflex** (Figure 14.14) – a convenient reflex for testing human sympathetic function.

External sensory receptors can affect heart rate and blood pressure

Cardiovascular responses are often evoked by receptors not concerned primarily with cardiovascular control. **Somatic pain** causes a tachycardia and hypertension. Severe **visceral pain** causes a bradycardia, hypotension and even fainting. **Ambient cold** causes a rise in blood pressure, which increases left ventricular work and can trigger angina in susceptible patients. The **special senses** too can influence the cardiovascular system. The alerting response, for example to a sudden loud noise or the

sight of a charging bull, produces a brisk tachycardia. Sexual stimulation evokes tachycardia and hypertension (Figure 8.13). Stimulation of facial receptors by cold water elicits a strong bradycardia, (diving reflex, Section 17.6).

16.7 Central pathways: role of the medulla oblongata

In 1854 the celebrated French physiologist, Claude Bernard, reported that transection of the cervical spinal cord causes a peripheral vasodilatation and an abrupt fall in blood pressure to ~40 mmHg. This shows that the normal, tonic activity of the sympathetic vasomotor fibres and their spinal neurons depends on a tonic, net excitatory drive from the brain (Figure 14.1). This pre-sympathetic excitatory drive comes from the medulla oblongata, the most caudal (tail-end) part of the brainstem (Figure 16.15). However, the medulla is by no means the only region involved in cardiovascular regulation; the hypothalamus, limbic system, periaqueductal grey area, cerebellum and cerebral cortex all play a role, though the pathways are as yet incompletely understood.

The traditional notion that the medulla has a dorsal 'vasomotor centre' is no longer tenable. The modern view emphasizes transverse traffic between

Figure 16.16 Schematic transverse section through the medulla, showing reflex pathways and relative positions of cardiovascular nuclei in dorsoventral plane. Dashed lines indicate inhibitory pathways. The various neuron groups occur at different rostrocaudal levels, so in reality they would not all be seen in a single anatomical section.

a number of different regions of the medulla, and up-and-down traffic between the medulla and higher regions, as follows.

Nucleus tractus solitarius receives and integrates all cardiovascular receptor traffic

The dorsomedial region of the medulla contains an elongated grouping of neurons called the **nucleus tractus solitarius** (Figures 16.15 and 16.16). Virtually all the cardiovascular afferents – baroreceptors, cardiopulmonary afferents, muscle mechano- and metaboreceptors, arterial chemoreceptors and pulmonary stretch receptors – terminate in the nucleus tractus solitarius. Consequently, destruction of this nucleus causes a sustained hypertension. Muscle work receptors also project to the lateral reticular nucleus and to the periaqueductal grey matter of the pons (midbrain), which are regions that help organize the exercise pressor response.

The processing of sensory information begins in the nucleus tractus solitarius. An individual neuron receives many different inputs, so its output is influenced by many different signals. This is called **sensory integration**. The integrated information is then **relayed** by nucleus tractus solitarius neurons to other regions, as follows.

Nucleus tractus solitarius relays integrated, afferent information to other regions

The nucleus tractus solitarius relays information to the hypothalamus, cerebellum and other parts of the medulla (Figure 16.15). Within the medulla a polysynaptic path projects to the **nucleus ambiguus**, which contains the vagal cardiac motor neurons. Another path projects to the **caudal vasodepressor area of the medulla**, located in the caudal ventrolateral medulla (CVLM), which influences sympathetic output (Figure 16.16). The **hypothalamus** receive projections to the vasopressin-producing **magnocellular neurons** of the supraoptic and paraventricular nuclei; and to the sympathetic-regulating **parvocellular neurons of the paraventricular nucleus** (Figure 16.15). The **cerebellum** receives projections to the **fastigial nuclei** and **vermal cortex**, which are important during exercise.

Nucleus ambiguus generates tonic vagal parasympathetic outflow to the heart

The cell bodies of the vagal parasympathetic fibres controlling the heart rate are located chiefly in the **nucleus ambiguus** of the brainstem, and to a lesser extent in the dorsal motor nucleus (Figures 16.15 and 16.16). These vagal nuclei used to be known collectively as the 'cardio-inhibitory centre'. Their activity is regulated by inputs from the nucleus tractus solitarius, the inspiratory neurons and the hypothalamus.

Rostral vasopressor area generates a tonic presympathetic outflow to the spinal cord

If the anaesthetic pentobarbitone is applied to the surface of the **rostral ventrolateral medulla (RVLM)**, there is a sharp fall in blood pressure, similar to that produced by cervical cord transection. Conversely, stimulation of this area raises blood pressure. These observations revealed a zone of tonically active vasomotor neurons, the **rostral vasopressor area**. The neurons are glutaminergic (excitatory), and ~70% are also adrenergic (C1 neurons). The vasopressor neurons may be organized organotopically, with some neurons controlling renal sympathetic activity, others controlling the output to the heart, muscle and so on. This allows independent control of the sympathetic activity to different organs. The vasopressor neurons send **bulbospinal fibres** down the dorsolateral funiculus of the spinal cord to synapse with the barosensitive sympathetic preganglionic neurons of the **thoracic spinal cord**, providing a tonic, excitatory drive (Figure 16.16). (Thermosensitive-type spinal sympathetic neurons, by contrast, are regulated from the hypothalamus via the rostroventral medial medulla, RVMM.) The spinal sympathetic neurons also receive a descending inhibitory input from **raphe nuclei** near the brainstem midline. The raphe nuclei receive an excitatory input from the nucleus tractus solitarius.

The tonically active, rostral vasopressor neurons are regulated, indirectly, by the nucleus tractus solitarius. The nucleus tractus solitarius sends an excitatory projection to the **caudal vasodepressor area** in the **caudal ventrolateral medulla (CVLM)**, and the caudal vasodepressor area sends a tonically inhibitory input, mediated by γ-aminobutyric acid (GABA), to the rostral vasopressor area, restraining its output (Figure 16.16).

The blood–brain barrier is absent in the **area postrema** on the floor of the fourth ventricle (dorsal surface of medulla). Here, circulating emetics and **angiotensin II** gain access to area postrema neurons, increasing their activity. Projections from the area postrema to the RVLM boost vasomotor presympathetic outflow. Thus a rise in circulating angiotensin II increases sympathetic vasomotor activity (Figure 14.12).

16.8 Central pathways: role of higher regions

Many central areas of the brain contribute to specific, organized cardiovascular response (Figure 16.15). The central long axis of the brain, the limbic system, the hypothalamus, the cerebellum and the cerebral cortex contribute as follows.

The central long axis organizes the alerting response

'Alerting' is a stereotyped pattern of responses to a sudden, unusual environmental stimulus, such as a sudden noise or danger – a vital response for survival in the wild. The alerting response has a behavioural component (head raised, ears pricked in dog and cats) and a cardiovascular component that prepares the animal for action. The alerting response was described by Cannon in 1929, and is often called the defence or **fear–fight–flight response**; but alerting response seems a better description in humans, since the cardiovascular manifestations can be elicited by quite mild stimuli, such as performing mental arithmetic to the beat of a metronome. The human cardiovascular alerting response is illustrated in Figures 14.7 and 14.14 and comprises:

- **tachycardia** and increased cardiac output;
- **skeletal muscle vasodilatation**;
- sympathetic-mediated **vasoconstriction** of the cutaneous, splanchnic and renal circulations, along with cutaneous venoconstriction;
- **a rise in blood pressure**, accompanied by central inhibition of the baroreflex.

The vasodilatation in skeletal muscle is mediated partly by circulating adrenaline, partly by reduced sympathetic vasoconstrictor activity to the muscle, and in many non-primates by sympathetic cholinergic nerves (Section 14.3).

Brain stimulation experiments show that the alerting response is generated by an extensive system of neurons distributed along the **central long axis** of the brain. The neurons are located in three zones, namely the amygdala, which is part of the **limbic system** (the generator of emotional behaviour patterns); the dorsomedial, perifornical, region of the **hypothalamus**; and the **periaqueductal grey matter** of the pons (Figure 16.15). Electrical

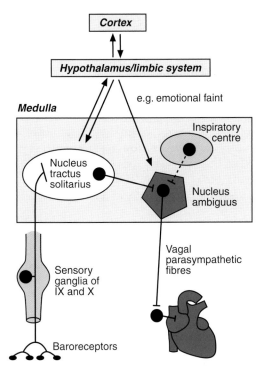

Figure 16.17 Central pathways by which baroreflex regulates vagal parasympathetic drive to heart. Inspiratory inhibition (dashed line) generates sinus arrhythmia. Inputs from muscle work receptors (exercise pressor reflex) and face (diving reflex) not shown. (Based on Spyer KM. *Journal of Physiology* 1994; **474**: 1–19, with permission from Wiley-Blackwell.)

stimulation of the periaqueductal grey matter evokes characteristic cardiac and vasomotor alerting responses and also, in conscious animals, the behavioural manifestations of fear and rage, such as spitting, snarling and piloerection. The central long axis is itself influenced by inputs from the cortex. The output of the central long axis modulates the nucleus tractus solitarius, cardiac vagal motor neurons and rostral vasopressor neurons to produce the characteristic tachycardia and increased blood pressure of the alerting responses.

Hypertensive humans show a greater renal vasoconstriction to a mental stress test than normal subjects, and less habituation to repeated stress. This led to the suggestion that an overdeveloped alerting response may contribute to the development of some forms of clinical hypertension (neurogenic hypertension).

The limbic system also co-ordinates the 'playing dead' response

The opossum, famously, and many other young creatures play dead when faced with danger.

This entails a profound **bradycardia** and **hypotension**, and as such is the opposite of the alerting response. The response originates in the **cingulate gyrus of the limbic system** (Figure 16.15). It is thought that **human emotional fainting** in response to an intolerable psychological stimulus ('swooning') is a manifestation of the same response, namely the avoidance of a threatening situation by collapse.

The hypothalamus influences temperature control, vasopressin secretion, the baroreflex and sympathetic outflow

In addition to the dorsomedial nucleus and adjacent perifornicular region of the hypothalamus (see 'alerting response' above), several other parts of the hypothalamus contribute to cardiovascular regulation, including:

- the temperature-regulating area
- vasopressin-secreting magnocellular neurons and
- sympathetic-regulating parvocellular neurons in the paraventricular nuclei (Figure 16.15).

The **temperature-regulating area** in the anterior hypothalamus receives information from peripheral and core temperature receptors. Its output controls the sympathetic vasodilator and sudomotor outflow to skin (Section 15.3), partly via the RVMM neurons.

The **magnocellular neurons** in the supraoptic and paraventricular nuclei synthesize vasopressin. They have two main inputs: baroreceptor information, transmitted by the nucleus tractus solitarius–CVLM pathway; and osmolarity information transmitted by local osmoreceptors (Figure 14.11). The magnocellular neurons respond with appropriate changes in vasopressin output via the pituitary gland.

The **paraventricular nucleus** contains not only magnocellular neurons but also small, glutaminergic **parvocellular neurons**, which regulate sympathetic activity. Baroreceptor and venoatrial receptor information is relayed to the parvocellular neurons by the nucleus tractus solitarius. The parvocellular neurons project to the RVLM and spinal cord to modulate sympathetic outflow. For example, increased parvocellular neuron activity in heart failure contributes to the excessive renal and cardiac sympathetic activity, which in turn contributes substantially to the pathophysiology. Parvocellular

Figure 16.18 Sympathetic drive to heart and blood vessels (red neurons) and regulatory pathways. Dashed lines denote inhibitory pathways; excitatory arterial chemoreceptors are not shown. CVLM, RVLM, caudal and rostral ventrolateral medulla, containing caudal vasodepressor area and rostral vasopressor areas respectively; IML, intermediolateral horns of thoracic spinal cord with sympathetic preganglionic neurons. PAG, periaqueductal grey matter of pons.

neurons also mediate the selective activation of renal sympathetic fibres by venoatrial volume receptors.

The cerebellum co-ordinates cardiovascular changes during exercise

The main function of the cerebellum is to co-ordinate movement, and it also co-ordinates the cardiovascular changes of exercise. Muscle afferents relay in the lateral reticular nucleus, which projects to the cerebellar fastigial nucleus and the associated vermal cortex, as does the nucleus tractus solitarius (Figure 16.15 and 16.18). Destruction of the fastigial nucleus reduces the tachycardia and the pressor response to exercise in dogs. Stimulation of the vermal cortex in laboratory animals elicits renal vasoconstriction and muscle vasodilatation, the characteristic pattern observed during exercise. Such observations indicate that projections from the cerebellum to the medullary cardiovascular areas help co-ordinate the cardiovascular response to exercise.

The cerebral cortex provides 'central command' during exercise

To explain the rapid onset of the cardiovascular response to exercise, Krogh and Lindhard postulated in 1913 that the cerebral cortex not only initiates muscular exercise, but also initiates cardiovascular responses through 'cortical irradiation' to the brainstem (Figure 16.15). This is now called the central command hypothesis. The hypothesis is supported by the finding that electrical stimulation of several areas of cerebral cortex, including the prefrontal cortex, insular cortex and cingulate cortex, elicits multiple cardiovascular changes. Moreover, if the arm muscles are paralysed by anaesthetizing the motor nerve, voluntary attempts to carry out handgrip exercise cause an immediate rise in heart rate and blood pressure. Recordings in the periaqueductal grey of conscious humans asked to anticipate (but not perform) exercise show potential changes coincident with changes in heart rate and blood pressure. The role of the periaqueductal grey, which also receives muscle work receptor information, may be to integrate feedback from exercising muscle and feedforward from the cortex.

16.9 Overview of central control

Figures 16.17 and 16.18 offer a highly simplified overview of the central, cardiovascular-regulating pathways – those that regulate the vagal outflow to the heart, and those that regulate the sympathetic outflow to the heart and peripheral blood vessels.

Control of the vagal outflow to the heart

Two main pathways link the baroreceptor input to the vagal motor neurons, whose activity restrains the heart rate. One pathway, of short latency, remains within the medulla and passes from the nucleus tractus solitarius to the vagal motor nuclei, possibly via inter-neurons (Figure 16.17). The other, of longer latency, passes from the nucleus tractus solitarius to a hypothalamic depressor area (dorsal anterior hypothalamus) and from there to the vagal motor neurons.

The vagal nuclei also receive an important projection from the inspiratory centre of the brainstem. During **inspiration** the inspiratory neurons elicit hyperpolarization of the vagal cardiac motor neurons. This reduces the vagal neuron responsiveness to the baroreflex during inspiration, a process termed **gating** of the baroreflex. The resulting fall in vagal activity causes a tachycardia synchronous with inspiration, i.e. **sinus arrhythmia**. The inspiratory tachycardia helps to compensate for the fall in left ventricular stroke volume during inspiration, which is itself caused by the expansion of the pulmonary vascular capacity during inspiration.

Control of the sympathetic outflow

The baroreceptor-stimulated output of the nucleus tractus solitarius has a net inhibitory effect on the spinal sympathetic neurons, but the intermediate pathways are more complex and less well understood than the vagal pathway (Figure 16.18). One pathway passes via the hypothalamic paraventricular nuclei. Another projects from the nucleus tractus solitarius to the caudal vasodepressor area, which in turn inhibits the tonically active rostral vasopressor area (Figure 16.19). The net effect is that many rostral vasopressor neurons fall silent during the pulse. The baroreflex thus inhibits the descending excitatory drive from the rostral vasopressor area to the spinal preganglionic sympathetic neurons. The spinal neurons are also inhibited by bulbospinal fibres from the brainstem raphe nuclei, which are activated by the baroreflex.

Figure 16.19 Reflex control of vasopressor presympathetic neurons in rostral ventrolateral medulla (RVLM). (*Left*) Raising blood pressure by i.v. phenylephrine evokes a baroreflex inhibition of RVLM. (*Right*) Stimulation of the caudal vasodepressor area of the caudal ventrolateral medulla (CVLM) by a glutamate injection (excitatory neurotransmitter) inhibits the RVLM, leading to a fall in spinal sympathetic activity and blood pressure. This sequence mimics the baroreflex. (After Blessing WW. *News in Physiological Sciences* 1991; **6**: 139–41, with permission from the American Physiological Society.)

Blood pressure is labile in spinal patients

The activity of spinal, sympathetic, preganglionic neurons is determined chiefly by the descending excitatory and inhibitory bulbospinal fibres, and to a lesser degree by local inputs within the spinal cord. The net descending influence is normally excitatory, so cervical cord transection causes an abrupt hypotension, as demonstrated by Claude Bernard. Sherrington and others pointed out, however, that the **blood pressure gradually recovers following spinal transection**, over the course of several weeks, because local spinal pathways gradually take over the excitation of the sympathetic preganglionic neurons, once brainstem control is removed. Local spinal pathways also mediate a degree of reflex modulation of sympathetic activity in cervical transection patients; for example, a full bladder or somatic pain can cause a reflex rise in blood pressure. Although a spinal patient retains the baroreflex control of the heart rate via the vagus, the patient **lacks the vasomotor component of the baroreflex**. Consequently, they have an excessively labile blood pressure and are prone to postural hypotension during orthostasis – though some vascular compensation is provided by the myogenic constrictor response to dependency (Figures 8.6 and 11.5) and by angiotensin formation when renal artery pressure falls.

SUMMARY

- Heart rate, contractility, vascular tone and blood pressure are regulated by cardiovascular reflexes. The reflex can be **depressor** (pressure-lowering, e.g. baroreflex) or **pressor** (pressure-raising, e.g. arterial chemoreceptors, muscle metaboreceptors). The afferent input from the cardiovascular receptors relays in the brainstem and modifies the autonomic outflow to the heart and vessels.

- **Arterial baroreceptors** in the wall of the carotid sinus and aortic arch are dynamically sensitive stretch receptors that signal pulse pressure and mean pressure. The myelinated, low-threshold A-fibres and nonmyelinated, higher threshold C-fibres travel in the glossopharyngeal and vagal nerves to the medulla. Baroreceptor excitation elicits a depressor reflex comprising bradycardia, reduced contractility and relaxation of resistance vessels and some peripheral veins.

- During **hypovolaemia**, baroreceptor unloading elicits tachycardia, increased contractility, vaso- and venoconstriction, interstitial fluid absorption and renal fluid retention (mediated by renin–angiotensin–aldosterone and vasopressin). These responses help maintain arterial blood pressure.

- The baroreflex is thus a negative feedback loop that **stabilizes blood pressure** over seconds–minutes. '**Resetting**' enables the baroreflex to buffer the pressure around a higher level during exercise (central resetting) or clinical hypertension (peripheral resetting).

- **Cardiac receptors** fall into several classes. **Chemosensitive ventricular afferents** mediate ischaemic heart pain. **Myelinated veno-atrial stretch receptors** monitor atrial distension and evoke reflex tachycardia and diuresis, which reduces the cardiac distension and extracellular fluid volume. **Nonmyelinated mechanoreceptors** in the left ventricle, atria and pulmonary artery elicit a depressor reflex (vasodilatation), which is weak in dogs but may be important in humans.

- In humans, **increases in extracellular fluid volume and hence CVP** lead to increased cardiopulmonary and arterial baroreceptor activity. This elicits a reflex vasodilatation in skin, muscle and kidneys, reduced vasopressin secretion and reduced renin–angiotensin–aldosterone production. Atrial distension also stimulates atrial natriuretic peptide secretion.

- **Long-term homeostasis of arterial pressure** depends on the regulation of extracellular salt and water mass by the kidneys. Renal salt and water excretion is controlled by aldosterone, vasopressin and pressure natriuresis. Aldosterone and vasopressin levels are regulated reflexly by baroreceptor and cardiopulmonary receptors.

- **Muscle metaboreceptors** are group IV chemoreceptors that are excited by chemicals released locally within exercising muscle. Along with group III **muscle mechanoreceptors** they evoke the exercise pressor reflex (vasoconstriction and tachycardia). These 'work receptors' help to drive the cardiovascular response to exercise, especially isometric exercise.

- **Peripheral arterial chemoreceptors** in the carotid and aortic bodies are excited by hypoxia, acidosis, asphyxia, hyperkalaemia and underperfusion. Besides stimulating ventilation, they elicit hypertension through peripheral vasoconstriction. This supports the blood pressure during severe haemorrhage and asphyxiation. A reflex from **lung stretch receptors** elicits a concomitant tachycardia.

- The above afferent inputs relay in the **nucleus tractus solitarius** of the brainstem (medulla). The latter projects to the hypothalamus, cerebellum and other parts of the medulla, which modulate (i) cardiac vagal motor neuron activity in the **nucleus ambiguus**; and (ii) the presympathetic excitatory outflow from the **rostral vasopressor area** of the medulla.

- Higher regions mediate co-ordinated responses. The **central defence axis** elicits the alerting response (tachycardia, muscle vasodilatation, splanchnic, renal and cutaneous vasoconstriction) in preparation for fight or flight. The **hypothalamic temperature-regulating area** controls cutaneous sympathetic outflow. The **cerebral cortex** issues a 'central command' to raise heart rate and blood pressure rapidly at the start of exercise.

Further reading

Reviews and chapters

Andresen MC. Nucleus tractus solitarius – gateway to neural circulatory control. *Annual Reviews of Physiology* 1994; **56**: 93–116.

Biaggioni I. Autonomic/metabolic interactions modulating the exercise pressor reflex; the purinergic hypothesis. *Journal of Physiology* 2007; **578**: 5–6.

Brooks VL, Sved AF. Pressure to change? Re-evaluating the role of baroreceptors in the long-term control of arterial pressure. *American Journal of Physiology* 2005; **288**: R815–818.

De Burgh Daly M. *Peripheral Arterial Chemoreceptors and Respiratory–Cardiovascular Integration.* Oxford: Oxford Medical Publications, Oxford University Press (Monographs of The Physiological Society No. 46), 1997.

Eckberg DL, Fritsch JM. How should human baroreflexes be tested? *News in Physiological Sciences* 1993; **8**: 7–12.

Eckberg DL, Sleight P. *Human Baroreflexes in Health and Disease.* Oxford: Oxford University Press, 1992.

Foreman RD. Mechanisms of cardiac pain. *Annual Review of Physiology* 1999; **61**: 143–67.

Green AL, Paterson DJ. Identifying neurocircuitry controlling cardiovascular function in humans using functional neurosurgery: Implications for exercise control. *Experimental Physiology* 2008; **93**: 1022–8.

Guyenet PG. The sympathetic control of blood pressure. *Nature Reviews Neuroscience* 2006; **7**: 335–46. (Central sympathetic-regulating pathways)

Hainsworth R. Reflexes from the heart. *Physiological Reviews* 1991; **71**: 617–58.

Joyner MJ. Baroreceptor function during exercise; resetting the record. *Experimental Physiology* 2006; **91**: 27–36.

Marshall JM. Peripheral chemoreceptors and cardiovascular regulation. *Physiological Reviews* 1994; **74**: 543–94.

Marshall JM. Cardiovascular changes associated with behavioural alerting. In: Jordan D, Marshall J (eds). *Cardiovascular Regulation.* London: Portland Press, 1995: 37–60.

Smith JA, Mitchell JH, Garry MG. The mammalian exercise pressor reflex in health and disease. *Experimental Physiology* 2006; **91**: 89–102.

Spyer KM. Central nervous system mechanisms contributing to cardiovascular control. *Journal of Physiology* 1994; **474**: 1–19.

Wallin BG, Elam M. Insights from intraneural recordings of sympathetic nerve traffic in humans. *News in Physiological Sciences* 1994; **9**: 203–7.

Williams JL, Barnes KL, Brosnihan KB, Ferrario CM. Area postrema: A unique regulator of cardiovascular function. *News in Physiological Sciences* 1992; **7**: 30–34.

Research papers

See www.hodderplus.com/cardiovascularphysiology for a full list of Research papers for this chapter.

CHAPTER 17

Co-ordinated cardiovascular responses

Learning objectives

Regarding posture:
- Explain how orthostasis reduces cardiac output.
- Describe the compensatory reflexes that prevent postural dizziness.

Regarding the Valsalva manoeuvre:
- Explain how forced expiration affects cardiac output and blood pressure.

Regarding exercise and training:
- Explain how pulmonary O_2 uptake is increased during exercise.
- Explain how stroke volume and heart rate are raised during exercise.
- Outline how solute exchange is boosted between the active muscle and blood.
- Contrast the effects of static and dynamic exercise on blood pressure.
- State the roles of central command and peripheral reflexes during exercise.
- List the cardiovascular changes induced by endurance training.

Regarding feeding:
- State how a meal alters cardiac output, splanchnic and limb blood flow.

Regarding diving:
- List the three key features of the diving response and state the afferents responsible.

Regarding ageing:
- Define arteriosclerosis.
- State how mean, systolic and diastolic arterial pressure changes with ageing.
- Outline the changes in cardiac performance with ageing.

Regarding sleep and alerting:
- Contrast the cardiovascular responses to sleep and alerting (stress).

All the individual components of the circulation have been covered in the preceding chapters. As with a jigsaw puzzle, however, what really matters is how the components fit together to produce a functional whole. The purpose of this chapter is to show how the numerous components of the cardiovascular system respond in a co-ordinated way to the demands of everyday life. One general principle will emerge, the **principle of adaptation by integration**, i.e. each major response is achieved by the integration of several smaller responses. For example, a 13-fold increase in the rate of O_2 absorption by the pulmonary circulation during strenuous exercise is achieved, typically, by the combination of a one and a half-fold rise in stroke volume, a three-fold rise in heart rate and a three-fold increase in the arteriovenous concentration difference for O_2. Many further examples of adaptation by integration will be encountered in these last two chapters.

17.1 Posture (orthostasis)

Orthostasis causes an initial postural hypotension

Orthostasis, the adoption of an upright position, presents a serious challenge to the human circulation, because gravity causes a redistribution of our venous blood. Gravity increases the transmural pressure about ten-fold in the most dependent human veins (Figures 8.2 and 11.5), and the resulting venous distension increases the volume of blood in the lower body by ~500 ml (Figure 8.24). This reduces the intrathoracic blood volume by 20% over ~15 seconds and lowers central venous pressure from 5 to 6 mmHg (supine) to ~0 (upright). The resulting fall in cardiac contractile energy, mediated by the Frank–Starling mechanism (Figure 6.10b), lowers the stroke volume, initially by 30–40% (70 ml to 45 ml). This reduces the pulse pressure and also, prior to compensatory responses, the mean arterial pressure.

Although the mean arterial pressure is normally restored quickly by the baroreflex (see below), the hypotensive episode can be severe enough to impair cerebral perfusion transiently, resulting in dizziness and visual fading for a few seconds. Most healthy individuals will experience this postural giddiness occasionally. It is exacerbated by **warmth** (because the attendant cutaneous venodilatation lowers central venous pressure) and **prolonged bed-rest**. Postural hypotension only progresses to **postural syncope** (fainting) if the baroreflex is impaired, usually by drugs (e.g. α-adrenoceptor blockers) or autonomic neuropathy – or, in the case of returning astronauts, life under zero gravity.

Neuroendocrine reflexes quickly restore mean arterial pressure

The unloading of arterial baroreceptors and cardiopulmonary mechanoreceptors during orthostasis triggers reflexes that quickly restore mean arterial pressure in healthy subjects (Figure 17.1). **Carotid baroreceptor traffic** is reduced by a fall in both pulse pressure and mean sinus pressure. Being situated near the base of the skull, the carotid sinus is elevated 25 cm or so above heart level during orthostasis, reducing the carotid sinus pressure (Figure 8.2). **Cardiopulmonary receptor traffic** is reduced by the fall in cardiac blood volume. The reduced inputs to the nucleus tractus solitarius inform the brain of the gravity of the situation(!) and elicit a reduction in cardiac vagal outflow and increase in sympathetic outflow, with the following effects.

- **Heart rate increases** by 15–20 beats/min (Figure 17.2).
- **Stroke volume** remains depressed, despite a reflex increase in myocardial contractility and splanchnic venoconstriction. Pulse pressure therefore remains low for the duration of the orthostasis (Figure 17.2).
- **Cardiac output falls**, due to the low stroke volume; but the reflex tachycardia limits the fall to ~20%.
- **Peripheral resistance increases** by 30–40%, due to sympathetic-mediated vasoconstriction in the skeletal muscle, splanchnic and renal vascular beds.
- **Mean arterial pressure** is not only restored by the rise in peripheral resistance but is actually **raised** by 10–14 mmHg above the supine value (Figure 17.2).

These responses normally take less than a minute to complete. Over the next half-hour or so the orthostasis-induced rise in capillary filtration pressure in the lower body causes a **12–13% (375 ml) fall in plasma volume** (Section 11.9). This reduces the systolic pressure and elicits additional tachycardia. To compensate for the fall in plasma volume, the **excretion of salt and water is reduced** through sympathetic activation of the renin–angiotensin–aldosterone system and reflex vasopressin secretion.

The net result of the combined neuroendocrine responses is that the arterial blood pressure perfusing the brain is safe-guarded. It seems perverse that, despite all this physiological effort, the cerebral blood flow actually declines by 10–20% during orthostasis. The decline is caused by an increase in cerebral vascular resistance, brought about by multiple factors – reduced arterial P_{CO_2} due to increased ventilation during orthostasis; the gravitational collapse of the jugular veins in the neck; and a slight sympathetic-mediated cerebral vasoconstriction.

Figure 17.1 Reflex sympathetic response to orthostasis in humans. RVLM, rostro-ventro-lateral medulla (site of rostral vasopressor area).

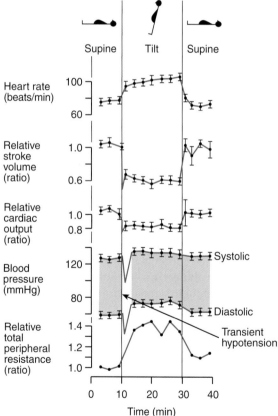

Figure 17.2 Response of young adults to a 20 min head-up tilt. Stroke volume, cardiac output and peripheral resistance are expressed as a fraction of the supine control values. Bars show standard error of mean. (From Smith JJ, Bush JE, Weideier VT, Tristani FE. *Journal of Applied Physiology* 1970; **29**: 133, with permission from the American Physiological Society.)

17.2 Valsalva manoeuvre

Valsalva was a noted eighteenth-century Italian physiologist. The eponymous manoeuvre is not, however, an ancient physiological rite but a natural event performed daily by all of us. It is a forced expiration against a closed or narrowed glottis, and this is a normal accompaniment to defecation, coughing, lifting heavy weights, singing a top A or playing the trumpet. Forced expiration creates a high intrathoracic pressure, which evokes a complex circulatory response with four phases (Figure 17.3).

- **Phase 1**. Arterial blood pressure increases as the thoracic aorta is compressed by the high intrathoracic pressure.
- **Phase 2**. Arterial pulse pressure and mean pressure begin to decline, because the high intrathoracic pressure impedes venous return, reducing stroke volume. Over the next 5–10 s, however, a reflex increase in sympathetic outflow causes **tachycardia** and **peripheral vasoconstriction**, which halts the fall in mean blood pressure (Figure 17.3a).
- **Phase 3**. On terminating the Valsalva manoeuvre, intrathoracic pressure falls to normal and the thoracic aorta is decompressed, so arterial blood pressure falls abruptly.
- **Phase 4**. The pulse pressure and mean pressure quickly increase from their depressed levels,

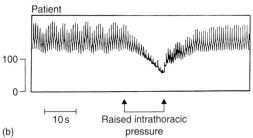

Figure 17.3 Effect of Valsalva manoeuvre on blood pressure and heart rate. (a) Normal subject. (b) Patient with idiopathic orthostatic hypotension, caused by an autonomic neuropathy. Pressure failed to stabilize in phase 2 and no reflex bradycardia in phase 4. SSA and MSA, skin and muscle sympathetic activity respectively. ((a) From Bannister Sir R. In: Sleight P (ed.). *Arterial Blood Pressure and Hypertension.* Oxford: Oxford University Press, 1980: 117–21; and Wallin BG, Elam M. *News in Physiological Sciences* 1994; **9**: 203–7; (b) from Johnson RH, Spalding JMK. *Disorders of the Autonomic Nervous System.* London: Blackwell, 1974, with permission from Wiley-Blackwell.)

because venous blood surges into the thorax as intrathoracic pressure falls to normal. The increased venous return distends the heart, causing an overshoot in the stroke volume, pulse pressure and mean arterial pressure. This in turn stimulates the baroreflex, causing a characteristic, transient **reflex bradycardia**.

The sudden bradycardia during phase 4 of the Valsalva response is used as a **clinical test of baroreflex competence** in humans. If the baroreflex is blocked by a neurological disorder such as autonomic neuropathy, the Valsalva test shows a continuing pressure fall in phase 2 and neither pressure overshoot nor bradycardia in phase 4 (Figure 17.3b). Individuals with such a response are very prone to postural hypotension.

17.3 Exercise

Probably the most important circulatory response for an animal's survival in the wild is the response to physical exercise. Exercise imposes three tasks on the circulation.

- **Pulmonary blood flow** must increase, to boost O_2 uptake and CO_2 removal.
- **Blood flow in active muscles** must increase, to boost O_2 and glucose delivery.
- **Arterial pressure** must be stabilized, despite the huge changes in cardiac output and peripheral vascular resistance occasioned by the above two requirements.

Raised pulmonary blood flow and reduced venous O_2 boost alveolar O_2 uptake

During exercise the O_2 uptake by pulmonary blood ($\dot{V}_{O_2}$) must increase, to satisfy the increased demands of active muscle. This is achieved partly through increased pulmonary blood flow, i.e. cardiac output (CO), and partly through an increase in the amount of O_2 that is added to each litre of pulmonary blood, since:

$$\dot{V}_{O_2} = CO(C_A - C_V)$$

where C_A and C_V are the O_2 contents of arterial and mixed venous blood respectively (**Fick principle**, Section 7.1). The cardiac output of an untrained human can increase about four-fold, from $5\,l/min$ at rest to $20\,l/min$ in heavy exercise. The O_2 uptake per litre of blood, ($C_A - C_V$), can increase around three-fold – not because there is any increase in arterial O_2, but because the mixed venous blood entering the lungs has a reduced O_2 content, due to the increased extraction by active muscle (Figure 17.4). The mixed venous O_2 (C_V) falls from $\sim 145\,ml\,O_2/litre$ at rest to $40\,ml\,O_2/litre$ during heavy exercise. The arterial O_2, $\sim 195\,ml\,O_2/litre$, is unchanged at most exercise intensities.

Substituting the above values into the Fick equation, we see that pulmonary oxygen uptake, $\dot{V}_{O_2}$, increases ~ 13-fold during maximal exercise in an untrained human; the basal level is 0.25 litre O_2/min and the maximum, termed $\dot{V}_{O_2\,max}$, is just over 3 litre O_2/min (Table 17.1). Oxygen uptake is widely used as a measure of work intensity; light work, such as level walking at $3\,km/h$, raises $\dot{V}_{O_2}$ to 0.4–$0.8\,l/min$; moderate work corresponds to

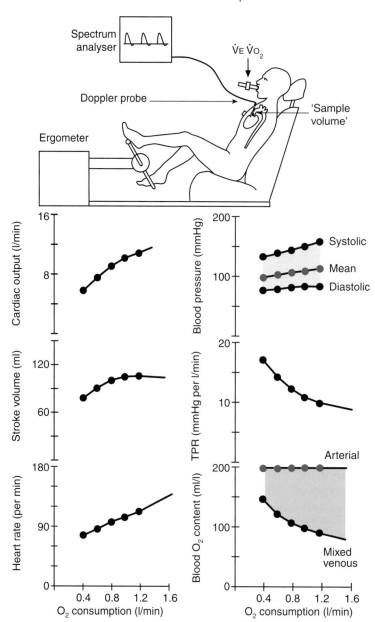

Figure 17.4 Human cardiovascular response to exercise, measured by pulsed Doppler method (Section 6.3) and expired gas analysis. (Adapted from Innes JA, Simon TD, Murphy K, Guz A. *Quarterly Journal of Experimental Physiology* 1988; **73**: 323–41, by permission.)

0.8–1.6 l/min, hard work to 1.6–2.4 l/min and severe work, such as running at 12 km/h, to 2.4–3.3 l/min.

Pulmonary blood flow is increased through changes in heart rate and stroke volume

Cardiac output, and hence pulmonary blood flow, increases in almost linear proportion to total O_2 consumption (Figure 17.4). This tight coupling implies that the brainstem regulatory centres receive information about O_2 consumption – but how this

is achieved is not well understood. The increased cardiac output is brought about mainly through an increase in heart rate, and to a lesser degree stroke volume.

Heart rate is a linear function of work rate, in the steady state (Figure 17.4). The tachycardia commences very rapidly, within a second or so of starting the exercise, then climbs to its steady-state level (Figure 16.13). The initial tachycardia is brought about by the withdrawal of the vagal inhibition of the pacemaker, under the direction of central command and the muscle group III mechanoreceptor

Table 17.1 Cardiovascular and pulmonary function during maximal exercise in five college students and six Olympic athletes[a]

	Exercising students			Olympic athletes
	Control	After bedrest	After training	
Maximal oxygen uptake $\dot{V}_{O_2\,max}$ (litre/min)	3.30	2.43	3.91	5.38[b]
Maximal voluntary ventilation (litre/min)	191.0	201.0	197.0	219.0
Lung transfer coefficient for O_2 ($ml\,min^{-1}\,mmHg^{-1}$)	96.0	83.0	86.0	95.0
Arterial O_2 capacity (ml O_2/100 ml blood)	21.9	20.5	20.8	22.4
Maximal cardiac output (litre/min)	20.0	14.8	22.8	30.4[b]
Maximal stroke volume (ml)	104.0	74.0	120.0	167.0[b]
Maximal heart rate (beats/min)	192.0	197.0	190.0	182.0
Max. systemic arteriovenous O_2 difference (ml O_2/100 ml blood)	16.2	16.5	17.1	18.0

[a]Age, height and weight similar.
[b]Significantly different from trained college students, $P < 0.05$.
(After Blomqvist CG, Saltin B. *Annual Review of Physiology* 1983; **45**: 169–89.)

reflex. Later, sympathetic drive to the pacemaker adds to the tachycardia. Maximum heart rate is $180-200\,min^{-1}$ in a young, human adult.

Stroke volume is raised partly through increased **filling pressure**, which increases the ventricular end-diastolic volume (EDV), and partly through increased **ejection fraction**, which reduces the end-systolic volume (ESV) (Figure 6.24 and Table 17.2).

Right ventricle filling pressure, i.e. central venous pressure, rises by ~1 mmHg during moderate, sustained, upright exercise. The rise is brought about by the skeletal muscle pump and sympathetically mediated splanchnic venoconstriction. During an explosive burst of cycling, however, the muscle pump can raise right atrial pressure by 12 mmHg transiently. Increases in EDV thus make a greater contribution in sudden, maximal effort than in sustained, moderate exercise. Increases in EDV are also relatively more important in the elderly; see 'Ageing'.

Ejection fraction increases because cardiac sympathetic activity increases. This raises ventricular contractility, which reduces the ESV and thus increases stroke volume. Ejection fraction can exceed 80% during heavy exercise. Ischaemic heart disease, however, prevents such increases in ejection fraction, leading to a poor cardiac output during exercise (Table 17.2).

The contribution of increased stroke volume depends very much on whether the exercise is upright or supine (Table 17.3). In **supine exercise**, central venous pressure and EDV start from a high resting value, and stroke volume increases at most by 10–20%, brought about mainly by a reduction in ESV. The increased cardiac output is thus due almost entirely to tachycardia. In **upright exercise**, by contrast, the stroke volume starts from a lower value, because central venous pressure is low, and can increase by 50–100% due to a combination of increased EDV and reduced ESV. Most of this increase in stroke volume occurs at low work rates (Figure 17.4).

Blood flow to active muscle is increased by metabolic vasodilatation

Blood flow increases in the active skeletal muscles (Figure 17.5). In a fit man the total muscle blood flow can increase from 1 l/min at rest (20% of cardiac output) to ~19 l/min during heavy dynamic exercise (>80% of cardiac output). Many muscle groups are used only lightly, even in heavy exercise (e.g. arm muscles during running), so the blood flow to the most active muscles probably increases as much as 40-fold. This is brought about primarily by the dilatation of the local resistance vessels (arterioles and terminal arteries) in the active muscle. The fall in vascular resistance enhances O_2 and glucose delivery specifically to the active muscle. It also permits cardiac output to increase optimally, because without a fall in peripheral resistance the rising cardiac output would cause severe hypertension, which would limit the cardiac output (see 'Afterload', Section 6.9).

The hyperaemia of active muscles is brought about chiefly by **metabolic vasodilatation**, aided by the calf muscle pump during upright exercise (Figure 15.8). Metabolic dilatation of the resistance vessels increases **flow**, and also causes **capillary recruitment**. Capillary recruitment greatly increases

Table 17.2 Ventricular volume during upright, submaximal bicycle exercise in normal subjects and patients with multiple coronary artery disease

	Normal		Coronary disease	
	Rest	Exercise	Rest	Exercise
Cardiac output (litre/min)	6.0	17.5	5.7	11.3
Heart rate (beats/min)	81	170	75	119
Stroke volume (ml)[a]	76	102	76	96
End-diastolic volume (ml)[a]	116	128	138	216
End-systolic volume (ml)[a]	40	26	62	120
Ejection fraction[a]	0.66	0.8	0.6	0.46

[a]Left ventricle dimensions determined by radionuclide angiocardiography. (After Rerych SK, Scholz PM, Newman GE et al. Annals of Surgery 1978; **187**: 449–58.)

Table 17.3 Supine versus upright exercise in eight healthy subjects

	Stroke volume (ml)	Heart rate (beats/min)	Cardiac output (litre/min)
Supine			
Rest	111	60	6.4
Exercise	112	91	9.7
Upright			
Rest	76	76	5.6
Exercise	92	95	8.4

Response to pedalling at 30% of maximum oxygen consumption, $\dot{V}_{O_2 max}$. Stroke volume was measured by the aortic Doppler flow technique. (After Loeppky JA, Green ER, Hoekenga DE et al. Journal of Applied Physiology 1981; **50**: 1173–82.)

the rate of gas and nutrient diffusion between the blood and active muscle fibres, by increasing the surface area available for exchange and by shortening the diffusion distance (Figure 10.14). The increases in O_2 and glucose and transport are described more fully in Sections 10.10 and 10.11.

The arteriolar dilatation of metabolic hyperaemia raises not only blood flow but also capillary pressure (Figure 11.4). This, along with the hyperosmolarity of the interstitial fluid in active muscles, increases the capillary filtration rate. As a result, **plasma volume falls** – by as much as 600 ml during prolonged heavy exercise (Section 11.9). The attendant haemoconcentration modestly increases the O_2-carrying capacity of the blood. This counteracts a slight fall in arterial O_2 saturation (Figure 15.17), which is caused by the Bohr shift (increased acidity and temperature), short pulmonary capillary transit times and shunts. As a result, the arterial O_2 content changes little during sustained heavy exercise in non-athletes, though it can fall in athletes.

As emphasized above, the vasodilatation inside active muscles is induced by intrinsic metabolic control, not by extrinsic autonomic control. If mental stress is involved (e.g. start of a race), the alerting response too is evoked. **Feedforward** by the alerting response leads to an anticipatory, autonomic-mediated tachycardia and muscle vasodilatation (Figure 14.7).

Blood flow to other tissues is altered during exercise: the 'diversion' misconception

Blood flow is also readjusted in most other tissues of the body during exercise; it is raised in some and reduced in others, as follows (Figure 17.5).

- **Coronary blood flow** increases in proportion to cardiac work, due to local metabolic vasodilatation (Figure 15.4).
- **Respiratory muscle perfusion** increases, due to the increased work of breathing. This can account for up to 16% of the cardiac output during heavy exercise.
- **Skin** is a battleground of conflicting demands. Initially, the cutaneous vessels are constricted; but as core temperature rises, the thermoregulatory role of skin supervenes and dilatation ensues (Figure 15.10a,b). This requires a further increase in cardiac output. Moreover, since the cutaneous venodilatation reduces cardiac filling pressure, the stroke volume tends to decline during prolonged hard exercise, so the heart rate increases further to compensate.
- Sympathetic vasoconstrictor outflow to the **splanchnic, renal** and **non-exercising muscle vascular beds** increases substantially during exercise, due to baroreflex resetting by central command, muscle work receptors and arterial chemoreceptors. During leg exercise, for example, vascular resistance increases in forearm muscles. The vasoconstriction of the inactive vascular beds is needed to maintain blood pressure; without it, the vasodilatation in active muscles, myocardium and skin would lower blood pressure by 12–40 mmHg during intense exercise. Increased sympathetic activity also constrains the metabolic vasodilatation in the contracting muscle in order to maintain blood pressure.

Textbooks commonly state that the vasoconstriction in the resting tissues 'diverts' blood to working muscle, but a simple audit of the changes in Figure 17.5 shows that the diverted flow, 0.6 l/min, makes a trivial contribution to the active hyperaemia. The true importance of the sympathetic vasoconstrictor

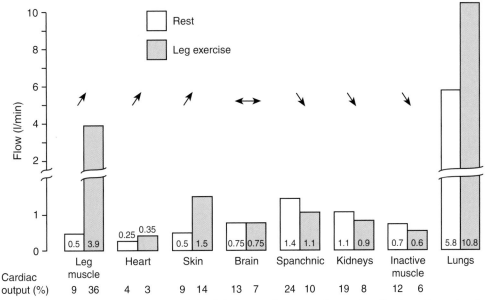

Figure 17.5 Redistribution of human cardiac output during light leg exercise at room temperature. Number at base of each column is blood flow in litre/min. (Based in part on data from Wade OL, Bishop JM. *Cardiac Output and Regional Blood Flow.* Oxford: Blackwell, 1962, with permission from Wiley-Blackwell.)

response lies in adjusting the total peripheral resistance so as to maintain arterial blood pressure.

Static exercise raises arterial pressure more than dynamic exercise

Mean arterial blood pressure normally increases during exercise. The size of the increase depends on the exercise intensity (Figure 17.4), duration, muscle mass involved, and especially the type of exercise – whether dynamic or isometric (Figure 17.6).

Dynamic exercise is exercise in which a muscle alternately shortens and lengthens, under a relatively low load. The rise in mean arterial blood pressure is quite moderate, because the rise in cardiac output is almost offset by the fall in total peripheral resistance. Typically, the mean arterial pressure rises by 20 mmHg or less, and rarely exceeds 120 mmHg. Systolic pressure and pulse pressure increase much more than the mean pressure, because the ejection velocity and stroke volume increase; indeed, systolic pressure can reach 200 mmHg. Diastolic arterial pressure increases relatively little (Figure 17.5), and may even fall, due to increased runoff through the increased peripheral conductance (Figure 17.6, right panel). During the **post-exercise period**, arterial pressure is depressed by ~6 mmHg for up to 30 min. The post-exercise hypotension is caused by the persistence of the increased vascular conductance and by a temporary resetting of the baroreflex to a lower level.

Figure 17.6 Effect of static exercise compared with dynamic exercise. Static exercise caused a bigger increase in arterial blood pressure. Dynamic exercise caused a bigger rise in pulse pressure and heart rate. MVC, maximal voluntary static contraction; arrowed numbers refer to oxygen consumption. (From Lind RA, McNicol GW. *Canadian Medical Association Journal* 1967; **96**: 706.)

Static exercise, such as a sustained handgrip, causes a much bigger increase in arterial blood pressure than dynamic exercise (Figure 17.6, left panel). For example, supporting a 20 kg suitcase for 2–3 min can raise diastolic pressure by 30 mmHg, due chiefly to a rise in total peripheral resistance. Isometric contraction compresses the intra-muscle blood vessels. This attenuates the fall in muscle vascular resistance and causes a relative under-perfusion, which strongly activates the muscle metaboreflex, i.e. exercise pressor reflex (Section 16.6). Since arterial pressure dominates the work of the left ventricle, isometric exercise is best avoided by patients with ischaemic heart disease.

Resistive exercise is a combination of static and heavily loaded dynamic exercise, e.g. weightlifting. Blood pressures up to 350/250 mmHg (truly!) have been recorded in young adults during maximum effort. Such high pressures are the result of the Valsalva phase 1 (aortic compression by a raised intrathoracic pressure), exercise pressor reflex and intra-muscle vessel compression. Fortunately, a concomitant rise in cerebrospinal fluid pressure protects cerebral vessels during these extreme exertions. Nevertheless, hard resistive exercise is best avoided by subjects with ischaemic heart disease.

Pulmonary arterial pressure increases substantially during exercise (Figure 15.17). Indeed, in percentage terms the rise is bigger than in the systemic circulation, because there is no active vasodilatation in the pulmonary circulation (Table 15.1).

Circulating catecholamines help transplanted hearts respond to exercise

Under normal circumstances the increased cardiac output during exercise is driven chiefly by the cardiac autonomic nerves. Nevertheless, animals and humans with transplanted, denervated hearts still increase their cardiac output during exercise, owing to a **redundancy of control mechanisms**. The chief back-up mechanisms are the circulating catecholamines and the skeletal muscle pump.

The contribution of **circulating catecholamines** was demonstrated in racing greyhounds subjected to chronic cardiac denervation. Exercise still causes a tachycardia in these animals, albeit of smaller magnitude and slower onset (Figure 17.7). The tachycardia is mediated by a rise in plasma adrenaline and noradrenaline, due to which the greyhound's track speed is only 5% slower than normal. If the back-up catecholamines are blocked by a β-adrenoceptor antagonist, however, the exercise tachycardia is abolished, track speed falls markedly and the greyhound becomes exhausted (Figure 17.7b). During strenuous human exercise the **plasma noradrenaline** increases from ~1 nM to 10–20 nM, due chiefly to spillage from peripheral sympathetic vasomotor terminals. **Plasma adrenaline** shows little change

Figure 17.7 Greyhound heart rate, monitored by telemetry (radio transmitter) during a race: (a) normal; (b) after cardiac denervation. Red lines show effect of β-adrenoceptor blockade by propranolol. Response of denervated heart depends on circulating catecholamines. Arrows show time to 5/16th mile mark. (From Donald DE, Ferguson DA, Milburn SE. *Circulation Research* 1968; **22**: 127–33, by permission.)

during light to moderate exercise (0.2 nM), but rises to 2–5 nM during maximal dynamic exercise, due to adrenal medulla secretion. The positive inotropic action of the catecholamines more than offsets the negative inotropic effects of exercise-induced hyperkalaemia (up to 8 mM) and lactic acidosis (plasma pH as low as 6.9).

Cardiac transplant patients also benefit from back-up by the **skeletal muscle pump**. This raises the cardiac filling pressure during upright exercise, which in turn raises the stroke volume by the Frank–Starling mechanism. These examples of redundant mechanisms illustrate a general principle enunciated by the respiratory physiologist, Julius H Comroe: if a job is worth doing, the body generally has more than one way of doing it.

What initiates the circulatory adjustments in exercise?

With the major exception of metabolic vasodilatation, the cardiovascular responses to exercise are brought about by the autonomic nervous system. But what induces the brainstem cardiovascular centres to change the autonomic outflow? Two main hypotheses have been put forward – the central command hypothesis and the peripheral reflex hypothesis. Both processes seem to contribute.

Central command
The central command hypothesis, proposed by Krogh and Lindhard in 1913, states that parts of the cerebral cortex (insular cortex, anterior cingulate cortex) and/or related motor regions of the thalamus and basal ganglia, not only initiate voluntary movement but also command the cardiovascular and respiratory centres of the medulla. This is supported by several observations.

- The heart rate increases at the first beat after the onset of exercise (Figure 16.13) – so early that it implies 'feedforward' by the central nervous system; there is insufficient time for feedback to operate.
- After partial neuromuscular blockade by curare, voluntary attempts to contract the partially paralysed muscle require an exaggerated central command signal, and this is accompanied by an enhanced tachycardia, bigger pressor response and greater resetting of the baroreflex (Figure 16.7).

Although central command can account for the early cardiac response, it less readily explains the quintessential feature of the steady-state response, namely the linear relation between cardiac output and total O_2 consumption (Figure 17.4). This coupling is underpinned by information from the active muscle itself, telling the brain about the work rate.

Muscle work receptors link cardiac output to work rate
Group III muscle mechanoreceptors and the group IV muscle metaboreceptors reflexly increase the heart rate and blood pressure during exercise (Figures 16.13 and 16.14). The mechanoreceptors contribute to the initial vagal inhibition and rapid onset of tachycardia. The local accumulation of interstitial chemicals then activates the metaboreceptors and helps drive the further increases in heart rate and blood pressure that occur over in the initial 1–2 min (Figure 17.6).

Thus **central command feedforward** and **work receptor feedback** together drive the cardiac response to exercise. The central command and muscle mechanoreceptors produce the initial, rapid-onset tachycardia by suppressing the cardiac vagal motor neurons; and the muscle metaboreflex contributes to the subsequent slower, sympathetically mediated rise in cardiac output and peripheral

vasoconstriction. **Joint mechanoreceptors** too contribute slightly, perhaps 10%, to the increased reflex drive to the heart.

17.4 Physical training and performance

Brief **power events**, such as sprinting or shot-putting, are not critically dependent on cardiovascular performance, because aerobic muscle metabolism is not essential for a brief burst of power. Power training nevertheless evokes left ventricular wall hypertrophy, probably in response to the strong exercise pressor response (see below).

In an **endurance event**, such as a medium-distance race, the continuous work depends on aerobic muscle metabolism. Consequently, performance is influenced by the maximum rate of O_2 transport from the lungs to the muscle mitochondria. This depends on (i) $\dot{V}_{O_2max}$, the maximum rate of O_2 uptake by pulmonary blood, (ii) muscle perfusion and (iii) the diffusive resistance from muscle capillary to mitochondrion. All three aspects are enhanced by endurance training; a rise in maximum cardiac output improves $\dot{V}_{O_2max}$, and changes in the skeletal muscle arteries and capillaries optimize local perfusion and gas exchange.

Endurance training improves maximum cardiac output and $\dot{V}_{O_2max}$
$\dot{V}_{O_2\,max}$ is determined by maximum cardiac output and haematocrit, and can increase from ~3 l/min in an untrained student to >5 l/min in an endurance-trained Olympic athlete (Table 17.1). This is achieved mainly through a rise in maximal **cardiac output**, from ~20 l/min (untrained) to 30–36 l/min in athletes. At such high outputs, a red cell's residence time in the alveolus is so short as to curtail gas equilibration, and arterial O_2 saturation can fall to ~90%.

It is interesting to compare humans with athletic animals such as dogs and horses. Unlike humans, many athletic animal species have a contractile spleen that pumps red cells into the circulation during exercise, raising the **haematocrit**. In a galloping racehorse, the spleen can inject several litres of red cells into the circulation, raising the haematocrit by 50%, to 0.65. Selective breeding in racehorses has increased the heart size disproportionately, relative to the lungs, reducing the pulmonary transit time. This leads to a fall in arterial O_2 saturation to ~77% during maximum effort. Moreover the huge pulmonary blood flow in a galloping racehorse generates an alarmingly high pulmonary artery pressure,

~120 mmHg, which can lead to pulmonary haemorrhage during extreme exertion.

Endurance training boosts stroke volume: eccentric versus concentric hypertrophy

Endurance training

Big hearts win long races! Dynamic, endurance training leads to:

- ventricular enlargement and increased stroke volume;
- bradycardia at rest;
- a 5–10% increase in blood volume, raising the central venous pressure;
- increased myocardial vascularity.

Endurance training enlarges the cavities of both the right and left ventricles. New sarcomeres are added in series within each myocyte, increasing the myocyte length but not width. Consequently, the ventricle expands, with little increase in wall thickness. This growth pattern is called **eccentric hypertrophy**. It is driven by local growth factors such as IGF (insulin-like growth factor), and can increase the left ventricle mass by 20%. Myocyte contractility increases too, at least in endurance-trained rats. The eccentric hypertrophy is accompanied by increases in the number of capillaries and arterioles, and by an increase in coronary artery calibre.

Resting ventricular EDV in endurance-trained athletes increases from ~120 ml to 160–220 ml, due to eccentric hypertrophy, an increase in blood volume and an increase in central venous pressure. **Resting stroke volume** increases from 70–80 ml to 100–125 ml. **Resting cardiac output** is unchanged, because the high stroke volume is offset by a **resting bradycardia** of 40–50 min^{-1}, or in extreme cases 35 min^{-1}. The resting bradycardia is brought about by three factors: increased tonic vagal activity; increased local acetylcholine release (mediated by a nitric oxide pathway in the fibre terminals); and a fall in the intrinsic pacemaker rate. Sinus arrhythmia is enhanced by the increased vagal tone. A third and fourth heart sound may be audible, along with a benign systolic ejection murmur. The ECG shows a resting bradycardia. Mean blood pressure is little changed.

During **maximal exercise**, endurance-trained athletes achieve up to 60% bigger stroke volumes than untrained subjects (Table 17.1). The maximal heart rate is unaltered, 180–190 min^{-1}; but as athletes have lower resting heart rate, they can achieve a proportionately greater increase in rate, e.g. 4.5-fold from 40 min^{-1} to 180 min^{-1} (cf. untrained 2.6-fold, from 70 min^{-1} to 180 min^{-1}). As a result of these adaptations, endurance-trained athletes can increase the right and left ventricular output up to seven-fold, substantially improving $\dot{V}_{O_2 max}$ (Table 17.1). Maximal cardiac outputs as high as 35 l/min have been recorded in some individuals.

Strength training

An increase in cardiac chamber size is specific to endurance training. Strength training (isometric exercise), by contrast, causes short bouts of greatly raised blood pressure (Figure 17.6), which evokes left ventricular wall hypertrophy (thickening), with no increase in internal chamber diameter. This growth pattern is called **concentric hypertrophy**. Some training disciplines (e.g. triathletes) evoke both concentric and eccentric hypertrophy. Concentric hypertrophy also occurs in **hypertensive patients**. It arises from the fact that sarcomeres are replicated in parallel, in order to normalize the stress on them (stress = tension/thickness). Severe myocardial hypertrophy predisposes the ventricle to arrhythmia, and may account for around half of **sudden deaths in young athletes**. The pro-arrhythmogenic changes include prolonged mid-myocardial and subepicardial action potentials, altered repolarization patterns (with ECG T-wave inversion in some cases) and frequent ventricular ectopics due to afterdepolarization.

Vascular changes enhance muscle blood flow capacity and gas exchange

Endurance training increases maximal muscle blood flow and local O_2 transport through two adaptations – local arterial expansion and increased number of capillaries. **Muscle conduit arteries** expand with training; the femoral artery of a trained human, for example, has a 7–9% wider lumen and thinner wall than in a sedentary subject. The **number density of arterioles** increases (it can double in endurance-trained rats), probably through the arterialization of capillaries. Such changes are driven, presumably, by the increases in endothelial shear stress during training. Basic regulatory processes such as the myogenic response and metabolic hyperaemia are not materially changed by training. **Capillary angiogenesis**, induced by vascular endothelial growth factor, increases the surface area for gas exchange and reduces diffusion distance – or, if the muscle fibre diameter hypertrophies, prevents an increase in diffusion distance. Muscle mitochondria become more abundant, especially at subsarcolemmal sites close to capillaries, and muscle myoglobin concentration increases.

17.5 Feeding, digestion and the splanchnic circulation

The splanchnic circulation comprises the gastrointestinal tract, spleen and pancreas, which are fed by the coeliac, superior mesenteric and inferior mesenteric arteries (Figure 1.6). The arrival of food in the gastrointestinal tract triggers **mucosal hyperaemia**, lasting 1–3 h. The hyperaemia is initiated partly by local hormones (gastrin, cholecystokinin), partly by digestive products (glucose, fatty acids) and partly by vagal parasympathetic activity. Also, parasympathetic-mediated **pancreatic hyperaemia** accompanies pancreatic secretion (Section 14.2). As a result of these changes, human splanchnic blood flow increases from a basal 1.5 l/min to 2.5 l/min after a carbohydrate meal. Conversely, sympathetic-mediated vasoconstriction can reduce the splanchnic blood flow to as little as 0.3 l/min during hypovolaemia.

The postprandial splanchnic vasodilatation elicits **tachycardia** and an **increase in cardiac output**, by ~1 l/min for 30–60 min after the meal. Carbohydrate meals cause the greatest hyperaemia and cardiac changes, and may cause **postprandial angina** in patients with severe ischaemic heart disease. **Reflex vasoconstriction** in other vascular beds (e.g. forearm, calf) normally prevents postprandial hypotension. Failure of this response and the reflex tachycardia in patients with autonomic dysfunction (e.g. diabetics) or some elderly subjects can result in **postprandial hypotension** after a carbohydrate meal or oral glucose.

Ethanol is absorbed rapidly from the gastrointestinal tract and causes cutaneous vasodilatation (facial flushing) and coronary vasodilatation; 0.2% ethanol (two and a half times the UK driving limit) doubles the coronary blood flow in guinea pigs. The vasodilatation is mediated by CGRP (calcitonin gene-related peptide), which is released from sensory terminals upon activation of capsaicin receptors (TRPV1). Moderate, daily ethanol consumption reduces deaths from coronary atheroma, but higher consumption contributes to hypertension, alcoholic cardiomyopathy and hepatic cirrhosis. The excessive flushing of many Chinese and Japanese people to alcohol is caused by two liver enzyme isoforms; one convert alcohol unusually rapidly into acetaldehyde and the other is unusually slow at degrading acetaldehyde.

17.6 Diving response

Diving animals such as the duck, seal and whale undergo remarkable cardiovascular changes during a dive. Humans too exhibit a diving response, albeit a less well-developed one. The diving response comprises three reflex changes, namely:

- apnoea
- intense bradycardia
- peripheral vasoconstriction.

The cardiovascular changes conserve O_2 for use by the heart and brain during prolonged dives (pearl divers 40–50 s, competitive free divers a few minutes, Weddell seals ≤70 min, whales ≤2 h – though feeding dives are usually shorter). The superior performance of seals and whales is due to their large store of O_2 in blood and muscle myoglobin (Figure 17.8, bottom), more extreme cardiovascular responses and greater toleration of asphyxia. The arterial gas values in a harbour seal after a prolonged dive, 10 mmHg O_2 and 100 mmHg CO_2, vastly exceed the human breath-hold breaking point and would probably kill us.

The diving response is initiated by cold water touching **trigeminal nerve facial receptors**, particularly around the eyes, nose and nasal mucosa. Immersion of the body but not the face, or immersion of the face wearing a breathing tube, fails to elicit the reflex. As the dive progresses, asphyxia develops and **arterial chemoreceptors** reinforce the cardiovascular responses.

Facial immersion causes bradycardia in humans

A seal's heart rate falls to ~20 min^{-1} during a dive, due to vagal inhibition of the pacemaker (Figure 17.8). Many humans likewise display a pronounced reflex bradycardia to facial immersion in cold water (Figure 17.9). Indeed, some patients find this simple procedure can terminate a supraventricular tachycardia. The reflex may contribute to sudden deaths associated with water or foreign bodies in the airways.

Peripheral vasoconstriction diverts blood to the heart and brain

Facial immersion triggers vasoconstriction in human skin and skeletal muscles, as in diving mammals (Figure 17.9, inset). Diving mammals show a profound,

Figure 17.8 Physiological adaptation of the seal to breath-hold diving. Heart rate response of a seal trained to perform voluntary head immersion is shown at top. (Various sources.)

Figure 17.9 Diving response in humans; bradycardia in a medical student following breath-hold facial immersion in cold water. The experiment was stopped in alarm when the heart rate fell to <40/min! (*Inset*) Concomitant vasoconstriction in forearm. (Courtesy of JR Henderson, unpublished). (Inset from Heistad DD, Abboud FM, Eckstein JW. *Journal of Applied Physiology* 1968; **25**: 542–49, with permission from the American Physiological Society.)

sympathetically mediated vasoconstriction of the splanchnic, renal and skeletal muscle circulations. Arteries upstream of local metabolic vasodilator agents contract strongly, overriding the usual metabolic hyperaemia. The peripheral vasoconstriction maintains arterial pressure despite the extreme bradycardia, and diverts the remaining cardiac output to the heart and brain. A large quantity of lactic acid accumulates in the swimming muscles, leading to a sharp vasodilatation when the animal resurfaces.

17.7 Ageing

Ageing is associated with changes in artery wall structure, a rise in blood pressure (especially systolic pressure), reduced baroreflex sensitivity and impaired cardiac performance during exercise. These changes are due to the ageing process, not atheroma.

Elastic arteries develop sclerosis of the tunica media (arteriosclerosis)

The elasticity of ageing elastic arteries is reduced by diffuse changes in the media. The elastic lamellae

(Figure 1.11) become thin, broken and disordered, due possibly to repetitive strain injury. This diffuse fracturing of elastic lamellae weakens the artery wall, leading to **structural dilatation**; the aorta, for example, dilates by ~50% between the ages of 40 and 70 years. As the elastin fragments and the wall stretches, wall stress is transferred to the **collagen fibres**. More collagen is laid down, and since collagen is much stiffer than elastin, the vessel becomes **stiffer**, as well as dilated (Figure 18.7). Calcium salts may also be deposited in the media, and there is intimal hyperplasia. These degenerative changes are called arteriosclerosis; 'sclerosis' means fibrous hardening, hence the common expression 'hardening of the arteries'. Arteriosclerosis affects primarily the elastic vessels, and is important because it raises the pulse pressure and cardiac work (see below).

Arteriosclerosis is not atheroma

Arteriosclerosis is distinct from atheroma (Section 9.9), both biochemically and pathologically. Confusingly, atheroma is often called 'atherosclerosis' – a self-contradictory term meaning 'porridge-like hardening'. Even worse, and generating maximum confusion, atheroma is sometimes called arteriosclerosis – in which case one has to look at the context to see which pathology the author really means. The differences are summarized in Table 17.4. They include **distribution** (arteriosclerosis is diffuse, atheroma forms plaques), **location** (media versus intima), **biochemistry** (elastin fragmentation versus subintimal cholesterol deposit), effect on **vessel diameter** (arteriosclerotic dilatation versus atheromatous narrowing), **pathological consequence** (raised pulse pressure in arteriosclerosis, distal ischaemia in atheroma) and **epidemiology** (loss of elasticity with ageing in all societies, cf. atheroma associated with Western diet).

Arterial blood pressure increases with age

The pattern of pressure change with age is the same in Eastern and Western populations, and has changed little from the early twentieth century to the present day; Figure 17.10, based on UK health statistics for 2003, shows the same pattern as the 1936 data in earlier editions of this book.

Mean arterial blood pressure increases moderately with age due to a rise in total peripheral resistance (Figure 17.10). This may be due partly to an increase in sympathetic vasomotor activity, as indicated by neural recordings and an enhanced dilator response to the α-adrenoceptor blocker phentolamine.

Systolic pressure increases much more than the mean pressure, because the compliance of the elastic vessels is reduced by arteriosclerosis. In the **brachial**

Table 17.4 Arteriosclerosis contrasted with atheroma (atherosclerosis)

	Arteriosclerosis of ageing	Atheroma
Epidemiology	All societies, West and East	Western lifestyle and diet
Distribution along artery	Diffuse	Focal
Layer primarily affected	Media	Intima
Key biochemical change	Elastin fragmentation and loss	Cholesterol plaque
Effect on lumen	Dilatation	Stenosis
Effect on blood flow	None	Impaired
Resulting pathophysiology	↑ systolic pressure ↑ ventricular O_2 consumption	Distal tissue ischaemia

Figure 17.10 Effect of ageing on brachial artery pressure in English population. Recent Australian and American surveys show the same pattern, as did the 1936 survey of South Wales. BP was measured by an automated cuff device (Section 8.5) (Public data from Department of Health National Statistics. *Health Survey for England 2003*, Vol 2 Risk Factors for Cardiovascular Disease.)

artery, where blood pressure is normally measured, systolic pressure increases steeply from childhood until age 20, levels off until age 30–40 and climbs steadily thereafter. The levelling-off of brachial systolic pressure between 20 and 40 years is caused by the gradual loss of distal pressure amplification with age (Figure 8.11). In the **aorta**, systolic pressure probably pursues a more steady climb; consequently, the afterload on the ventricular myocardium increases progressively with age.

Diastolic pressure, which drives most of the coronary blood flow (Figure 15.5), actually begins to decline beyond 60 years.

Systolic pressure rises due to reduced arterial compliance and rapid wave reflection

The systolic pressure and pulse pressure increase disproportionately with ageing due to two biomechanical consequences of arteriosclerosis, as follows.

1 Pulse pressure depends on stroke volume divided by arterial compliance (Section 7.4). Since arteriosclerosis reduces arterial compliance, the pulse pressure increases. Clinical hypertension has a similar effect, and has been likened to accelerated vascular ageing (Figure 18.7).

2 The velocity of propagation of the pulse depends on artery wall stiffness. In the aorta, where the increase in wall stiffness is greatest, the wave velocity more than doubles, from ~4 m/s at 25 years to ~10 m/s at 70 years. The wave now travels so fast that its reflected component returns to the aorta during late systole, adding to the late systolic pressure (Figure 8.10). This systolic augmentation is estimated to add ~25 mmHg to systolic pressure between age 30 and age 60.

High systolic pressures impair left ventricular performance

The systolic pressure in the aorta governs the afterload on the contracting left ventricle, and this affects cardiac performance (Figures 6.2 and 6.15). Also, by increasing cardiac work, a high systolic pressure raises myocardial O_2 demand. Arteriosclerosis can therefore contribute to heart failure in the elderly. The severity of cardiovascular disease is more closely related to systolic than diastolic pressure, and the incidence of cardiovascular disease is reduced by treating systolic hypertension.

Exercise-related cardiac performance and skeletal muscle hyperaemia are impaired by ageing

Ageing has little effect on resting heart rate or stroke volume, despite age-associated myocardial fibrosis. The fibrosis increases ventricular wall stiffness, which slows relaxation and early diastolic filling (diastolic dysfunction). Myocardial O_2 demand increases for reasons explained above. The major effect of ageing on the heart, however, emerges when it is stressed, for example by physical exercise. The ability to increase the cardiac output and muscle blood flow during exercise declines substantially with ageing, reducing $\dot{V}_{O_2 \, max}$ and exercise tolerance.

Maximum heart rate in exercise is impaired

The maximum attainable heart rate falls as we get older. As a rule-of-thumb, the maximum is $220 \, min^{-1}$ minus age (in years). The decline is caused by a fall in the responsiveness of the pacemaker to β_1-adrenoceptor stimulation (see below). Cardiac responsiveness to the baroreflex is reduced too.

Maximum stroke volume in exercise is impaired

The ability to reduce ESV, by raising the ventricular ejection fraction, declines with age. Although the stroke volume can still be increased, this is brought about chiefly by raising EDV (Frank–Starling mechanism) rather than by raising contractility to reduce ESV. The decline in maximum heart rate and ejection fraction are both due to an impaired response to β-adrenoceptor stimulation. There is ample sympathetic activity and catecholamine release, but the β_1-adrenoceptors trigger less of a rise in intracellular cAMP (reduced receptor coupling). In addition, counts of myocardial nuclei show that many millions of myocytes are lost each year – though there is some compensatory hypertrophy of the remaining myocytes.

Skeletal muscle active hyperaemia is impaired

Microvascular density in skeletal muscles appears to be maintained during ageing; but leg muscles nevertheless show ~20% less increase in blood flow in elderly humans than in young ones, for the same degree of exercise. This is due partly to a substantial, two- to three-fold increase in sympathetic vasoconstrictor activity in the elderly, and partly to a fall in endothelial NO availability (mediating shear-dependent vasodilatation of conduit arteries). Conducted vasodilatation of the feed arteries is reduced too, at least in mice.

17.8 Sleep and the alerting response

Sleep. During sleep, the metabolic rate and O_2 consumption decline. This is accompanied by a characteristic pattern of cardiovascular and respiratory changes, namely:

- bradycardia and a low cardiac output
- a fall in blood pressure (e.g. 80/50 mmHg, Figure 8.13)
- splanchnic vasodilatation
- reduced ventilation.

On first falling asleep, during the non-rapid-eye-movement phase (non-REM), bradycardia accounts for the fall in blood pressure. Later, during REM sleep, dilatation of the splanchnic circulation also contributes to the hypotension. Cerebral blood flow is increased in many parts of the brain despite the low blood pressure.

The alerting response. The response to an unusual or threatening environmental stimulus is in many respects the opposite of the sleep response, being characterized by:

- tachycardia
- a rise in blood pressure
- splanchnic, renal and cutaneous vasoconstriction
- muscle vasodilatation
- increased ventilation.

The alerting response is clearly an appropriate preparation for imminent physical action. It originates from the central long axis of the brain, and is described further in Section 16.8.

SUMMARY

Posture (orthostasis)

- During standing the distension of dependent veins by gravity redistributes ~500 ml blood from the thorax into the lower limbs. The reduced cardiac filling pressure leads, via the Frank–Starling mechanism, to a 30–40% fall in stroke volume and arterial pulse pressure. A transient fall in mean pressure can cause postural hypotension and dizziness in warm, venodilated subjects.

- The fall in pulse pressure and carotid sinus mean pressure reduce arterial baroreceptor activity. This evokes a reflex peripheral vasoconstriction, splanchnic venoconstriction and increase in heart rate by 15–20 beats/min, which together restore mean arterial pressure.

- Over a longer period, an increase in capillary filtration into the dependent limbs reduces the plasma volume by ~12%. Reflex increases in plasma vasopressin and renin–angiotensin–aldosterone reduce the excretion of salt and water.

Valsalva manoeuvre

- Forced expiration against a closed glottis raises intrathoracic and arterial pressure by mechanical compression (phase 1).

- The impeded venous return results in a fall in stroke volume and arterial pressure. The latter elicits a baroreflex tachycardia and peripheral vasoconstriction, leading to pressure stabilization (phase 2).

- On resumption of normal breathing, intrathoracic and arterial pressure immediately fall (phase 3).

- The inrush of accumulated peripheral venous blood raises the stroke volume (Frank–Starling mechanism). The resulting rise in pulse pressure triggers a baroreflex bradycardia (phase 4). This is used as a clinical test of autonomic function.

Exercise

- **Metabolic hyperaemia** in the active muscle (increased blood flow), along with **capillary recruitment** and **steepened diffusion gradients**, speed up O_2 and glucose delivery to active fibres. The increased blood flow is due chiefly to metabolic vasodilatation, aided by the muscle pump during upright exercise and by a relatively small rise in arterial pressure.

- **A rise in cardiac output** supplies the increased flow to active muscle, and also increases pulmonary gas exchange (Fick's principle). Output is proportion to muscle O_2 consumption and can increase $4\times$ to $\sim20\,l/min$ in untrained students. Pulmonary O_2 uptake can increase much more ($12-13\times$), because mixed venous O_2 content falls (Fick's principle).

■ **Tachycardia** (maximum $180-190\,min^{-1}$) is initiated quickly by withdrawal of vagal tone, followed by increased sympathetic activity. **Stroke volume** increases during upright, dynamic exercise; less so supine. Increases of 50–100% result from a rise in end-diastolic volume (due to muscle pump and peripheral venoconstriction) and a fall in end-systolic volume (due to sympathetic-mediated increased contractility).

■ The autonomic outflow that drives the cardiac response is elicited by **central command** from the forebrain (feedforward) and by a **pressor reflex from muscle mechano- and metaboreceptors** (feedback).

■ **Sympathetic-mediated vasoconstriction** in inactive circulations (splanchnic, renal, inactive muscles) counters the hypotensive effect of vasodilatation in active limb muscles, respiratory muscles, myocardium and, later, skin (heat dissipation). The baroreflex is reset, allowing mean arterial pressure to rise by $\sim20\%$ during hard dynamic exercise. Pressure climbs much higher during static (isometric) exercise, due to a stronger muscle metaboreflex; so isometric/resistive exercise is best avoided by patients with ischaemic heart disease.

Physical training and performance

■ Enhancement of cardiovascular performance by training is advantageous in dynamic, endurance events (cf. brief, strength events).

■ Endurance training enlarges the ventricular cavities through sarcomere addition. End-diastolic volume and stroke volume are increased at rest and in exercise.

■ Resting cardiac output is unaltered, because a vagus-mediated bradycardia ($40-50\,min^{-1}$) offsets the increased resting stroke volume. Since the maximum heart rate remains $180-190\,min^{-1}$, heart rate can increase $4\times$

(cf. normal two and a half-fold). Cardiac output can reach $30-35\,l/min$ in athletes.

■ Arterial changes and capillary angiogenesis in the endurance-trained muscle and myocardium raise the local maximum perfusion and facilitate solute exchange.

Feeding, digestion and splanchnic circulation

■ Mucosal hyperaemia is most pronounced after a carbohydrate meal, but more prolonged after a fatty meal. The hyperaemia is mediated by digestion products, local hormones (gastrin, vasoactive intestinal polypeptide) and vagal parasympathetic activity.

■ The hyperaemia, up to $1\,l/min$, necessitates a rise in cardiac output. Blood pressure is further supported by vasoconstriction in the limbs. If the latter fails, as in patients with autonomic neuropathy and some elderly subjects, post-prandial hypotension can develop.

Diving response

■ Stimulation of trigeminal facial and nasal mucosa afferents by cold water evokes a reflex bradycardia, peripheral vasoconstriction and apnoea.

■ As asphyxia develops, the arterial chemoreflex reinforces the bradycardia and vasoconstriction.

■ The cardiovascular changes conserve the O_2 store for the benefit of the brain and heart. In humans, dives of up to a few minutes are possible; in whales, up to $2\,h$.

Ageing

■ Arteriosclerosis is diffuse elastin fragmentation and fibrosis (collagen deposition) in the tunica media of ageing elastic arteries. The reduced compliance (increased stiffness) and early return of the reflected wave raise systolic arterial pressure and hence cardiac work.

■ Mean arterial pressure rises too, probably due to a sympathetic-mediated increase in total peripheral resistance.

■ The cardiac response to exercise is impaired. Maximum heart rate and the ability to raise the ejection fraction decline, due to impaired responsiveness to β_1-adrenoceptor stimulation (reduced coupling of receptors to cAMP production). Stroke volume is raised instead by increasing the end-diastolic volume.

■ Skeletal muscle maximum flow capacity declines, due to increased sympathetic vasoconstrictor activity and reduced endothelial NO production.

Sleep and the alerting response

■ Sleep evokes bradycardia, reduced cardiac output, reduced blood pressure, splanchnic vasodilatation and reduced ventilation.

■ The alerting response to stress is the opposite to sleep; it involves tachycardia, increased blood pressure, splanchnic, renal and cutaneous vasoconstriction, muscle vasodilatation and increased ventilation.

Further reading

Reviews and chapters

Posture (orthostasis)

Huisman HW, Pretorius PJ, Van Rooyen JM *et al.* Haemodynamic changes in the cardiovascular system during the early phases of orthostasis. *Acta Physiologica Scandinavica* 1999; **166**: 145–9.

Jacob G, Ertl AC, Shannon JR, Furlan R, Robertson RM, Robertson D. Effect of standing on neurohumoral responses and plasma volume in healthy subjects. *Journal of Applied Physiology* 1998; **84**: 914–21.

Smit AAJ, Halliwill JR, Low PA, Wieling W. Pathophysiological basis of orthostatic hypotension in autonomic failure. *Journal of Physiology* 1999; **519**: 1–10.

Wieling W, Halliwill JR, Karemaker JM. Orthostatic intolerance after space flight (Perspective). *Journal of Physiology* 2000; **538**: 1.

Valsalva

Smith ML, Beightol LA, Fritsch-Yelle JM, Ellenbogen KA, Porter TR, Eckberg DL. Valsalva's maneuver revisited: a quantitative method yielding insight into human autonomic control. *American Journal of Physiology* 1996; **271**: H1240–9.

Exercise, training, performance and stress

Coote JH, Bothams VF. Cardiac vagal control before, during and after exercise. *Experimental Physiology* 2001; **86**: 811–15.

Fletcher GF (ed.). *Cardiovascular Response to Exercise.* American Heart Association Monograph. New York: Futura, 1994.

Hart G. Exercise-induced cardiac hypertrophy: A substrate for sudden death in athletes? *Experimental Physiology* 2003; **88**: 639–44.

Jones JH, Linstedt SL. Limits to maximal performance. *Annual Reviews of Physiology* 1993; **55**: 547–69.

Rowell LB, Shepherd JT (eds). Exercise: Regulation and integration of multiple systems. *Handbook of Physiology*, Section 12. New York: Oxford University Press, 1996.

Williamson JW, Fadel PJ, Mitchell JH. (2006) New insights into central cardiovascular control during exercise in humans: A central command update. *Experimental Physiology* 2006; **91**: 51–58.

Feeding, digestion and splanchnic circulation

Kearney MT, Cowley AJ, MacDonald IA. The cardiovascular responses to feeding in man. *Experimental Physiology* 1995; **80**: 683–700.

Diving response

Butler PJ, Jones DR. Physiology of diving of birds and mammals. *Physiological Reviews* 1997; **77**: 837–99.

de Burgh Daly M. *Peripheral Arterial Chemoreceptors and Respiration–Cardiovascular Integration.* Oxford: Clarendon Press, 1997.

Ageing

Fleg JL. Effects of aging on the cardiovascular response to exercise. In: Fletcher GF (ed.). *Cardiovascular Response to Exercise.* New York: Futura, 1994: 387–404.

Folkow B, Svanborg A. Physiology of cardiovascular aging. *Physiological Reviews* 1993; **73**: 725–45.

Nichols WW, O'Rourke MF. *McDonald's Blood Flow in Arteries*, 5th edn. London: Arnold, 2005.

Olivertti G, Meissari M, Capasso JM, Anvers P. Cardiomyopathy of the aging human heart. *Circulation Research* 1991; **68**: 1560–8.

Payne GW, Bearden SE. The microcirculation of skeletal muscle in aging. *Microcirculation* 2006; **13**: 275–7. (Many related articles in same volume).

Sleep

Franzini C, Zoccoli G, Cianci T, Lenzi P. Sleep-dependent changes in regional circulations. *News in Physiological Sciences* 1996; **11**: 274–80.

Marshall JM. Cardiovascular changes associated with sleep. In: Jordan D and Marshall (eds). *Cardiovascular Regulation.* Londn: Portland Press, 1995: 61–76.

Research papers

See www.hodderplus.com/cardiovascularphysiology for a full list of Research papers for this chapter.

CHAPTER 18

Cardiovascular responses in pathological situations

Learning objectives

After reading this chapter you should be able to:

● State the key cardiovascular responses to hypoxia (18.1).
● List the principal causes of acute circulatory failure (clinical shock) (18.2).
● Describe the reflexes that support blood pressure during hypovolaemia (18.2).
● Explain the cardiovascular basis of fainting (18.3).
● Define 'clinical hypertension' and list its main ill-effects (18.4).
● Draw the hypertensive pressure pulse and explain (i) the rise in mean pressure; and (ii) the disproportionate increase in systolic pressure (18.4).
● Outline the chief aetiological theories for hypertension (18.4).
● Define chronic cardiac failure and sketch the altered ventricular function curve (18.5).
● Outline the changes in excitation–contraction coupling and electrophysiology of failing myocytes (18.5).
● List the changes in cardiac performance and peripheral circulation associated with heart failure (18.5).
● Explain dyspnoea and how oedema arises in heart failure (18.5).

The previous chapter described co-ordinated cardiovascular responses to the challenges of everyday life, and in this final chapter we consider how the circulation reacts to pathological situations. **Atheroma**, a major pathology of large arteries, was covered in earlier chapters (*pathogenesis*, Section 9.10; *risk factors*, Concept box 15.1; *distinction from arteriosclerosis*, Table 17.4; *myocardial infarction and angina*, Section 15.1; *intermittent claudication/gangrenous necrosis*, Section 15.2; *thrombo-embolic strokes*, Section 15.4). The present chapter opens with systemic hypoxaemia, a pathological situation encountered not only in chronic lung disease but also by healthy individuals at high altitude.

18.1 Systemic hypoxaemia

Systemic hypoxaemia is a subnormal partial pressure of O_2 in the arterial blood. It can be caused by high altitude, asphyxiation, lung pathology (chronic emphysema, pulmonary oedema) or right-to-left shunts through congenital heart defects. The following account focuses on high altitude hypoxaemia, which can be simulated in the laboratory by reducing the O_2 content of the inspired air (Figure 18.1).

Arterial P_{O_2} falls with increasing altitude

Atmospheric pressure at sea level is $\sim760\,$mmHg (100 kPa), and oxygen makes up 21% of the atmosphere; so the partial pressure of inspired oxygen, P_{O_2}, is 160 mmHg (21 kPa). Alveolar P_{O_2} is lower, 100 mmHg (13 kPa), because some of the oxygen has been extracted by the pulmonary blood. Arterial P_{O_2} is almost the same as alveolar P_{O_2}, because oxygen equilibrates across the pulmonary capillary wall. Arterial haemoglobin saturation is 97% at sea level.

Atmospheric pressure, inspired P_{O_2}, alveolar P_{O_2} and arterial P_{O_2} all fall with increasing altitude. Arterial saturation shows little fall up to 2000 metres, owing to the plateau on the oxyhaemoglobin

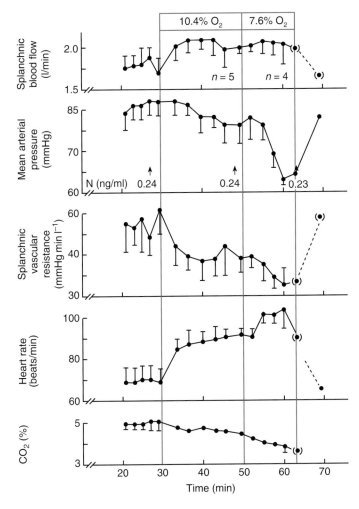

Figure 18.1 Human cardiovascular responses to hypoxaemia. Inspired O_2 of 21% at sea-level was reduced to 10.4% (equivalent altitude 5500 m), then 7.6% (equivalent to a major Himalayan summit). Arterial P_{O_2} fell from 100 mmHg to 27 mmHg. Hyperventilation reduced alveolar CO_2. N, noradrenaline. (After Rowell LB. *Human Circulation Regulation during Physical Stress*. New York: Oxford University Press, 1986, with permission from Oxford University Press and the American Physiological Society.)

dissociation curve (Figure 15.3). Saturation begins to fall significantly when arterial P_{O_2} falls below 60 mmHg (8 kPa), at 3000 m – an altitude commonly experienced by skiers, tourists and climbers. On a major Alpine summit (~4000 m), arterial P_{O_2} is less than half normal, ~45 mmHg (6 kPa). Even so, there is permanent human habitation up to 5000 m in the Andes, and acclimatized individuals have survived days without supplementary O_2 above 8000 m on Himalayan peaks.

Humans respond to arterial hypoxaemia with three primary compensatory changes: resting hyperventilation, increased cardiac output and peripheral vasodilatation, as follows.

Resting hyperventilation improves arterial P_{O_2}

The hypoxic stimulation of arterial chemoreceptors (Section 16.6) causes a reflex increase in resting ventilation. This raises alveolar P_{O_2} closer to the inspired P_{O_2}, and thus raises arterial P_{O_2}. The hyperventilation

also reduces alveolar and arterial P_{CO_2} (Figure 18.1). This shifts the haemoglobin dissociation curve to the left (reverse Bohr shift) and enables arterial blood to bind more O_2 at the prevailing P_{O_2}. The hypocapnia also attenuates peripheral and central chemoreceptor activity, so it limits the ventilatory response. (By contrast, in **asphyxiation** the arterial P_{CO_2} rises as P_{O_2} falls, thereby augmenting the chemoreceptor activity and ventilatory drive.)

Resting heart rate and cardiac output increase

An increase in resting cardiac output is necessary to maintain O_2 delivery to the cells of the body. Since arterial P_{O_2} is low, the blood-to-cell diffusion gradient for O_2 is reduced; so less O_2 diffuses out of each millilitre of blood, and the oxygen **arteriovenous difference falls**. For example, at 7.5% inspired O_2 (Himalayan hypoxia), the arterial O_2 content is 120 ml l^{-1} (normal 195 ml l^{-1}), mixed venous O_2 is 90 ml l^{-1} (normal 145 ml l^{-1}) and the $(A - V)_{O_2}$

is $30\,\mathrm{ml}\,\mathrm{l}^{-1}$ (normal $50\,\mathrm{ml}\,\mathrm{l}^{-1}$). An increase in resting cardiac output compensates for the fall in $(A - V)_{O_2}$, as dictated by the **Fick principle** (Section 7.1), so that tissue O_2 consumption is not impaired. In our example, a rise in resting cardiac output to just over $8\,\mathrm{l/min}$, when multiplied by the reduced $(A - V)_{O_2}$ of $30\,\mathrm{ml}\,\mathrm{l}^{-1}$, allows basal metabolism to proceed at its normal rate, $\sim250\,\mathrm{ml}$ $O_2\,\mathrm{min}^{-1}$.

The raised cardiac output is brought about by a **resting tachycardia** of up to $100\,\mathrm{min}^{-1}$, due to the withdrawal of vagal inhibition of the pacemaker (Figure 18.1). What drives vagal withdrawal is not entirely clear, since pacemaker hypoxia and the arterial chemoreflex cause bradycardia (Section 16.6); perhaps the cardiac vagal motor neurons are suppressed by the hyperactive inspiratory neurons (Figure 16.17).

Peripheral vasodilatation increases tissue perfusion

Arterial hypoxaemia causes dilatation of the systemic resistance vessels, particularly in the human coronary and splanchnic circulations (Figure 18.1). The resulting fall in peripheral resistance prevents systemic hypertension as cardiac output rises, and facilitates the increased peripheral perfusion. The hypoxaemic vasodilatation is mediated by adenosine and adrenaline. Vasodilatation is restrained by an increase in sympathetic vasomotor activity due to the arterial chemoreflex – as proved by enhanced hypoxic vasodilatation after α-adrenoceptor blockade. By contrast, the CO_2-sensitive cerebral vessels show little vasodilatation at altitude, because hyperventilation-induced hypocapnia has a counterbalancing vasoconstrictor effect (Figure 15.13).

Systemic arterial pressure falls; pulmonary arterial pressure rises

The hypoxic reduction of peripheral resistance outweighs the rise in cardiac output, so systemic arterial pressure falls (Figure 18.1). In the lungs, by contrast, pulmonary hypertension develops, due to the raised cardiac output and hypoxic pulmonary vasoconstriction (Section 15.5). Mean pulmonary artery pressure can double to $\sim30\,\mathrm{mmHg}$ at rest; and it trebled in one group of healthy mountaineers who climbed rapidly to $4560\,\mathrm{m}$. Pulmonary hypertension confers certain advantages, in that it improves apical perfusion in the upright position (Figure 15.20) and reduces ventilation–perfusion ratio inequality; but it is dangerous when prolonged, as in chronic emphysema or an extended stay at extreme altitude. The chronic increase in right ventricular workload, along with the negative inotropic effect of the hypoxaemia (Section 6.12), can lead to right ventricular failure.

Hypoxaemic exercise requires exaggerated cardiac outputs

During submaximal hypoxaemic exercise the cardiac output is higher than normal, for a given work rate and O_2 consumption. Blood flow to the active muscle is likewise higher than normal. During maximal hypoxaemic effort, however, the maximal heart rate and output are lower than at sea level, due to hypoxic depression of the pacemaker. Consequently, maximum O_2 transport rate $\dot{V}_{O_2\mathrm{max}}$ is reduced. This severely limits physical performance at high altitudes.

High altitude can cause mountain sickness and pulmonary oedema

Unacclimatized subjects who ascend too rapidly to $>3000\,\mathrm{m}$ ($10\,000\,\mathrm{ft}$) often experience **acute mountain sickness** after $8\text{–}24\,\mathrm{h}$. This is a cerebral disorder, comprising headache, dizziness, sweating, nausea, vomiting, sleeplessness and irritability. The symptoms are attributed to the effects of hypoxaemia and acute respiratory alkalosis (low P_{CO_2}) on cerebral neurons. Treatment includes descent to a lower altitude, supplementary O_2 and acetazolamide (to stimulate the renal excretion of bicarbonate, to counter the respiratory alkalosis). Severe cases receive the steroid dexamethasone, to reduce cerebral oedema.

Acute pulmonary oedema is distinct from acute mountain sickness. It can develop after a rapid ascent to high altitude, especially if the subject has a predisposing factor such as ischaemic heart disease. Pulmonary oedema is also common in climbers exposed for too long to extreme altitude.

Acclimatization to hypoxia follows chronic exposure

Slow, progressive exposure to moderately high altitudes over several days allows time for acclimatization and prevents acute mountain sickness. Acclimatization involves the following adaptations.

- There is a **further rise in resting hyperventilation**. This is traditionally attributed to correction of the respiratory alkalosis by the kidneys.

- The **O$_2$-carrying capacity of blood** is increased by a rise in the haematocrit, which can reach 0.6. The rise is due to increased bone marrow erythropoiesis, driven by renal erythropoietin. The attendant high viscosity increases the risk of a thrombo-embolic event such as a **high-altitude stroke**.
- The **haemoglobin dissociation curve** shifts to the right (Bohr shift, Figure 15.3), due to an increase in red cell 2,3-diphosphoglycerate. This improves O$_2$ unloading in the tissues.

18.2 Shock and haemorrhage

Clinical shock is acute circulatory failure

The term 'shock' is used by the medical profession and general public alike, but in very different senses. In general conversation, 'shock' means a psychological reaction to a traumatic experience, without organic pathology. Clinical shock, by contrast, is a **potentially fatal, pathophysiological disorder characterized by acute failure of the cardiovascular system to perfuse the tissues of the body adequately**. This results in the following characteristic signs:

- The skin is pale, cold, sweaty and venoconstricted.
- The pulse is rapid and weak, due to tachycardia and a reduced stroke volume.
- Mean arterial pressure may be reduced or normal, but pulse pressure is always reduced.
- Breathing is rapid and shallow.
- Urine output is reduced.
- There may be reduced mental awareness or confusion, muscular weakness and collapse.

Causes of clinical shock

These can be divided into four categories:

1 **Hypovolaemic shock** is caused by a fall in circulating blood or plasma volume, following haemorrhage, diarrhoea and vomiting, dehydration, extensive burns, crush injuries or pancreatitis.
2 **Cardiogenic shock** is caused by the acute impairment of cardiac function by myocardial infarction, myocarditis or an arrhythmia.
3 **Septic shock** is caused by cardiovascular toxins, such as endotoxin from a bacterial infection.
4 **Anaphylactic shock** is caused by an intense allergic reaction to antigens to which the patient has become sensitized, such as foodstuffs, insect bites, antibiotics.

Categories 1 and 2 are associated with a compensatory peripheral vasoconstriction, but categories 3 and 4 (septic and anaphylactic shock) show a loss of peripheral vascular tone. The pathophysiology thus varies to some degree. We will concentrate here on one of the commonest medical emergencies, namely acute haemorrhage leading to hypovolaemic shock.

Haemorrhagic shock triggers compensatory reflexes

A 10% blood loss (standard blood donation) is not a significant threat to the circulation. A rapid 20–30% blood loss causes clinical shock, but, given prompt treatment, is not usually life-threatening. A 30–40% blood loss reduces arterial pressure to 50–70 mmHg and causes severe, sometimes irreversible shock, with anuria and impaired cerebral and coronary perfusion.

The immediate effect of acute hypovolaemia is to reduce the central blood volume and thus the ventricular end-diastolic volume. This reduces the ventricular contractile energy through the **Frank–Starling mechanism**, so the stroke volume and pulse pressure decline. Note that the fall in arterial pressure is mediated by the Frank–Starling mechanism; it is in no way analogous to the loss of pressure in a punctured tyre!

Following the onset of hypovolaemia, reflexes are activated to maintain mean arterial pressure, and thus cerebral and myocardial perfusion. **Cardiopulmonary stretch receptor** and **arterial baroreceptor activity** decline (Figure 18.2). **Arterial chemoreceptor activity** increases, due partly to the metabolic acidosis caused by tissue underperfusion (Figure 18.3) and partly to reduced chemoreceptor perfusion (stagnant hypoxia). This drives the characteristic rapid breathing of shock.

The changes in afferent input to the nucleus tractus solitarius evokes a reflex increase in **sympathetic outflow** and **circulating vasoactive hormones** (adrenaline, noradrenaline, angiotensin II, vasopressin). If the blood loss is ≤20%, the increased neuroendocrine outflow can maintain mean arterial pressure at a near normal level (**compensated haemorrhage**). If the blood loss is >30%, however, a later phase of falling blood pressure can supervene (**decompensated haemorrhage**).

During compensated, non-hypotensive hypovolaemia, the body's defences operate over three time scales: rapid reflexes that take effect within seconds; intermediate responses that act over 5–60 min; and slow responses that act over days–weeks, as follows.

Figure 18.2 Single aortic baroreceptor fibre activity and aortic parameters before (left) and after (right) a slow, 20% blood volume loss in a dog. Pulse pressure fell (because stroke volume fell) but mean pressure was unchanged (compensated haemorrhage). The reduced baroreceptor activity is caused by the reduced pulse pressure and reduced aortic diameter (caused probably by catecholamines). (After Hartikainen, Ahonen, Nevalaines, Sikanen, Hakumaki. *Acta Physiologica Scandinavica* 1990; **140**: 181–90, with permission from Wiley-Blackwell.)

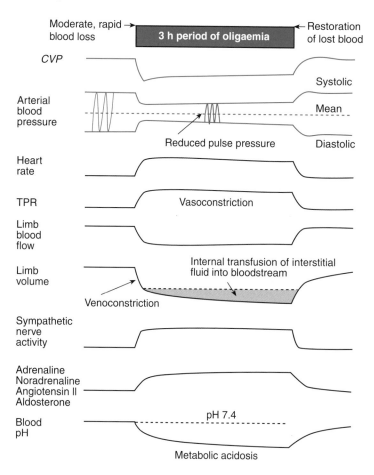

Figure 18.3 Compensated haemorrhage (blood loss <20%). Pulse pressure falls but mean blood pressure is preserved by tachycardia and peripheral vasoconstriction. The rapid, initial fall in limb volume is caused by venoconstriction; the slow fall (pink area) is caused by transcapillary absorption of interstitial fluid into circulation. A more severe blood loss reduces mean arterial pressure (decompensated phase). (Adapted from Chien S. *Physiological Reviews* 1967; **47**: 214–88, with permission from the American Physiological Society; Jacobsen J, Sofelt S, Sheikh S, Warberg J, Secher NH. *Acta Physiologica Scandinavica* 1990; **138**: 167–73, with permission from Wiley-Blackwell; and Länne T, Lundvall J. *Acta Physiologica Scandinavica* 1992; **146**: 299–306, with permission from Wiley-Blackwell.)

Rapid neurohumoral reflexes provide immediate support for the blood pressure

The reflex increase in sympathetic vasoconstrictor activity raises **vascular resistance** in the cutaneous, skeletal muscle, splanchnic and renal circulations. This provides immediate support to the arterial pressure. However, the **reduced tissue perfusion** also causes muscular weakness, lactic acidosis, oliguria (low urine flow) and skin pallor. Increased sympathetic cholinergic discharge to the skin causes sweating – hence the characteristic cold, clammy skin. In severe shock, white cell adhesion in microvessels contributes further to the poor tissue perfusion.

Sympathetic-mediated **venoconstriction** in the splanchnic and cutaneous circulations partially restores the thoracic blood volume and cardiac filling pressure. It also increases the difficulty of cannulating a vein for intravenous fluid replacement. Filling pressure remains subnormal despite the venoconstriction, so stroke volume remains low. The effect of this on cardiac output is partly counteracted by a reflex, sympathetic-mediated **tachycardia**.

The sympathetic-mediated vasoconstriction is reinforced by increased levels of **circulating vasoconstrictor hormones** (adrenaline, noradrenaline, angiotensin II, vasopressin). Catecholamine and angiotensin II levels increase substantially during compensated, normotensive haemorrhage. **Angiotensin II** contributes to peripheral vasoconstriction by both peripheral and central actions (Section 14.8), and accounts for ~30% of the initial recovery of arterial pressure in venesected dogs. **Vasopressin** only reaches high enough levels to cause vasoconstriction during severe, hypotensive haemorrhage (Figure 14.11).

Due to the increased peripheral resistance, reduced peripheral venous capacitance and increased cardiac performance, mean arterial pressure may be well maintained after a moderate haemorrhage. Consequently, **mean arterial pressure is not a reliable index of blood loss**.

Absorption by capillaries causes a slow, internal fluid transfusion

The fall in venous pressure, coupled with the sympathetic-mediated rise in pre- to postcapillary resistance ratio R_A/R_V, lowers capillary blood pressure (Figure 11.4). This enables plasma colloid osmotic pressure (COP) to establish a net absorption force across the capillary wall (Figure 11.11b). Consequently, there is a slow **absorption of interstitial fluid** into the depleted circulation, called the 'internal transfusion'. There is also increased lymphatic pumping. Up to 500 ml fluid can be transferred into the human circulation within an hour. This partially restores the depleted plasma volume and produces haemodilution. Consequently, haemorrhagic patients generally have a **reduced haematocrit** by the time they reach hospital. Although this reduces the O_2-carrying capacity of blood, it also reduces its viscosity, and thus improves tissue perfusion. The internal transfusion ceases within an hour, due to the attendant fall in interstitial fluid pressure, rise in interstitial COP and fall in plasma COP (haemodilution) (Figure 11.11c).

The transfusion of interstitial fluid into the circulation is helped by fluid translocation from the much bigger **intracellular fluid compartment** into the interstitial compartment. Circulating adrenaline and glucagon stimulate hepatic glycogenolysis, which increases glucose concentration and extracellular fluid osmolarity by up to 20 milliosmolar. This draws fluid osmotically from the large intracellular compartment into the smaller interstitial compartment, allowing capillary absorption to continue for 30–60 min. It is estimated that about half of the internal transfusion comes, indirectly, from the intracellular compartment.

Long-term renal and biosynthetic responses restore blood volume

The above responses preserve cardiac and cerebral perfusion over the short term in compensated shock. Over the following days–weeks the lost water, salts, plasma proteins and red cells are gradually made good. First the water and salt deficit is corrected through increased fluid intake and reduced renal excretion. **Glomerular filtration rate** is reduced by a sympathetic-mediated contraction of the afferent arterioles. **Salt and water reabsorption** are stimulated by circulating aldosterone and vasopressin. Circulating angiotensin II stimulates not only aldosterone secretion but also **thirst,** by activating the subfornical organ of the brain. The increase in water intake, coupled with oliguria, quickly replenishes body water mass. The normal dietary intake of 2–10 g salt per day, along with renal salt retention, restores body salt mass in a few days.

Albumin synthesis by the liver gradually restores the plasma protein mass over a week or so. **Red cell production** by the bone marrow is stimulated by erythropoietin secreted by the kidney. Erythropoiesis restores the haematocrit to normal in a few weeks, given an adequate dietary iron intake.

Decompensated (hypotensive) shock leads to organ failure

The above account describes reversible, compensated shock. If the blood loss is >30% and external fluid transfusion is delayed >3–4 h, shock enters a second, decompensated stage, which is often irreversible despite subsequent blood transfusion. In this phase, the arterial pressure falls, leading to myocardial under-perfusion and possibly death. The 'golden hour' for transfusion is thus soon after the initial haemorrhage.

Figure 18.4 ECG recorded during a faint (vasovagal attack) in a healthy medical student. The student had received the vasodilator nitroglycerine and was then tilted from supine to upright. There was a period of 8 s asystole during the faint. The wobbly baseline is a movement artefact.

The collapse of blood pressure in the decompensated phase is due primarily to a **fall in peripheral resistance** (except in skin), caused by reduced sympathetic vasoconstrictor outflow. The latter may be triggered by a central **depressor opioid pathway**. Endogenous opioids (enkephalins, β-endorphins) acting on δ and κ opiate receptors may depress the medullary vasopressor region. In support of this hypothesis, the administration of the opioid antagonist **naloxone** into the fourth ventricle of the brain helps to restore the sympathetic outflow and prevent decompensation.

As arterial pressure falls, the attendant fall in coronary perfusion and increasing metabolic acidosis impair myocardial contractility. This reduces cardiac output, which further reduces arterial pressure and coronary perfusion. Thus **acute cardiac failure** sets in and establishes a deleterious **positive feedback loop**.

Decompensated shock can damage the kidneys, heart and other organs. Ischaemic damage to the renal tubules, called **acute tubular necrosis,** can cause acute renal failure; so urine output is monitored closely. In patients with pre-existing ischaemic heart disease, **myocardial infarction** can be precipitated by the reduced coronary pressure and **increased blood coagulability**. The latter can create numerous micro-thrombi in small vessels, which further impairs tissue perfusion. **Acute cardiac failure** may develop even without pre-existing coronary disease, due to the low perfusion pressure, micro-thrombi and white cell adhesion in microvessels. The condition can progress to **multi-organ failure** in severe cases.

18.3 Fainting (syncope)

Syncope is a sudden, transient loss of consciousness resulting from an abrupt fall in arterial pressure, sufficient to halve cerebral blood flow. The critical, mean cerebral artery pressure is ~40 mmHg, which corresponds to ~70 mmHg at heart level during orthostasis. Fainting can be initiated by haemodynamic stresses, such as severe hypovolaemia, postural hypotension (Figure 18.4), paroxysmal coughing (impaired venous return to thorax) or exercise combined with aortic valve stenosis (Clinical case 5). Fainting can also be triggered by emotional stress, such as fear, pain or horror (Figure 18.5). The sight of blood, especially one's own, often induces emotional fainting in young adults. Fainting occurs almost exclusively when upright, i.e. it requires a low CVP, so a person feeling faint should be advised to lie down.

Psychogenic, emotional fainting (the 'swoon' of Victorian novels) is usually preceded by the alerting response (tachycardia, muscle vasodilatation, cutaneous vasoconstriction, sweating). During this pre-faint period, the subject looks pale and sweaty, hyperventilates and, very characteristically, yawns. Then a sudden increase in vagal outflow causes **a profound bradycardia**; in the medical student of Figure 18.4, for example, there was no heartbeat for 8 seconds. The bradycardia is accompanied by a sudden **peripheral vasodilatation,** due to an abrupt fall in peripheral sympathetic vasoconstrictor activity. As a result, mean arterial pressure falls precipitously (Figure 18.5), cerebral perfusion falls below the autoregulation range, and loss of consciousness follows within seconds.

The above sequence is sometimes called a '**vasovagal attack**'. The pathways that cause the sudden changes in vasomotor and vagal activity are not clear, but the brainstem **depressor opioid pathway** may be involved (Section 18.2). Psychogenic fainting is thought to be related to the 'playing dead' response of small animals, which emanates from the cingulate gyrus (Section 16.8). Orthostatic and posthaemorrhagic syncope used to be attributed to a reflex from ventricular mechanoreceptors in a near-empty heart; but recent echocardiography shows no pre-syncopal fall in cardiac volume; moreover, fainting can occur in cardiac transplant patients with denervated ventricles.

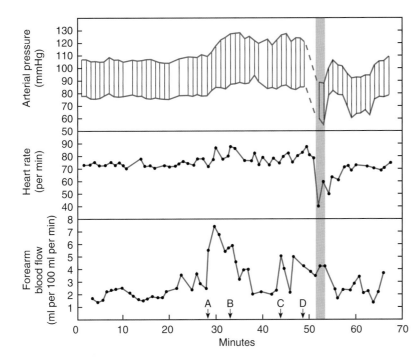

Figure 18.5 Circulatory changes in a male student during an emotional faint. The student showed forearm vasodilatation (alarm response) while watching the preparation for venepuncture (A) and the venepuncture of a colleague (B) – but did not faint as the experimenter intended. Insertion of a needle into his arm (C) again produced vasodilatation, but no faint. The subject was therefore asked to drink some of the blood taken from his colleague (D). He became pale, yawned, said 'I'm going' and fainted (tinted area). No heart beat was detected by ECG for 11 s and heart rate then averaged 37 min⁻¹. Forearm blood flow remained above resting level despite the slump in blood pressure, showing that vasodilatation had occurred. Consciousness was regained after 2 min. (From Greenfield ADM. *The Lancet* 1951; 1303, with permission from Elsevier.)

Recovery. The patient should not be propped up, because the collapsed, supine position raises the intrathoracic blood volume and filling pressure, which increases the stroke volume by the Frank–Starling mechanism. As the bradycardia fades and vascular tone returns, cardiac output and arterial pressure are restored. Consciousness is regained in ~2 min.

18.4 Hypertension

What exactly is hypertension?

Clinical hypertension is the commonest chronic disease, affecting an estimated billion individuals worldwide. It might be defined, simplistically, as a chronic, usually progressive, raised arterial blood pressure – but this begs the question 'how high does the pressure have to be to be deemed "raised"?' This is a non-trivial problem, because arterial pressure is distributed unimodally across the population. A pragmatic, partial solution is to adopt a clinical criterion, namely evidence of substantial, treatable harm. Clinical hypertension is therefore **defined** as a rise in arterial blood pressure sufficient to raise the incidence of strokes, myocardial infarction, heart failure and renal failure. On this basis, hypertension is diagnosed when repeated measurements of resting brachial artery pressure exceed 140/90 mmHg in a patient under 50 years old, or 160/95 mmHg in

older patients. Hypertension thus defined is associated with ~7 million early deaths per year worldwide, from heart disease and strokes. The relation between blood pressure and disease, however, is a continuous one; so humans with a systolic pressure of 130 mmHg, although not formally hypertensive, have a demonstrably higher risk of cardiac disease and strokes than humans with a systolic pressure of 120 mmHg. In England the prevalence of pressures above 140/90 mmHg in 1998 was 4% and 16% at age 16–24 years (females and males respectively), rising to 78% and 74% at 75 years.

Classification of clinical hypertension

Essential or **primary hypertension** is hypertension without an obvious predisposing organic cause. It was called 'essential' because it was thought that the rise in pressure was essential to maintain tissue perfusion. Essential hypertension follows one of two courses. **Benign essential hypertension** is the usual form. Being almost symptomless, it generally comes to light though a routine check-up. Otherwise, it may present much later through its serious consequences (heart disease, renal failure, strokes). Predisposing factors include high dietary salt intake, obesity, excessive alcohol consumption, stress and lack of exercise. In the rarer **malignant hypertension**, pressure increases rapidly, leading to cardiac failure, peripheral oedema, renal damage with proteinuria, hypertensive encephalopathy (brain oedema, papilloedema) and hypertensive retinopathy.

Secondary hypertension has an identifiable pathological cause and is uncommon, except for pre-eclamptic toxaemia.

- **Pre-eclamptic toxaemia** is a brachial artery blood pressure of ≥140/90 mmHg during pregnancy, with a proteinuria of >0.3 g/day, resolving post-partum. It occurs in the third trimester of 2–6% of pregnancies. Failure of the placental spiral arteries to dilate normally results in placental ischaemia and the release of toxins into the maternal circulation. The toxins impair endothelial NO and prostacyclin production, and raise circulating endothelin, leading to peripheral vasoconstriction, reduced renal excretion and hypertension. Untreated, the hypertension may progress rapidly and cause cerebral oedema and fits (eclampsia).

- In **primary hyperaldosteronism** (Conn's syndrome), excessive secretion of aldosterone by an adrenal tumour stimulates renal salt and water retention, leading to hypertension (Figure 16.12). Excessive adrenal glucocorticoid secretion (Cushing's disease) can likewise cause hypertension.

- **Renal artery stenosis** and certain other renal diseases activate the renin–angiotensin–aldosterone (RAA) system, leading to hypertension (Figure 16.12).

- A **phaeochromocytoma** is a rare, catecholamine-secreting tumour, usually in the adrenal medulla. Vascular α-adrenoceptor activation causes the hypertension.

In ~95% of non-pregnant hypertensives no organic cause is found and the disorder is classed as essential hypertension. The changes in arterial pressure arise from pathological alteration in the walls of both **small arterial resistance vessels** and **large elastic vessels**, as follows.

Small artery narrowing raises peripheral resistance and mean arterial pressure

Mean arterial blood pressure equals cardiac output × peripheral resistance (Section 8.5). In the earliest stage of the disease, when the hypertension is marginal and labile, the cardiac output is raised and the peripheral resistance is only slightly above normal. In established hypertension, however, the cardiac output is normal or slightly reduced, so the elevated mean pressure must be caused by a rise in peripheral resistance (Figure 18.6). Vascular resistance

Figure 18.6 Changes in resistance vessels of the hand in hypertensive patients (red) relative to normal subjects (grey). (*Upper panel*) In the hypertensive patients, vascular resistance is raised at rest and after maximum vasodilatation; and the vasoconstrictor response to noradrenaline is increased. (Results of Sivertsson R, Olander B. *Life Science* 1968; **7**: 1291–7.) (*Lower panel*) Hypertension narrows the lumen and increases the wall thickness of human gluteal and subcutaneous small arteries. This is inward eutrophic remodelling – total wall area is unchanged. The changes were reversed by ACE inhibitors, but not by β-blockers. (Results of Thybo NK, Stephens N, Cooper A, Aalkjaer C, Heagerty AM, Mulvany MJ. *Hypertension* 1995; **25**: 474–81.)

increases in virtually every organ, including the kidney, due to a narrowing of the small resistance arteries and rarefaction.

Rarefaction, a reduction in the number of vessels per unit tissue volume, has been demonstrated in the retina, skin and intestine. In the skin the capillary density falls by ~21% in established hypertension.

The core feature of hypertension, however, is a **narrowing of proximal resistance arteries**. This is visible in retinal vessels as 'silver wiring'. In the early stages the narrowing is caused by an increase in vascular tone, and is fully reversible by vasodilator drugs. As time passes, however, the structure of the tunica media changes. In mild hypertension a rearrangement of the vascular myocytes, along with a modest increase in extracellular matrix, narrows the lumen by ~10%, with little change in wall area (**inward eutrophic remodelling;** little hypertrophy). The ratio of wall thickness to internal radius increases by around 30%. Even maximal vasodilatation now fails to rectify the abnormal resistance (Figure 18.6). In severe human hypertension (and hypertensive rats), there is also hypertrophy of the vascular myocytes, which increases the vascular wall area. The wall changes are thought to be triggered by increases in wall stress, angiotensin II and plasma Na^+. Angiotensin II is not only a vaso-constrictor agent but also a growth factor, stimulating vascular hypertrophy (increased cell size) and hyper-plasia (increased cell numbers). When the RAA sys-tem is stimulated by clipping a rat renal artery, the tunica media throughout the body remodels and hypertrophies in days–weeks.

The **baroreflex** remains functional in hyperten-sive patients, but its sensitivity is reduced by the stiffening of the artery wall, and it operates around a higher set point due to peripheral resetting (Section 16.2). It is accepted that the baroreflex changes are a consequence of the hypertension, not a cause.

Large artery stiffening exacerbates systolic hypertension

Although small artery narrowing is the primary pathology, secondary changes in the large, elastic arteries exacerbate the rise in systolic pressure and pulse pressure. This is important, because morbidity and mortality correlate more closely with **systolic hypertension** than diastolic hypertension. The elastic arteries show elastin fragmentation, dilatation and increased wall stiffness (reduced compliance) – the picture is, in effect, one of **accelerated ageing** (Section 17.7). The structural deterioration raises systolic pressure through two effects.

- **Arterial stiffness** (elastance) is increased; com-pliance is reduced. Since pulse pressure depends on stroke volume $\times$ elastance, a rise in elastance raises the pulse pressure (Figure 18.7). Conse-quently, systolic pressure increases much more than diastolic pressure.
- **Pulse wave velocity** increases due to the increased wall stiffness (Section 8.4). Conse-quently, the reflected wave arrives back in the ascending aorta at an earlier time (Figure 8.10c). Moreover, the degree of reflection is enhanced by the raised peripheral resistance. The early return of a bigger reflected pressure wave greatly augments the original or 'incident' systolic pres-sure wave (Figure 18.8). This **systolic aug-mentation** can add as much as 50 mmHg to the systolic pressure in a hypertensive patient.

Aortic systolic hypertension is thus the product of three biophysical mechanisms, namely an increase in peripheral resistance, a fall in central artery com-pliance and the rapid return of a larger, reflected

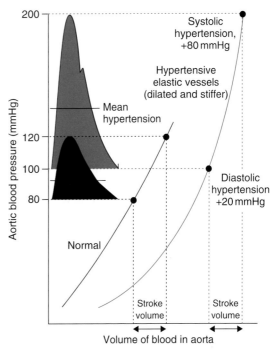

Figure 18.7 Increased stiffness of elastic vessels contributes to systolic hypertension. The central elastic arteries are dilated, because elastin fragments with ageing and hypertension. They are stiffer (steeper slope) due to collagen deposition and stress at the raised pressure. The same stroke volume causes a bigger pulse pressure and systolic pressure, due to the increased slope (elastance, 1/compliance). Diastolic pressure was raised 20 mmHg by increased peripheral resistance, but systolic pres-sure increased by 80 mmHg, due to the reduced compliance, even neglecting augmentation by wave reflection. (Based on Nichols WW, O'Rourke MF. *McDonald's Blood Flow in Arteries*. London: Arnold, 2005.)

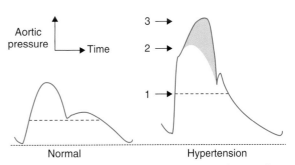

Figure 18.8 Changes in the aortic pressure wave in hypertension. Arrow 1 and dashed lines show the increase in mean pressure, caused by the increased resistance of small arterial vessels. Arrow 2 highlights the effect of reduced aortic compliance, namely a dis-proportionate increase in the systolic incident wave (clear area). Arrow 3 shows the augmentation of pressure in late systole by the early return of a large reflected wave (pink area). Augmentation can account for as much as half the systolic hypertension. (Based on Nichols WW, O'Rourke MF. *McDonald's Blood Flow in Arteries*. London: Arnold, 2005.)

pressure wave. The first two mechanisms increase the incident wave (Figure 18.7) and the third increases the degree of systolic augmentation by wave reflection (Figure 18.8).

The left ventricular wall hypertrophies and may fail eventually

The high systolic pressure increases the work of the left ventricle, leading to **concentric hypertrophy** (as with strength training, Section 17.4). The addition of sarcomeres in parallel within the cardiac myocytes can increase ventricular wall thickness (w) up to about three-fold. This normalizes the stress S on the individual cardiac myocyte, since by Laplace's law $S = (P/2w) \times$ radius (eqn 6.2), where P is systolic pressure (afterload). Hypertrophy thus enables the ventricle to maintain a normal ejection fraction, despite the increased systolic pressure (afterload). The hypertrophy may be driven by wall stress, angiotensin II and possibly plasma Na^+ changes (see below).

Eventually, however, the left ventricle begins to fail (**decompensated hypertrophy**). The cardiac myocytes begin to degenerate and die by necrosis and apoptosis, possibly because the increased diffusion distance into the thickened myocytes causes intracellular hypoxia. The loss of myocytes leads to a dilated cardiomyopathy. As ventricle radius increases and w decreases, wall stress S increases (Laplace's law), which exacerbates the myocyte death rate. This is one of several reasons for treating systolic hypertension. ACE inhibitors and calcium channel blockers are particularly effective at reducing hypertensive left ventricle hypertrophy.

What initiates the resistance vessel pathology?

The answer to this key question remains incomplete, but both genetic and environmental factors are involved. Impaired renal salt handling (possibly genetic), coupled with a high dietary salt intake (environmental) is pivotal in many patients.

Genetic factors account for distinct familial and racial tendencies towards hypertension. For example, blood pressure correlates better between monozygotic twins than adopted siblings; the response of blood pressure to a standard intravenous or dietary salt load reveals salt-sensitive families; and hypertension is commoner in black than white humans. Only rarely is a single gene defect responsible, e.g. the renal Na^+ channel gene in Liddle's syndrome. Generally, multiple genes are implicated.

Most of the hypertension-susceptibility genes identified to date, such as angiotensinogen and ACE gene variants, affect renal Na^+ handling. We may have protective genes too; a gain-of-function mutation in the human vascular smooth muscle BK_{Ca} channel promotes hyperpolarization and vasorelaxation, and is associated with a reduced incidence of hypertension. About 30–60% of blood pressure variation is estimated to be genetic (cf. environmental).

Environmental factors. Both epidemiological and direct, interventional studies show a link between hypertension and **high dietary NaCl intake, low dietary K^+, obesity, stress** and **alcohol consumption**. This has led to a number of causative theories, amongst which high dietary salt intake and impaired renal salt handling are pivotal.

Salt imbalance renal hypothesis

High salt intake. The natural diet of primates is low in salt (NaCl) and rich in K^+, so the kidney has evolved powerful Na^+-retaining mechanisms. The salt hypothesis proposes that a small but sustained discrepancy between the high, modern dietary Na^+ intake and renal Na^+ excretion raises the body salt mass, which then causes hypertension through multiple mechanisms (see later). Epidemiological studies and direct, interventional studies of humans, primates, dogs and rats show a strong association between a high-salt diet ($>10\,g/day$) and hypertension. Salt-sensitivity evidently has a genetic component, since it often runs in families; and the salt-sensitive Dahl strain of rats develops hypertension on a salt intake that is harmless to ordinary rats.

Low K^+ intake. Hypertension correlates even better with the dietary Na:K ratio than with salt intake *per se*. The ratio is >2.5 for a typical Western diet (e.g. ham, 8). Given a fixed daily salt intake, K^+ supplementation by fruit and vegetables (Na:K ~0) lowers blood pressure. Conversely, reducing the K^+ intake raises blood pressure, because it promotes renal tubular Na^+ reabsorption.

How does salt overload cause hypertension? Plasma $[Na^+]$ increases by $\sim2\,mM$ in hypertensive patients. The **cardiac hypothesis** proposes that an increase in salt mass, acting via the central osmoreceptor–ADH pathway and thirst centre, raises the extracellular fluid volume at an early stage (Figure 16.12). The attendant rise in the plasma volume increases the cardiac filling pressure, stroke volume and arterial blood pressure, which in turn provokes tunica media remodelling and a rise in peripheral resistance.

However, contrary to the cardiac hypothesis, extracellular fluid volume and plasma volume are not consistently raised in hypertensives – so researchers have sought additional mechanisms. There is some evidence that a small, chronic increase in plasma $[Na^+]$ directly affects vascular tone and remodelling. Also, a high Na^+ intake stimulates the adrenal cortex and brain to release a steroidal, **endogenous digitalis-like factor** (ouabain, or its stereoisomer). Circulating digitalis-like factor is raised in 40–50% of hypertensives, and its action is to inhibit the electrogenic $3Na^+–2K^+$ pump of vascular myocytes (Figure 12.5). The resulting partial depolarization increases the L-type Ca^{2+} channel open probability; and the rise in intracellular $[Na^+]$ reduces Ca^{2+} expulsion by the $3Na^+–Ca^{2+}$ exchanger. Consequently, intracellular Ca^{2+} increases, raising vascular tone.

What causes the kidneys to retain too much salt? Normally, a high Na^+ intake triggers a fall in circulating renin – angiotensin II – aldosterone (Figure 14.12). This reduces distal tubular Na^+ and water reabsorption, and thus maintains Na^+ balance. What disturbs renal Na^+ regulation in hypertension? (i) **High RAA subgroup.** A subgroup of hypertensives (particularly white patients under 55) have raised RAA levels. This presumably explains the renal salt retention in these individuals. (ii) **Renal defect subgroup.** Not all hypertensives have raised RAA levels and ~25% have low renin levels. Excessive renal Na^+ reabsorption in such cases may be due to an acquired dysfunction or genes encoding renal ion channels and transporters. In keeping with the renal defect hypothesis, normal rats develop hypertension when transplanted with kidneys from spontaneously hypertensive rats with narrow afferent renal arterioles.

Endothelin can contribute to hypertension

Endothelin levels are high in pre-eclamptic toxaemia, but are generally only slightly raised in essential hypertension, though a subgroup of severe hypertensives over-express the endothelin-1 gene in subcutaneous small arteries. The endothelin receptor blocker bosentan reduces blood pressure by ~5 mmHg in patients with essential or pulmonary hypertension.

Neurogenic or stress hypothesis

The neurogenic hypothesis proposes that an exaggerated alerting response causes an excessive sympathetic outflow in response to stress, causing bouts of reversible hypertension. These repeated periods of hypertension induce remodelling of small vessel walls, which perpetuates the hypertension. In support, the repeated exposure of laboratory animals to psychogenic stress can indeed cause chronic hypertension; and increasing the sympathetic outflow by experimental lesions of the nucleus tractus solitarius leads to chronic hypertension. Also, recordings of sympathetic activity in mixed peripheral nerves show elevated activity in many human hypertensives.

Multifactorial hypothesis

The long-term regulation of blood pressure involves complex interactions between dietary, neural, hormonal and renal mechanisms (Section 16.5), and hypertension may only develop when one or more of the regulatory processes is disturbed in a genetically susceptible individual. Whatever the initial cause, the process is self-perpetuating once media remodelling develops; a rise in arterial pressure evokes media remodelling/hypertrophy, which normalizes the wall stress but raises the resistance and arterial pressure, which evokes further wall changes, and so on.

Clinical sequelae and therapeutic strategies

Hypertension itself is virtually symptomless; contrary to popular belief, it rarely presents with nose bleeds or headaches. Untreated, however, hypertension (and especially systolic hypertension) damages the heart, brain, retina and kidneys, leading to:

- hypertensive heart failure;
- coronary artery atheroma and myocardial infarction;
- cerebrovascular accidents (strokes);
- hypertensive retinopathy;
- chronic renal failure.

It is important, therefore, to treat hypertension. Six types of lifestyle change have been shown to reduce blood pressure, namely reduction of dietary salt to 5 g daily (-4 mmHg), increased fruit and vegetable intake (-5 mmHg at 7 portions/day), reduction of obesity (-2 mmHg per kg lost), reduction of fat intake, limitation of alcohol consumption, and $\geqslant 30$ min dynamic exercise three times per week. Further reduction is achieved through a graded pharmacological approach, the **A–C–D** regime.

- **'A'. ACE inhibitors/Angiotensin receptor blockers.** Captopril, enalapril and ramipril block angiotensin-converting enzyme (ACE) and therefore reduce the circulating levels of angiotensin II and aldosterone. This reduces vascular tone and extracellular fluid volume. A common side effect is a dry cough, due to the concurrent inhibition of bradykinin breakdown. Losartan and valsartan block the AT_1 receptor and avoid the above side effect. Aliskiren binds to and inhibits renin. RAA inhibitors are the first choice treatment for white patients under 55, because this subgroup often has high renin levels.

- **'C'. Calcium-channel blockers** (nifedipine, amlodipine) are peripheral vasodilators and thus lower the peripheral resistance. Alpha$_1$-adrenoreceptor inhibitors (prazosin, long-acting doxazosin) reduce sympathetic vasoconstrictor tone, but this often results in postural hypotension, so they are used less often. Either calcium blockers (C) or diuretics (D) are the recommended initial treatment for white patients over 55 and all black patients.
- **'D'. Diuretics.** Thiazide diuretics (e.g. bendrofluazide) reduce the extracellular fluid volume and have a poorly explained vasodilator action. If treatment A or C/D proves inadequate, the next stage is A+C/D, followed if necessary by A+C+D. The remaining major anti-hypertensive drugs, used less frequently these days, are the β-blockers.
- **Beta-adrenoceptor blockers** (propranolol, atenolol, metoprolol) reduce the cardiac output, so are not ideal in those over 55. They also reduce the sympathetic outflow and the activation of the juxtaglomerular apparatus (renin secretion), leading to a gradual lowering of blood pressure over several days.

The aim is to reduce systolic pressure to 135–145 mmHg and diastolic pressure to 85 mmHg. This reduces the incidence of strokes by 38% and cardiovascular deaths by 21%. Untreated, ~50% of patients develop heart failure, 25% renal failure and 25% cerebral complications (retinopathy, encephalopathy, strokes).

18.5 Chronic cardiac failure

Chronic or congestive cardiac failure (CCF) is a chronic inability of the heart to maintain adequate tissue perfusion at a normal filling pressure. Starling, working with the isolated heart–lung preparation, observed that when the heart begins to fail, it requires a higher filling pressure and higher end-diastolic volume to maintain its stroke volume (Figure 18.9). At a normal filling pressure, the stroke

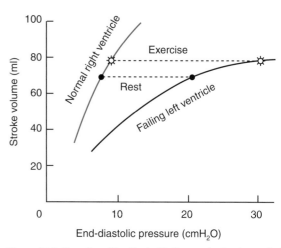

Figure 18.9 Operation of the Frank–Starling mechanism in a patient with a failing left ventricle but still normal right ventricle. The left ventricle function curve is depressed. Under resting conditions (filled circles), the left ventricle requires an elevated filling pressure to match the right ventricle stroke volume. During exercise (open symbols), the disparity in filling pressure becomes extreme owing to the near-plateau on the function curve of the failing left ventricle. The attendant pulmonary congestion will cause severe exertional dyspnoea.

volume would decline. Thus the immediate cause of cardiac failure is a fall in the energy of contraction at a given end-diastolic volume (preload). In other words, **cardiac failure is an abnormal fall in myocardial contractility**.

Causes & clinical course

In many but not all patients, a recognizable pathology initiates the cardiac failure. The commonest **causes of chronic left ventricular failure** are (i) diffuse coronary artery disease, (ii) reduced myocardial mass due to an infarct (two-thirds of cases have a history of ischaemic heart disease), (iii) excessive work (afterload) due to clinical hypertension or aortic valve disease and (iv) cardiomyopathy. (v) Cardiac failure in the elderly, not attributable to the above causes, is thought to be an idiopathic myopathy, arising from myocytes senescence and death.

The commonest **causes of chronic right ventricular failure** are (i) pulmonary hypertension due to chronic lung disease or high altitude and (ii) left ventricular failure, which increases the pressure work of the right ventricle. Biventricular failure is therefore common.

The clinical features of left and right ventricular failure are summarized in Table 18.1. The commonest presenting features are **exercise intolerance**, i.e. excessive fatigue during moderate exercise; or **breathlessness (dyspnoea),** especially on lying down (orthopnoea) and at night (nocturnal

Table 18.1 Characteristic signs and symptoms of chronic left- or right-sided heart failure[a]

Left ventricular failure	Right ventricular failure
Shortness of breath (dyspnoea)	Oedematous swelling of feet, ankles and legs (sacrum if bed-bound)
Orthopnoea (dyspnoea on lying down)	Hepatomegaly (enlarged, palpable, tender liver)
Paroxysmal nocturnal dyspnoea	Ascites (fluid in abdominal cavity)
Pulmonary congestion and oedema (crackles)	Excessive nocturnal urination (caused by oedema fluid excretion)
Exercise intolerance	Raised jugular venous pressure (JVP)
	Exercise intolerance

[a]It is common for both left and right ventricular failure to co-exist. Additional diagnostic signs include a laterally displaced, weak apex beat and chest X-ray abnormalities, such as a cardiothoracic ratio of >0.5.

dyspnoea), due to left ventricular failure; or **ankle swelling** (peripheral oedema), due to right ventricular failure. The mortality rate is 50% over 5 years, and the cause of death is usually **pump failure** or **ventricular arrhythmia**. The cellular basis of the pump failure and arrhythmia is described next, followed by the pathophysiological changes in the heart and circulation.

Reduced Ca^{2+} transients impair contractility

Cardiac myocytes from failing ventricles show multiple transporter and channel abnormalities, namely:

- reduced Ca^{2+} pumping into the sarcoplasmic reticulum (SR);
- impaired, leaky SR Ca^{2+} release channels (ryanodine receptors);
- upregulation of the sarcolemmal Na^+-Ca^{2+} exchanger;
- downregulation of K^+ channels (inward rectifier, K_{ir}; transient outward current (i_{to}), $K_v4.3$).

Systolic contractile failure arises primarily from the first two of these cellular abnormalities, as follows.

The reduced contractility of failing myocytes is due primarily to a **reduced, slow, systolic Ca^{2+} transient**. This is caused by a fall in the size of the SR Ca^{2+} store, and probably impaired Ca^{2+} release too (Figure 18.10). The fall in store size is the result of a reduced expression and activity of the SR Ca^{2+} pumps, exacerbated by a diastolic leak of Ca^{2+} out of altered Ca^{2+} release channels. The diastolic Ca^{2+} leak, coupled with slow Ca^{2+} reuptake in early diastole by the reduced SR pump, impairs diastolic relaxation. The failing ventricle thus displays diastolic dysfunction (stiffness), as well as systolic dysfunction. The slow diastolic relaxation impairs ventricular filling and is sometimes called '**diastolic failure**'.

Several additional factors contribute to the systolic dysfunction, namely a fall in the sensitivity of

troponin to Ca^{2+}, wall fibrosis, dilatation (see later) and, in severe failure, impaired energy supply. Creatine kinase, which transfers high energy phosphate from creatine phosphate to ADP to maintain ATP availability, declines not only in the myocardium but also in the skeletal muscles – a factor that may contribute to the characteristic exercise intolerance. In advanced failure there is a switch from fatty acids to glucose as the chief energy substrate.

Multiple electrophysiological abnormalities cause arrhythmia

Ventricular arrhythmia is a common cause of death in cardiac failure patients. Ventricular arrhythmia is often triggered by a **delayed afterdepolarization** (DAD, Figure 3.16). DADs occur when the SR Ca^{2+} store discharges spontaneously during diastole, stimulating the depolarizing $3Na^+$–Ca^{2+} exchanger current, $i_{Na–Ca}$ (Section 3.10). Due to the **upregulation of the Na^+–Ca^{2+} exchanger** (more inward, depolarizing current) and **downregulation of the inward rectifier K^+ channel** (less outward, polarizing current), a relatively modest SR Ca^{2+} discharge can generate a DAD of sufficient size to trigger an action potential and arrhythmia. The SR discharge in diastole may be the result of Ca^{2+} overload (driven by the raised **sympathetic activity of** heart failure) and leakiness of the Ca^{2+} release channels due to channel phosphorylation. Excessive sympathetic activity is a prominent feature of moderate heart failure and predisposes to arrhythmia. Consequently, β-blockers can reduce the risk of arrhythmia in moderate heart failure. In the later stages of failure, myocardial responsiveness to $β_1$ stimulation deteriorates, so arrhythmias become less common.

Another pro-arrhythmogenic change is **action potential prolongation** in severe failure (Figure 18.10). This is caused by the **downregulation of $K_v4.3$ channels**, which carry the early

Figure 18.10 Changes in cardiac myocyte Ca^{2+} cycle, ionic currents and action potential in chronic heart failure. Dashed line is normal action potential. CICR, calcium-induced calcium release (Section 3.7). (Based on information in Sipido KR, Eisner D. *Cardiovascular Research* 2005; **68**: 167–74; and Bers DM. *Physiology* 2006; **21**: 380–7).

repolarizing current i_{to}. The delayed rectifier (K_v) is often downregulated too. Repolarization depends on the outward K^+ currents exceeding the (increased) inward current i_{Na-Ca}; so the plateau is prolonged. This is seen as an increased QT interval in the ECG. The lengthening of the plateau, and hence the refractory period, is greater in some myocytes than others. This heterogeneity increases the likelihood of **re-entry circuits** developing, and hence ventricular tachycardia or fibrillation (Figure 5.10).

To summarize, the upregulation of the Na^+–Ca^{2+} exchanger and the heterogeneous downregulation of K^+ channels contribute to the high incidence of arrhythmia in failing hearts, because these changes facilitate (i) the development of the DADs that trigger arrhythmia and (ii) the re-entry circuits that sustain arrhythmia.

Resting cardiac output may/may not be reduced substantially; compensatory rise in filling pressure

A fall in myocardial contractility depresses the ventricular function curve (Figure 18.9) and pump

function curve (stroke volume versus arterial pressure; Figure 6.15). In **moderate failure**, however, there is surprisingly little reduction in the resting stroke volume, owing to a compensatory rise in ventricular filling pressure to $>12\,cmH_2O$ (see below). This raises both end-diastolic volume (EDV) and end-systolic volume (ESV), so there is **ventricular dilatation** throughout the cardiac cycle (Figure 18.11). Consequently, the **cardiothoracic ratio** (cardiac shadow width/thoracic cavity width in chest radiogram) exceeds its normal value of 0.5 (Figure 18.12). The increase in the filling pressure and EDV shifts the ventricle up the depressed ventricular function curve, restoring contractile energy through the Frank–Starling mechanism (Figure 18.9). Due to this interaction, resting stroke volume and cardiac output can be almost normal in moderate failure (Figure 6.13). The ejection fraction, by contrast, is always reduced (Figure 18.11). In **severe failure** the ventricular function curve is so depressed that the stroke volume falls despite the increased EDV. The **ejection fraction**, measured by echocardiography, falls from its normal resting value of 66% to as little as 10–20%.

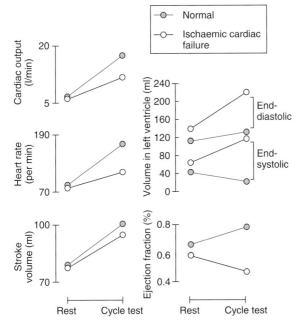

Figure 18.11 Effect of chronic cardiac failure on cardiac performance at rest and during a standard exercise test, submaximal bicycle ergometry. Data from Table 17.2.

thorax. A third factor is **increased renal salt and water retention** (see later). This expands the extracellular fluid compartment by up to 30%, and the attendant increase in plasma volume helps raise the cardiac filling pressure.

Cardiac output fails to increase normally during exercise

An **exercise test** reveals cardiac failure even when the output is compensated at rest. Figure 18.11 shows that a standard exercise test raised cardiac output in normal subjects to 18 l/min, whereas in heart failure the output increased to only 11 l/min. The inadequate output during exercise is due to two factors: stroke volume impairment and, surprisingly, impaired tachycardia (Figure 18.11).

Stroke volume fails to increase adequately for several reasons. (i) Stroke volume is less responsive than normal to the exercise-induced rise in the filling pressure (preload), because the slope of the ventricular function curve is reduced (Figure 18.9). (ii) Stroke volume is more susceptible to depression by the raised arterial pressure (afterload) of exercise, because the pump function curve is depressed (Figure 6.15). (iii) The β_1-adrenoceptor pathway, which normally raises contractility and ejection fraction during exercise, is impaired in heart failure (see below). (iv) Diastolic relaxation is impaired by the slow reuptake of Ca^{2+} into the SR, so diastolic filling is impaired ('diastolic failure').

The impaired **heart rate response** is due partly to a fall in tyrosine hydroxylase activity in cardiac sympathetic terminals, leading to noradrenaline depletion. Also, β_1-adrenoceptors are downregulated in failing cardiac myocytes, due to increased phosphorylation by receptor kinase. The phosphorylated receptors become uncoupled from adenylate cyclase and internalized.

The puzzle of exercise intolerance

Excessive fatigue during moderate exercise is a common presenting symptom of cardiac failure. Surprisingly, patients often experience fatigue at low work levels, that call for little increase in cardiac output – so exercise intolerance is not fully explained by the limited rise in cardiac output or by the exertional dyspnoea. It appears that Ca^{2+} handling is abnormal in the skeletal muscle fibres, as well as cardiac fibres. Slow skeletal muscle fibres and cardiac myocytes express the same isoform of SR Ca^{2+}–ATPase; and in animal models of heart failure, skeletal muscle fibres show reduced Ca^{2+} reuptake, slow relaxation and impaired fatigue resistance.

To summarize, the resting cardiac output can be within the normal range in **compensated failure** (Figure 18.11) or subnormal in **decompensated failure**. In either case, ventricular filling pressure is raised and the heart is dilated throughout the cardiac cycle.

How is the filling pressure raised in heart failure?

The compensatory increase in ventricular filling pressure is responsible for most of the clinical features of heart failure, including cardiac dilatation, pulmonary congestion (causing dyspnoea), jugular venous pressure elevation and ankle oedema (Table 18.1). But how does ventricular dysfunction raise the filling pressure? Multiple mechanisms are involved. The first is the **sump pump effect** (Figure 6.12). The cardiac pump removes blood from the feed line (the sump – central veins/pulmonary veins) and transfers it into the outflow line (pulmonary artery, aorta). If the pump becomes less effective, returning blood is removed less quickly from the feed line, so pressure builds up there. Haemodynamic modelling indicates, however, that the sump pump effect cannot account for the entire rise in filling pressure. A second factor is **increased sympathetic venomotor activity**, which causes marked peripheral venoconstriction and thereby shifts peripheral venous blood into the

There is also evidence of reduced mitochondrial function and creatine kinase levels. Changes in the skeletal muscle themselves thus contribute to exercise intolerance during heart failure.

Compensatory mechanisms to support the failing heart cause many problems

Chronic cardiac failure evokes responses in other tissues/organs that can be a mix of helpful and harmful. The chief responses are:

- compensatory influences on the heart;
- sympathetic redistribution of the cardiac output amongst the peripheral tissues;
- renal retention of salt and water;
- pulmonary congestion and oedema;
- peripheral oedema.

This section deals with the first of these – compensatory influences on the heart. The output of the failing heart is supported by an increase in **filling pressure**, as described earlier, and also by an increase in **adrenergic stimulation** by circulating catecholamines and sympathetic activity. The resulting compensation is effective in mild failure at rest, but not during exercise or severe failure. Moreover, the compensatory mechanism can have harmful side effects, such as dyspnoea.

Circulating catecholamine concentration rises but β_1-adrenoceptors are downregulated

Plasma adrenaline and noradrenaline concentration increases markedly in heart failure, though the cardiac sympathetic terminals become depleted of noradrenaline in severe failure. During mild failure the inotropic action of the catecholamines helps to support the stroke volume. As the disease progresses, however, the uncoupling and downregulation of myocardial β_1-adrenoreceptors vitiates the inotropic effect.

Raised filling pressure: friend or foe?

In mild failure the rise in filling pressure and diastolic dilatation improves the contractile energy by the Frank–Starling mechanism, so resting stroke volume is almost normal (Figure 18.9). As failure worsens, however, the ventricular function curve becomes flatter, so increases in filling pressure and cardiac dilatation achieve little increase in stroke volume; rather, they cause serious problems, as follows.

- Cardiac dilatation impairs the **mechanical efficiency** of systole, as dictated by **Laplace's law** (eqn 6.1, Section 6.8). That is to say, the

contractile force needed to generate systolic pressure increases with ventricular radius (Figure 6.14). Cardiac dilatation thus increases the energy cost of systole.

- In a grossly dilated heart, **tricuspid/mitral valve leakage** may occur during systole due to the widened atrioventricular orifices and separation ('lateralization') of the papillary muscles, which pull on the free margins of the valve leaflets through the chordae tendineae. If the free margins cannot meet and seal properly, regurgitation reduces the effective stroke volume. Tricuspid regurgitation can also cause a palpable liver pulsation during systole.
- The high filling pressures associated with left ventricular failure causes **pulmonary vascular congestion** (Figure 18.12) and **extra-alveolar oedema**. The stiffened lungs require more effort to inflate, generating a sensation of difficulty in breathing called **dyspnoea**.
- The high central venous pressures associated with right ventricular failure causes **peripheral oedema**, a visibly **raised jugular venous pressure** and **hepatomegaly**.

There are thus many reasons for reducing the cardiac filling pressure and dilatation therapeutically (see below).

Sympathetic-mediated peripheral vasoconstriction redistributes cardiac output and supports blood pressure

The limited cardiac output is preferentially distributed to the coronary, cerebral and skeletal muscle circulations through intense vasoconstriction of other tissues (Figure 18.13). In the cutaneous, renal and splanchnic vascular beds, resistance vessels and veins are constricted by **increased sympathetic vasomotor activity**, along with increased circulating **catecholamines**, **angiotensin II** and **endothelin-1**. Increased sympathetic activity is a pronounced feature of heart failure, driven perhaps by the hypothalamic paraventricular nucleus and baroreflex. Resistance vessel vasoconstriction maintains the arterial pressure, which would otherwise be threatened by a low cardiac output; and venoconstriction contributes to the rise in cardiac filling pressure. In mild failure these responses can be beneficial. In severe failure, however, the venoconstriction contributes to the excessive cardiac dilatation; and the afterload created by the maintained arterial pressure curtails the stroke volume of the enfeebled ventricle (Figure 6.15).

Figure 18.12 Anteroposterior radiograph of chest. *(Left)* Normal subject; cardiothoracic ratio 0.45. *(Right)* Patient with left ventricular failure; cardiothoracic ratio 0.72. Asterisk marks grossly dilated left ventricle. Arrow, septal line caused by interstitial oedema (Kerley B lines). Radiating opacities due to pulmonary interstitial oedema are present in the left lung field (Kerley A lines). Also note 'air bronchogram' (the outlining of the major bronchi by surrounding oedema) and blunting of the costophrenic angle images by oedema. (Courtesy of Dr A Wilson, St George's Hospital, London.)

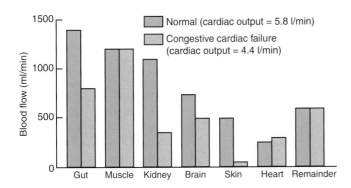

Figure 18.13 Redistribution of cardiac output in a resting patient with chronic cardiac failure and an output of 4.4 l/min (grey columns). Note the reduced perfusion of the kidney, gut and skin, caused by a high sympathetic activity. (From Wade OL, Bishop JM. *Cardiac Output and Regional Flow.* Oxford: Blackwell, 1962, by permission.)

Renal salt and water retention expands the extracellular fluid compartment, contributing to oedema

During cardiac failure the kidneys retain salt and water. The resulting expansion of the extracellular fluid compartment, by up to 30%, contributes to the cardiac dilatation and oedema formation. The salt and water retention is caused by the **increased renal sympathetic activity,** which causes **renal vasoconstriction** (Figure 18.13) and activates the **renin–angiotensin–aldosterone** system. Circulating aldosterone is raised further through reduced degradation in the congested, under-perfused liver. Circulating **natriuretic factors** (NF) too are raised, due to ANF secretion by the distended atria and a big increase in BNF secretion by the

distended ventricles. The NF may have a beneficial role in attenuating the excessive renal retention of salt and water.

Pulmonary congestion, pulmonary oedema and/or peripheral oedema occur in heart failure

Pulmonary congestion, oedema and dyspnoea result from left ventricular failure

Ischaemic failure affects the left ventricle primarily. If the left ventricle transiently pumps out less blood than the right, blood accumulates in the lungs, raising pulmonary venous pressure ('sump pump' effect, see earlier) until the Frank–Starling mechanism restores left–right equality (Figure 18.9). The resulting pulmonary congestion (vascular distension) is obvious in chest radiographs (Figure 18.12). The congestion reduces lung compliance, making them stiffer and harder to inflate, thus **increasing the work of breathing**. The unpleasant sensation of having to work inappropriately hard to draw each breath is called **dyspnoea** (difficulty in breathing). Dyspnoea is a major symptom of left ventricular failure (Table 18.1).

Since capillary pressure is higher than venous pressure, the increased pulmonary venous pressure raises pulmonary capillary pressure, which increases transcapillary filtration. This leads to **pulmonary oedema**. In moderate pulmonary oedema the excess fluid collects in the pulmonary interstitium and inside the bronchi, causing basal crackles (**crepitations**) during breathing, audible through a stethoscope. In severe pulmonary oedema, fluid accumulates in the alveoli too, impairing O_2 transport, with potentially fatal results.

The pulmonary vascular congestion and interstitial oedema become worse on lying down, due to the shift of blood into the thorax. Consequently, cardiac dyspnoea becomes worse on lying down (**orthopnoea**). The pulmonary oedema gradually increases as the night wears on, awakening the patient with an attack of **paroxysmal nocturnal dyspnoea**. Consequently, patients in failure tend to sleep propped up by several pillows.

Peripheral oedema results from right ventricle failure

When the right ventricle fails, central venous pressure is raised by the sump pump effect, peripheral venoconstriction and renal salt and water retention. The rise in central venous pressure raises venous pressures throughout the systemic circulation; for example, pressure in the venous limb of human skin capillaries at heart level rises to 20–40 mmHg (normal 12–15 mmHg). Also the plasma colloid osmotic pressure falls by ~7 mmHg, due to the increase in plasma volume caused by salt and water retention. The altered Starling forces increase the transcapillary filtration rate, leading to peripheral oedema (Section 11.10). The oedema is usually located in a dependent region (feet, ankles, leg; Figure 11.16), or over the sacrum in bed-ridden patients. The combination of **distended jugular veins** and **pitting peripheral oedema** points strongly to right ventricular failure.

Failure occurs not infrequently in both the right and left ventricles, so patients may have both peripheral and pulmonary oedema.

Treatment is based on physiological principles

The treatment of cardiac failure is an exercise in applied physiology, aimed at relieving the symptoms and improving the condition of the heart. Specifically, the objectives are to:

1 reduce myocardial O_2 demand, by reducing cardiac work;
2 improve stroke volume, by reducing arterial blood pressure (afterload);
3 improve mechanical efficiency, by reducing cardiac dilatation (Laplace's law);
4 reduce pulmonary congestion/oedema, by reducing plasma volume and filling pressure;
5 prevent arrhythmias;
6 improve myocardial contractility.

These objectives are addressed as follows.

1. Cardiac work can be reduced by bed-rest, arterial pressure reduction (afterload) and filling pressure reduction (preload). **Arterial pressure** can be reduced by peripheral vasodilators, such as angiotensin-converting enzyme inhibitors (captopril, enalapril), the endothelin antagonist bosentan, α_1-adrenoceptor blockers (e.g. prazosin), or in severe failure hydralazine. **Filling pressure** can be reduced by venodilators (oral nitroglycerine, intravenous nitroprusside, ACE inhibitors). An **ACE inhibitor** is usually the drug of first choice, because it has multiple actions, namely relaxation of resistance and capacitance vessels, reduction of sympathetic activity and reduction of renal fluid retention. **Angiotensin receptor blockers** (losartan, valsartan) are more expensive alternatives, if ACE inhibitors cause persistent coughing (due to increased bradykinin).

2. Stroke volume and ejection fraction can be markedly improved by reducing the pressure opposing ejection, using the peripheral vasodilators discussed above. Due to the steepness of the pump function curve, a small reduction in arterial pressure can improve the stroke volume substantially; see Figure 6.15, point 4.

3 and 4. Cardiac dilatation, pulmonary congestion and **oedema** can be reduced by **diuretics,** such as furosemide (frusemide), which reduce extracellular fluid and plasma volume. **ACE inhibitors/ AT_1 receptor blockers** also help, by reducing aldosterone levels. If necessary, the aldosterone receptor antagonist **spironolactone** can also be added. These various pharmacological interventions reverse physiological compensations that have been overdone in cardiac failure.

5. Arrhyhmia, an important cause of mortality in cardiac failure patients, is reduced by prophylactic, low to moderate doses of β-**adrenoceptor blockers** (propranolol, atenolol, metoprolol). Beta-blockers also slow the heart rate, which reduces cardiac work, increases the diastolic interval for coronary perfusion (Figure 15.5) and helps compensate for slow relaxation (diastolic dysfunction). Beta-blockers can only be used in mild/moderate failure, however, and with caution, since they also reduce contractility.

6. Myocardial contractility can be partially restored by **digoxin**, which remains the only relatively safe inotropic drug for oral use. The discovery of digoxin by William Withering in 1785 is a nice example of the roles of chance and a prepared mind in scientific discovery. Dr Withering was journeying through Shropshire when he was asked to see a woman suffering from severe dropsy (cardiac failure). He could do little for her and on his return journey was astonished to find her not only alive but much improved. On enquiring he discovered that she had been taking a local folklore remedy, an infusion of the leaves of the foxglove, *Digitalis purpurea*. The efficacy of the digitalis infusion is illustrated in Figure 3.15. Digoxin boosts the intracellular Ca^{2+} store (Section 3.8). Unfortunately, this can trigger afterdepolarizations and arrhythmia (coupled beats, called bigeminy; ventricular tachycardia; ventricular fibrillation) – so plasma digoxin must be carefully monitored and maintained at 1–2.6 nM. Digoxin toxicity is increased by loop diuretics such as furosemide, which lower plasma $[K^+]$; K^+ and digoxin compete for the same Na–K–ATPase binding site. Due to these complications, digoxin is not as widely prescribed as formerly. Digoxin is now used mainly when there is concomitant **atrial fibrillation**, because digoxin enhances parasympathetic activity through a central action, slowing atrioventricular node conduction and thus improving the irregular ventricular tachycardia.

Other inotropic drugs, such as the phosphodiesterase III inhibitor **milrinone** and the β₁-agonists **dobutamine** and **dopamine**, are used to provide short-term, emergency support for the heart during acute failure. Milrinone increases mortality if used chronically. Temporary support can also be provided by a mechanical system called intra-aortic balloon counterpulsation.

Given this extensive pharmacological armoury, where does one start? It is usual to commence therapy with an ACE inhibitor, and to add a loop diuretic if there is persisting pulmonary or peripheral oedema. ACE inhibitors, spironolactone and low-dose β-blockers (where appropriate) have each been shown to prolong life; other treatments, such as digoxin, improve the symptoms and quality of life, but do not significantly prolong it.

SUMMARY

Systemic hypoxaemia

- Systemic hypoxaemia can be caused by high altitude, asphyxiation, chronic emphysema and severe pulmonary oedema.

- Increased arterial chemoreceptor activity drives a reflex hyperventilation, which improves arterial P_{O_2} but causes hypocapnia and a reversed (left) Bohr shift.

- Tachycardia increases the resting cardiac output, to maintain O_2 delivery in the face of reduced arterial O_2 saturation. Increased peripheral perfusion is also promoted by vasodilatation – except in the cerebral circulation, where the vasoconstrictor effect of hypocapnia offsets hypoxic vasodilatation.

- In the lungs, hypoxic pulmonary vasoconstriction causes pulmonary hypertension, which promotes apical perfusion – but can also lead to right ventricular failure.

- Maximum cardiac output and arterial O_2 saturation fall, so $\dot{V}_{O_2max}$ and exercise performance are impaired.

- Acclimatization to altitude involves a correction of the respiratory alkalosis, a further increase in resting ventilation, increased haematocrit and a right Bohr shift that facilitates peripheral O_2 unloading.

Shock and haemorrhage

- Acute circulatory failure, or clinical shock, is caused by hypovolaemia (e.g. haemorrhage), acute cardiac failure, septicaemia and anaphylaxis.

- Hypovolaemia reduces central venous pressure, which reduces stroke volume and pulse pressure (Frank–Starling mechanism). Reduced cardiopulmonary and baroreceptor activity, along with increased arterial chemoreceptor activity, evoke a reflex increase in sympathetic outflow, circulating catecholamines, angiotensin II and, in severe cases, vasopressin.

- If the hypovolaemia is <20%, mean blood pressure is maintained near normal (compensated, non-hypotensive phase), due to reflex tachycardia, increased cardiac contractility, increased peripheral resistance and venoconstriction. Pulse pressure is reduced. The skin is pale, cold and sweaty. Hyperventilation is driven by arterial chemoreceptor, stimulated by lactic acidosis.

- Over 30–60 min the reduced capillary pressure allows plasma oncotic pressure to draw ~500 ml interstitial fluid into the circulation. This 'internal transfusion' is facilitated by a shift of intracellular fluid into the interstitial compartment.

- The kidneys conserve salt and water, due to increases in renal sympathetic activity, aldosterone II and vasopressin (ADH). Fluid intake is increased by angiotensin II-stimulated thirst. Extracellular fluid volume is thereby restored over a few days. Plasma proteins and red cells are re-synthesized more slowly.

- In severe hypotensive haemorrhage, with delayed transfusion, an irreversible, decompensated phase sets in. Peripheral vessels relax, causing blood pressure to collapse. Poor coronary perfusion sets up a positive feedback leading to acute cardiac failure. Poor renal perfusion leads to acute renal failure, signalled by anuria.

Fainting

- Emotional stress, hypovolaemia or prolonged orthostasis can cause an abrupt, profound bradycardia (vagally mediated) and peripheral vasodilatation (vasovagal attack).

- As mean arterial pressure falls below ~70 mmHg, a fall in cerebral perfusion causes a loss of consciousness. The collapsed, supine position raises stroke volume, and the heart rate soon picks up. Consciousness is regained in ~2 min.

Essential hypertension

- Resting blood pressures of >140/90 mmHg increase the incidence of myocardial infarction, heart failure, strokes, retinopathy and renal failure. Systolic hypertension in particular is harmful.

- The rise in mean pressure is caused by an increase in peripheral resistance, due to a narrowing and rarefaction of the small resistance arteries. Narrowing is caused initially by reversible vasoconstriction, then by inward eutrophic remodelling of the media and finally by myocyte hypertrophy.

- Systolic pressure increases more than diastolic pressure. This is due to (a) reduced aortic compliance, which raises the pulse pressure; and (b) systolic augmentation by an early reflected wave, caused by the increased wave conduction velocity.

- Essential hypertension is caused by an interaction between susceptibility genes (probably affecting aldosterone or endothelin secretion in some subgroups) and environmental factors, notably high salt intake, low potassium intake, stress and obesity.

- Hypertension can be controlled by the A–C–D regime – ACE inhibitors/AT_1 receptor blockers, Ca^{2+}-channel blockers (peripheral vasodilatation) and diuretics. Beta-adrenoceptor blockers can be added to reduce cardiac output.

Chronic cardiac failure

- Chronic cardiac failure is a reduced ventricular contractility secondary to ischaemic heart disease, pulmonary or systemic hypertension, valve defects or cardiomyopathy. Failure results in exercise intolerance, dyspnoea and pulmonary/peripheral oedema. Death arises from pump failure or arrhythmia.

- The pump weakness is due primarily to a small, sluggish, systolic Ca^{2+} transient and reduced Ca^{2+} store. The small store is caused by downregulation of the SR Ca^{2+} pump, leaky Ca^{2+}-release channels and upregulation of the sarcolemmal Na^+–Ca^{2+} exchanger.

- Fatal arrhythmia is due to delayed afterdepolarization (DAD) and heterogeneity of the refractory period caused by increased action potential duration. Action potentials are prolonged by K^+ channel downregulation. Large DADs are the result of $3Na^+$–Ca^{2+} exchanger upregulation, K^+ channel downregulation, leaky Ca^{2+}-release channels and high sympathetic activity.

- The ventricular function (Starling) curve, pump function curve and ejection fraction are depressed. The heart is swollen (cardiothoracic ratio >0.5), due to a raised filling pressure. In mild, compensated failure the stroke volume and output are almost normal at rest, due to the raised filling pressure (Starling's law) and raised plasma catecholamines. In severe failure the output is low even at rest, due to further Starling curve depression, mechanical inefficiency caused by dilatation (Laplace's law; mitral/tricuspid regurgitation) and β_1-adrenoceptor downregulation.

- During exercise the heart rate and stroke volume both fail to increase adequately, due to cardiac sympathetic noradrenaline depletion, β_1-adrenoceptor downregulation and the low slope of the depressed Starling curve. Exercise intolerance is due to the poor cardiac output, dyspnoea and altered skeletal muscle Ca^{2+} handling.

- In the cutaneous, splanchnic and renal circulations, constriction of resistance vessels supports the arterial blood pressure. Venoconstriction contributes to the elevated CVP. Constriction is driven by increased peripheral sympathetic-activity and raised plasma angiotensin II, endothelin and catecholamines.

- The kidneys retain fluid, due to high aldosterone levels and renal vasoconstriction. The plasma volume expansion, along with venoconstriction and the sump pump effect, raise ventricular filling pressure. In right ventricular failure, the increased central venous pressure raises systemic capillary pressure, leading to oedema of the legs/sacrum. In left ventricular failure the increased pulmonary venous pressure causes pulmonary congestion, pulmonary oedema and dyspnoea.

- ACE inhibitors, often supplemented by diuretics and spironolactone, reduce arterial pressure and cardiac work, promote renal fluid excretion, reduce cardiac dilatation and improve stroke volume. Alpha-blockers, hydralazine and nitrodilators can reduce cardiac work further. In mild failure, β-adrenoceptor blockers reduce the incidence of arrhythmia. Contractility can be increased by the inotropic drug digoxin.

Further reading

Reviews and chapters

Hypoxaemia

Longhurst J. Exercise in hypoxic environments: the mechanisms remains elusive. *Journal of Physiology* 2003; **550**: 335.

Marshall JM. The integrated response to hypoxia: From circulation to cells. *Experimental Physiology* 1999; **84**: 449–70.

Savard GK, Areskog N-H, Saltin B. Cardiovascular responses to exercise in humans following acclimatization to extreme altitude. *Acta Physiologica Scandinavica* 1995; **154**: 499–509.

Wilkins BW, Pike TL, Marting EA, Curry TB, Ceridon ML, Joyner MJ. Exercise intensity-dependent contribution of β-adrenergic receptor-mediated vasodilatation in hypoxic humans. *Journal of Physiology* 2008; **586**: 1195–205.

Shock and haemorrhage

Frithiof R, Eriksson S, Rundgren M. Central inhibition of opioid receptor subtypes and its effect on haemorrhagic hypotension in conscious sheep. *Acta Physiologica* 2007; **191**: 25–34.

Länne T, Lundvall J. Mechanisms in man for rapid refill of the circulatory system in hypovolaemia. *Acta Physiologica Scandinavica* 1992; **146**: 299–306.

Schadt JC, Ludbrook J. Hemodynamic and neurohumoral responses to acute hypovolaemia in conscious mammals. *American Journal of Physiology* 1991; **260**: H305–18.

Fainting

Jardine DL, Melton IC, Crozier IG *et al.* Decrease in cardiac output and muscle sympathetic activity during vasovagal syncope. *American Journal of Physiology* 2002; **282**: H1804–9.

Julu POO, Cooper VL, Hansen S, Hainsworth R. Cardiovascular regulation in the period preceding vasovagal syncope in conscious humans. *Journal of Physiology* 2003; **549**: 299–311.

Novak V, Honos G, Schondorf R. Is the heart empty at syncope? *Journal of Autonomic Nervous System* 1996; **60**: 83–92.

Hypertension

Adrogué HJ, Madias NE. Sodium and potassium in the pathogenesis of hypertension. *New England Journal of Medicine* 2007; **356:** 1966–78.

Binder A. A review of the genetics of essential hypertension. *Current Opinion in Cardiology* 2007; **22:** 176–84.

Diwan A, Dorn GW. Decompensation of cardiac hypertrophy: Cellular mechanisms and novel therapeutic targets. *Physiology* 2007; **22:** 56–64.

Feihl F, Liaudet L, Levy BI, Waeber B. Hypertension and microvascular remodelling. *Cardiovascular Research* 2008; **78:** 274–85.

Gilbert JS, Ryan MJ, LaMarca BB, Sedeek M, Murphy SR, Granger JP. Pathophysiology of hypertension during preeclampsia: Linking placental ischemia with endothelial dysfunction. *American Journal of Physiology* 2008; **294:** H541–50.

Iwamoto T. Na^+/Ca^{2+} exchanger; implications for the pathogenesis and therapy of salt-dependent hypertension. *American Journal of Physiology* 2006; **290:** R536–45.

Meneton P, Jeunemaitre X, de Wardener HE, MacGregor GA. Links between dietary salt intake, renal salt handling, blood pressure and cardiovascular diseases. *Physiological Reviews* 2005; **85:** 679–715.

Nichols WW, O'Rourke MF. *McDonald's Blood Flow in Arteries.* London: Arnold, 2005.

Ramsay LE, Williams B, Johnston GD *et al.* Guidelines for management of hypertension: Report of the third working party of the British Hypertension Society. *Journal of Human Hypertension* 1999; **13:** 569–92.

Schiffrin EL, Touyz RM (2004) From bedside to bench to bedside: Role of renin–angiotensin–aldosterone system in remodelling of resistance arteries in hypertension. *American Journal of Physiology* 2004; **287:** H435–46.

Chronic cardiac failure

Bers DM. Altered cardiac myocyte Ca regulation in heart failure. *Physiology* 2006; **21:** 380–7.

Ikeda Y, Hoshijima M, Chien KR. Towards biologically targeted therapy of calcium cycling defects in heart failure. *Physiology* 2008; **23:** 6–16.

Li YF, Patel KP. Paraventricular nucleus of the hypothalamus and elevated sympathetic activity in heart failure: The altered inhibitory mechanisms. *Acta Physiologica Scandinavica* 2003; **177:** 17–26.

Sipido KR, Eisner D. Something old, something new: Changing views on the cellular mechanisms of heart failure. *Cardiovascular Research* 2005; **68:** 167–74.

Ventura-Clapier R, Garnier A, Veksler V. Energy metabolism in heart failure. *Journal of Physiology* 2004; **555:** 1–13.

Winaver J, Hoffman A, Abassi Z, Haramati A. Does the heart's hormone ANP help in congestive heart failure? *News in Physiological Sciences,* 1995; **10:** 247–53.

Research papers

See www.hodderplus.com/cardiovascularphysiology for a full list of Research papers for this chapter.

The end but not the end

'Begin at the beginning', said the King, very gravely, to the White Rabbit, 'and go on till you come to the end: then stop'. Heart failure seems to offer a natural ending to this text, but the scientific investigation of the circulation is far from at an end – too many mysteries remain unsolved. The discerning reader will have recognized the superabundance of unresolved problems from the frequent use of 'may be', 'probably', 'is thought to' and so on. Our subject began essentially with the work of William Harvey over three centuries ago, yet a comment by Harvey still makes an apt conclusion to today's textbook: 'I see a field of such vast extent – that my whole life perchance would not suffice for its completion'.

(Mallock A. *William Harvey*. New York: Hoeber, 1929)

CLINICAL CASES

for problem-based learning

CASE 1 The elderly man with a murmur

A 70-year-old man, keen on keeping fit, visited his doctor because he experienced a tight, constricting band across his chest during exercise, relieved by rest. He also complained of excessive breathlessness and dizziness on exercise, and had recently fainted while exercising.

On examination, his pulse was regular but slow-rising and of small amplitude. His brachial blood pressure, 115/80 mmHg, confirmed a low pulse amplitude for his age. On palpation, the apex beat was in the fifth interspace, mid-clavicular line; but a 'thrill' (vibration) was palpable during systole. Auscultation revealed a systolic crescendo–decrescendo murmur (diamond-shaped murmur, Figure 2.8), loudest over the aortic area. The second heart sound was soft, with reversed splitting, i.e. splitting on expiration.

A chest X-ray showed a normal cardiothoracic ratio, but dilated ascending aorta. An ECG showed left axis deviation, ST-segment depression and T-wave inversion. An echocardiogram showed left ventricular concentric hypertrophy and poorly mobile, calcified aortic valve cusps. Cardiac catheterization revealed a left ventricular systolic pressure of 170 mmHg, but 115 mmHg in the aorta. The patient was referred for replacement of the stenosed aortic valve. In the meantime, he was advised against over-exertion and given a β-blocker, atenolol, to prevent angina.

Questions

1 Which valves create the second heart sound and why was it soft here?

2 What is the structure of the aortic valve and what orifices lie just behind the cusps?

3 Explain the reversed splitting of the second sound.

4 Does inspiration/expiration affect stroke volume and/or heart rate?

5 How big is the pressure gradient across the normal aortic valve during (i) ejection and (ii) diastole. Why was the systolic gradient increased here?

6 What is a typical arterial pressure for a healthy 70-year-old?

7 How does the coronary circulation normally respond during exercise?

8 How is systolic coronary blood flow affected by a rise in ventricular systolic pressure?

9 Can exercise induce angina in the absence of coronary artery stenosis?

10 How does left ventricular hypertrophy affect pulmonary venous pressure, and could this contribute to the exercise dyspnoea?

11 How might aortic valve stenosis lead to dizziness and fainting on exercise?

12 How does aortic valve stenosis cause a murmur and thrill?

13 Does a systolic murmur always indicate a valve lesion?

14 In electrocardiography, why is the ST segment normally isoelectric, and why is the T wave normally upright?

15 What does 'electrical axis' mean, and how does left ventricular hypertrophy affect it?

16 How does myocardial ischaemia depress the ST segment?

17 How does a β-blocker help to relieve exercise-induced angina?

Answers

1 The second heart sound is caused by the vibration of the aortic and pulmonary valve cusps on closing. When the cusp mobility is impaired by calcification, as here, there is less vibration and a softer sound.

2 A normal aortic valve has three cusps, but aortic stenosis often develops in a congenitally bicuspid valve. Each cusp is a thin sheet of fibrous tissue covered by endothelium. The openings of the right and left coronary arteries lie immediately behind the valve cusps, in the sinuses of Valsalva (Figure 1.4).

3 Normally, the aortic component of the second sound precedes the pulmonary component (Figure 2.4). The 'splitting' normally increases during inspiration, because a transient increase in systemic venous return raises right ventricular filling, which prolongs ejection (Figure 8.27) and, at the same time, pulmonary vascular expansion reduces flow into the left ventricle, shortening left ventricular ejection. In aortic stenosis the aortic component comes second, due to the increased resistance to left ventricular ejection. This 'reversed splitting' is amplified by expiration, because expiration transiently reduces systemic venous return and thus shortens right ventricular ejection.

4 Expiration slows the heart rate by increased vagal inhibition (sinus arrhythmia, Figures 5.4a and 16.17). Expiration also reduces right ventricular stroke volume and increases left ventricular stroke volume – see (3) above.

5 The systolic pressure gradient across the aortic valve is normally only a few mmHg, because the wide aperture offers little resistance to flow (Figure 2.4). The large systolic pressure gradient in the patient, 55 mmHg, is caused by the high resistance of the narrowed valve (Figure 2.8). In diastole the gradient across the closed valve is large, namely diastolic aortic pressure (80 mmHg) minus diastolic left ventricular pressure (5–10 mmHg).

6 Ageing raises blood pressure to ~140/75 mmHg for a 70-year-old white male (Figure 17.10). The exaggerated rise in pulse pressure and systolic pressure is due to arteriosclerosis, which reduces arterial compliance (Figure 18.7) and increased systolic augmentation by wave reflection (Figure 18.8).

7 During exercise the coronary blood flow normally increases in proportion to the increased myocardial O_2 consumption, due to metabolic vasodilatation (Figure 15.4).

8 Coronary blood flow normally declines sharply in systole, because the tense myocardium compresses intramural coronary vessels (Figure 15.5). An exaggerated increase in ventricular systolic pressure, 170 mmHg here, further curtails the systolic perfusion.

9 Yes. Ischaemic myocardial pain occurs whenever myocardial O_2 supply fails to meet demand. In this patient the myocardial O_2 demand is excessive (because the ventricle is pumping through a narrowed outlet) and at the same time the increased ventricular wall tension impedes systolic coronary flow (see (8) above).

10 Since the ventricle wall is hypertrophied, it is stiffer than normal, so filling requires a higher diastolic pressure. The attendant increased left atrial pressure raises pulmonary venous pressure, which congests the lungs and makes them stiffer. Lung stiffness causes dyspnoea, as in Case 5.

11 During exercise, arterial pressure is normally maintained by the increased cardiac output, despite the fall in peripheral resistance caused by the muscle metabolic vasodilatation (Figure 17.5); mean arterial pressure = cardiac output × peripheral resistance. Severe aortic stenosis prevents an adequate increase in cardiac output, so arterial pressure falls during exercise. If pressure falls below the limit of cerebral autoregulation (Figure 15.13), cerebral hypoperfusion leads to dizziness or even fainting on exercise.

12 Aortic valve stenosis creates turbulent flow, which sets up the vibrations heard as a crescendo–decrescendo murmur (Figure 2.8) or felt as a thrill. Turbulence is favoured by the abrupt change in diameter at the stenosed valve exit, and by the high Reynolds number (fluid velocity × diameter × density/viscosity) generated by the high velocity of blood in the narrowed valve.

13 No. If the aortic Reynolds number exceeds ~2000 during peak systolic flow, turbulence can develop, creating a benign systolic murmur. This is

particularly common in pregnancy, owing to the increased cardiac output and moderate anaemia (low viscosity).

14 The ST segment corresponds to the plateau of the ventricular myocyte action potential. Since all the ventricle myocytes are at approximately the same potential, no current flows between them and the EGC is isoelectric (baseline). The T wave is upright because subepicardial myocytes have shorter plateaux than subendocardial myocytes (Figure 5.3), and therefore repolarize first (Figure 5.8).

15 The electrical axis is the direction of the largest dipole during ventricular depolarization (Figure 5.7). The axis depends on the physical angle of the heart and on left ventricular muscle mass relative to the right ventricular mass. Left ventricular hypertrophy increases the magnitude of left-side current, shifting the electrical axis to the left.

16 Ischaemia is most severe in the subendocardium of the hypertrophied ventricle, where compressive stress is highest. This reduces the size of the subendocardial resting potentials and action potentials. The potential difference between the ischaemic and non-ischaemic regions generates an injury current, which displace the ST segment (Figure 5.11).

17 Blockage of the cardiac β_1-adrenoceptors reduces the tonic effect of the cardiac sympathetic nerves on rate and contractility, lowering cardiac output. This reduces myocardial work and O_2 demand, and increases the diastolic period, during which coronary perfusion is highest. These changes help prevent angina.

CASE 2 The man with chest pain

A collapsed 60-year-old bus driver was brought into Casualty complaining of a severe, sustained crushing pain in a band across the chest, spreading into the arms. Previously he had been well, but smoked ten cigarettes a day.

On examination, he was pale, with cold, sweaty skin. His pulse was weak, with occasional extrasystoles (ventricular ectopics). His arterial blood pressure was 95/70 mmHg. Heart sounds were normal. An ECG revealed large Q waves and ST segment elevation. He was admitted with a provisional diagnosis of myocardial infarction. Plasma analysis showed raised cardiac enzymes (lactic dehydrogenase, creatine phosphokinase, aspartate aminotransferase) and cholesterol.

He was given O_2 and morphine. A streptokinase infusion was set up to lyse the coronary thrombus. He was started on regular, low-dose aspirin.

Questions

1 Name the major coronary arteries and their territories; define 'functional end-artery'.

2 What is the likely coronary artery pathology here and how does endothelial dysfunction contribute to it?

3 Which afferents mediate ischaemic cardiac pain?

4 Since the left ventricle contains oxygenated blood, why is the left ventricle wall ischaemic?

5 If the patient's arterial blood contained 190 ml O_2 per litre, mixed venous blood 90 ml O_2 per litre and his O_2 consumption was 300 ml/min, what was the cardiac output? Name the principle involved.

6 How do you account for the low blood pressure?

7 What makes the skin pale, cold and sweaty (clammy)? Of what general response is this a characteristic?

8 Draw a normal lead II ECG and show how it aligns with a ventricular action potential. What feature correspond with the ST segment?

9 What causes ST-segment displacement in myocardial ischaemia?

10 How does low-dose aspirin improve the prognosis?

11 What are the roles of lactic dehydrogenase and creatine phosphokinase?

12 What are the dangers of abruptly restoring blood flow to a tissue after prolonged ischaemia?

13 What is a ventricular ectopic beat, how does it affect stroke volume and what might cause it?

Answers

1 The left coronary artery supplies mainly the left ventricle and septum. The right coronary artery

supplies mainly the right ventricle. A functional end artery is one with insufficient arterial anastomoses to maintain tissue viability if the main vessel is obstructed (Figure 15.6).

2 A thrombus (organized blood clot) forms on an atheromatous plaque. Atheroma originates with the transendothelial passage of lipoproteins, fibrinogen and monocytes (Section 9.9). Endothelial NO, an inhibitor of platelet aggregation, is low in atheromatous regions, enabling platelets to aggregate and initiate thrombosis.

3 Chemosensitive sympathetic afferents in the myocardium mediate cardiac ischaemic pain (Figure 16.10). Convergence with pathways from the arms in the spinal column may explain the 'referred pain'.

4 The left ventricle wall is ~1 cm thick. The time needed for O_2 diffusion increases as distance squared, so diffusion is too slow to support myocyte metabolism beyond ~100 μm from the chamber lumen (Table 1.1).

5 For an $(A–V)_{O_2}$ of 100 ml/l (i.e. 190–90) and an O_2 uptake of 300 ml/min, the cardiac output must be 3 litre/min (i.e. 300/100). This is the Fick principle (Section 6.1). Cardiac output is depressed.

5 Ischaemia impairs contractility (Figures 6.22 and 6.23). This reduces the stroke volume and blood pressure.

6 The skin is pale and cold due to sympathetic-mediated veno- and vaso-constriction, respectively (Section 15.3). The 'clamminess' (cold sweat) is due to sympathetic sudomotor activity. The patient is in cardiogenic shock (Section 18.2).

7 See Figure 5.3. The ST segment corresponds to the plateau of the action potential.

8 The ST segment is displaced by injury currents (Figure 5.11b). Injury currents develop because the action potential of ischaemic myocytes is less positive than that of the neighbouring normal myocytes and the resting potential is less negative than normal.

9 The primary event of thrombosis is platelet aggregation. This is promoted by platelet thromboxane, which is synthesized through cyclo-oxygenase (Section 13.5). Low doses of aspirin inhibit platelet cyclo-oxygenase, helping prevent a recurrence.

10 Myocardial lactic dehydrogenase oxidizes circulating lactate, an important myocardial energy source (Section 7.14). Creatine phosphokinase transfers high-energy phosphate from creatine phosphate to ADP to form ATP (the Lohmann reaction).

11 There is reperfusion injury, due to contracture (caused by cytosolic Ca^{2+} overload), white cell activation and free oxygen radical generation (Sections 6.12 and 13.9).

12 A ventricular ectopic beat is a premature systole triggered from within the ventricle (Figure 5.4b). The trigger is often a delayed after-depolarization (Figure 3.16). Excitation does not follow the normal route, so the contraction is ill co-ordinated and generates little output. The pulse appears to miss a beat.

CASE 3 The haemorrhagic alcoholic

A 60-year-old civil servant, known to be a regular, heavy drinker, with a deteriorating work performance, collapsed after vomiting copious fresh blood (haematemesis). When examined in the Emergency Department he was confused, with a pale, clammy skin. His pulse was regular, but weak and rapid (120 min^{-1}). Recumbent blood pressure was 100/75 mmHg. When the patient was sat up, he felt faint and pressure dropped to 80/65 mmHg. His history of alcoholism, coupled with a firm, palpably enlarged liver and characteristic skin changes, indicated hepatic cirrhosis. Rectal examination revealed black 'tarry' stools characteristic of melaena (old blood from a bleed high in the gastrointestinal tract). Endoscopy revealed bleeding oesophageal varices (distended veins in the lower oesophagus), the result of portal vein hypertension caused by alcoholic cirrhosis.

A cannula was inserted into the small, constricted dorsal vein of the hand (with difficulty), to infuse a plasma substitute (Gelatin 40 g/l; molecular mass 30 000 daltons, colloid osmotic pressure 36 mmHg), while awaiting cross-matched blood. A tube inserted into the internal jugular vein recorded a central venous pressure (CVP) of −4 cmH$_2$O (subatmospheric). This line was used to infuse vasopressin. Haematocrit was 0.36 on admission, and haemoglobin 11.8 g/dl. Urine output was 20 ml/hour, and the patient complained of thirst.

Rehydration and blood transfusion was followed by the injection of a sclerosant solution into the gastro-oesophageal varices to induce local thrombosis. On discharge, the patient was prescribed daily propranolol.

Questions

1 What is a 'portal circulation'? Sketch the blood supply to the liver.

2 Why does hepatic cirrhosis cause oesophageal bleeding?

3 Was the CVP normal? Was stroke volume affected? (Hint: consider the pulse pressure.)

4 What was the recumbent patient's mean blood pressure? Was he severely hypotensive when supine?

5 Why was the arterial pressure also measured in orthostasis and why did the pressure fall?

6 Which class of blood vessel regulates mean blood pressure? Did the skin provide any evidence of vascular regulation?

7 Is the peripheral venoconstriction (obvious when venipuncture was attempted) likely to be of benefit?

8 What cardiac responses helped to maintain mean arterial pressure, and what induced them?

9 Identify three types of afferent receptor that drive the cardiovascular responses to hypovolaemia.

10 What accounts for the low haematocrit and haemoglobin concentration on admission, assuming that the values were normal previously?

11 Would you expect an artificial colloid solution to be of greater benefit than 0.15 molar saline?

12 Why was the urine output monitored?

13 What mechanism might account for the patient's thirst?

14 How might the vasopressin infusion be of benefit?

15 What is propranolol and how might it help?

Answers

1 A portal circulation is one downstream of, and in series with, another circulation; the tissue receives venous blood from the upstream organ (Section 1.8). The liver has a dual blood supply – a small arterial supply from the hepatic artery and a much larger portal supply, namely intestine-derived venous blood in the portal vein (Figure 1.5). The hepatic vein drains the liver.

2 Hepatic cirrhosis distorts the liver and raises its vascular resistance. This raises portal vein pressure (normally 5–6 mmHg). The portal vein is linked to the lower oesophageal veins by venous collaterals, so swollen oesophageal veins (varices) develop. Being very superficial, they bleed readily.

3 The patient's CVP, $-4\,cmH_2O$, was low (normal $\sim 4\,cmH_2O$), due to hypovolaemia. The low CVP reduced stroke volume (Starling's law), as shown by the low pulse pressure, 25 mmHg (systolic minus diastolic). Pulse pressure depends on stroke volume (Figure 7.4), and on arterial compliance.

4 Mean brachial artery blood pressure is diastolic pressure plus one-third of the pulse pressure (eqn 8.4). The recumbent mean was 83 mmHg, i.e. normotensive. The patient was therefore in compensated haemorrhagic shock (Figure 18.3).

5 The doctor was assessing the severity of the hypovolaemia, which is not apparent from the compensated supine value. Orthostasis causes peripheral venous blood pooling, lowering CVP and stroke volume further, so the pulse pressure fell to 15 mmHg.

6 Resistance vessels (arterioles, terminal arteries) regulate mean blood pressure (Section 1.6). The low skin temperature and pallor indicated cutaneous vaso- and venoconstriction, respectively, caused by increased sympathetic activity, circulating catecholamines, angiotensin II and vasopressin.

7 Peripheral venoconstriction displaces blood into the thorax and thus limits the fall in CVP and stroke volume.

8 Sympathetic-mediated tachycardia $(120\,min^{-1})$ and increased contractility helped to maintain cardiac output and therefore arterial pressure. The tachycardia is also aided by reduced vagal parasympathetic activity.

9 (i) The activity of carotid sinus and aortic arch baroreceptors is reduced by the fall in pulse pressure (Figure 18.2). (ii) Cardiopulmonary receptor input is reduced by the reduced central venous pressure. (iii) Peripheral arterial chemoreceptor activity is increased by hypoperfusion and metabolic acidosis (Figure 18.3). The altered input into the nucleus tractus

solitarius triggers a reflex increase in sympathetic activity (Figure 16.18).

10 The patient's haemodilution is caused by an 'internal transfusion' of interstitial fluid into capillary and venular blood (Figure 18.3). Capillary pressure is reduced by the venous hypotension and precapillary resistance vessel contraction (Figure 11.4). This allows plasma colloid osmotic pressure to predominate and draw water into the circulation (Starling principle of fluid exchange). The interstitium is topped up with water drawn osmotically from the intracellular compartment by extracellular fluid hyperglycaemia (Section 18.2).

11 Saline expands the plasma volume temporarily, but it reduces plasma colloid osmotic pressure, and thus enhances fluid filtration (Section 11.3). This is avoided by the use of a colloid solution.

12 Urine output was monitored because acute renal failure, caused by acute tubular necrosis, is a potentially fatal complication of severe hypotension.

13 Thirst is stimulated by the action of angiotensin II on the subfornical organ near the hypothalamus. Angiotensin levels are high due to the renal secretion of renin, in response to the increased sympathetic activity, low perfusion pressure and low tubular salt load (Figure 14.12).

14 Vasopressin contracts the splanchnic resistance vessels feeding the portal vein. This temporarily reduces portal vein pressure.

15 Propranolol is a non-selective β-adrenoceptor blocker. It reduces heart rate and cardiac output by blocking cardiac β_1-receptors, and it raises splanchnic vascular resistance by blocking vascular β_2-receptors. Together, these effects reduce portal vein pressure.

CASE 4 The hypertensive fainter

A 45-year-old travelling salesman, attending a local Casualty department after a minor accident, was told his blood pressure was 180/110 mmHg. His general practitioner subsequently recorded supine brachial artery pressures of 185/110 and 165/105 mmHg on two visits. On the last visit, the pressure during standing was 155/110 mmHg and heart rate increased from 75 (supine) to 85/min (standing). The patient was obese and admitted to a regular, moderately heavy alcohol intake. Cardiac signs were normal. After checking the retina, the doctor made a provisional diagnosis of essential hypertension. He started the patient on prazosin (an odd first choice) and advised the patient to lose weight, avoid added salt and salty processed foods, and reduce his alcohol intake.

After a few days on prazosin, the patient returned, because he felt faint and dizzy on standing up, and on one occasion had collapsed for a few minutes. Exercise too made him feel faint and dizzy. The doctor recorded a supine pressure of 145/95 mmHg, falling to 90/65 mmHg on standing, with faintness and fading vision that made the patient lie down again. The doctor stopped the prazosin and started the patient on captopril, which resolved the problem.

Questions

1 How is brachial arterial blood pressure measured in humans?

2 What were the mean pressure and pulse pressure on the first visit to the GP? Why did the GP insist on a second visit?

3 At what systolic/diastolic pressure is hypertension usually diagnosed?

4 What two parameters determine mean blood pressure. Which one is responsible for established hypertension?

5 Why should the patient reduce his salt intake?

6 What structural changes occur in peripheral resistance vessels in hypertension?

7 What are the principal factors regulating vascular tone?

8 What changes occur in elastic arteries in hypertension? Which aspects of arterial blood pressure does this affect?

9 How might mental stress contribute to hypertension?

10 What are the long-term effects of systemic hypertension on the heart?

11 Since most drugs have side effects, why treat symptomless hypertension?

12 Prazosin is an α_1-adrenoceptor antagonist. What is the role of α_1-adrenoceptors in vascular control?

13 Explain how prazosin caused dizziness (i) on standing and (ii) on exercise.

14 How does captopril act?

15 Name three other classes of drug used to treat essential hypertension, and state their modes of action.

Answers

1 Brachial BP is traditionally measured by sphygmomanometry, with auscultation of the Korotkoff sounds (Figure 8.12). Automatic cuff devices are increasingly used today.

2 The pulse pressure was 75 mmHg ($185 - 110$). The mean pressure was 135 mmHg (diastolic + one-third pulse pressure). The alerting response (Section 16.8) often raises pressure during the initial visit to the doctor (white-coat hypertension), hence the repeat visit.

3 Brachial artery pressure in normal 45-year-old white males averages 130/78 mmHg (Figure 17.10) and is a little higher in Afro-Caribbeans. Systolic pressures above 140 mmHg and diastolic pressures above 90 mmHg in young to middle-aged subjects substantially increase the risk of strokes, ischaemic heart disease, cardiac failure and renal failure, so 140/90 is considered the diagnostic level.

4 Mean blood pressure = cardiac output × total peripheral resistance. In established hypertension, cardiac output is normal. The hypertension is therefore due to increased vascular resistance.

5 Hypertension correlates strongly with salt intake (Figure 16.12). Hypertension may be due to an imbalance between salt intake and defective renal salt excretion.

6 The media thickens and the lumen narrows (eutrophic inward remodelling, later hypertrophy; Figure 18.6). Resistance is inversely proportional to the fourth power of lumen radius (Poiseuille's law), so a 10% narrowing raises resistance by 46%.

7 *Intrinsic factors* include the myogenic response (Section 13.2), shear stress-mediated vasodilatation by endothelial NO (Section 13.3), other endothelial products (prostacyclin, EDHF, endothelin), tissue products mediating metabolic vasodilatation (Section 13.4), and autacoids. *Extrinsic factors* are the ubiquitous sympathetic noradrenergic vasoconstrictor fibres (Section 14.1), and circulating vasoactive hormones, notably adrenaline, angiotensin II and vasopressin.

8 Hypertension ages the elastic vessels prematurely, causing elastin fragmentation, dilatation and increased stiffness. The reduced compliance raises pulse pressure and systolic pressure (Figure 18.7). The rapid return of the reflected wave adds further to the systolic hypertension (Figure 18.8).

9 Stress evokes the alerting response, which comprises tachycardia, muscle vasodilatation, vasoconstriction in the renal, splanchnic and cutaneous circulations, and increased blood pressure (Section 16.8). An exaggerated alerting response and the attendant repeated episodes of transient hypertension may contribute to resistance vessel remodelling.

10 Systemic hypertension increases left ventricular work (Section 7.5), the tension-time index (Section 7.14) and O_2 demand. The left ventricle myocytes hypertrophy, thickening the wall (concentric hypertrophy). Eventually left ventricular failure may develop.

11 Treatment is justified by the increased morbidity and mortality from strokes, ischaemic heart disease, cardiac failure and renal failure.

12 Alpha$_1$-adrenoceptors mediate the vasoconstriction evoked by sympathetic activity and circulating catecholamines (Sections 12.5 and 12.6). Consequently, α_1-blockers reduce blood pressure.

13 (i) On standing, the blood pressure falls initially, because venous pooling in the legs reduces cardiac filling pressure and therefore stroke volume (Starling's law of the heart). The resulting postural hypotension reduces cerebral blood flow, leading to dizziness. Prazosin (which should not be the drug of first choice) blocks the compensatory, sympathetic-mediated contraction of resistance vessel. (ii) During exercise, metabolic vasodilatation in the active muscles lowers total peripheral resistance, but blood pressure is maintained by sympathetic vasoconstriction in inactive tissues, along with increased cardiac output. Also, increased sympathetic drive to the active muscle prevents excessive metabolic dilatation. When these effects are blocked by prazosin, exercise can cause hypotension, cerebral hypoperfusion and giddiness.

14 The A–C–D therapeutic regime is considered best practice. 'A' is for ACE inhibitors, such as captopril, which reduce angiotensin II formation. Angiotensin II raises blood pressure by direct vasoconstriction, peripheral neuromodulation,

central presympathetic stimulation, thirst and aldosterone secretion. If side effects (cough) are a problem, angiotensin receptor blockers are used instead.

15 (i) The 'C' of A–C–D refers to Ca^{2+}-channel blockers, e.g. nifedipine. This reduce Ca^{2+} entry into vascular myocytes and thus relax the resistance vessels, lowering blood pressure. Sympathetic neurotransmission is not impaired, so postural hypotension is not a problem.

(ii) The 'D' of A–C–D refers to diuretics, such as the thiazide bendrofluazide. These cause salt and water excretion, and dilate resistance vessels (mechanism uncertain), lowering blood pressure.
(iii) β-adrenoceptor blockers, such as propranolol, reduce cardiac output and hence blood pressure. They also reduce the sympathetic stimulation of the renin–angiotensin–aldosterone system and act centrally to reduce sympathetic outflow.

CASE 5 The breathless woman

A 70-year-old woman complains that she can no longer do her housework or climb the stairs without frequent rests; and she gets very breathless. At night she wakes up struggling to breathe, and finds that sleeping propped up by several pillows helps. Her ankles swell as the day progresses, but improve after a night's rest.

On examination the doctor notes that her breathing is rapid. Chest auscultation reveals fine, basal crackles (crepitations). The pulse is regular and arterial blood pressure is within the normal range, but the neck veins are distended even in the upright position. The doctor estimates the central venous pressure to be about 18 cmH_2O. The apex beat is palpable faintly in the anterior axillary line of the fifth intercostal space. Examining the puffy ankles, he presses on the skin over the tibia for a minute and observes that a deep pit forms.

A chest X-ray shows a cardiothoracic ratio of 0.69, congested pulmonary vessels and the thin horizontal lines of interseptal oedema. ECG is normal. A diagnosis of biventricular cardiac failure is made. She is treated initially with captopril and furosemide, supplemented later by digoxin.

Questions

1 How is central venous pressure (CVP) estimated, using inspection of the jugular veins?
2 What is the relation between CVP and stroke volume?
3 What are the chief roles of Starling's law in humans?
4 Which factors govern the size of the CVP?
5 Can cardiac distension be disadvantageous?
6 Might lowering the arterial pressure help the failing heart?
7 What key intracellular parameter triggers cardiac contraction and how is it changed in cardiac failure?
8 Draw a pair of ventricular function curves to illustrate the meaning of 'impaired contractility'.
9 What factors can raise contractile energy besides Starling's law?
10 How can cardiac contractility be assessed in humans?

11 What is the link between pulmonary vessel distension and dyspnoea?
12 What causes crepitations (crackles) in the lungs?
13 Why was the dyspnoea worse at night (paroxysmal nocturnal dyspnoea), and why did sleeping propped up help?
14 Why is the pitting test negative in normal tissues?
15 What factors govern the distribution of fluid between the vascular and interstitial compartment and how are they changed in cardiac oedema?
16 Why did the ankle swelling get worse during the day?
17 What might account for the patient's poor exercise tolerance?
18 How does digoxin act?

Answers

1 The jugular vein is as a valveless tube connected to the right atrium (Figure 8.23). A vein collapses when its luminal pressure is below atmospheric

pressure. If the point of jugular vein collapse (pressure equal to atmosphere) is, say, 18 cm vertically above the right atrium, atrial pressure (CVP) must be atmospheric pressure plus 18 cm of fluid.

2 CVP determines right ventricle diastolic distension, which governs the energy of contraction and stroke volume (Section 6.4, Figures 6.10 and 6.19).

3 (i) Starling's law equalizes the outputs of the right and left ventricles. (ii) It helps raise stroke volume during exercise. (iii) It can cause postural hypotension (Section 17.1). (iv) It mediates the arterial hypotension of hypovolaemia (Section 18.2).

4 CVP depends on blood volume and distribution. Blood distribution between the thoracic and peripheral veins depends on posture (effect of gravity), movement (muscle pump) and peripheral sympathetic venous tone.

5 As the ventricular function curve flattens, distension no longer raises contractile energy significantly, but it impairs the conversion of wall tension into luminal pressure (Laplace's law; Figure 6.14), and may cause functional incompetence of the atrioventricular valves.

6 If arterial pressure is lowered, less energy is used in raising ventricular pressure. This leaves more energy to eject the stroke volume; see the 'pump function curve' (Figure 6.15).

7 Release of the SR Ca^{2+} store generates a systolic Ca^{2+} transient that, via the troponin–tropomyosin complex, triggers myosin head–actin interaction and the sliding filament process (Sections 3.2 and 3.5). In heart failure the Ca^{2+} transient is small and sluggish.

8 See Figure 18.9. Impaired contractility is a reduced force of contraction for a given filling pressure or cardiac distension.

9 Sympathetic noradrenaline activates β_1-adrenoceptors which, via the adenylate cyclase–cAMP–protein kinase A pathway, increase the plateau Ca^{2+} current, Ca^{2+} store and systolic Ca^{2+} transient, raising contractility (Section 6.10). Beta$_1$-adrenoceptor downregulation weakens this mechanism in advanced cardiac failure (Section 18.5).

10 Human ventricular contractility is assessed by (i) the ejection fraction measured by echocardiography or radionuclide angiography (normally $\geqslant 66\%$) and (ii) ventricular dP/dt_{max}

measured through an intracardiac catheter (Figure 2.5).

11 The pulmonary vessels are distended because left atrial pressure is raised by left ventricle failure, renal salt and water retention and peripheral venoconstriction. Congestion and oedema stiffen the lungs, increasing the work of breathing.

12 Crepitations indicate oedema of the conducting airways, caused by increased pulmonary capillary pressure, secondary to the raised left atrial pressure.

13 The supine position redistributes peripheral venous blood into the thorax (Figure 8.24). This exacerbates pulmonary congestion and oedema. Movement of oedema fluid from the legs into the circulation overnight exacerbates the problem. Sleeping propped up helps prevent these gravity-based problems.

14 Normal interstitial fluid does not pit readily because the glycosaminoglycan matrix offers a high resistance to flow (Figure 11.9). In oedema, the glycosaminoglycans are diluted, so fluid is easily displaced.

15 The Starling principle of fluid exchange describes the factors (Section 11.1). Capillary pressure is increased by the raised venous pressure (Figure 11.5). Also, dilution of plasma proteins by renal salt and water retention lowers plasma colloid osmotic pressure moderately.

16 Gravity raises leg capillary pressure (Figure 11.5). Oedema improves overnight because lower limb capillary pressure falls in the supine position, allowing lymphatic drainage to outpace fluid filtration.

17 The exercise intolerance is caused by the impaired responses of heart rate and stroke volume to exercise (Figure 18.11), dyspnoea and increased skeletal muscle fatigability.

18 Digoxin partly restores contractility by increasing the Ca^{2+} store. It achieves this by partially inhibiting the sarcolemmal Na^+–K^+ pump, thus reducing the Na^+ gradient driving the Na^+–Ca^{2+} exchanger and Ca^{2+} expulsion.

Further reading

Kumar P, Clark M. *Clinical Medicine*, 6th edn. London: Elsevier, 2007.

Lille LS (ed.). *Pathophysiology of Heart Disease*, 3rd edn. Baltimore, MD: Williams and Wilkins, 2003.

APPENDIX 1

Human cardiovascular parameters

Values refer to young, resting human adult at heart level unless specified otherwise.

Aortic parameters

Cross-sectional area at root	$4-5\,\mathrm{cm}^2$
Reynolds number at peak flow	~4600
Stroke distance	15–20 cm
Stroke volume, rest	$70-80\,\mathrm{cm}^3$
Stroke volume, exercise	$110-120\,\mathrm{cm}^3$
Velocity of blood, peak ejection	70 cm/s
Velocity, mean during ejection	50 cm/s
Velocity, mean over whole cycle	20 cm/s
Velocity, mean during ejection in heavy exercise	250 cm/s

Area

Body surface, 70 kg adult	$1.8\,\mathrm{m}^2$
Capillary endothelium of lungs (combined)	$90\,\mathrm{m}^2$
Capillary endothelium, all skeletal muscles	$280\,\mathrm{m}^2$

Arterial parameters (systemic and pulmonary)

Brachial artery pressure at age 30 years	125/70 mmHg
Foot artery, standing, mean	183 mmHg
Compliance, elastic arteries at 30 years	$1.5\,\mathrm{ml\,mmHg}^{-1}$
Pulse velocity, young	$4-5\,\mathrm{m\,s}^{-1}$
Pulse velocity, elderly	$10-15\,\mathrm{m\,s}^{-1}$
Pulmonary artery pressure, supine	25/12 mmHg
Pulmonary artery pressure, standing	22/9 mmHg
Pulmonary artery pressure, heavy exercise	40/24 mmHg

Blood biophysical parameters

Blood volume, total	5 litre
Blood volume, venous	~3 litre
Blood volume, pulmonary	0.6 litre
Density, ρ	$1.06\,\mathrm{g\,cm}^{-3}$
Haematocrit, female	0.40
Haematocrit, male	0.45
Oxygen content, see *Oxygen*	
Relative viscosity, blood/water	~4
Relative viscosity, plasma/water	1.7
Viscosity, water at 37°C	0.69 mPa s

Blood flow and velocity

Cerebral, grey matter	$100\,\mathrm{ml\,min}^{-1}100\,\mathrm{g}^{-1}$
Coronary, resting subject	$70-80\,\mathrm{ml\,min}^{-1}100\,\mathrm{g}^{-1}$
Coronary, maximum	$300-400\,\mathrm{ml\,min}^{-1}100\,\mathrm{g}^{-1}$
Skeletal muscle, rest (phasic)	$3-5\,\mathrm{ml\,min}^{-1}100\,\mathrm{g}^{-1}$
Skeletal muscle, rest (postural)	$15\,\mathrm{ml\,min}^{-1}100\,\mathrm{g}^{-1}$
Skeletal muscle, maximum	$100-200\,\mathrm{ml\,min}^{-1}100\,\mathrm{g}^{-1}$
Skin, thermoneutral	$10-20\,\mathrm{ml\,min}^{-1}100\,\mathrm{g}^{-1}$
Skin, maximum	$150-200\,\mathrm{ml\,min}^{-1}100\,\mathrm{g}^{-1}$
Transit time, coronary circulation	15 s
Transit time, systemic capillary bed	0.5–2.0 s
Transit time, left ventricle to left ventricle	1 min
Velocity, aortic, peak	$70\,\mathrm{cm\,s}^{-1}$
Velocity, capillary	$0.05-0.1\,\mathrm{cm\,s}^{-1}$

Cardiac parameters

Cardiac index	$3\,\mathrm{litre\,min}^{-1}\mathrm{m}^{-2}$
Cardiac output, rest	$4-7\,\mathrm{litre\,min}^{-1}$
Cardiac output, maximum	$20-35\,\mathrm{litre\,min}^{-1}$
Electrical axis	$-30°$ to $+110°$
Weight of heart	300–350 g

Timing

Cardiac cycle, typical, rest	0.9 s
ECG, P wave duration	0.08 s

ECG, PR interval	<0.2 s
ECG, QRS wave	<0.1 s
ECG, ST segment	0.2–0.4 s
Heart rate, rest	50–100 min^{-1}
Heart rate, maximum	180–200 min^{-1}
Intrinsic pacemaker rate	105 min^{-1}
Isovolumetric contraction	0.05 s
Isovolumetric relaxation	0.08 s
Ventricular filling	0.5 s
Ventricular systole	0.35 s
Ventricular ejection	0.30 s

Pressure, relative to atmospheric (760 mmHg)

Central venous pressure	0–10 mmHg
L. ventricle, end–diastole, supine	9 mmHg
L. ventricle, end–diastole, standing	4–5 mmHg
L. ventricle, peak systolic	~125 mmHg
R. ventricle, end–diastole, supine	4 mmHg
R. ventricle, end–diastole, standing	0 mmHg (atmospheric)
R. ventricle, peak systolic, supine	25 mmHg
R. ventricle, peak systolic, standing	22 mmHg

Volume, resting subject

End–diastolic volume, ventricle	120 ml
End–systolic volume	40–50 ml
Ejection fraction	67%
Stroke volume	70–80 ml
Stroke work	1 joule

Cellular/subcellular dimensions

Contractile filament, myocardial actin (thin)	6 nm diam, 1.05 μm long
Contractile filament, myosin (thick)	11 nm diam, 1.6 μm long
Desmosome gap (cadherin)	25 nm
Gap junction (nexus, connexon)	2–4 nm
Muscle, cardiac myocyte	10–20 μm diam, 50–100 μm long
Muscle, cardiac Purkinje fibre	40–80 μm diam
Muscle, skeletal fibre (typically)	50 μm diam
Muscle, vascular myocytes	4 μm diam, 20–60 μm long
Red cell	8 μm diam
Sarcomere length, normal diastole	1.8–2.0 μm
Sarcomere, maximum stretch	2.2–2.3 μm

Density at 20°C

Blood	1.06 g ml^{-1}
Mercury	13.55 g ml^{-1}
Water	1.00 g ml^{-1}

Diameter

Aortic root	2.5 cm
Arteriole	10–100 μm
Arteriovenous anastomosis	20–130 μm
Artery, large named (e.g. iliac)	1–2 cm
Artery, medium to small named (e.g. radial, cerebral, coronary)	0.2–0.5 cm
Artery, resistance vessel	100–500 μm
Capillary	4–8 μm
Postcapillary (pericytic) venule	15–40 μm
Venule	50–200 μm

Distance and thickness

Aortic valve to iliac bifurcation	0.5 m
Capillary to parenchymal cell	10–20 μm
Capillary wall	0.2–0.3 μm
Sympathetic neuromuscular gap	0.1 μm
Wall of L. ventricle	1.0 cm
Wall of R. ventricle	0.5 cm

Electrophysiology

Cardiac resting potential	−80 to −90 mV
Cardiac action potential	+20 to +30 mV
Cardiac pacemaker potential	−50 to −70 mV
Cardiac plateau potential	0 to −20 mV
Cardiac action potential duration	200–400 ms
Conduction velocity, atrial	1 m s^{-1}
Conduction velocity, AV node	0.05 m s^{-1}
Conduction velocity, Purkinje	3–5 m s^{-1}
Conduction velocity, ventricle wall	0.5–1.0 m s^{-1}
Equilibrium potential, Ca^{2+}	+124 mV
Equilibrium potential, Cl^- (vascular)	−23 mV
Equilibrium potential, K^+	−94 mV
Equilibrium potential, Na^+	+70 mV
Vascular myocyte, basal	−50 to −60 mV

Ionic and other concentrations

ATP, intracellular	~5 mM
Ca^{2+}, free ions, extracellular	1.2 mM
Ca^{2+}, cardiac cytosol, diastole	0.1 μM
Ca^{2+}, cardiac cytosol, systole	2 μM
Cl^-, extracellular	120–134 mM
Cl^-, intracellular (vascular muscle)	54 mM

HCO_3^-, extracellular	27 mM
HCO_3^-, intracellular	10 mM
K^+, extracellular	3.5–5.5 mM
K^+, intracellular	140 mM
Myoglobin, cardiac	$3.4\,g\,l^{-1}$
Na^+, extracellular	135–145 mM
Na^+, intracellular	10 mM
pH, extracellular	7.4
pH, intracellular	7.0–7.1

Mass of soft tissue in 70 kg human

Blood	5 kg
Brain	1.5 kg
Gastrointestinal tract and liver	4 kg
Heart	0.35 kg
Kidneys	0.3 kg
Lungs	1 kg
Skeletal muscle	40 kg
Skin	2–3 kg

Oxygen (rest)

Blood content, arterial	$195\,ml\,O_2\,l^{-1}$
Blood content, mixed venous	$150\,ml\,O_2\,l^{-1}$
Extraction, whole body	25%
Extraction from coronary blood	65–75%
Consumption, basal, 70 kg adult	$250\,ml\,min^{-1}$
Consumption, maximal $(\dot{V}_{O_{2max}})$	$\sim3000\,ml\,min^{-1}$
Partial pressure, inspired	160 mmHg (21 kPa)
Partial pressure, arterial	100 mmHg (13 kPa)
Partial pressure, mixed venous	40 mmHg
Partial pressure, cardiac myocyte	5–20 mmHg
Saturation, arterial	97%
Saturation, mixed venous	72%

Pressure

See also *Arterial parameters*, *Venous pressure*, *Cardiac parameters* and Table 15.1 (*Pulmonary circulation*)

Capillary, arterial limb, heart level	32–36 mmHg
Capillary, venous limb, heart level	12–25 mmHg
Capillary, foot during standing	95 mmHg
Pulmonary capillary, supine	13 mmHg
Pulmonary capillary, upright	9 mmHg
Mean circulatory pressure (arrested)	7 mmHg
Pressure drop across capillary bed	20–30 mmHg
Pressure drop across resistance vessels	40–50 mmHg

Resistance

Pulmonary circulation	$0.003\,mmHg\,min\,ml^{-1}$
Systemic circulation, rest	$0.02\,mmHg\,min\,ml^{-1}$

Venous pressure

Antecubital or femoral vein, heart level	8–10 mmHg
Foot vein, standing	90 mmHg
Pulmonary vein, supine	9 mmHg
Pulmonary vein, standing	5 mmHg
Systemic venule, heart level	12–20 mmHg
Venoatrial junction	0–10 mmHg

Volume

Water as % body weight (male, female)	60% (m), 55% (f)
Total water, 70 kg male, 55 kg female	42 litre (m), 30 litre (f)
Intracellular water (two-thirds)	28 litre (m), 20 litre (f)
Extracellular water, (one-third)	14 litre (m), 10 litre (f)
Interstitial water,	11 litre (m), 8 litre (f)
Plasma volume	3 litre (m), 2 litre (f)
Blood volume	5 litre (m), 3.5 litre (f)

Cardiac volumes, see *Cardiac parameters*

Stroke volume, rest	$70\text{–}80\,cm^3$
Stroke volume, exercise	$110\text{–}120\,cm^3$

APPENDIX 2

Biophysical parameters and physiological mechanisms

Units are based mainly on the standard international (SI) system (metre, kilogram, second).

Acidosis and vasodilatation Acidosis causes vasodilatation by multiple mechanisms (Wray S. *Journal of Physiology* 1997; **503**: 235). (1) Intracellular acidosis hyperpolarizes the vascular myocytes, probably because K_{ATP} channels respond to pH. Hyperpolarization closes voltage-sensitive Ca^{2+} channels, leading to vasodilatation. (2) If vascular myocyte are depolarized by raising external K^+, acidosis still reduces cytosolic Ca^{2+} – perhaps because acidosis reduces the open probability of Ca^{2+} channels. (3) CO_2 causes endothelium to release NO in the mesentery, but less certainly in the brain (Carr *et al. Pfluger's Archiv* 1993; **423**: 343–5; You *et al. Acta Physiologica Scandinavica* 1994; **152**: 391–8). Lactate by contrast has a non-endothelium dependent action (McKinnon *et al. Journal of Physiology* 1996; **490**: 783–792).

Adenosine-induced vasodilatation Adenosine is formed by the action of 5-nucleotidase on extracellular AMP in hypoxic myocardium, skeletal muscle and cerebral tissue. Adenosine causes vasodilatation through multiple pathways. (1) A_{2A} receptors on vascular myocytes activate the adenylate cyclase–cAMP–protein kinase cascade (Chen CW, Chang HY, Hsiue TR. *American Journal of Physiology* 2000; **279**: H2210–17). (2) A_1 receptors are coupled to K_{ATP} channels, leading to hyperpolarization-mediated relaxation (Dart C, Standen NB. *Journal of Physiology* 1993; **471**: 767–86). (3) Adenosine binds to receptors on sympathetic varicosities to reduce noradrenaline release (neuromodulation, Figure 14.2).

Arterial input impedance Resistance is the ratio of fall in mean pressure to mean unit flow. Over a timescale of a second, however, arterial pressure and flow oscillate out of phase. Consequently, the pressure:flow ratio changes from instant to instant. To take account of this, the concept of 'impedance' has been adapted from the theory of alternating electrical currents. Arterial input impedance is a measure of the opposition of the circulation to an oscillating input, i.e. the stroke volume. Input impedance depends on peripheral vascular resistance, arterial viscoelastic compliance and oscillation frequency (heart rate).

Avogadro's number (N, N_A) is the number of molecules in 1 mole (1 gram-molecule), namely 6.0×10^{23} molecules per mole.

Brownian motion The random movements of particles in water was first observed in a pollen suspension by the Scottish botanist Robert Brown in 1828. The movement is caused by the kinetic, diffusive motion of water molecules, as Einstein showed in 1905. This was a turning point in the acceptance of the molecular theory of matter.

Capillary solute concentration and extraction Under idealized conditions of uniform permeability and uniform or zero interstitial solute concentration (C_i), capillary solute concentration decays exponentially with axial distance, and mean solute concentration = $C_i + [(C_a \times C_v)/\ln((C_a - C_i)/(C_v - C_i))]$, where C_a, C_v are arterial and venular concentrations (Figure 10.8). Substitution into the permeability equation (eqn 10.3) and Fick principle (eqn 10.4) gives the Renkin–Crone extraction equation: extraction $E = 1 - \exp(-PS/\dot{Q})$ for $C_i = 0$ (eqn 10.6). This tells us that the extraction of solute from capillary blood, defined as $(C_a - C_v)/C_a$, varies non-linearly with permeability and capillary blood flow.

Density ρ (rho) Density is mass per unit volume. See Appendix 1 for values.

Diffusion **Fick's first law of diffusion** (1855) states that diffusion rate dm/dt (mass transferred per unit time) across a body of liquid of area A over a short distance dx equals $-DA(dC/dx)$, where dC/dx is the concentration gradient and D is the diffusion coefficient. The **diffusion coefficient** or diffusivity (Table 10.1) is a measure of the solute's intrinsic velocity in the solvent. Due to friction, D

varies inversely with solvent viscosity and is inversely proportional to the cube root of solute molecular weight. D is often measured to assess the effective radius a of a molecule, idealized as a sphere; see **Stokes–Einstein radius**.

In narrow pores (radius r), the diffusivity D is restricted by increased **hydrodynamic drag** (Figure 10.6b). The 'restricted' diffusion coefficient D_{res} equals $D \times [1 - 2.1a/r + 2.09(a/r)^3 - 0.95 (a/r)^5]$. Diffusion across a narrow pore is also reduced by **steric exclusion** (Figure 10.6a); if the pore is cylindrical, the space available for solute diffusion is reduced by the factor, $(r - a)^2/r^2$. For a neutral solute, $(r - a)^2/r^2$ equals the solute **partition coefficient** ϕ (phi). If the membrane has a surface area S and pore area A_p, the fractional area available for diffusion is $\phi A_p/S$. The effective diffusion coefficient through a pore, D_m, relative to free diffusivity D, is the product of steric exclusion and hydrodynamic restriction, as stated by the **Renkin equation** (solid line, Figure 10.6) $D_m/D = [(r - a)^2/r^2] \times [1 - 2.1a/r + 2.09(a/r)^3 - 0.95(a/r)^5]$.

Taking into account the increased pathlength $\Delta x'$ caused by the obliquity of the pore through a membrane of thickness Δx, Fick's law of diffusion (eqn 10.1) takes the following form for diffusion through a porous membrane.

$$J_S = D_{res}\phi A_p \Delta C/\Delta x'$$

Comparing this with the permeability equation $J_S = PS\Delta C$ (eqn 10.3), we see that the **membrane permeability** P equals $D_{res}/\Delta x' \phi(A_p S)$. In other words, membrane permeability is governed by the restricted intrapore diffusivity, pore length, fractional pore area A_p/S, and partition coefficient ϕ.

Electrical conductance G of a membrane permeable to ions The electrical conductance of a membrane, G, depends on its permeability to ions, P.

$$G = \frac{P(V_m CF)}{(RT/F)^2(1 - \exp(-V_m F/RT))}$$

where V_m is the membrane potential, R the gas constant, F the Faraday constant, T the absolute temperature and C is ion concentration.

Equilibrium A system is in equilibrium when its components have the same free energy level. For example, two solutions containing a neutral solute at the same concentration or, more accurately, the same chemical potential, are in chemical equilibrium. Equilibrium should **not** be confused with **steady state**, a non-equilibrium situation (see below).

Extraction, E Extraction is defined as the fraction of solute removed as plasma passes through the capillary bed. The rate of delivery of solute to the capillary bed equals plasma flow $\dot{Q} \times$ arterial concentration C_a. The rate at which solute emerges into the veins is $\dot{Q} \times$ venous concentration C_a. The rate of transendothelial solute escape is therefore $\dot{Q}C_a - \dot{Q}C_v$ or $\dot{Q}(C_a - C_v)$ – the Fick principle. From the definition of extraction, $E = \dot{Q}(C_a - C_v)/\dot{Q}C_a$ or $E = (C_a - C_v)/C_a$. The transcapillary solute flux J_s equals $\dot{Q}C_a E$.

Faraday's constant, F F is the charge carried by one mole of monovalent ion, namely 96 484 coulombs/ mole. 1 volt is defined as 1 joule of energy per coulomb charge. The term RT/F in the **Nernst equation** equals 26.7 mV at 37°C (310°K).

Flux Flux is, strictly, the rate of movement of a material, such as a diffusing solute, across unit area of surface. In physiology the word is often used rather loosely to mean simply rate of movement, omitting the 'per unit area of surface' consideration.

Force, work, energy and power A **force** of 1 newton (N) is one that accelerates 1 kg mass at 1 m s^{-2}. The outdated c.g.s. unit of force, the dyne (1 g cm s^{-2}), is 10^{-5} N. **Work** is force $\times$ distance moved. **Energy** is the capacity to do work and has the same units as work. One joule of work or energy (J) equals a force of 1 newton displaced over 1 metre (1 N-m). One joule is 10^7 ergs, the c.g.s unit of energy (1 dyne-cm). **Power** is rate of work or rate of change of energy. Its unit, the watt W, is 1 J s^{-1}.

Free radicals In most molecules the chemical bonds between the atoms consist of a pair of electrons. A free radical is a molecule with an odd number of electrons – effectively a half-bond. The **superoxide radical** O_2^- is an O_2 molecule that has gained an extra electron, making it highly reactive. For example, O_2^- reacts with NO to form peroxynitrite, $ONOO^-$, destroying NO in the process. Superoxide is formed during oxidative metabolism. Superoxide can also be formed slowly by the reaction of O_2 with the ferrous Fe^{2+} of haemoglobin; the Fe^{2+} donates an electron to O_2 and becomes ferric Fe^{3+}, turning haemoglobin into useless **methaemoglobin**. A scavenger enzyme, **superoxide dismutase**, protects tissues against superoxide by catalysing its conversion to hydrogen peroxide, which is then degraded by catalase and glutathione peroxidase.

Gas constant, R The fundamental gas law states that, for 1 mole of gas, the pressure $P \times$ volume V divided by temperature T is a constant; $PV/T = R$. R is thus the pressure $\times$ volume of one mole of gas per unit absolute temperature (degrees Kelvin, °K). The volume occupied by 1 mole of gas at 1 atmosphere (1.01×10^5 Pascal) and 273°K (zero degrees Centigrade or Celsius) is 22.4 litre (RT). Therefore R is 0.08205 litre-atmospheres °K^{-1} mole^{-1}. Since the product PV has the units of energy (N-m – as in the ventricle pressure-volume loop of Figure 6.11), R is also the energy of one mole of gas per degree Kelvin, namely 8.314 joules °K^{-1} mole^{-1}.

Goldman's constant field equation The potential V_m across a membrane that is permeable to multiple monovalent ion species depends on the permeability to each ion species and on the ion concentrations inside (subscript i) and outside (subscript o).

$$V_m = (RT/F) \ln \left[\frac{P_K[K]_o + P_{Na}[Na]_o + P_{Cl}[Cl]_i}{P_K[K]_i + P_{Na}[Na]_i + P_{Cl}[Cl]_o} \right].$$

An analogous, but more complex expression applies to mixtures of monovalent and divalent ions.

Gravity, g The acceleration due to the force of gravity varies with latitude and altitude. It is $9.81 \, \text{m s}^{-2}$ at latitude 50° North (e.g. Land's End in Cornwall, UK).

Hypoxia and vascular tone This is a complex topic! In **systemic resistance vessels**, local hypoxia causes vasodilatation. In *isolated vessels/myocytes*, free from any influence by blood or tissue, hypoxic vasorelaxation is brought about **hyperpolarization** (Figure 12.1), which closes L-type Ca^{2+} channels. The hyperpolarization is mediated partly by K_{ATP} channels, activated by increasing intracellular ADP and H^+ levels (Dart C, Standen NB. *Journal of Physiology*, 1995; **483**: 29–39), and partly by K_{ir} channel, activated through the cAMP–PKA path (Park WS *et al. American Journal of Physiology* 2005; **289**: H2461–7). Hypoxic vasodilatation can also occur, however, with little fall in cytosolic Ca^{2+} (Figure 13.5) (Taggart MJ, Wray S. *Journal of Physiology* 1998; **509**: 315–25), due to **reduced Ca^{2+} sensitivity** (Soloviev MJ, Basilyuk S. *Experimental Physiology* 1993; **78**: 395–402). Ca^{2+} sensitivity is reduced by reducing myosin light chain phosphorylation, through the inhibition of rho kinase (Gu *et al. Journal of Physiology* 2005; **562**: 839–46). In addition, changes in the pentose phosphate pathway and NADPH:NADP ratio may

contribute to hypoxic vasodilatation (Larsen BT, Gutterman DG. *American Journal of Physiology* 2006; **290**: H2169–71 and Gupte SA, Wolin MS. *American Journal of Physiology* 2006; **290**: H2228–38).

In *intact tissues*, paracrine agents too contribute to hypoxic vasodilatation. Hypoxic myocardium, skeletal muscle and brain produce the vasodilator, **adenosine** (Skinner MR, Marshall JM. *Journal of Physiology* 1996; **495**: 553–60). Also, hypoxia reduces the production of the vasoconstrictor 20-HETE (Frisbee JC, Lombard JH. *Microvascular Research* 2002; **63**: 340–3). Furthermore, in blood-perfused tissues, the deoxygenation of haemoglobin may release the vasodilator nitric oxide, which is bound reversibly to a cysteine group of oxyhaemoglobin as S-nitrosothiol (Allen BW, Piantadosi CA. *American Journal of Physiology* 2006; **291**: H1507–12).

In **large systemic arteries**, such as ischaemic coronary arteries, severe hypoxia can cause vasospasm (Siegel *et al. Journal of Vascular Medicine and Biology* 1991; **3**: 140–9). The vasospasm is due to the release of noradrenaline from hypoxic sympathetic fibres, and the local release of autacoid vasoconstrictors, such as platelet activating factor.

In the lungs, hypoxia causes vasoconstriction of the pulmonary resistance vessels – **hypoxic pulmonary vasoconstriction** (HPV) (Section 15.5). HPV has been studied in isolated pulmonary vessel and whole lung. There is growing agreement that hypoxia is 'sensed' by the vessel mitochondria, which generate reactive oxygen species (Archer S, Michelakis E. *News in Physiological Sciences* 2002; **17**: 131–7); but how this leads to vasoconstriction is not fully understood (Aaronson PI *et al. Journal of Physiology* 2006; **570**: 53–8). One mechanism involves myocyte depolarization as K^+ channels are inhibited (a K_V isoform and TASK). A second mechanism is SR Ca^{2+} store release and Ca^{2+} entry through store-operated channels – a process shown to be critical for early HPV. Over the next 20–40 min, the HPV increases further, but cytosolic $[Ca^{2+}]$ does not, indicating a third, slower mechanism, Ca^{2+} sensitization. The slow phase is partly endothelium dependent and is mediated by the Ca^{2+}-sensitizing kinase, rho kinase (Section 12.5). Sustained HPV is largely blocked by inhibitors of rho kinase.

Love's equation for tension in a thick-walled tube Love's equation for mechanical equilibrium in a thick-walled tube is analogous to Laplace's law, which, strictly speaking, applies to infinitely thin-walled tubes. For a real tube, of internal radius r_i and external radius r_o, Love's equation is derived by similar reasoning to that in Figure 8.17. Love's equation states $T = P_i r_i - P_o r_o$, where T is the *absolute* circumferential tension (force) in the wall. In physiology we are more interested in the *increase* in tension as P_i (blood pressure) rises above atmospheric pressure P_o. For this purpose Laplace's law (eqn 8.8) is a convenient approximation.

Osmole An osmole can be defined as the mass of solute that, in solution, yields 1 mole of particles (Avogadro's number of particles). Since NaCl in solution dissociates into two particles ideally, 0.3 moles of NaCl provides 0.6 osmoles of Na^+ and Cl^-. An osmole can also be defined, more practically, as the amount of solute that, when dissolved in 22.4 kg of solvent at 0°C, exerts an osmotic pressure of 1 atmosphere (760 mmHg, 1030 cmH$_2$O). A 1 **osmolal** solution contains 1 osmole per kilogram of solvent. A 1 **osmolar** solution contains 1 osmole per litre of solution. A litre of plasma contains only ~0.95 kg water. Mammalian body fluids contain ~0.3 osmole per kg water (300 milliosmolal, 300 mOs), and exert a potential osmotic pressure of 5800 mmHg at 37°C (310°K). (See **van't Hoff's law**; $\pi = 22.4$ atmos × 310/273 × 0.3 = 7.6 atmospheres = 5800 mmHg.) By contrast, human plasma proteins (60 − 80 g l^{-1}) exert a far smaller osmotic pressure, 25–28 mmHg.

Potassium and vasodilatation Normal extracellular [K$^+$] is ~4 mM. Physiological increases, namely up to ~10 mM, cause vasodilatation. Pharmacological concentrations, >20 mM, cause contraction. A plot of vascular tone versus extracellular K$^+$ is thus U-shaped. **Pharmacological** K$^+$ levels depolarize the myocyte; see the Nernst equation, Section 3.1. This activates voltage-sensitive Ca^{2+} channels, leading to contraction. **Physiological** rises in extracellular K$^+$ hyperpolarize the cell (paradoxically), leading to Ca^{2+} channel closure and relaxation. The hyperpolarization is due to (1) stimulation of the electrogenic 3Na$^+$–2K$^+$ pump by extracellular K$^+$. The pump inhibitor ouabain attenuates the vasodilator response to K$^+$. (2) Increased extracellular K$^+$ increases the open-state probability of inward rectifying K$^+$ channels (K_{ir}), which shifts the membrane potential closer to the Nernst E_K, i.e. hyperpolarizes the cell (eqn 3.4).

Pressure Pressure is the force exerted by a gas or liquid upon unit area of surface. Unlike stress, which has the same units, pressure acts equally in all directions. The SI unit of pressure, the Pascal (Pa), is 1 newton per square metre (N m^{-2}). One atmosphere pressure is 101 325 Pa (101.3 kPa, kilopascals).

This pressure will support a column of mercury 760 mm high in a barometer, so 1 atmosphere = 760 mmHg pressure. Body fluid pressures are always expressed relative to atmospheric pressure, so a venous pressure of '0 mmHg' is really an absolute pressure of 760 mmHg; and an interstitial pressure of '−5 mmHg' is an absolute pressure of 755 mmHg. 1 mmHg = 133 Pa = 1.36 cmH$_2$O at 20°C. The extra pressure at the bottom of a column of fluid in a gravitational field (e.g. blood in the feet) equals fluid density (ρ) × gravity (g) × height (h) (ρgh). A 1 cm column of water (1 cmH$_2$O) at 20°C exerts a pressure of 98.1 Pa on earth (981 dynes/cm^2).

Quantity of ions exchanged during a cardiac myocyte action potential A cylindrical myocyte (length ~10^{-2} cm, radius 10^{-3} cm) has a volume of 3.14 × 10^{-8} cm^3 and a surface area of 6.28 × 10^{-5} cm^2. To shift the cell's potential by 1 volt, each cm^2 of cell membrane requires 1 microcoulomb of charge (**membrane capacitance**). An action potential of 0.1 volts (from −80 mV to +20 mV) thus requires a net transfer of 6.28 × 10^{-6} microcoulomb per cell. One mole of monovalent ion carries 96 500 coulomb of charge (Faraday's constant), so the quantity of ions that must be transferred is 6.51 × 10^{-17} moles or, applying Avogadro's number, 3.9 × 10^7 ions. From the cell volume and intracellular concentrations in Table 3.1, the cell actually contains 1.9 × 10^{11} Na$^+$ ions and 2.6 × 10^{12} K$^+$ ions. The fractional change in intracellular ion concentration after a single action potential is thus tiny (Na$^+$ increase, 0.02%; K$^+$ decrease, 0.002%).

Reflection coefficient, σ (sigma) The reflection coefficient σ is a measure of the difficulty that a solute experiences in entering a pore (Figure 10.7). This depends on steric exclusion (Figure 10.6a). For a spherical neutral solute of radius a entering a cylindrical pore of radius r, the available pore space is $(r - a)^2/r^2$. It can be shown that σ equals the square of the excluded space: $\sigma = [1 - (r - a)^2/r^2]^2$. Measurements of σ can thus be used to estimate pore size. For albumin ($a = 3.6$ nm) and an endothelial pore of radius 4 nm, σ is 0.975.

Solute transport by convection (wash along or 'solvent drag') depends on σ, filtration rate J_v and bulk solute concentration C. The convective transport through a pore equals $J_v(1 - \sigma)C$. This expression does not, however, take account of diffusive transport. At low flows, diffusive transport can dominate, whereas at high flows convective transport can dominate.

Sodium–calcium exchanger; forward and reverse modes The sarcolemmal exchanger swaps three Na^+ ions for one Ca^{2+} ion and can operate in either direction. For most of the cardiac cycle the exchanger removes Ca^{2+} from the sarcoplasm and adds Na^+ to it (**forward mode**), with an attendant net inward positive current. Being electrogenic, the exchanger is influenced by membrane potential, as well as concentration gradient. For ion species X, the driving force is $(V_m - E_x)$, where V_m is intracellular potential and E_x is the ion's Nernst equilibrium potential, which depends on the ion concentrations (Section 3.3). Due to the 3:2 charge ratio, the force driving the net exchanger current i_{Na-Ca} is $3(V_m - E_{Na}) - 2(V_m - E_{Ca})$. During **diastole** V_m is $-80\,mV$, E_{Na} is $69\,mV$ and E_{Ca} is $130\,mV$ (Table 3.1), so the force on the exchanger is equivalent to an internal potential of $-27\,mV$, drawing a net positive charge into the cell, (forward mode) and expelling Ca^{2+}. Immediately after **depolarization**, the exchanger switches briefly into **reverse mode**, i.e. Ca^{2+} entry – because an action potential $+20\,mV$ changes the net force on the exchanger to $+73\,mV$ (i.e. $3(20 - 69) - 2(20 - 130)$). The brief, exchanger-mediated Ca^{2+} entry makes a small contribution to the early systolic Ca^{2+} transient and calcium-induced calcium release. During the **plateau** of the cardiac action potential, the cytosolic Ca^{2+} is high, reducing E_{Ca}, and the membrane potential falls to around zero. The balance of forces now causes the exchanger to revert to **forward mode**, i.e. Ca^{2+} expulsion.

If intracellular Na^+ is raised, e.g. by inhibiting the Na–K pump with digoxin, E_{Na} declines. The net force driving the exchanger therefore falls; Ca^{2+} expulsion declines, the SR Ca^{2+} store increases and contractility improves.

Steady state When two components at different energy levels are brought into contact, material or energy can flow from the higher to the lower level. When the transfer occurs at a steady rate, and without changing the energy level at either end, the system is said to be in a steady state. This should not be confused with an equilibrium state (no difference in free energy, see earlier). For example, a flowing river may be in a steady state (steady flow from a constant, high-level water source, such as a dam, to a constant low-level sink, such as the sea) but it is not at equilibrium – the energy levels are not the same at any two points along its course. If there is in reality a very slow, almost negligible change in the feeder and downstream energy levels, the system is said to be in a quasi steady state (Latin *quasi*, 'as if').

Stokes–Einstein radius (a, r_{se}) The hydrodynamic resistance that a solute particle experiences as it diffuses through a solvent depends on the particle's size and shape. Although the particle may not be spherical, it is commonly represented by an 'equivalent sphere', i.e. a sphere that would generate the same resistance and diffusion rate as the particle. The radius of the equivalent sphere is called the particle's diffusion radius/hydrodynamic radius/Stokes–Einstein radius. Stokes and Einstein showed that the solute free diffusion coefficient D is inversely proportional to its radius a:

$$a = \frac{RT}{D N_A 6\pi\eta}$$

where η (eta) is the solvent viscosity and T is absolute temperature. Thus, the radius of a solute can be determined simply by measuring its diffusivity.

Strain and stress When a solid body is subjected to a force, the force per unit cross-sectional area of material is called the **stress** ($N\,m^{-2}$). Although the units of stress are the same as pressure, stress has a specific direction, whereas pressure is a property of a fluid and acts equally in all directions. One should not talk of 'solid pressure' in science, although we do in everyday usage. The change in size of a solid object caused by a given stress is usually expressed as a fraction of the original size, and this dimensionless fraction is called the **strain**. The ratio of stress to strain, called **Young's modulus of elasticity**, is a measure of stiffness. Note that this is the opposite of our everyday use of the term 'elastic' to mean easily stretched.

Work See *Force*.

van't Hoff's law (crystalloid osmotic pressure) Osmotic pressure is a 'colligative' property, like freezing point depression, i.e. it depends primarily on solute concentration, not chemical identity. The osmotic pressure π of an ideal solution is described by van't Hoff's law, namely $\pi = RTC$ (R, gas constant; T, absolute temperature; C, molal concentration). RT is 25.4 atmospheres for a 1-molal solution at 37°C (22.4 atm at 0°C). Since the concentration of ions (crystalloids) in plasma and extracellular fluid is ~ 0.3 molal, the van't Hoff osmotic pressure is 7.6 atmosphere, or 5800 mmHg. This **crystalloid osmotic pressure** acts across the cell membranes and is the primary force distributing water between the intracellular and extracellular compartment. Crystalloid osmotic pressure does not generally influence water movement across the capillary wall because (1) the endothelial cleft is highly permeable to electrolytes (except in the brain), so the plasma and interstitial concentrations are almost identical and (2) the reflection coefficient of endothelial clefts to electrolytes is very small. By contrast, the plasma proteins or 'colloids', at a mere 0.001 molar concentration, exert a sustained osmotic pressure across the capillary wall (25–28 mmHg), because the wall is relatively impermeable to plasma proteins.

Plasma protein osmotic pressure is nonideal, i.e. it greatly exceeds the value predicted by van't Hoff's law (Figure 11.7). The excess COP is partly due to the large self-volume of protein molecules (partial molar volume, 0.7 ml/g), which increases the effective concentration per ml of solution, and partly to the charge on plasma proteins. An albumin molecule has a net negative charge of -17 units at pH 7.4. This attracts a slight excess of Na^+ ions into the plasma (the **Gibbs–Donnan distribution**). These ions are retained electrostatically in the plasma, so they are effective osmotically and account for approximately one-third of albumin's osmotic pressure.

Viscoelasticity When a perfectly elastic body, such as a spring, is subjected to a stress, such as suspended weight, the strain is linearly proportional to the stress and does not change with time. On removing the stress, the original conformation is immediately restored. Biological materials, such as the artery wall, behave differently. Stress causes an initial rapid elastic deformation, which is followed by a slower, ever-decreasing deformation as time passes (**creep**). On removal of the stress, the recovery of shape follows a non-symmetrical pathway (**hysteresis**), due to energy dissipation. Viscoelasticity can be modelled by viscous, flowing elements (dashpots) arranged in parallel with elastic elements (springs).

Viscosity Viscosity is the friction between two moving planes of fluid. Formally, viscosity is the shear stress needed to generate one unit of shear rate. **Shear stress** is the sliding force applied to unit area of contact between two laminae ($N\,m^{-2}$), and is proportional to the pressure gradient along a blood vessel. **Shear rate** is the change in velocity per unit distance radially; its units are (m/s)/m, which is, bizarrely, s^{-1}. The viscosity of water at 20°C is 0.001 N-s/m^2, or 1 mPa-s (1 centiPoise) and this falls to 0.69 mPa.s at 37°C. The viscosity of a fluid relative to water is easily measured in a capillary viscometer. The time taken for the fluid to drain between two marks in a capillary tube is simply divided by the time for water under the same pressure head. The albumin and globulins in plasma raise its viscosity by 70% to 1.2 mPa.s at 37°C.

INDEX